Pediatrics: Pathophysiology, Diagnosis and Clinical Management

Pediatrics: Pathophysiology, Diagnosis and Clinical Management

Edited by Jimmy Taylor

hayle
medical

New York

Hayle Medical,
750 Third Avenue, 9th Floor,
New York, NY 10017, USA

Visit us on the World Wide Web at:
www.haylemedical.com

ISBN: 978-1-63241-431-1

The publisher's policy is to use permanent paper from mills that operate a sustainable forestry policy. Furthermore, the publisher ensures that the text paper and cover boards used have met acceptable environmental accreditation standards.

Trademark Notice: Registered trademark of products or corporate names are used only for explanation and identification without intent to infringe.

Printed in the United States of America.

Cataloging-in-Publication Data

Pediatrics : pathophysiology, diagnosis and clinical management / edited by Jimmy Taylor.
p. cm.
Includes bibliographical references and index.
ISBN 978-1-63241-431-1
1. Pediatrics. 2. Children--Diseases--Diagnosis. 3. Physiology, Pathological. 4. Clinical medicine.
5. Children--Health and hygiene. I. Taylor, Jimmy.
RJ45 .P43 2017
618.92--dc23

Table of Contents

Preface

This book aims to highlight the current researches and provides a platform to further the scope of innovations in this area. This book is a product of the combined efforts of many researchers and scientists from different parts of the world. The objective of this book is to provide the readers with the latest information in the field.

Pediatrics as a study, deals with the healthcare and physical maintenance of children and infants. The body of a child is different from that of an adult, therefore, the treatments used to treat their organs and other diseases are different as well. Pediatricians examine, treat and prevent disorders affecting infants and children. This book elucidates new techniques and their applications in a multidisciplinary approach. It strives to provide a fair idea about this discipline and to help develop a better understanding of the latest advances within this field. Students, researchers, pediatricians and all associated with pediatrics will benefit alike from this text. It includes contributions of experts and scientists which will provide innovative insights into this field.

I would like to express my sincere thanks to the authors for their dedicated efforts in the completion of this book. I acknowledge the efforts of the publisher for providing constant support. Lastly, I would like to thank my family for their support in all academic endeavors.

Editor

The Cost of Autism Spectrum Disorders

Chiara Horlin[1], Marita Falkmer[1,2], Richard Parsons[1], Matthew A. Albrecht[3], Torbjorn Falkmer[1,4,5]*

1 School of Occupational Therapy & Social Work, CHIRI, Curtin University, Perth, Australia, 2 School of Education and Communication, CHILD Programme, Institute of Disability Research, Jönköping University, Jönköping, Sweden, 3 School of Psychology, CHIRI, Curtin University, Perth, Australia, 4 Rehabilitation Medicine, Department of Medicine and Health Sciences (IMH), Faculty of Health Sciences, Linköping University & Pain and Rehabilitation Centre, Linköping, Sweden, 5 School of Occupational Therapy, La Trobe University, Melbourne, VIC, Australia

Abstract

Objective: A diagnosis of an autism spectrum disorders is usually associated with substantial lifetime costs to an individual, their family and the community. However, there remains an elusive factor in any cost-benefit analysis of ASD diagnosis, namely the cost of *not* obtaining a diagnosis. Given the infeasibility of estimating the costs of a population that, by its nature, is inaccessible, the current study compares expenses between families whose children received a formal ASD diagnosis immediately upon suspecting developmental atypicality and seeking advice, with families that experienced a delay between first suspicion and formal diagnosis.

Design: A register based questionnaire study covering all families with a child with ASD in Western Australia.

Participants: Families with one or more children diagnosed with an ASD, totalling 521 children diagnosed with an ASD; 317 records were able to be included in the final analysis.

Results: The median family cost of ASD was estimated to be AUD $34,900 per annum with almost 90% of the sum ($29,200) due to loss of income from employment. For each additional symptom reported, approximately $1,400 cost for the family per annum was added. While there was little direct influence on costs associated with a delay in the diagnosis, the delay was associated with a modest increase in the number of ASD symptoms, indirectly impacting the cost of ASD.

Conclusions: A delay in diagnosis was associated with an indirect increased financial burden to families. Early and appropriate access to early intervention is known to improve a child's long-term outcomes and reduce lifetime costs to the individual, family and society. Consequently, a per symptom dollar value may assist in allocation of individualised funding amounts for interventions rather than a nominal amount allocated to all children below a certain age, regardless of symptom presentation, as is the case in Western Australia.

Editor: Jennifer Gladys Mulle, Emory University School Of Medicine, United States of America

Funding: This study was funded by the Department of Social Services (DSS), formerly the Department of Families, Housing, Community Services and Indigenous Affairs (FaHCSIA), with in-kind support of the Autism CRC, established and supported under the Australian Government's Cooperative Research Centres Program. The research was also conducted in collaboration with Disabilities Services Commission Western Australia (DSC). DSS had no active role in the design, implementation, data collection, analysis or interpretation of the study. DSC collaborated with the authors and assisted in data collection by in-kind contribution of its employee's time in some aspects of the study. Writing of the report and the decision to submit this manuscript were solely the role and responsibility of the authors. However, approval to submit this study for publication was sought from CRC Living with Autism Spectrum Disorders, DSS and DSC. All researchers are independent from both DSS and DSC and take full responsibility for the integrity of the data and the accuracy of the analyses. (DSS grant number - RES-HEA-CRD-TB-50940 http://www.dss.gov.au/)

Competing Interests: The authors have declared that no competing interests exist.

* Email: T.Falkmer@curtin.edu.au

Introduction

A diagnosis of an Autism Spectrum Disorder (ASD) results in an estimated annual national cost to Australia of $4.5–7.2 billion [1] that is borne by the individuals themselves, their families, their community, and by government. Costs of autism can peak during the periods when a diagnosis is being assessed and when treatments are being administered, but many costs are ultimately on-going and constitute a life-long burden. The accurate identification of ASDs necessarily relies on assessing observable behaviours using timely, accurate, reliable and valid diagnostic procedures. At present, the "gold standard" diagnosis of autism is a lengthy and time consuming process that requires a suitably qualified multi-disciplinary team (MDT) to assess behavioural,

historical and parental report information to determine a definitive diagnosis [2–4]. This is discouraging since failing to accurately identify, or prolonging the identification of, children as having ASD will delay access to apposite intervention and support services [5,6]. This issue is compounded by the possible 25 fold increase in the recent diagnosis rates of ASD in Australia [1], and resultant pressing demand for delivery of diagnostic services and intervention.

It is possible that the delay in treatment and support for children with ASD results in significant costs. Recently, the estimated annual adjusted costs for an adult and a child with autism have been calculated as follows (all dollar values are in AUD and rounded to the nearest dollar):

$$(P + SP + S + M + C_{MD}) \times 250$$

where, P = production loss of the individual and family with an ASD diagnosis, SP = support costs, S = school costs, mainly addition and specialist staff, M = medical costs, and C_{MD} = missed diagnosis. It is important to note that several assumptions are made regarding productivity costs that we do not feel fully encompass the impact of a child's diagnosis on parent employment resulting in what appears to be a very low estimate of the financial impact (e.g., time taken out from current employment for treatment visits is accounted for, but reduced employment of parents so that they can care for a child with ASD is not taken into account). Notably, estimates for the parameter C_{MD} (missed diagnosis) have not been made and, as a result, the true benefit of a diagnosis of ASD could not be calculated. It seems plausible that an early diagnosis of autism may reduce the cost of ASD because diagnosis leads to early intervention, which results in better outcomes [7,8], improved social behaviour [9,10], and less reliance on specialised education support classes [7,9]. These improvements may, in turn, have knock-on benefits to families and society more broadly, as well as increased productivity for parents and the individual themselves later in life. These gains are usually accomplished when intervention is commenced very early, between the ages of 2 and 4 [11,12].

However, the complication here is clear: those individuals remaining undiagnosed are, for that very reason, inaccessible to service providers and researchers alike. The next closest approximation that can be made for parameter C_{MD} is therefore the difference in costs between those children identified and treated early in their development and those not identified and/or treated until later in childhood or even adolescence and adulthood. One method of estimating this cost is to identify a subgroup of children who receive a diagnosis of ASD shortly after their parents suspect their child's development is atypical, and then compare costs for these children with a subgroup of children who had their diagnosis formally confirmed much later. However, one possible offset of the cost of early diagnosis is the long-term accumulated cost of interventions and special services. Therefore, the potential added cost associated with a later diagnosis may not be substantially higher than an earlier diagnosis.

Research into the impact of receiving an early diagnosis and on a family's financial burden is limited [4]. In Australia, state and territory governments are primarily responsible for supporting disability, including ASD, rather than the Commonwealth. However, families with a child diagnosed with an ASD receive a finite amount of Commonwealth funding up to the child's seventh birthday (the so-called "Helping Children with Autism "-funding) for the purposes of early intervention. From this point onwards, ongoing therapies and services outside of school are largely parent-funded on top of other medical and non-medical costs. Aside from the obvious cost to families of missing this early opportunity for government funding, the current study also seeks to determine whether a delayed diagnosis results in inflated costs, reduced incomes and increased financial stresses to families on a long-term basis when compared to families of individuals with a more immediate the immediate diagnosis. Thus it will be possible to estimate an accessible proxy of the parameter C_{MD}.

Methods

Participants and Procedures

With the assistance of the Disabilities Services Commission (DSC) Western Australia, a questionnaire was distributed to families with children registered as having an ASD on their client register. Only families with diagnosed children currently under the age of 18 years were included. This decision was made in line with recommendations from the DSC based on the likelihood of correct/valid information being extractable from the register. At the time of the mail out, 3,965 children were registered with DSC from 3,723 families. Of the packages mailed out, 3,494 were sent to families with one child with ASD, 217 packages sent to families with two diagnosed children, 11 packages sent to families with three diagnosed children and one package sent to a family with four children diagnosed with ASD. Families with more than one child under 18 received one questionnaire for each child with ASD. Of the 3,723 questionnaire packs (covering 3,965 children) sent out by DSC, 192 were returned as "address unknown". In total, 521 questionnaires were returned, resulting in a response rate of 15%.

Questionnaire Development. Development of the full parent-report questionnaire was informed by anecdotal reports from clinical experts and families, the current research literature and insurance reports. Firstly, the general areas of interest were listed and all financial aspects were itemised and categorised to cover as many potential expenses that were a consequence of having a child with ASD. The questionnaire also attempted to gather and summarise information on all possible direct medical, direct non-medical and indirect costs associated with having a child with an ASD. The areas of expense addressed in the questionnaire are listed in Table 1 and specific items relevant to each area are presented in the final questionnaire in the Appendix S1 in the provided Supporting Information.

Questions were then devised to gather the information conveniently and efficiently, which would lead to clear and relevant summary reports whilst taking into account the heterogeneity of families with ASD. A pilot version of the questions and response formats were sent for comments to a number of clinical psychologists, neuropsychologists, developmental psychologists, social workers, occupational therapists, and other clinicians and service providers.

A full version of the questionnaire was then piloted on three families who have children with ASD. Based on their comments and feedback the questionnaire was adjusted to its final version (Appendix S1) and comprised a total of 73 items on demographic information, the child's diagnosis, developmental history, treatment history, education, child care and qualitative questions about the child and families' quality of life.

The final page of the questionnaire included a diagnostic checklist of DSM-IV-TR/ICD-10 items [13]. The checklist consists of 20 symptom characteristics divided into 4 sections addressing the traditional symptom domains of;

-Impairments in social interaction (five symptom characteristics),
-Impairments in communication (seven symptom characteristics),
-Restricted, repetitive and stereotyped patterns of behaviour, interest or activities (seven symptom characteristics),
-The presence of impairments in at least one of the above before the age of three (one characteristic).

Parents were asked to indicate whether any of these characteristics currently previously applied to their child.

Data Collection. Questionnaire packs were prepared by the authors before being delivered to the DSC. To maintain confidentiality of the DSC's client register, all printing of cover letters and addressing of envelopes was handled by the DSC's staff and at no time did any of the researchers have access to this register. As per the DSC's records, packs were sent to the primary contact, the default for which was the diagnosed child's father.

Table 1. Areas of expense for families with children with ASD addressed in the questionnaire.

Direct Medical	Direct Non-Medical	Indirect
Physicians/dentists	Childcare	Caregiver lost productivity
Pharmaceuticals	Respite care	Family quality of life
Therapeutic services/interventions	Home improvement	
Alternative/complimentary therapies	Special education	
Emergency room/hospitals	Support services for other family members	
Home healthcare		
Treatment-related travel		

The questionnaire pack included the questionnaire itself and a reply paid return envelope. All questionnaires were de-identified and asked for no identifying information.

After a period of one month, reminders to complete the questionnaire were published online, in newspapers, DSC newsletters and on community radio. Upon receiving deidentified and completed questionnaires, a unique anonymous identifier was allocated to each questionnaire. Responses were then entered into a data file using IBM SPSS version 20 and analysed using the SAS version 9.2 statistical software.

Data analysis

Treatment-related travel costs. Direct costs associated with travel for medical, therapeutic and complimentary/alternative treatments were calculated as a function of the reported frequency of average visits per month (questions 19, 28 and 36 respectively) and distance from these services (questions 18, 27 and 35 respectively). Round trip costs were calculated based on doubling the median kilometre distance from services and the average per kilometre cost of running a small car (approximated at $0.65AUD per kilometre by the most recent Royal Automobile Club figures).

Individual cost estimates were calculated for medical visits relating to a child's ASD diagnosis, therapeutic visits relating to an ASD diagnosis and complimentary/alternative visits undertaken as part of ASD treatment. These were summed to create a monthly cumulative total, which was then adjusted to create an annual estimate of treatment related travel costs according to the following formula:

$$\text{Travel Cost (\$AUD)} = 12 \times \sum (0.65 \times (V_{Medical} \cdot D_{Medical} + V_{Therapy} \cdot D_{Therapy} + V_{Comp} \cdot D_{Comp}))$$

where V equals the number of visits per month, D equals the distance in km to the service. 'Medical', 'Therapy' and 'Comp' refer to medical professional services, other therapeutic services and complementary and alternative services respectively.

Out of pocket treatment costs. The reported annual out-of-pocket costs to families in relation to ASD- specific medical, therapeutic and complimentary/alternative treatment services (questions 22, 33 and 37) were summed to create a total direct treatment cost variable. All three questions had seven potential response options representing intervals of dollar amounts. These options were then converted to the mid-point of each interval to create a single dollar amount for analysis. These recoded variables were then summed to create a cumulative total of the out of pocket

costs associated with ASD-specific medical, therapeutic and complimentary/alternative treatments.

Loss of income from employment reduction. The productivity loss associated with having a child diagnosed with ASD was calculated based on self-reported impact of their child's diagnosis on the parent/caregiver ability to work (question 51) and, if employment status was affected, the size of this reduction as a function of hours in the average work week (question 52). Those responding to question 51 by selecting options one, two or three, as presented in Table 2, then indicated the reduction in hours in question 52. This reduction was thereafter converted to a proportion of full-time equivalent (FTE) employment. Those indicating that either one or both parents could not work at all at this time due to the needs of their ASD child were converted to an FTE reduction of 1 or 2 units, respectively. Parents indicating that their employment status was unaffected were coded as 0. This variable was then multiplied with the median full-time income for 2010–2011 as reported by the Australian Taxation Office (the latest figures made available), which was $48, 864.

Cumulative cost of having a child diagnosed with ASD. To create a single estimate of direct and indirect expenses to each family that were specifically related to having a child diagnosed with ASD, the costs associated with treatment-related travel, out-of-pocket treatment expenses and loss of income/productivity were summed.

'Immediate' versus 'delayed' diagnosis. A dichotomous 'immediate' versus 'delayed' diagnosis variable was created based on cross-tabulations between questions 10 (age at first suspicion of something not being quite right) and 12 (age at which a formal diagnosis was received). This variable was intended to capture the chronological difference between those receiving early or more immediate diagnosis (and presumably treatment and intervention) and a later or delayed diagnosis (often after the optimal developmental window for treatment and period at which early intervention would take place). Those children with a zero or one step chronological difference between questions 10 and 12 were coded as 'immediate' and those with a two or more step difference between these questions were coded as 'delayed'. A further, stricter, division of 'immediate' and 'delayed' was also conducted by retaining only those with a zero step difference between questions 10 and 12 ('immediate') and those with a three or more step difference ('delayed'). These divisions are delineated in Table 3.

Cumulative presence of ASD symptoms. The total number of ASD symptoms was estimated by a cumulative total of the positive indications from the presence of symptoms within the four domains listed on the DSM-IV/TR-ICD-10 checklist. Positive indications were coded as one and responses in domain one to

Table 2. Questions 51 and 52 and the coding of responses used to estimate proportions of FTE reductions.

Question 51: How much has your child's diagnosis affected the employment status of your household?		
1	Both parents must work less hours	
2	One parent (of a two-parent household) must work less hours	
3	Single parent must work less hours	
4	One parent cannot work at this time	**1** FTE reduction
5	Both parents cannot work at this time	**2** FTE reduction
6	Unaffected	**0** FTE reduction
Question 52: If your employment status has been affected, please estimate by how many hours in an average week your employment load has been reduced.		
−99	Not relevant	**0** FTE reduction
1	<7 hours	**.2** FTE reduction
2	7–14 hours	**.4** FTE reduction
3	15–21 hours	**.6** FTE reduction
4	22–28 hours	**.8** FTE reduction
5	29–35+hours	**1** FTE reduction

three were summed to create a total for each child. The fourth domain comprised one single developmental history question and was excluded from this total, since this characteristic was regarded as a prerequisite for receiving a diagnosis of ASD.

Analysis of non-respondents. Six months after the initial mail-out, a random sample of 405 families registered with the DSC were contacted for a telephone follow-up. Given the confidentiality of the DSC register and the de-identified nature of the returned questionnaires, it was not known which families on the register had or had not completed the long-form questionnaire. Thus, the random sample of 405 families would include those that had completed and returned a questionnaire and those that had not. Non-respondents were then asked to answer an abbreviated form of the questionnaire over the phone. This short-form phone questionnaire consisted of twenty questions taken from the original questionnaire for the purposes of a later drop-out analysis. Those questions included in the short-form are shown in italics in Appendix S1. For the purposes of comparisons between those that did and did not respond to the long-form questionnaire that was sent out via mail, independent samples *t*-tests were used to compare the ages of children, chi-square tests were used to compare categorical demographic variables and Mann-Whitney U tests were conducted to compare calculated cost variables. Due to the shortened nature of the short-form questionnaire, only the out of pocket treatment costs and the loss of income from employment

reduction variables could be calculated for both respondents and non-respondents. The response categories of some demographic variables (question 10 and 12 specifically) were collapsed to ensure validity of the chi-square test.

Ethical approval

Ethical approval was obtained from the Curtin University Human Research Ethics Committee (HR 138/2012) and the internal ethical review board of the DSC in Western Australia. Questionnaire packs were sent to the DSC's clients with a cover letter from the Director General of DSC explaining the nature and purpose of the study as well as an information sheet inviting families to complete and return the questionnaire. Completed and returned questionnaires were taken as consent to participate in the study.

Results

The characteristics of the included 521 children with ASD are presented in Table 4. Descriptive statistics for all cumulative cost estimates and the cumulative presence of ASD symptoms are presented in Table 5. An additional total cost of ASD variable for families with only one child diagnosed with ASD was calculated to express the costs of ASD without the compounding effect of having multiple children with ASD and the implications this may have to

Table 3. Division of children receiving 'immediate' (N = 250) versus 'delayed' (N = 266) diagnoses.

		Q12: How old was your child when she/he was formally diagnosed with an ASD?				
		12–18 months*(2)*	**19–24 months***(3)*	**2–6 years***(4)*	**6–12 years***(5)*	**13–18 years***(6)*
Q10; How old	<12 months*(1)*	6	15	*65*	*34*	6
was your child	12–18 months*(2)*	*5*	22	91	*28*	*2*
when you or	19–24 months*(3)*	-	*7*	74	19	*3*
someone else noticed	2–6 years*(4)*	-	-	*93*	32	3
something was different	6–12 years*(5)*	-	-	-	*10*	-
or not quite right?	13–18 years*(6)*	-	-	-	-	*1*

Numbers in bold indicate the stricter division of 'immediate' (N = 116) versus 'delayed' (N = 138).

Table 4. Characteristics of the children with ASD and their families.

	N	%		
Total	521			
Male	431	83		
Female	90	17		
Age (months)	**Mean** (SD) 119 (50)	**Median** 113.5		
Respondent				
Biological mother	421	81		
Biological father	87	17		
Grandparent	5	.96		
Foster parent	4	.77		
Step parent	1	.2		
Other	1	.2		
ASD diagnosis				
Autism	272	52.60		
High-functioning autism	128	24.70		
Asperger Syndrome	36	7		
PDD-NOS	76	14.70		
CDD	2	.40		
Other	7	1.40		
How many children with ASD have one or more ASD sibling?				
0 (only child with ASD)	355	71		
1 sibling	121	24		
2 siblings	15	3		
3 siblings	9	2		
Presence of CD/ID				
Yes	371	72		
No	144	28		
Presence of other mental health/psychological conditions				
Yes	408	79		
No	108	21		
Presence of other medical conditions				
Yes	341	66.70		
No	170	33.30		
How old was your child when you first noticed something wasn't right?				
<12 months	126	24		
12–18 months	150	29		
19–24 months	103	20		
2–6 years	128	24.70		
6–12 years	10	2		
13–18 years	2	.3		
How old was your child when formally diagnosed?				
<12 months	0	0		
12–18 months	11	2.10		
19–24 months	44	8.50		
2–6 years	325	62.70		
6–12 years	123	23.70		
13–18 years	15	2.90		
Parent's highest education	**N**	**%**	**N**	**%**
	Mother		Father	
Completed year 10	72	14	74	15
Completed year 12	60	12	42	8.5

Table 4. Cont.

	N	%		
Completed certificate at TAFE (or similar)	135	26.40	87	17.60
Apprenticeship	13	2.50	94	19
Some university education but did not complete	46	9	36	7.60
Completed university undergraduate degree	103	20.10	85	17.20
Completed university postgraduate degree	82	16	75	15.20
Household composition	**N**	**%**		
Two-parent	396	76.90		
Single parent	72	14		
Only extended family (grandparents etc)	4	.80		
Two-parent plus extended	22	4.30		
Single parent plus extended	10	2		
Foster situation	3	.60		
Other	8	1.50		
Combined annual income				
<$25,000	55	10.50		
$25,000–$50,000	56	10.70		
$50,000–$75,000	68	13		
$75,000–$100,000	90	17.30		
$100,000–$125,000	59	11.30		
$125,000–$150,000	65	12.50		
$150,000–$200,000	57	11		
>$200,000	50	9.60		
Unknown	21	4		

Percentage values are rounded to two decimal places where possible.

reductions in FTE employment. The cumulative 'Cost of ASD' variable predominantly consisted of loss of income of the parents and caregivers (89%) with ASD-related travel costs (3%) and treatment costs (8%) making smaller contributions.

The cost of ASD as a function of 'immediate' versus 'delayed' diagnosis or frequency of ASD symptoms

A regression analysis was conducted with cost of ASD as the dependent variable. Independent variables included: 'immediate' (coded as 1) versus 'delayed' (coded as 2) diagnosis, ASD symptom frequency (as continuous numeric), age of child in years, number of siblings (0, 1, 2 or 3+), number of siblings with ASD (0, 1, or 2+), combined income (in $AUD), age of diagnosis of child with autism (1 = 0–12 months, 2 = 12–24 months, 3 = 2–6 years, 4 = 6–12 years, 5 = 12–18 years) and highest education of the mother and father (1 = year 10, 2 = year 12, 3 = TAFE, 4 = Apprenticeship, 5 = some university, 6 = Bachelor degree, 7 = postgraduate degree). The residuals from the regression analysis were plotted (histogram and density plots) and followed a normal distribution. The R^2 values for the two models evaluating the different criteria for immediate versus delayed diagnosis (i.e., loose and strict cut off) below were 21% and 31%, respectively, as shown in Table 6.

Table 5. Descriptive statistics for all estimated cost variables (rounded to nearest dollar) and cumulative presence of ASD symptomatology.

	N	Mean (SD)	Median	Quartiles		
				1st	2nd	3rd
ASD-related travel	521	$1,500 ($1,200)	$860	$620	$860	$2,000
Out of pocket treatment	370	$4,800 ($5,000)	$2,600	$1,000	$2,600	$7,500
Loss of income	474	$30,000 ($20,300)	$29,200	$19,500	$29,200	$48,700
Cost of ASD	**339**	**$37,60 ($21,700)**	**$37,800**	**$22,000**	**$37,800**	**$52,800**
Cost of ASD (1 ASD child per household)	**223**	**$35,100 ($20,300)**	**$34,900**	**$20,700**	**$34,900**	**$51,700**
Frequency of ASD symptoms	508	12.4 (4.2)	13	10	13	16

Table 6. Regression model of symptom frequency and delay from first identifying a problem to ultimate diagnosis and the total cost including covariates.

	Full available sample (final N = 332)						Strict immediate vs delayed sub-sample (final N = 152)					
	df	F	p^a	Contrast	Coefficient	95% CI	df	F	p^a	Contrast	Coefficient	95% CI
Immediate/Delayed diagnosis	1	0.13	0.72	1 vs 2	$-1500	-6000, 3100^b	1	0.17	0.68	1 vs 2	$2100	-6200, 10500^b
Cumulative symptom presence	1	33.0	<0.0001	slope	$1400^c	860, 1900	1	15.36	<0.0001	slope	$1500^c	630, 2400
Age group	4	2.77	0.028	1 vs 5	$730	-15000, 16000	4	1.58	0.18	1 vs 5	$-2200	-28300, 23900
				2 vs 5	$720	-15000, 16000				2 vs 5	$-80	-25300, 25200
				3 vs 5	$-340	-16000, 15000				3 vs 5	$-1900	-27400, 23600
				4 vs 5	$-6900	-22000, 8300				4 vs 5	$-9100	-34200, 15900
Number of Siblings	3	2.33	0.075	0 vs 3+	$4300	-4700, 13200	3	1.88	0.14	0 vs 3+	$15600	685, 30600
				1 vs 3+	$-4000	-11300, 3100				1 vs 3+	$2100	-8800, 13000
				2 vs 3+	$-4800	-12300, 2700				2 vs 3+	$1600	-9400, 12700
Number of Siblings with ASD	2	5.34	0.005	0 vs 2+	$-29500	-46000, -13000	1	5.24	0.007	0 vs 2+	$-44500	-71700, -17400
				1 vs 2+	$-24600	-35600, -13600				1 vs 2+	$-35300	-52100, -18500
Income	1	2.24	0.14	slope	$-800	-1900, 290	1	3.34	0.07	slope	$-1400	-3100, 270
Age of Diagnosis	4	0.18	0.95	1 vs 5	$9000	-12800, 30800	4	0.26	0.90	1 vs 5	$18800	-14100, 51800
				2 vs 5	$5300	-10800, 21500				2 vs 5	$12400	-15200, 39900
				3 vs 5	$5600	-9100, 20300				3 vs 5	$11200	-9500, 31900
				4 vs 5	$3900	-11300, 19100				4 vs 5	$9400	-11500, 30200
Education (Max of M/D)	7	0.31	0.95	1 vs 8	$17700	-5700, 41200	7	0.41	0.90	1 vs 8	$21600	-39300, 46000
				2 vs 8	$10300	-1100, 21700				2 vs 8	$8200	-5300, 27000
				3 vs 8	$1300	-7500, 10100				3 vs 8	$8800	-24200, 10500
				4 vs 8	$2800	-4300, 9800				4 vs 8	$5500	-12200, 9700
				5 vs 8	$2100	-5200, 9400				5 vs 8	$5900	-16500, 7000
				6 vs 8	$1400	-7200, 10000				6 vs 8	$7600	-15800, 14300
				7 vs 8	$1700	-4500, 8000				7 vs 8	$4900	-13300, 5900

^{a}The p-value was obtained from a regression model using the square root of the total cost as dependent variable (because of skewness in this variable).
^{b}This is the CI for the difference in cost between early and late.
^{c}This is the amount by which the cost increases (dollars) per unit increase on the symptom score.

Regardless of whether the strict or loose definition of the 'immediate 'versus 'delayed' diagnosis variable was used, neither was found to be significantly associated with the of cost of ASD. However, in both regression models, the number of ASD symptoms present was a significant predictor. In both models, costs were increased by approximately $1,400 per ASD symptom reported for the loose and strict criteria models. Models with fewer covariates were also fitted yielding similar estimates for the cost of immediate versus delayed diagnosis and the cumulative presence of ASD symptoms.

Mediation analysis

A delay in diagnosis and treatment may have an indirect effect on costs associated with ASD by increasing the number of symptoms present. In order to test this hypothesis, a mediation analysis was conducted. Firstly, it was confirmed that a delay in diagnosis was statistically significantly associated with an increased number of symptoms (number of increased symptoms associated with delay = 1.56, p = 0.001, 95% CI = 0.63, 2.49). Following this, two models were constructed and contrasted: 1) total costs were modelled as a function of delay in diagnosis alone, with the direct effect of diagnostic delay denoted as c, and 2) total costs were modelled as a function of delay in diagnosis and cumulative symptom count, with the parameter estimate for delay in diagnosis with the effect attributable to cumulative symptom count partialled out denoted c'. The final mediated effect was calculated by subtracting c' from c (i.e., mediated effect $= c - c'$). To produce 95% CIs around the mediated effect, 10,000 bootstrapped samples were taken and the quantiles representing 2.5% and 97.5% of the $c - c'$ distribution calculated. Bootstrapping the estimate of the mediated effect has been recommended for mediation analysis because the technique offers acceptable statistical power properties, directly estimates the mediated effect, and does not rely on many of the assumptions necessary for other tests [14,15].

The mediation analysis was supportive of this hypothesis. A statistically significant reduction in the effect associated with diagnostic delay of $2,110 (95% CI = 820, 3700) was observed when symptom count was included in the model. This was despite the delay in diagnosis not being statistically significantly associated with total cost directly (see above). The mediation analysis was repeated with all covariates included in the original model (age of child, number of siblings, number of siblings with ASD, combined income, age of ASD diagnosis, and highest education of mother and father) and a similar effect was found (mediated effect $c - c' = $1,770$, 95% CI = 360, 3340).

Analysis of non-respondents

Contact was established with 267 of the 405 families who did not return a completed questionnaire, and, of these, 148 agreed to complete the short-form questionnaire. Sixty-four families had already completed the long-form questionnaire. Fifty-two families (13%) declined to participate in the phone questionnaire. Incorrect phone numbers and no answer were the main reasons for failures to contact. A complete breakdown of the telephone sample is shown in Figure 1. Two of the 148 families that agreed to participate did not have a child with ASD. From the 146 families with children with ASD that agreed to complete the short- form questionnaire, data were collated for 171 individual children.

As shown in Table 7, there were few noteworthy differences between respondents and non- respondents. Demographically, respondents were slightly more likely to have a male child and to have noticed developmental atypicality earlier. Respondents also received a formal diagnosis of ASD earlier than non-respondents.

Respondents reported higher treatment costs than non-respondents. However, there were no differences in reported income loss.

Discussion

ASD-related costs were strongly associated with the cumulative presence of the child's symptoms. This builds upon previous research that has found that having a child with ASD is associated with significant financial strain [16–19]. The association between increased costs and ASD symptom severity suggests that effective and early interventions that result in the reduction of expressed symptoms may have a significant impact on improving a family's productivity and their resultant financial situation.

Contrary to expectations, there was no statistically significant differences in costs related to receiving the diagnosis of ASD whether soon or late after suspicion. We suggest two possible reasons for this. Firstly, given the above finding that increasing symptomatology is directly related to the cost of ASD, the more immediate identification of ASD may create a situation where improvement in outcomes and the effect on associated symptomatology measures dwarfs the influence of delay to diagnosis on the final cost of ASD. This interpretation appears to be consistent with the mediation analysis, whereby an indirect effect of diagnostic delay on costs appeared to be mediated by an association between increased symptomatology and increased diagnostic delay. Secondly, families with a child with ASD may adapt their work-family balance regardless of whether the child has a diagnosis or not. This is reflected by the finding that the largest cost reported by parents was a loss of income from reduced working hours. This is consistent with a previous report stating that a loss of approximately 14% of family income is often the consequence of having a child with ASD [16], equalling $7,200 (based on the median income and average exchange rate of 2008). The results from the present study suggest a substantially higher (29%) loss of combined household income.

From a family and societal perspective, support that allows family members to work may more effectively assist families with children with ASD by lessening the financial burden and improving well-being of all family members. Furthermore, the long-term consequence of high costs associated with having a child who has a diagnosis of ASD is not well researched. A study reporting on the distribution of societal costs of ASD distributed throughout the lifespan estimated that fathers of children with moderate to severe autism were unemployed 20% of a full time equivalent [20], whereas 60% of mothers were unemployed and 30% worked part time of a full time equivalent [20]. If these estimates are indeed accurate, the family income may therefore be severely impacted through the lifespan as a result of having a child with ASD [20]. The largest direct life time cost is to provide care for adults with ASD [20,21]. Consequently, parents of adults with ASD may face an even larger financial strain when having to provide services for their adult children whilst having had less opportunity to save or accumulate superannuation funds due to reduced possibilities to work full time [20].

Limitations

There are several limitations to the cost analysis presented here: 1) The return rate of 15% observed in the present study is quite poor in comparison to similar studies. This may be because client details registered with the DSC are maintained sporadically and a number of records contained incomplete or inaccurate entries. Furthermore, distributed questionnaires were addressed only to the fathers of the registered child for some families due to a DSC database error. Given reports of higher than normal divorce rates

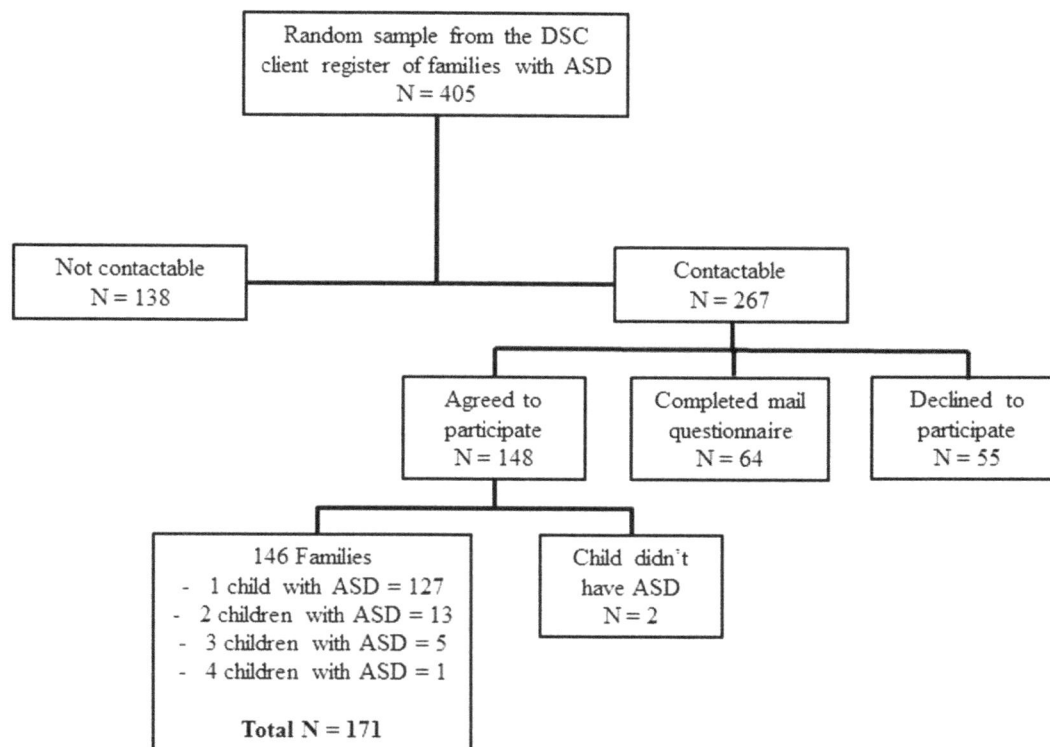

Figure 1. Breakdown of the non-respondent sample for the purposes of the short-form telephone questionnaire. A full representation of a random sample of families registered as having received or currently receiving service provision for the purposes of an analysis of non-respondents. From a random sample of 405 families, 146 families (totalling 171 children with ASD) agreed to participate in the telephone questionnaire

in families with children with ASD [22], this may be another reason for a lower than usual return rate reflected by the higher than expected number of respondents reporting being in two-parent households compared to non-respondents. 2) There are multiple reasons why a child might not be diagnosed until later in development, giving rise to a number of caveats with respect to the 'delayed' diagnostic group. For example, some of those diagnosed later in development may present with symptomatology that is either more complex or reduced in severity compared to those children with evident and more severe symptoms from an early age. However, this influence appeared to be relatively small as the effect of the variable "Age of diagnosis" was not a statistically significant contributor to cost, or may be reflected more by the cumulative presence of ASD symptomatology measure. 3) Requesting estimates of current costs may not be representative of historical costs as current expenses are dependent on the child's stage of development, time since diagnosis, and current stage of treatment or intervention. However, one aspect for which our estimates are robust is their specification of only ASD-related expenses for medical, behavioural or complimentary/alternative therapies. 4) In contrast to most parents that had reduced their hours due to the needs of their child with ASD, a small number of parents were seeking *more* work due to the expenses of having a child with ASD. This is not often considered when calculating the costs and productivity losses associated with a diagnosis of ASD. 5) A number of parents reported low treatment costs because they had exhausted all funded avenues and could not afford to independently fund treatment for their children. 5) Lastly, the present study does not address all aspects of how an immediate or

delayed diagnosis may impact families and their financial situation. The processes that parents undergo in order to access a proficient diagnosis are reported as being extremely stressful [23] and may result in health related consequences difficult to estimate in any cost benefit analysis [18]. Consequently, health related consequences and costs for family members and society in relation to early/late diagnosis may warrant further scrutinising.

Conclusions

The median family cost of ASD was estimated to be AUD $34,900 per annum (IQR $20,700 - $51,700; based on median income from wages), with almost 90% of the sum ($29,200) due to loss of income from employment. While there was no statistically significant direct effect on the cost depending on the timeliness of the diagnosis (immediate versus delayed) the cumulative presence of ASD symptoms had a significant impact on the costs and a delay in diagnosis could indirectly increase costs by neglecting symptoms that may respond to more immediate intervention. For each additional symptom reported, a $1,400 cost for the family per annum was added. These findings take on a great deal of significance when considered within a regional context as funding amounts vary across states and countries. The financial burden of families of children with ASD is correlated with the existing societal financial safety net [17]. In an Australian context, families may miss out on the most widely available financial support for early intervention if the diagnosis is received after the age of six [24]. If the family is expected to carry a substantial share of the cost needed to support the development of children with ASD, this may have detrimental consequences for the wellbeing of the child

Table 7. Comparison between respondents (N = 521) and non-respondents (N = 171) on demographics and two main study variables that can be derived from the short-form telephone questionnaire.

	Non-Respondents (N = 171)	Respondents (N = 521)
Age (months)	Mean (SD) 122 (50)	Mean (SD) 119 (50)
	Median 120	Median 113.50
		t (678) = .53, p = .60
	Proportion (%)	**Proportion (%)**
Sex of diagnosed child		
Male	75.50	83
Female	24.50	17
		χ^2(1, N = 689) = 4.41, p = .04
ASD diagnosis		
Autism	47.40	52.60
HFA	25.10	24.70
Asperger Syndrome	11.10	7
PDD-NOS	15.80	14.70
CDD	.60	.40
Other	-	1.40
		χ^2(6, N = 703) = 4.31, p = .64
How old was your child when you first noticed something was not right?		
<12 months	24.10	24
12–18 months	17.10	29
19–24 months	18.20	20
2–6 years	35.30	24.70
6–18 years*	5.30	2.30
		χ^2(4, N = 704) = 15.38, p < .05
How old was your child when formally diagnosed?		
<12–24 months*	10.30	10.60
2–6 years	50.10	62.70
6–18+ years*	38.70	26.60
		χ^2(2, N = 698) = 9.61, p < .01
Household composition		
Two-parent	73.70	76.90
Single parent	22.20	14
Only extended family (grandparents etc)	.60	.80
Two-parent plus extended	2.30	4.3
Single parent plus extended	1.20	2
Foster situation	-	.6
Other	-	1.5
-		χ^2(6, N = 702) = 10.94, p = .09
Out-of-pocket treatment costs	Mean (SD) $2,300 ($2,900)	Mean (SD) $4,800 ($5,000)
-	Median $1,000	Median $2,600
-		Z = −16.95, p < .001, r = −.76
Loss of income	Mean (SD) $25,400 ($21,000)	Mean (SD) $30,000 ($20,300)
-	Median $29,300	Median $29,200
-		Z = −.94, p = .35, r = −.04

Categorical demographic variables are presented as proportions due to missing data in some variables.
* These variables have been collapsed across categories for the purposes of chi-square analyses.

with ASD, as well as for other family members, especially for low income families that may not seek services at all for financial reasons [17].

Acknowledgments

Aoife McNally, Kirsty Oehlers, Mandy Richards, Geoff Cole, Susan Peden, staff at Disabilities Services Commission, Caitlin Axford, Fiona Choi, Helen Weldergergish, Rachel Owens, Rex Parsons, Stephen Lawrie, Gal Rose, Tim Parkin and the AIM employment AAWA.

Authorship statement& transparency declaration

The final manuscript has been seen and approved by all authors and they have taken due care to ensure the integrity of the work. The work is original and has not been published elsewhere and is currently not under consideration by another journal. All authors have had full access to the data, analysis and writing and editing has jointly been done.

The lead author affirms that this manuscript is an honest, accurate, and transparent account of the study being reported; that no important aspects of the study have been omitted; and that any discrepancies from the study as planned (and, if relevant, registered) have been explained.

Author Contributions

Conceived and designed the experiments: CH MF MA TF. Performed the experiments: CH MF. Analyzed the data: CH RP MA TF. Wrote the paper: CH MF RP MA TF.

References

1. Consulting SE (2007) Economic Costs of ASD in Australia. Synergies Economic Consulting.
2. Le Couteur A, Haden G, Hammal D, McComachie H (2008) Diagnosing Autism Spectrum Disorders in pre-school children using two standardised assessment instruments: The ADI-R and the ADOS. Journal of Autism and Developmental Disorders 38: 362–372.
3. Woolfenden S, Sarkozy V, Ridley G, Williams K (2012) A systematic review of the diagnostic stability of Autism Spectrum Disorder. Research in Autism Spectrum Disorders 6: 345–354.
4. Shattuck PT, Grosse SD (2007) Issues related to the diagnosis and treatment of autism spectrum disorders. Mental Retardation and Developmental Disabilities Research Reviews 13: 129–135.
5. Sikora D, Hall T, Hartley S, Gerrard-Morris A, Cagle S (2008) Does Parent Report of Behavior Differ Across ADOS-G Classifications: Analysis of Scores from the CBCL and GARS. Journal of Autism and Developmental Disorders 38: 440–448.
6. South M, Williams B, McMahon W, Owley T, Filipek P, et al. (2002) Utility of the Gilliam Autism Rating Scale in Research and Clinical Populations. Journal of Autism and Developmental Disorders 32: 593–599.
7. McEachin JJ, Smith T, Lovaas OI (1993) Long-term outcome for children with autism who received early intensive behavioral treatment. American Journal on Mental Retardation 97: 359–372.
8. Rogers S (1996) Brief report: Early intervention in autism. Journal of Autism and Developmental Disorders 26: 243–246.
9. Lovaas OI (1987) Behavioral treatment and normal educational and intellectual functioning in young autistic children. Journal of Consulting and Clinical Psychology 55: 3–9.
10. Remington B, Hastings RP, Kovshoff H, degli Espinosa F, Jahr E, et al. (2007) Early Intensive Behavioral Intervention: Outcomes for Children With Autism and Their Parents After Two Years. American Journal on Mental Retardation 112: 418–438.
11. Harris SL, Handleman JS (2000) Age and IQ at Intake as Predictors of Placement for Young Children with Autism: A Four- to Six-Year Follow-Up. Journal of Autism and Developmental Disorders 30: 137–142.
12. Fenske EC, Zalenski S, Krantz PJ, McClannahan LE (1985) Age at intervention and treatment outcome for autistic children in a comprehensive intervention program. Analysis and Intervention in Developmental Disabilities 5: 49–58.
13. Matson JL, Wilkins J, Boisjoli JA, Smith KR (2008) The validity of the autism spectrum disorders-diagnosis for intellectually disabled adults (ASD-DA). Research in Developmental Disabilities 29: 537–546.
14. Hayes AF (2009) Beyond Baron and Kenny: Statistical mediation analysis in the new millennium. Communication Monographs 76: 408–420.
15. MacKinnon DP, Fairchild AJ, Fritz MS (2007) Mediation analysis. Annual Review of Psychology 58: 593.
16. Montes G, Halterman JS (2008) Association of Childhood Autism Spectrum Disorders and Loss of Family Income. Pediatrics 121: e821–e826.
17. Parish SL, Thomas KC, Rose R, Kilany M, Shattuck PT (2012) State Medicaid Spending and Financial Burden of Families Raising Children with Autism. Intellectual and Developmental Disabilities 50: 441–451.
18. Phelps KW, Hodgson JL, McCammon SL, Lamson AL (2009) Caring for an individual with autism disorder: A qualitative analysis*. Journal of Intellectual and Developmental Disability 34: 27–35.
19. Sharpe D, Baker D (2007) Financial Issues Associated with Having a Child with Autism. Journal of Family and Economic Issues 28: 247–264.
20. Ganz ML (2007) THe lifetime distribution of the incremental societal costs of autism. Archives of Pediatrics & Adolescent Medicine 161: 343–349.
21. Ganz M (2006) The Costs of Autism. Understanding Autism: CRC Press. pp. 475–502.
22. Hartley SL, Barker ET, Seltzer MM, Floyd F, Greenberg J, et al. (2010) The Relative Risk and Timing of Divorce in Families of Children with an Autism Spectrum Disorder. Journal of Family Psychology 24: 449–457.
23. Keenan M, Dillenburger K, Doherty A, Byrne T, Gallagher S (2010) The Experiences of Parents During Diagnosis and Forward Planning for Children with Autism Spectrum Disorder. Journal of Applied Research in Intellectual Disabilities 23: 390–397.
24. Australian Government (2013) Helping Children with Autism. Department of Families, Housing, Community Services and Indigenous Affairs.

2

The Clinical Impact of Chromosomal Microarray on Paediatric Care in Hong Kong

Victoria Q. Tao[1], Kelvin Y. K. Chan[2], Yoyo W. Y. Chu[1], Gary T. K. Mok[1], Tiong Y. Tan[1,3], Wanling Yang[1], So Lun Lee[1], Wing Fai Tang[4], Winnie W. Y. Tso[1], Elizabeth T. Lau[4], Anita S. Y. Kan[2], Mary H. Tang[4], Yu-lung Lau[1], Brian H. Y. Chung[1,4]*

1 Department of Paediatrics and Adolescent Medicine, LKS Faculty of Medicine, The University of Hong Kong, Hong Kong Special Administrative Region, China, 2 Department of Obstetrics and Gynecology, Queen Mary Hospital, Hong Kong Special Administrative Region, China, 3 Victorian Clinical Genetics Service, Murdoch Children's Research Institute, Royal Children's Hospital, Department of Paediatrics, University of Melbourne, Melbourne, Australia, 4 Department of Obstetrics and Gynecology, LKS Faculty of Medicine, The University of Hong Kong, Hong Kong Special Administrative Region, China

Abstract

Objective: To evaluate the clinical impact of chromosomal microarray (CMA) on the management of paediatric patients in Hong Kong.

Methods: We performed NimbleGen 135k oligonucleotide array on 327 children with intellectual disability (ID)/ developmental delay (DD), autism spectrum disorders (ASD), and/or multiple congenital anomalies (MCAs) in a university-affiliated paediatric unit from January 2011 to May 2013. The medical records of patients were reviewed in September 2013, focusing on the pathogenic/likely pathogenic CMA findings and their "clinical actionability" based on established criteria.

Results: Thirty-seven patients were reported to have pathogenic/likely pathogenic results, while 40 had findings of unknown significance. This gives a detection rate of 11% for clinically significant (pathogenic/likely pathogenic) findings. The significant findings have prompted clinical actions in 28 out of 37 patients (75.7%), while the findings with unknown significance have led to further management recommendation in only 1 patient (p<0.001). Nineteen out of the 28 management recommendations are "evidence-based" on either practice guidelines endorsed by a professional society (n = 9, Level 1) or peer-reviewed publications making medical management recommendation (n = 10, Level 2). CMA results impact medical management by precipitating referral to a specialist (n = 24); diagnostic testing (n = 25), surveillance of complications (n = 19), interventional procedure (n = 7), medication (n = 15) or lifestyle modification (n = 12).

Conclusion: The application of CMA in children with ID/DD, ASD, and/or MCAs in Hong Kong results in a diagnostic yield of ~11% for pathogenic/likely pathogenic results. Importantly the yield for clinically actionable results is 8.6%. We advocate using diagnostic yield of clinically actionable results to evaluate CMA as it provides information of both clinical validity and clinical utility. Furthermore, it incorporates evidence-based medicine into the practice of genomic medicine. The same framework can be applied to other genomic testing strategies enabled by next-generation sequencing.

Editor: Michael Edward Zwick, Emory University School Of Medicine, United States of America

Funding: The study was funded by SK Yee Medical Foundation 2011 (#211203), SK Yee Medical Foundation 2012 (#212210), and SK Yee Medical Research 2012 (#20006551) applied by BHYC.(http://www.skyeemedicalfoundation.org/). TYT was funded by an Overseas Training Fellowship (#607431) provided by the National Health and Medical Research Council of Australia. The funders had no role in study design, data collection and analysis, decision to publish, or preparation of the manuscript.

Competing Interests: The authors have declared that no competing interests exist.

* Email: bhychung@hku.hk

Introduction

Chromosomal microarray (CMA) has emerged as a major tool to identify unbalanced chromosomal aberrations in children for its higher resolution compared to conventional cytogenetics and is recommended as the first-tier investigation for intellectual disability (ID)/developmental delay (DD), autism spectrum disorders (ASD) and multiple congenital anomalies (MCAs). [1–9] Balanced rearrangements and low-level mosaicism are generally not detectable; however, these are relatively infrequent causes of abnormal phenotypes in patients (<1%). [2] Large-scale studies in Asian populations have revealed similar detection rates compared to studies conducted in Europe and Northern America. [10–13]

While the clinical interpretation of microarray anomalies remains an ongoing challenge, the impact of CMA results on clinical management is not well studied. Surveys of physicians showed changes in management in 70% patients with positive CMA results [14]. Multiple case reports have demonstrated the usefulness of CMA in identifying the genetic causes in patients with unknown diagnoses and in uncovering cancer susceptibility.

[15–17] In a cohort of 1792 patients with ID, ASD and/or MCAs, management recommendations were made in 54% patients with clinically significant CMA results and 34% with findings of possible significance. [18] Riggs et al. compiled a list of 146 genomic disorders which would be detected by CMA for which there are published evidence supporting management recommendation and identified that 7% of all cases in the ISCA (International Standards for Cytogenomic Arrays) Consortium database are "clinically actionable". [19] In a review based on 46298 cases in the laboratory database, Ellison et al found that 35% of the cases with positive CMA results were established microdeletion/microduplication syndromes, conditions with increased cancer susceptibility or other actionable conditions associated with dosage-sensitive genes. [20] Henderson et al. found that 55% of the positive CMA results prompted clinical actions in their cohort of 1780 cases. [21]

Despite the growing evidence of its diagnostic yield and cost-effectiveness [22], CMA has not yet been implemented as a first-tier diagnostic test for the above mentioned conditions for children in Hong Kong. The objective of this study is to evaluate the clinical impact of CMA on the medical management of the paediatric patients in whom CMA was applied as first-tier clinical testing in Hong Kong. We study the clinical impact of CMA by evaluating the detection rate of pathogenic/likely pathogenic findings and the proportion of these findings that are clinically actionable, and the level of evidence supporting these recommendations.

Materials and Methods

Patients and Samples

From January 2011, we started to offer CMA to paediatric patients in 2 university-affiliated hospitals: Queen Mary Hospital (QMH) and the Duchess of Kent Children's Hospital (DKCH). Indications for CMA included unexplained ID/DD, ASD, or multiple MCAs after review by a clinical geneticist. Clinically recognizable syndromic conditions, e.g. Down syndrome, were confirmed by conventional cytogenetic (e.g. karyotype)/molecular tests (e.g. rapid aneuploidy detection by QF-PCR and fluorescent in-situ hybridization, FISH) instead of "first-tiered" CMA, and referred for CMA when conventional investigation showed negative results. Written informed consent for CMA was obtained from all parents/legal guardians. Clinicians or geneticists counseled the parents/guardians about the indication for the CMA, benefits and limitations of the test, methodology, reporting time and possible outcomes upon recruitment. Patients who had received prenatal CMA testing or parents who opted not to receive test result were excluded.

CMA testing and interpretation

For each patient, 3 ml of peripheral blood in EDTA bottle was sent to Prenatal Diagnostic Laboratory, Tsan Yuk Hospital (TYH). All samples were tested by NimbleGen CGX-135K arrays designed by Signature Genomics (Roche NimbleGen, Inc., Madison, WI, USA) following manufacturer's instructions. The coverage of the array has an average resolution of 140 kb across the genome and 40 kb or less in regions of clinical relevance. It evaluates over 245 known genetic syndromes and over 980 gene regions of functional significance in human development. Data were analyzed by Genoglyphix software (Signature Genomics, Spokane, USA). Genomic coordinates were based on genome build hg18.

Detected copy number variants (CNVs) were systematically evaluated for its clinical significance by comparing the CNVs to information in the Signature Genomics' proprietary Genoglyphix Chromosome Aberration Database (Signature Genomics, Spokane, WA, USA), internal laboratory database at TYH and public databases [Database of Genomic Variant (DGV), International Standards for Cytogenomic Arrays Consortium Database (ISCA), Children Hospital of Philadelphia database (CHOP), Database of Chromosomal Imbalance and Phenotype in Humans using Ensembl Resources (DECIPHER)]. Categorization of CNVs was based on available phenotypes and comparison of phenotypes with genes in the region of copy gain or loss. This was done through searching Online Mendelian Inheritance in Man (OMIM), PubMed, RefSeq, the University of California Santa Cruz (UCSC) genome browser. [23] Confirmatory FISH/qPCR/conventional karyotype was performed as indicated. Parental testing was offered to aid further interpretation and classification. CNVs were classified as pathogenic, likely pathogenic, unknown/uncertain significance, or benign according to the 2011 American College of Medical Genetics (ACMG) practice guideline. [24] Only pathogenic and likely pathogenic CNVs are regarded as clinically significant.

Management actions based on clinically significant CMA result

We identified 327 patients that fulfilled our inclusion criteria on whom we have performed CMA from the period January 2011 to May 2013. Retrospective medical record review was performed in September 2013 when all the abnormal CMA results had been disclosed to the patients/families in the post-test genetic counseling session. We analyzed the detection rate of clinically significant CMA results (pathogenic or likely pathogenic) and the medical management recommendations directly based on these findings. Since the interpretation of CNVs can evolve with new evidence over a short period of time, we also evaluated CNVs classified as "benign" and "unknown significance" for comparison.

A recommendation for clinical action was defined as any management recommendations prompted by CMA results including recurrent surveillance (S), specialist referral/assessment (R), diagnostic investigation (D) such as laboratory tests, ECG, diagnostic imaging studies etc., medical/surgical procedure (P), drug administration (M) (such as indication/contraindication for drug treatment), lifestyle recommendation (L) and other interventions (O) such as alternative therapies etc. [18,19] Information on the clinically actionable genomic regions and the level of supporting evidence (Level 1 to 4) proposed by Riggs et al. [19] was used to analyze our findings. We did not include genetic counseling (for advice on reproductive options and/or prenatal diagnosis), confirmatory karyotype/QF-PCR/FISH, or parental testing which was done to clarify CNVs inheritance as countable clinical action.

Statistical Analysis

Unpaired t-test was used for comparing CNVs size between pathogenic or likely pathogenic group and unknown clinical significance group. Fisher's exact tests were used to examine any potential association between CMA outcome and patients' characteristics including age group, gender and indications for CMA. Statistical analysis was carried out using IBM SPSS Statistics software version 19. A two-tailed p-value of less than 0.05 was treated as statistically significant.

Ethics Statement

Approval was obtained from the Institutional Review Board of the University of Hong Kong and Hospital Authority of Hong

Kong West Cluster. The title of the approved study is "Comparative study in prenatal/postnatal diagnostic detection using microarray technology and conventional cytogenetic analysis", under the reference number UW10-226. Written informed consent was obtained from all parents/legal guardians.

Results

Three hundred and twenty seven patients had CMA testing in the 29 months period and all were included in our analysis. Thirty-three patients were found to have pathogenic CNVs; 4 with likely pathogenic CNVs; 40 with CNVs of unknown significance, while the rest had benign CNVs. The detection rate of clinically significant CNVs (pathogenic or likely pathogenic) was 11.3% (37/327). In the group with clinically significant findings, 22 patients had copy number loss (deletions), 9 had copy number gain (duplications), and 6 patients had both deletion and duplication. There were a total of 45 clinical significant CNVs and 6 CNVs of unknown clinical significance found in these 37 patients. Of the group with CNVs of unknown clinical significance, 11 were deletions, 26 were duplications, and 3 were both deletion and duplication. There were a total of 45 CNVs of unknown clinical significance in these 40 patients. (See Table 1 for characteristics of the patients, Table 2 for CNVs types and numbers in clinically significant CNVs and CNVs with unknown significance group.)

Patients with clinically significant CNVs were younger (age <12 months old, p<0.001, by Fisher's exact test), more likely to be female (p<0.001, by Fisher's exact test) and also more frequently had MCA/dysmorphism as indications for CMA (p<0.001, by Fisher's exact test), compared to others (Table 1). The mean size of clinical significant CNVs (9.20 Mb±4.56 Mb, mean±95% C.I.) was larger than that of CNVs of unknown significance

(0.53 Mb±0.19 Mb) (p<0.001, by unpaired t-test). Copy number loss was found more frequently in clinically significant CNVs than in CNVs of unknown clinical significance (64.4% compared to 31.1%, p = 0.003, by Fisher's exact test).

Within the group of patients with clinically significant CNVs, there were patients with well-known genomic disorders including 1p36 deletion (n = 1), Wolf-Hirschhorn syndrome (n = 2), Cri du Chat syndrome (n = 2), Klinefelter syndrome (n = 1), 22q11.2 deletion (n = 2), and Williams syndrome (n = 3). CMA was offered to these patients either because their clinical features did not allow definitive diagnosis of the condition, or because they were atypical deletions or duplications that could not be detected by standard cytogenetic methods e.g. 22q11.2 deletion. [25] A few patients with interesting clinical/CMA findings in this cohort have been reported previously. [26–28]

Recommendations for clinical management were made in 75.7% (28 out of 37) patients with significant CNVs (Table 3), and in 2.5% (1 in 40) patients with unknown significance (see discussion section for detail of this case) respectively (p<0.001 by Fisher's exact test). Specific clinical actions for the patients with significant CNVs include 19 recommendations for surveillance (S), 24 specialist referrals (R), 25 diagnostic tests (D), 7 medical/surgical procedures (P), 15 recommendations regarding drug administration (M), 12 recommendations for lifestyle modification (L). According to the criteria by Riggs et al. [19], in nine of these patients, recommendations were based on Level 1 evidence, i.e. from practice guideline endorsed by a professional society; 10 were based on Level 2 evidence, i.e. from peer-reviewed publication describing medical management recommendations; 8 were based on Level 3 evidence, i.e. from peer-reviewed publications not regarding management but implying potential management based on clinical judgment; 1 was based on Level 4 evidence, i.e. could

Table 1. Patients' characteristics and CMA findings.

	[A] Number of patients with Pathogenic or Likely Pathogenic CNVs (%)	[B] Number of patients with CNVs of Unknown Clinical Significance (%)	[C] Number of patients with Benign CNVs (%)	[A] vs [B+C] comparison (by Fisher's exact test)
Total	37/327 (11.3%)	40/327 (12.2%)	250/327 (76.5%)	
Age				p<0.001
<12 m	20/37 (54.1%)	4/40 (10.0%)	34/250 (13.6%)	
1 – 5 y	10/37 (27.0%)	27/40 (67.5%)	164/250 (65.6%)	
6 – 10 y	2/37 (5.4%)	6/40 (15.0%)	28/250 (11.2%)	
11 – 18 y	4/37 (10.8%)	2/40 (5.0%)	20/250 (8.0%)	
>18 y	1/37 (2.7%)	1/40 (2.5%)	4/250 (1.6%)	
Gender				p<0.001
Male	15/37 (40.5%)	32/40 (80.0%)	172/250 (68.8%)	
Female	22/37 (59.5%)	8/40 (20.0%)	78/250 (31.2%)	
Indications (Number of total cases)				p<0.001
Neurodevelopmental disorders (DD/ID/ASD) (215 cases)	9/37 (24.3%)	28/40 (70.0%)	178/250 (71.2%)	
	9/215 (4.2%)*	28/215 (13.0%)*	178/215 (82.8%)*	
MCA/Dysmorphism ± neurodevelopmental disorders (105 cases)	26/37 (70.3%)	12/40 (30.0%)	67/250 (26.8%)	
	26/105 (24.8%)*	12/105 (11.4%)*	67/105 (63.8%)*	
Others (7 cases)	2/37 (5.4%)	0/40 (0%)	5/250 (2.0%)	
	2/7 (28.6%)*	0/7 (0%)*	5/7 (71.4%)*	

* = detection rate based on referring indications. Abbreviations: MCA = Multiple Congenital Anomalies; DD = Developmental Delay; ID = Intellectual Disability; ASD = Autism Spectrum Disorders; m = months old, y = years old.

Table 2. CNVs type in patients with clinically significant CNVs and patients with CNVs of unknown clinical significance.

CNVs type	Patients with clinically significant CNVs (n = 37)	Patients with CNVs of unknown clinical significance (n = 40)
One deletion	21/37	11/40
Two deletions	1/37	0
One duplication	8/37	24/40
Two duplications	1/37	2/40
Deletion and Duplication	6/37	3/40

be managed symptomatically regardless of underlying diagnosis. Of the 28 patients with recommendations made based on the CMA result, 21 of them have findings overlapping with the clinically actionable genomic regions reported by Riggs et al. in 2013. [19] In the other 7 patients, management recommendations were made for one patient with Klinefelter syndrome (Level 1 evidence), one with trisomy X syndrome (Level 2 evidence) while in the rest the recommendations were based on case series/case reports (Level 3 evidence). The overall diagnostic yield of clinically actionable abnormal CMA findings is 8.6% (28/327).

Case Illustration

Level 1 evidence for clinical action: 47,XXY/Klinefelter syndrome (Case 37 in Table 3)

A 3 year old boy presented with speech delay and autistic features. He was born preterm following a spontaneous monochorionic diamniotic twin pregnancy. CMA showed arr(1-22,X)×2,(Y)×1 (confirmed by karyotype). He was referred to the endocrinology clinic, where he was managed according to existing protocols for Klinefelter syndrome with other various recommendations (R,D,P,S,M,L). [29,30] His otherwise healthy twin was also confirmed to have Klinefelter Syndrome. Their mother was pregnant when the diagnosis of Klinefelter syndrome was disclosed and parental karyotype was offered due to their anxiety. The karyotype of their father was normal while that of their mother (30 years old) showed low level mosaicism of 47,XXX[1]/46,XX[29]. Sex chromosome aneuploidy is recognized to be a normal phenomenon in culture lymphocytes from women of different ages and specifically it was reported that 4% of women between 23 to 34 years of age can have X chromosome gain. [31] This low frequency of aneuploid cells does not signify an increased risk of prenatal diagnosis of sex chromosomal aneuploidy in the fetus and this was explained to the parents in subsequent session of genetic counseling.

Level 2 evidence for clinical action: 1p36 deletion (Case 1 in Table 3)

A newborn girl was diagnosed to have Ebstein anomaly. She developed a generalized seizure shortly after cardiac surgery on day 3 of life. CMA showed diagnosis of 1p36 microdeletion syndrome (OMIM #607872). Neurodevelopmental and feeding assessment (R), eye assessment (S), EEG (D), brain MRI (D), USG kidney (D), and thyroid function test (S) were recommended. [32] Thyroxine replacement (M) and antiepileptic therapy (M) were prescribed subsequently. Parents were provided with extensive counseling on the prognosis and management of the condition. The patient had a prolonged hospital stay and died at 20 months of age after an acute deterioration without identifiable cause.

Level 3 evidence for clinical action: 1q44 deletion (Case 3 in Table 3)

A full term baby with pulmonary atresia, ventricular septal defect and thyroid agenesis was referred for genetic evaluation at 2 months of age. She had a history of intrauterine growth restriction and exhibited failure to thrive. CMA showed 1q44 deletion [arr 1q44(241,821,041–247,174,728) ×1]. Her clinical features were consistent with the phenotype associated with 1q44 deletion (OMIM #612337). Seizures and abnormal corpus callosum are commonly reported. [33–35] Our patient was recommended to have brain MRI which showed a hypoplastic corpus callosum. Upon our recommendation, she was followed by the neurologists and confirmed to have severe DD. She later developed seizures and required antiepileptic treatment.

No recommendation for clinical action: submicroscopic unbalanced translocation (Case 2 in Table 3)

A 24 year-old female being followed in the paediatric clinic was referred for evaluation of developmental delay and dysmorphic features. She had a past history of being small for gestational age, short stature, scoliosis, hypotonia and resolved tremor/head shaking. All her previous investigations, including brain MRI (hypoplastic inferior vermis), karyotype, FISH for Williams syndrome, 7 blood tests and 2 urine tests for metabolic diseases, spine MRI, nerve conduction velocity/electromyography, Tensilon test, muscle biopsy, were non-diagnostic. CMA showed terminal 1p36.33p36.32 duplication and terminal 10q26.2q26.3 deletion, suggesting an unbalanced translocation. The unbalanced translocation was then confirmed by FISH. Patients with 10q26 deletion are reported to share similar features of ID/DD, dysmorphic features, as well as behavioral problems. [36–38] Although there was no clinical action prompted in this patient, this case showed how first-tier CMA testing might have avoided 15 unnecessary investigations (including the invasive muscle biopsy) and ended the diagnostic odyssey.

Discussion

A growing body of evidence demonstrates the superior diagnostic yield of CMA compared to conventional karyotype, and CMA has been endorsed by various professional organizations as a first-tier investigation for children with unexplained DD/ID/ASD and/or MCAs. [2,3] However in the States, the evidence has not been sufficient to support coverage of CMA by many health insurance providers. The decision of which often depends on the evidence of whether a test will influence medical management and result in improvement in health outcome. In Hong Kong where most medical expenses are publicly funded, similar decisions have to be made by the government for supporting new testing and

Table 3. Management recommendations for clinically significant CNVs and recommendation according to the level of evidence.

Case no.	Age/Sex	Indication	Genomic coordinates (hg18) of CNVs	CNV size and type/syndrome or locus	Parental Testing	Clinical action	Level of evidence
1*	1m/F	MCA/dys	chr1: 825,513–6,489,818	5.6 Mb terminal copy loss at 1p36.33–p36.31/1p36 deletion	De novo	R,D,S,M	level 2
2*	24y/F	MCA/dys +DD	chr1: 825,513–3,930,371; chr10: 129,188,065–135,253,240	3.1 Mb copy gain at 1p36.33–p36.32 and 6 Mb copy loss at 10q26.2–q26.3/unbalanced translocation	N	no	no
3*	2m/F	MCA	chr1: 241,821,041–247,174,728	5.3 Mb terminal copy loss at 1q44/1q44 deletion	N	R,D	level 3
4*	18y/M	MCA+DD, cytogenetic diagnosis	chr3: 76,277–8,720,170; chr10: 102,474,001–135,246,402	8.6 Mb terminal copy loss at 3p26.3–p25.3; 32.7 Mb terminal copy gain at 10q24.31–q26.3/unbalanced translocation	N	no	no
5*	3y/F	MCA+cytogenetic diagnosis	chr4: 33,860–15,640,617	15.6 Mb copy loss at 4p16.3–p15.32/Wolf–Hirschhorn syndrome	N	R,D,P,M	level 2
6*	4m/M	MCA	chr5: 108,368–133,485; chr15: 20,372,901–37,603,955	25.1 kb copy loss (UCS) at 5p15.33; 17.2 Mb copy loss at 15q11.2–q14, karyotyping showed loss of chromosome 15 segment proximal to 15q15: karyotype 45,XY,der(5)t(5;15)(p15.3;q15)dn, –15/Expanded Prader–Willi syndrome	De novo	R,D,S,M,L for PWS; R,D for 15q13.3 del	level 1 for PWS, level 2 for 15q13.3 del
7*	6d/F	MCA	chr5: 108,467–17,723,107	17.6 Mb terminal copy loss at 5p15.33–p15.1/Cri du Chat syndrome	De novo	R,D,S	level 2
8*	7m/F	MCA	chr5: 108,467–1,237,565; chr5: 1,255,929–27,782,119	1.13 Mb terminal copy gain at 5p15.33; 26.5 Mb copy loss at 5p15.33–p14.1/Cri du Chat syndrome	N	R,D,S	level 2
9*	10m/F	MCA+DD+ASD	chr5: 108,467–1,597,323; chr11: 115,190,302–134,434,130	1.5 Mb terminal copy loss at 5p15.33; 19.2 Mb terminal copy gain at 11q23.2–q25/unbalanced mat. translocation t(5;11)(p15.3;q23)	Mat	R,D,S	level 2
10*	2m/F	MCA	chr5: 58,860,944–59,124,691; chr7: 72,382,850–73,776,237	263.7 kb copy loss (UCS) at 5q11.2–q12.1; 1.4 Mb copy loss at 7q11.23/Williams syndrome	N	R,D,S,M,L	level 1
11^	3.1y/M	ASD	chr6: 162,541,977–163,015,824	473 kb copy gain at 6q26	De novo	no	no
12*	9m/F	MCA	chr7: 72,382,850–73,776,237	1.4 Mb copy loss at 7q11.23/Williams syndrome	N	R,D,S,M,L	level 1
13*	6d/M	MCA	chr7: 72,382,850–73,776,237; chr20: 34,118,917–34,173,592	1.4 Mb copy loss at 7q11.23; 54.6 kb copy loss (UCS) at 20q11.23/Williams syndrome	N	R,D,S,M,L	level 1

Table 3. Cont.

Case no.	Age/Sex	Indication	Genomic coordinates (hg18) of CNVs	CNV size and type/syndrome or locus	Parental Testing	Clinical action	Level of evidence
14*	5y/M	ASD	chr7: 110,765,432–111,124,405; chr15: 82,433,250–89,427,223	358.9 kb copy loss (paternal) at 7q31.1; 6.9 Mb copy loss at 15q25.2–q26.1/15q deletion	De novo	no	no
15*	6y/F	MCA+DD	chr9: 199,254–1,532,084; chr9: 1,544,692–29,980,935	1.3 Mb terminal copy loss at 9p24.3; 28.4 Mb copy gain at 9p24.3–p21.1/complex imbalanced 9p: karyotype 46,XX,der(9)[p21.1–>p24.3::p24.3–>qter)dn	De novo	no	no
16*	2m/F	MCA	chr9: 95,929,405–96,708,956; chr22: 46,600,315–49,522,658	779.5 kb copy gain (UCS) at 9p22.32; 2.9 Mb copy loss at 22q13.31–q13.33/ring chr22 with 22q13 microdeletion (including SHANK3)	N	R,D,S,L	level 3
17*	4y/F	MCA+DD	chr10: 125,911,563–135,253,240	9.3 Mb terminal copy loss at 10q26/10q26 deletion	De novo	D	level 3
18*	2m/M	MCA	chr16: 14,957,300–16,195,404	1.2 Mb copy loss at 16p13.11/16p13.11 microdeletion	N	R,D,P	level 3
19^	2.5y/M	ASD	chr16: 15,033,259–16,195,404	1.2 Mb copy gain at 16p13.11/16p13.11 duplication	Mat	D	level 3
20^	8y/M	ASD+DD	chr16: 15,033,259–16,195,404	1.2 Mb copy gain at 16p13.11/16p13.11 duplication	N	D	level 3
21*	1y/M	ASD	chr16: 28,395,992–28,953,785	558 kb copy loss at 16p11.2/16p11.2 (SH2B1 gene) microdeletion	De novo	R,S	level 2
22*	11y/M	Dys+DD	chr16: 54,476,646–58,816,939	4.3 Mb copy loss at 16q12.2–q21/16q12.2 deletion	De novo	D	level 4
23*	1m/M	MCA/dys	chr17: 740,287–1,530,746	790 kb copy gain at 17p13.3/17p13.3 duplication	N	R,S	level 3
24*	7m/M	MCA	chr17: 2,520,702–3,680,586	1.16 Mb copy loss at 17p13.3–p13.2/17p13.3p13.2 (LIS1 intragenic deletion)	De novo	no	no
25*	4m/F	MCA/dys	chr17: 26,140,621–27,346,744	1.2 Mb copy gain at 17q11.2/17q11.2 NF1 duplication	N	R,S	level 3
26*	8m/F	MCA	chr17: 43,878,156–45,719,328; chr17: 62,047,278–62,372,365	1.8 Mb copy loss at 17q21.32–q21.33; 325 kb copy gain (UCS) at 17q24.2/17q21.32–q21.33 deletion	N	R,D,P,M,L	level 2
27*	2m/F	MCA+cytogenetic diagnosis	chr18: 30,273,585–62,939,673	32.6 Mb copy gain at 18q12.1–q22.1/inverted duplication 18q12.1–q22.1	Only mother tested, not mat.	no	no
28*	1m/F	MCA	chr22: 17,299,469–19,790,658	2.5 Mb copy loss at 22q11.21/22q11 deletion	De novo	R,D,S,M,L	level 1
29*	3y/M	ASD	chr22: 17,299,469–19,790,658	2.5 Mb copy loss at 22q11.21/22q11 deletion	De novo	R,D,S,M,L	level 1

Table 3. Cont.

Case no.	Age/ Sex	Indication	Genomic coordinates (hg18) of CNVs	CNV size and type/syndrome or locus	Parental Testing	Clinical action	Level of evidence
30^	4.9y/M	ASD	chrX: 22,857,404–22,980,069	122 kb copy loss at Xp22.11 involving deletion of the DDX53 gene	Mat	no	no
31*	2m/F	MCA, cytogenetic diagnosis	chrX: 71,010,717–154,881,514	83.9 Mb terminal copy gain at Xq13.1–q28/functional partial monosomy 15 and Trisomy Xq, karyotype 46,XX,der(15)t(X;15)(q13.1;p10)dn	N	R,D,S,M,L	level 2
32*	13y/F	other	chrX: 107,539,632–107,750,773; chrX: 107,759,164–108,180,837	211.1 kb copy loss at Xq22.3; 421.6 kb copy gain at Xq22.3/X-linked Alport plus diffuse leiomyomatosis syndrome	Only mother tested, not mat.	R,D,S,M	level 2
33*	9m/F	Dys+DD+ cytogenetic diagnosis	chrX: 134,459,007–134,901,914; chr4: 33,860–11,295,959	442.9 kb copy loss (UCS) at Xq26.3; 11.2 Mb terminal copy loss at 4p16.3–p15.33/Wolf-Hirschhorn syndrome	De novo	R,D,P,M	level 2
34*	3y/F	ASD	chrX: 216,519–4,031,220	3.8 Mb copy loss at Xp22.33/Xp22.33 (SHOX) deletion Léri-Weill dyschondrosteosis syndrome	N	R,D,P,S,M,L	level 1
35*	12y/F	other, genetic diagnosis	chrX: 216,519–39,315,013	39.1 Mb terminal copy loss at Xp22.33–p11.4/Xp22.33p11.4	De novo	R,D,P,S,M,L	level 1
36*	9m/F	MCA+DD	chrX: 369,190–886,653; 18: 3,404,569–3,886,147	517.4 kb copy gain (maternal) at Xq28; 481.5 kb copy gain at 18p11.31/18p11.31 duplication	Mat	no	no
37*	3y/M	ASD	chrX	47,XXY (gain of chrX)/Klinefelter syndrome	Inconclusive; Karyotype of mother: mos 47,XXX[1]/46,XX[29]	R,D,P,S,M,L	level 1

Abbreviations: MCA = Multiple Congenital Anomalies; DD = Developmental Delay; ASD = Autism Spectrum Disorders; Dys = Dysmorphism; UCS = Uncertain Clinical Significance.

Abbreviations: S = Surveillance; R = specialist Referral/assessment; D = Diagnostic testing; P = medical/surgical Procedure; M = Medication administration; L = Lifestyle recommendation; O = Other interventions.

* = pathogenic CNVs, ^ = likely pathogenic CNVs.

N = not tested; Mat = maternal inheritance; Pat = paternal inheritance.

therefore it is also our interest to study whether a genetic test can significantly affect clinical management and patient outcome.

To evaluate the degree to which CMA can impact clinical management of our patient population, we retrospectively reviewed the medical records of 327 patients tested in a single laboratory and managed in a single paediatric unit (2 teaching hospitals) over a 29-month period. We included only patients in whom the CMA results had been disclosed and management recommendations have been suggested in a post-test genetic counseling session. We had full access to the medical records of all patients and the latest recruited patient had at least 3-month follow-up period for the evaluation of outcome after the recommendation. It was noted that parental testing rate was 56.8% in the 37 patients with significant CMA results, due to either parental refusal.

Compared to 4 previous studies on clinical utility of CMAs [18–21], we found a detection rate of 8.6% for clinically actionable CNVs, which was comparable if not slightly higher than the reported number of 3.6%~7% (Table 4). There are significant differences in the design in previous studies and we have adopted the approach used by Riggs et al. [19] We grouped the recommendations into various categories (S, R, D, P, M, L, O) and linked them to the current level of evidence. This standardized approach allows better comparison with other studies and re-evaluation of our own finding with new evidence after a certain period of time. [39]

We observed a good correlation between the clinical significance and the clinical actionability of the CMA findings. Clinical management changes were recommended in 75.7% of patients with clinically significant CNVs; in 2.5% of patients with CNVs of unknown significance and in 0% with benign findings respectively. The clinically significant findings are larger in size and were more likely to be deletions than duplications. Interestingly, in those with clinically significant CNVs, management recommendations were made in 22/26 patients (84.6%) with MCA/dysmorphism as an indication for CMA, compared to 4/9 patients (44%) in those with neurodevelopmental disorders only. This lower clinical actionability rate for CNVs found in patients with isolated neurodevelopmental disorders was also observed in previous studies. [18,21] Young age was associated with clinical significant CNVs in our study, which was also observed in the study of Coulter et al (2011). [18]

Only 1 investigation was ordered in 1 patient with CNV of unknown significance, referred for non-syndromic ASD. The recommendation (an ECG) was based on the finding of the same 20p12.3 duplication in a single case report on a patient with familial Wolf-Parkinson-White syndrome. [40] Parents agreed for ECG on the child because the non-invasive nature of the investigation and the availability of potential treatment if WPW was identified. In this patient, the ECG was normal. Similarly we have made a level 4 recommendation (brain MRI) for another patient with DD, epilepsy and a 16p12 deletion based on positive

Table 4. Comparison of clinically actionable abnormal CMA findings in published studies.

Study (published year)	Coulter et al (2011)	Ellison et al (2012)	Riggs et al (2014)	Henderson et al (2014)	Our study
Study design	Retrospective review of medical records	Retrospective laboratory database review (Signature Genomics)	Retrospective laboratory database review (ISCA)	Retrospective review of electronic medical records	Retrospective review of medical records
Number of subjects	1,792	46,298	28,256	1,780	327 (first-tiered testing and with specific indications)
Study period	1 y (2009–2010)	7.5 y (2004–2011)	As in March 2012	3 y (2009–2012)	29m (2010–2013)
CMA platforms used	Not specified	Multiple BAC-based and oligo-arrays. (only those with oligo-arrays counted to evaluate clinical actionability)	Multiple platforms (not specified)	2 high resolution SNP array platforms	NimbleGen 135k oligonucleotide array
Definition of clinically actionable results	Findings that prompt specialist referral, imaging, diagnostic test or medication prescription.	1. Established microdeletion/microduplication syndromes; 2. Conditions with increased cancer susceptibility; 3. Other actionable conditions associated with dosage-sensitive genes.	Conditions diagnosable by CMA for which referral, diagnostic testing, surgical/interventional procedure, surveillance, medical and lifestyle changes would be recommended. The recommendations were stratified according to the level of evidence.	Findings that prompt recommendations of further action such as pharmacologic treatment, cancer-related screening, contraindications, additional evaluation or referrals.	Criteria by Riggs et al.
Diagnostic yield of significant results	235/1,792 (13.0%)	15.4% for the oligo-array (based on previous study from the same group)	4,125/28,256 (14.6%)	227/1,780 (12.7%)	37/327 (11.0%)
Clinical actionability in those with significant CMA results (%)	34.0–54.0%	35.0%	46.0% (66.0% for deletion cases and 11.0% for duplication cases)	54.7% (42.1% for patients referred for isolated neurodevelopmental disorders)	75.7% (44.0% for patients referred for isolated neurodevelopmental disorders)
Clinically actionability in the whole cohort (%)	3.6%	5.4%	7.0%	5.4%	8.6%

finding of bilateral frontoparietal polymicrogyria (BFPP) in a patient reported with a similar deletion. [41] In our patient, brain MRI did not show BFPP. This illustrates that with our study design we are able to evaluate not only the recommendations we made based on the CMA findings but the actual clinical outcomes of patients. This will be important especially for CNVs with clinical actions based on low level of evidence.

There are multiple advantages of reaching a genetic diagnosis in patients. First of all, making a diagnosis allows estimation of recurrence risk and informed decisions about future pregnancies for the parents. As illustrated by case 37 (with Level 1 evidence), the clinical utility of CMA in the proband can extend beyond the affected individuals and familial testing can reveal diagnosis in a sibling (normal development but with Klinefelter syndrome) with less obvious clinical manifestations. Secondly, for some like patient 2, a diagnosis of submicroscopic unbalanced translocation helps to end the 24 years of diagnostic odyssey. If the test is being offered as first-tier testing in a similar patient at the current time, it may help to avoid a lot of unnecessary investigations including the more invasive ones. The direct benefits to clinical management have been demonstrated by previous studies. [18–21] Our study was able to confirm that a significant CMA finding influenced medical management in 75% of our patients. Although our study involves a smaller number of patients, we were able to study at least the short-term direct clinical outcomes in our patients who have received recommendations based on their CMA findings. Future goals will be the long-term study of the impact on clinical outcomes for a larger cohort of patients with significant CMA findings and how the changing interpretation of CMA over time may change the clinical management of patients with different categories of findings. We advocate the use of diagnostic yield of clinically actionable results in the evaluation of CMA testing as this allows the clinicians to consider both clinical validity and clinical utility of CMA under the ACCE framework [42–47] and it provides a link between the practice of medical genetics and evidence-based medicine.

Acknowledgments

We thank all the patients and families, participating doctors and nurses of Department of Paediatrics, HKU and laboratory staff of Prenatal Diagnostic Laboratory, Tsan Yuk Hospital, O&G, HKU.

Author Contributions

Conceived and designed the experiments: KYKC ETL ASYK MHT YLL BHYC. Performed the experiments: KYKC WFT ETL. Analyzed the data: VT KYKC YWYC GTKM TYT WLY SLL WWYT ETL BHYC. Contributed reagents/materials/analysis tools: ETL ASYK MHT BHYC. Wrote the paper: VT KYKC GTKM TYT SLL WWYT YLL BHYC.

References

1. Hochstenbach R, van Binsbergen E, Engelen J, Nieuwint A, Polstra A, et al. (2009) Array analysis and karyotyping: workflow consequences based on a retrospective study of 36,325 patients with idiopathic developmental delay in the Netherlands. Eur J Med Genet 52: 161–169.
2. Miller DT, Adam MP, Aradhya S, Biesecker LG, Brothman AR, et al. (2010) Consensus statement: chromosomal microarray is a first-tier clinical diagnostic test for individuals with developmental disabilities or congenital anomalies. Am J Hum Genet 86: 749–764.
3. Manning M, Hudgins L (2010) Array-based technology and recommendations for utilization in medical genetics practice for detection of chromosomal abnormalities. Genet Med 12: 742–745.
4. Sagoo GS, Butterworth AS, Sanderson S, Shaw-Smith C, Higgins JP, et al. (2009) Array CGH in patients with learning disability (mental retardation) and congenital anomalies: updated systematic review and meta-analysis of 19 studies and 13,926 subjects. Genet Med 11: 139–146.
5. Shen Y, Dies KA, Holm IA, Bridgemohan C, Sobeih MM, et al. (2010) Clinical genetic testing for patients with autism spectrum disorders. Pediatrics 125: e727–735.
6. Edelmann L, Hirschhorn K (2009) Clinical utility of array CGH for the detection of chromosomal imbalances associated with mental retardation and multiple congenital anomalies. Ann N Y Acad Sci 1151: 157–166.
7. Stankiewicz P, Beaudet AL (2007) Use of array CGH in the evaluation of dysmorphology, malformations, developmental delay, and idiopathic mental retardation. Curr Opin Genet Dev 17: 182–192.
8. Kang JU, Koo SH (2012) Evolving applications of microarray technology in postnatal diagnosis (review). Int J Mol Med 30: 223–228.
9. Battaglia A, Doccini V, Bernardini L, Novelli A, Loddo S, et al. (2013) Confirmation of chromosomal microarray as a first-tier clinical diagnostic test for individuals with developmental delay, intellectual disability, autism spectrum disorders and dysmorphic features. Eur J Paediatr Neurol 17: 589–599.
10. Wu Y, Ji T, Wang J, Xiao J, Wang H, et al. (2010) Submicroscopic subtelomeric aberrations in Chinese patients with unexplained developmental delay/mental retardation. BMC Med Genet 11: 72.
11. Lee CG, Park SJ, Yun JN, Ko JM, Kim HJ, et al. (2013) Array-based comparative genomic hybridization in 190 Korean patients with developmental delay and/or intellectual disability: a single tertiary care university center study. Yonsei Med J 54: 1463–1470.
12. Park SJ, Jung EH, Ryu RS, Kang HW, Ko JM, et al. (2011) Clinical implementation of whole-genome array CGH as a first-tier test in 5080 pre and postnatal cases. Mol Cytogenet 4: 12.
13. Byeon JH, Shin E, Kim GH, Lee K, Hong YS, et al. (2014) Application of array-based comparative genomic hybridization to pediatric neurologic diseases. Yonsei Med J 55: 30–36.
14. Saam J, Gudgeon J, Aston E, Brothman AR (2008) How physicians use array comparative genomic hybridization results to guide patient management in children with developmental delay. Genet Med 10: 181–186.
15. Mroch AR, Flanagan JD, Stein QP (2012) Solving the puzzle: case examples of array comparative genomic hybridization as a tool to end the diagnostic odyssey. Curr Probl Pediatr Adolesc Health Care 42: 74–78.
16. Adams SA, Coppinger J, Saitta SC, Stroud T, Kandamurugu M, et al. (2009) Impact of genotype-first diagnosis: the detection of microdeletion and microduplication syndromes with cancer predisposition by aCGH. Genet Med 11: 314–322.
17. Adam MP, Justice AN, Schelley S, Kwan A, Hudgins L, et al. (2009) Clinical utility of array comparative genomic hybridization: uncovering tumor susceptibility in individuals with developmental delay. J Pediatr 154: 143–146.
18. Coulter ME, Miller DT, Harris DJ, Hawley P, Picker J, et al. (2011) Chromosomal microarray testing influences medical management. Genet Med 13: 770–776.
19. Riggs ER, Wain KE, Riethmaier D, Smith-Packard B, Faucett WA, et al. (2014) Chromosomal microarray impacts clinical management. Clin Genet 85: 147–153.
20. Ellison JW, Ravnan JB, Rosenfeld JA, Morton SA, Neill NJ, et al. (2012) Clinical utility of chromosomal microarray analysis. Pediatrics 130: e1085–1095.
21. Henderson LB, Applegate CD, Wohler E, Sheridan MB, Hoover-Fong J, et al. (2014) The impact of chromosomal microarray on clinical management: a retrospective analysis. Genet Med.
22. Regier DA, Friedman JM, Marra CA (2010) Value for money? Array genomic hybridization for diagnostic testing for genetic causes of intellectual disability. Am J Hum Genet 86: 765–772.
23. Kan AS, Lau ET, Tang WF, Chan SS, Ding SC, et al. (2014) Whole-Genome Array CGH Evaluation for Replacing Prenatal Karyotyping in Hong Kong. PLoS One 9: e87988.
24. Kearney HM, Thorland EC, Brown KK, Quintero-Rivera F, South ST (2011) American College of Medical Genetics standards and guidelines for interpretation and reporting of postnatal constitutional copy number variants. Genet Med 13: 680–685.
25. Verhagen JM, Diderich KE, Oudesluijs G, Mancini GM, Eggink AJ, et al. (2012) Phenotypic variability of atypical 22q11.2 deletions not including TBX1. Am J Med Genet A 158a: 2412–2420.
26. Ho AC, Liu AP, Lun KS, Tang WF, Chan KY, et al. (2012) A newborn with a 790 kb chromosome 17p13.3 microduplication presenting with aortic stenosis, microcephaly and dysmorphic facial features - is cardiac assessment necessary for all patients with 17p13.3 microduplication? Eur J Med Genet 55: 758–762.
27. Liu AP, Tang WF, Lau ET, Chan KY, Kan AS, et al. (2013) Expanded Prader-Willi syndrome due to chromosome 15q11.2–14 deletion: report and a review of literature. Am J Med Genet A 161a: 1309–1318.
28. Tsang JS, Tong DKH, Chung BHY, Tang MHY, Lau ET, et al. (2013) Alport's syndrome: case of a giant esophageal tumor. Esophagus 10: 114–117.
29. Aksglaede L, Link K, Giwercman A, Jorgensen N, Skakkebaek NE, et al. (2013) 47,XXY Klinefelter syndrome: clinical characteristics and age-specific recommendations for medical management. Am J Med Genet C Semin Med Genet 163c: 55–63.

30. Groth KA, Skakkebaek A, Host C, Gravholt CH, Bojesen A (2013) Clinical review: Klinefelter syndrome-a clinical update. J Clin Endocrinol Metab 98: 20–30.

31. Nowinski GP, Van Dyke DL, Tilley BC, Jacobsen G, Babu VR, et al. (1990) The frequency of aneuploidy in cultured lymphocytes is correlated with age and gender but not with reproductive history. Am J Hum Genet 46: 1101–1111.

32. (1993) GeneReviews. Seattle (WA): University of Washington, Seattle.

33. Orellana C, Rosello M, Monfort S, Oltra S, Quiroga R, et al. (2009) Corpus callosum abnormalities and the controversy about the candidate genes located in 1q44. Cytogenet Genome Res 127: 5–8.

34. van Bon BW, Koolen DA, Borgatti R, Magee A, Garcia-Minaur S, et al. (2008) Clinical and molecular characteristics of 1qter microdeletion syndrome: delineating a critical region for corpus callosum agenesis/hypogenesis. J Med Genet 45: 346–354.

35. Caliebe A, Kroes HY, van der Smagt JJ, Martin-Subero JI, Tonnies H, et al. (2010) Four patients with speech delay, seizures and variable corpus callosum thickness sharing a 0.440 Mb deletion in region 1q44 containing the HNRPU gene. Eur J Med Genet 53: 179–185.

36. Iourov IY, Vorsanova SG, Kurinnaia OS, Zelenova MA, Silvanovich AP, et al. (2012) Molecular karyotyping by array CGH in a Russian cohort of children with intellectual disability, autism, epilepsy and congenital anomalies. Mol Cytogenet 5: 46.

37. Courtens W, Wuyts W, Rooms L, Pera SB, Wauters J (2006) A subterminal deletion of the long arm of chromosome 10: a clinical report and review. Am J Med Genet A 140: 402–409.

38. Lukusa T, Fryns JP (2000) Pure distal monosomy 10q26 in a patient displaying clinical features of Prader-Willi syndrome during infancy and distinct behavioural phenotype in adolescence. Genet Couns 11: 119–126.

39. Palmer E, Speirs H, Taylor PJ, Mullan G, Turner G, et al. (2014) Changing interpretation of chromosomal microarray over time in a community cohort with intellectual disability. Am J Med Genet A 164a: 377–385.

40. Mills KI, Anderson J, Levy PT, Cole FS, Silva JN, et al. (2013) Duplication of 20p12.3 associated with familial Wolff-Parkinson-White syndrome. Am J Med Genet A 161a: 137–144.

41. Borgatti R, Marelli S, Bernardini L, Novelli A, Cavallini A, et al. (2009) Bilateral frontoparietal polymicrogyria (BFPP) syndrome secondary to a 16q12.1–q21 chromosome deletion involving GPR56 gene. Clin Genet 76: 573–576.

42. Hastings R, de Wert G, Fowler B, Krawczak M, Vermeulen E, et al. (2012) The changing landscape of genetic testing and its impact on clinical and laboratory services and research in Europe. Eur J Hum Genet 20: 911–916.

43. Burke W, Atkins D, Gwinn M, Guttmacher A, Haddow J, et al. (2002) Genetic test evaluation: information needs of clinicians, policy makers, and the public. Am J Epidemiol 156: 311–318.

44. Haddow JE, Palomaki GE (2004) ACCE: a model process for evaluating data on emerging genetic tests. Human genome epidemiology: A scientific foundation for using genetic information to improve health and prevent disease: 217–233.

45. Wald N, Cuckle H (1989) Reporting the assessment of screening and diagnostic tests. Br J Obstet Gynaecol 96: 389–396.

46. U.S. Department of Health and Human Services, Secretary's Advisory Committee on Genetic Testing (2000) Request for public comment on a proposed classification methodology for determining level of review for genetic tests. Federal Register 65: 76643–76645.

47. Dierking A, Schmidtke J (2014) The future of Clinical Utility Gene Cards in the context of next-generation sequencing diagnostic panels. Eur J Hum Genet.

3

Tobacco Smoke and Risk of Childhood Acute Non-Lymphocytic Leukemia: Findings from the SETIL Study

Stefano Mattioli[1]*, **Andrea Farioli**[1], **Patrizia Legittimo**[2,3], **Lucia Miligi**[4], **Alessandra Benvenuti**[4], **Alessandra Ranucci**[5], **Alberto Salvan**[6], **Roberto Rondelli**[7], **Corrado Magnani**[5] **on behalf of the SETIL Study Group**[¶]

1 Department of Medical and Surgical Sciences (DIMEC), University of Bologna, Bologna, Italy, 2 Unit of Occupational Medicine, S.Orsola-Malpighi University Hospital, Bologna, Italy, 3 Occupational and Environmental Epidemiology Unit, ISPO Cancer Prevention and Research Institute, Florence, Italy, 4 Occupational and Environmental Epidemiology Unit, ISPO Cancer Prevention and Research Institute, Florence, Italy, 5 Cancer Epidemiology Unit - Department of Translational Medicine, CPO Piemonte and University of Eastern Piedmont, Novara, Italy, 6 Currently retired, IASI-CNR, Rome, Italy, 7 Paediatric Oncology-Haematology "Lalla Seràgnoli", Policlinico S.Orsola-Malpighi, Bologna, Italy

Abstract

Background: Parental smoking and exposure of the mother or the child to environmental tobacco smoke (ETS) as risk factors for Acute non-Lymphocytic Leukemia (AnLL) were investigated.

Methods: Incident cases of childhood AnLL were enrolled in 14 Italian Regions during 1998–2001. We estimated odds ratios (OR) and 95% confidence intervals (95%CI) conducting logistic regression models including 82 cases of AnLL and 1,044 controls. Inverse probability weighting was applied adjusting for: age; sex; provenience; birth order; birth weight; breastfeeding; parental educational level age, birth year, and occupational exposure to benzene.

Results: Paternal smoke in the conception period was associated with AnLL (OR for ≥11 cigarettes/day = 1.79, 95% CI 1.01–3.15; P trend 0.05). An apparent effect modification by maternal age was identified: only children of mothers aged below 30 presented increased risks. We found weak statistical evidence of an association of AnLL with maternal exposure to ETS (OR for exposure>3 hours/day = 1.85, 95%CI 0.97–3.52; P trend 0.07). No association was observed between AnLL and either maternal smoking during pregnancy or child exposure to ETS.

Conclusions: This study is consistent with the hypothesis that paternal smoke is associated with AnLL. We observed statistical evidence of an association between maternal exposure to ETS and AnLL, but believe bias might have inflated our estimates.

Editor: Pal Bela Szecsi, Gentofte University Hospital, Denmark

Funding: The SETIL study was financially supported by research grants received by AIRC (Italian Association on Research on Cancer), MIUR (Ministry for Instruction, University and Research, PRIN Program), Ministry of Health (Ricerca Sanitaria Finalizzata Program), Ministry of Labour and Welfare, Associazione Neuroblastoma, Piemonte Region (Ricerca Sanitaria Finalizzata Regione Piemonte Program), Liguria Region, Comitato per la vita "Daniele Chianelli"- Associazione per la Ricerca e la Cura delle Leucemie, Linfomi e Tumori di Adulti e Bambini, (Perugia). The funders had no role in study design, data collection and analysis, decision to publish, or preparation of the manuscript.

Competing Interests: The authors have declared that no competing interests exist.

* Email: s.mattioli@unibo.it

¶ Membership of the SETIL Study Group is provided in the Acknowledgments.

Introduction

Acute leukemia is the most common childhood cancer; acute lymphoblastic leukemia (ALL) accounts for 75–80% of total cases of childhood leukemia, acute non-lymphocytic leukemia (AnLL) for about 20%. [1] Established risk factors, such as exposure to ionizing radiations and genetic syndromes, explain no more than 10% of cases; [2] Suggested risk factors include: car exhaust fumes, pesticides, non-ionizing radiation, pets, antiepileptic drugs, maternal alcohol consumption, maternal illicit drug use (*cannabis sativa*), maternal age, paternal age, breast feeding, birth order, chemical contamination in drinking water, both viral and bacterial infections, and parental cigarette smoking. [3–5] Alongside occupational exposure to benzene, [6] active tobacco smoking is

an established risk for adult myeloid leukemia. [7] According to the International Agency for Research on Cancer (IARC), the available body of evidence suggests a consistent association of childhood leukemia with preconception and with combined paternal and maternal smoking. [7] Conversely, studies on maternal tobacco smoking often showed modest increases in risk, or null or inverse associations. [7] Only one study was included on second hand smoke and leukemia (namely chronic lymphocytic leukemia) reporting a positive association. [7] Most of the evidence on the relationship between cigarette smoking and childhood leukemia regards ALL, [8], while there is scant evidence for AnLL. [7,9] As shown in supplemental Table S1, several studies highlighted that paternal smoking around the time of conception is a risk factor for childhood ALL. A meta-analysis of heavy paternal smoking (20+ cigarettes/day) highlighted a substantial increase in the risk of childhood leukemia (OR 1.44, 95%CI 1.24–1.68) [8].

Our aim was to investigate parental cigarette consumption and second-hand smoke exposure as risk factors for childhood AnLL, using data collected in a large case-control study primarily designed to evaluate the role of physical agents (including electromagnetic fields), parental occupation and environmental exposure in childhood hematopoietic malignancies. [10–11]

Methods

Study population

SETIL (*Studio sulla Eziologia dei Tumori Infantili Linfoemopoietici*, study on the etiology of childhood lympho-hematopoietic malignancies) is a population-based case-control study conducted in Italy between 1998 and 2003. Details of the study have been given elsewhere. [10–11] Thanks to the support of the Italian Association of Pediatric Hematology and Oncology almost all incident cases of childhood acute leukemia (aged between 0 and 10) in 14 Italian Regions were collected; [12] second primary neoplasms were excluded. Cases were individually matched for date of birth, sex and residence area with 2 population controls randomly drawn from Local Health Authority registries. Parents of eligible cases were contacted through the pediatric oncologist, parents of controls through their general practitioner; eligible subjects were asked to participate in a direct interview (non responders were 8% among cases and 29% among controls). During the study period 82 cases of AnLL, 601 cases of ALL and 1,044 controls (128 matched to AnLL cases and 916 matched to ALL cases) were enrolled.

Information was collected from parents of cases and controls in a direct interview using a standardized questionnaire that was constructed to collect data on many putative causes of childhood leukemia, including personal characteristics and exposure to physical, chemical and biological agents. For practical reasons, interviewers were not blinded to the case or control status of the child.

In the present analysis of AnLL, we broke the individual matching, and included the 82 cases of AnLL and all 1,044 sampled controls (irrespectively of individual matching with AnLL or ALL cases). Matching was retained in additional sensitivity analyses.

The SETIL study was conceived to investigate the etiology of hematopoietic malignancies. Findings on the association between tobacco smoke and risk of childhood acute lymphoblastic leukemia have been recently reported. [13] Queries about collaborations and access to the data can be addressed to the principal investigator of the SETIL Study (Prof. Corrado Magnani; email: magnani@med.unipmn.it). The SETIL study participated in the Childhood Leukemia International Consortium (CLIC, https://clic.berkeley.edu/about). [14]

The SETIL study was authorized by the ethics committee for the Piedmont Region (authorization n.2886, on 15/2/1999; letter n. 1852/28.3 on 17/2/1999) and later by the corresponding board of each participating research unit. Written informed consent was obtained from all participating subjects. The ethics committee approved the consent procedure.

Exposure variables and covariates

An English language translation of the smoking sections of the SETIL questionnaire is presented in appendix S1. Available information on paternal smoking status in the period of conception enabled us to classify fathers in four categories: never a smoker; former smoker; smoker, 1 to 10 cigarettes per day; and smoker, 11 or more cigarettes per day. Based on preliminary analyses, never smokers and former smokers were merged, creating the category of non-smokers with reference to the period of conception. Information on the smoking status of fathers (smoker or non-smoker) was also available for the pregnancy and the period between birth and diagnosis. As expected, an excellent agreement (Cohen's kappa = 0.96) was found between paternal smoking status in the conception period and smoking status after the child's birth.

For maternal smoking, information was available separately for each trimester of pregnancy. Since the consumption of cigarettes tended to be stable across the pregnancy (Cohen's kappa between first and third trimester = 0.92), smoking status was classified according to the first trimester of pregnancy. After a preliminary analysis and considering the small numbers of active smokers — only three mothers of cases declared they had smoked more than 10 cigarettes/day — a dichotomous variable was created: non-smoker (never a smoker or former smoker); smoker. Mothers were asked to declare how many hours per day they had been exposed to Environmental Tobacco Smoking (ETS) during pregnancy. A three-level variable was created using the collected information: never exposed to passive smoking, and two levels of exposure based on the median of exposure to passive smoking among controls' mothers.

Exposure of children to ETS, measured in cigarettes per day, was collected for every year of life; Hence, we created a cumulative exposure index equal to the number of cigarettes to which the children had been exposed (ETS). Again, a three-level variable was created: never exposed to ETS, and two levels of exposure based on the median of exposure to passive smoking among controls.

Possible confounders were selected *a-priori* and included: sex, age group (less than two years; between two and four years; between four and six years; more than six years), residence area (part of Italy: North, except Lombardy; Lombardy; center; South and islands), birth order; birth weight; duration of breastfeeding; maternal and paternal age at child's birth; maternal and paternal education level; and parental occupational exposure to benzene. Exposure to benzene was assessed by industrial hygienists on the basis of information gathered with a job specific questionnaire. Detailed methods for the evaluation of exposure to benzene were presented in Miligi et al. [10]

Statistical Analysis

Unmatched analyses were performed in order to avoid the loss of cases (9 cases were in matching strata without controls). To increase statistical power, considering that the sampling procedure and collection of information were the same for controls matched to AnLL and to ALL cases, we included all the 1,044 enrolled controls in the analysis and not only the 128 individually matched with AnLL cases. Unmatched analyses models always included age, gender and residence area. Matching was retained in additional sensitivity analyses.

In contingency tables, statistical independence of variables was tested using χ^2 test or Fisher exact test, according to Cochran rule. [15] We examined associations between AnLL and each of the aforementioned sources of exposure to tobacco smoke. Odds Ratios (OR) and relative 95% Confidence Intervals (95% CI) were obtained with unconditional logistic regression models. Linear trends for ordinal exposure variables were evaluated using the Wald test, treating the variable as a continuous variable (introduced in the model with 1 degree of freedom). To test for possible interactions on a multiplicative scale, product terms for the interaction between the exposure variable and the proposed effect modifier were created and likelihood ratio tests were used to compare models with and without the interaction terms.

The limited number of cases (n = 82) did not allow the direct inclusion of all covariates in multivariate logistic regression models. To deal with the small number of events per parameter, we performed two separate sets of analyses. Firstly, we adjusted for putative confounders (parameterized as presented in Table 1) via inverse probability weighting (IPW). [16] Then the conditional probability of being exposed given the individual covariates were estimated by fitting probit (for dichotomous exposure) or multinomial probit (for categorical exposure) regression models and we calculated robust standard error for the inference. [16–18]. A second set of regression models including covariates selected based on the change-in-estimates methods were fitted, using a threshold for inclusion of a 10% change in the odds ratios of interest [19]. All analyses were performed using Stata 12.1 SE (Stata corporation, Texas, TX) and all tests were 2 sided. A p-value of 0.05 or less was considered statistically significant.

Results

Characteristics of study participants by case-control status are reported in Table 1. The entire sample of controls, mainly consisting of subjects matched to ALL cases, has a different age distribution compared to AnLL cases and their matched controls. The duration of breastfeeding was comparable in AnLL cases and their matched controls; conversely, long breastfeeding periods were more frequent in the control sample. Parents of cases usually had a lower educational level than controls' parents. All other considered characteristics seemed to have comparable distribution among cases and controls.

The ORs for the association between exposures to tobacco smoke and risk of AnLL are presented in Table 2. Estimates for both the matched and unmatched analyses are reported. In the unmatched analysis, ORs were estimated with reference to the subpopulation with complete data on putative confounders. Depending on the studied exposure, this restriction determined the exclusion of 33–39 controls and, only for paternal smoking in the conception period, of one case. Estimates based on the entire sample were consistent with those presented in Table 2.

As shown in table 2, in matched analysis, paternal smoking in the conception period presented signs of association with the risk of AnLL (OR of smokers, 1–10 cigarettes/day = 1.95, 95%CI 0.76–5.04; OR of smokers, 11 or more cigarettes/day = 1.76, 95%CI 0.91, 3.41; P for trend 0.09). Unmatched analysis of paternal smoking produced similar estimates (adjusted OR of smokers, 1–10 cigarettes/day = 1.34, 95%CI 0.65–2.76; OR of smokers, 11 or more cigarettes/day = 1.79, 95%CI 1.01, 3.15; P for trend 0.05). Although supported by very weak statistical evidence ($P = 0.18$), the study of the interaction between paternal smoking and maternal age at child's birth showed interesting estimates (Figure 1). Apparently, paternal smoking affected the risk of childhood AnLL only among children born from mothers aged below 30 years, a cut-off selected a priori based on median maternal age. In the multivariable model selected with the change-in-estimate method and including age at diagnosis and maternal educational level, the adjusted OR for moderate smokers (1–10 cigarettes/day) was 2.61 (95%CI0.92–7.36), while the OR for heavy-smoker fathers (11 or more cigarettes/day) was 2.99 (95%CI1.40–6.37). Estimates for children born from mothers aged above 30 years were close to the unit (adjusted OR of smokers, 1–10 cigarettes/day = 1.13, 95%CI0.44–2.92, OR of smokers, 11 or more cigarettes/day = 1.16, 95%CI0.53–2.53). Of note, almost no evidence was found of an interaction between

paternal age and paternal smoking during the conception period (at multivariate analysis p interaction = 0.40, data not shown).

Maternal smoking during the first trimester of pregnancy did not show clear signs of association with the risk of childhood AnLL (Table 2). However, in unmatched analysis, marginal evidence of an association of AnLL with high levels of maternal exposure to ETS during the pregnancy (adjusted OR of mothers exposed more than 3 hours/day = 1.85, 95%CI 0.97–3.52; P for trend = 0.07) were observed. However, the exclusion of active-smoker mothers (n = 117) from the analysis determined a decrease of the estimates (adjusted OR of mothers exposed more than 3 hours/day = 1.42, 95%CI 0.69–2.95). The further adjustment by paternal smoking (an exposure that is likely to be associated with maternal exposure to ETS) caused a modest increase of the estimates (adjusted OR of mothers exposed more than 3 hours/day = 1.61, 95%CI 0.73–3.53).

As shown in Table 2, no evidence supported an association between the exposure of the child to ETS and the risk of AnLL (for children exposed to 4,000 or more cigarettes, OR adjusted through IPW = 1.15, 95%CI 0.45–2.95; P for trend = 0.77).

Discussion

In this analysis of data from a population-based case-control study moderate evidence supporting the hypothesis that children of fathers who smoked in the period of conception have an increased risk of AnLL was found. Interestingly, an apparent effect modification by maternal age was also identified. Indeed, only children of mothers aged below 30 years at the delivery presented an increased risk. We also found weak signs of an association between maternal exposure to second-hand smoke and risk of childhood AnLL. No sign of association was found for maternal smoking during pregnancy. Finally, we did not find any evidence supporting an association between child exposure to second-hand smoke and risk of AnLL.

Plausibility of the results and evidence from previous studies

An association between paternal smoking before the pregnancy and risk of childhood leukemia has already been reported. [7–9,20] However, most of the positive findings regarded ALL, while only limited evidence supports the association between AnLL and paternal smoking. [7] It should be considered that studies on AnLL and paternal smoking are all case-control studies and they are often underpowered, due to the rarity of the disease. Since tobacco smoke is an established leukemogenic in adults, [7] the biological plausibility of an association with childhood AnLL is high. Furthermore, the possible effect of exposure to tobacco smoke of the gametes or the embryo/fetus in utero on the risk of childhood AnLL is in line with the "two hits" model proposed by Greaves. [21] Moderate/weak evidence of a possible interaction between paternal smoking and maternal age at delivery was observed. Possible explanations of the observed interaction could be chance or a strong pattern of confounders differentially acting in the two maternal age strata. However, further investigations should be carried out before excluding causality, since during pre-implantation embryogenesis complex interactions exist between paternal and maternal factors and the biochemical environment. [22]

Our analysis did not produce evidence supporting an association between maternal tobacco smoking and risk of childhood AnLL. Results were broadly in line with those of previous studies. [7] However, one should consider our sample only included 19 women (3 cases and 16 controls) who declared having smoked

Table 1. Characteristics of Acute Non-Lymphocytic Leukemia Cases and Controls in the SETIL Case-Control Study, Italy, 1998-2003.

	AnLL cases No.	%	Controls matched to AnLL cases No.	%	All sampled controls No.	%	P value[a]
Gender[d]							
Female	39	47.6	62	48.4	482	46.2	Na
Male	43	52.4	66	51.6	562	52.8	
Age at study reference date (years)[d]							
≤1	21	25.6	35	27.3	156	14.9	Na
2–3	13	15.9	18	14.1	351	33.6	
4–5	13	15.9	15	11.7	233	22.3	
≥6	35	42.7	60	46.9	304	29.1	
Residence area (part of Italy)[d]							
North (except Lombardy)	22	26.8	33	25.8	250	24.0	Na
Lombardy	16	19.5	32	25.0	260	24.9	
Center	17	20.7	23	18.0	257	24.6	
South and islands	27	32.9	40	31.2	277	26.5	
Birth order							
First born	39	47.6	68	53.1	551	52.8	0.49[b]
Second born	31	37.8	39	30.5	379	36.3	
Third born and others	12	14.6	21	16.4	113	10.8	
Birth weight (g)							
<3,000	19	23.2	31	24.2	239	22.9	0.89[b]
3,000–3,299	18	22.0	28	21.9	246	23.6	
3,300–3,599	23	28.0	29	22.7	254	24.4	
≥3,600	22	26.8	40	31.2	304	29.2	
Duration of breastfeeding (months)							
0	12	14.6	26	20.5	232	22.3	0.04[b]
1–3	32	39.0	32	25.2	267	25.7	
4–6	19	23.2	37	29.1	233	22.4	
>6	19	23.2	32	25.2	308	29.6	
Maternal age at child's birth (years)							
≤24	14	17.1	23	18.1	140	13.4	0.65[b]
25–29	25	30.5	41	32.3	382	36.7	
30–34	30	36.6	44	34.6	359	34.5	
≥35	13	15.8	19	15.0	160	15.4	
Birth year of the mother							
<1960	15	18.3	22	17.3	145	13.9	

Table 1. Cont.

	AnLL cases		Controls matched to AnLL cases		All sampled controls		P value[a]
	No.	%	No.	%	No.	%	
1960–1964	27	32.9	32	25.2	328	31.5	
1965–1969	22	26.8	53	31.7	373	35.8	
≥1970	18	22.0	20	15.8	195	18.7	0.36[b]
Maternal educational level							
Less than high school	46	56.1	45	35.2	400	38.4	
High school	26	31.7	64	50.0	503	48.3	
University	10	12.2	19	14.8	139	13.3	<0.01[b]
Paternal age at child's birth (years)							
≤24	3	3.7	6	4.7	33	3.3	
25–29	18	22.2	29	22.8	241	23.8	
30–34	3	40.7	45	35.4	385	38.0	
≥35	27	33.3	47	37.0	353	34.9	0.96[b]
Paternal educational level							
Less than high school	47	58.0	54	42.2	463	44.6	
High school	24	29.6	59	46.1	424	40.9	
University	10	12.4	15	11.7	151	14.6	0.06[b]
Parental occupational exposure to benzene							
Absent	80	97.6	126	98.4	1,009	96.7	
Present	2	2.4	2	1.6	35	3.3	0.65[c]

Abbreviations: AnLL, acute non-lymphocytic leukemia; NA, not appropriate.
[a]Comparison between cases and all controls sampled in the SETIL study (AnLL controls + ALL controls).
[b]P values from χ2 test.
[c]P values from Fisher exact test.
[d]Matching variables.

Table 2. Association Between Acute non-Lymphocytic Leukemia and Sources of Exposure to Tobacco Smoke. The SETIL Study, Italy, 1998–2003.

Exposure	Matched analysis[a]				Unmatched analysis										
					Crude estimates				Models adjusted by sex, age and residence area		Models selected through change-in-estimates strategy		Models weighted by the inverse probability of exposure[f]	
	Ca	Co	OR	95%CI	Ca	Co	OR	95%CI	OR	95%CI	OR	95%CI	OR	95%CI
Paternal smoking in the conception period														
Non smoker	38	80	1.00	Ref.	38	612	1.00	Ref.	1.00	Ref.	1.00[b]	Ref.[b]	1.00	Ref.
Smoker, 1–10 cigs/day	12	15	1.95	0.76–5.04	12	123	1.57	0.80–3.09	1.74	0.87–3.48	1.59[b]	0.80–3.18[b]	1.34	0.65–2.76
Smoker, ≥11 cigs/day	30	33	1.76	0.91–3.41	30	264	1.83	1.11–3.02	1.90	1.14–3.17	1.79[b]	1.07–3.00[b]	1.79	1.01–3.15
P_{trend}				0.09				0.02		0.01		0.02		0.05
Maternal smoking in the 1st trimester of pregnancy														
Non smoker	71	115	1.00	Ref.	70	893	1.00	Ref.	1.00	Ref.	1.00[c]	Ref.[c]	1.00	Ref.
Smoker	11	14	1.22	0.47–3.12	11	111	1.26	0.65–2.46	1.35	0.68–2.66	1.30[c]	0.66–2.56[c]	0.83	0.38–1.81
Maternal exposure to ETS during the pregnancy														
Not exposed	49	84	1.00	Ref.	48	692	1.00	Ref.	1.00	Ref.	1.00[d]	Ref.[d]	1.00	Ref.
≤3 hours/day	15	22	0.99	0.43–2.29	15	188	1.15	0.63–2.10	1.03	0.55–1.92	1.04[d]	0.56–1.92[d]	0.89	0.46–1.72
>3 hours/day	17	19	1.69	0.78–3.64	17	115	2.13	1.18–3.83	1.94	1.06–3.54	2.12[d]	1.16–3.86[d]	1.85	0.97–3.52
P_{trend}				0.23				0.02		0.06		0.03		0.07
Cumulative exposure of child to ETS														
Not exposed	52	89	1.00	Ref.	52	718	1.00	Ref.	1.00	Ref.	1.00[e]	Ref.[e]	1.00	Ref.
<4000 cigs	15	20	1.33	0.57–3.07	15	151	1.37	0.75–2.50	1.27	0.69–2.36	1.18[e]	0.64–2.18[e]	1.25	0.63–2.48
≥4000 cigs	15	20	1.59	0.65–3.87	14	130	1.49	0.80–2.76	1.51	0.78–2.92	1.33[e]	0.69–2.57[e]	1.15	0.45–2.95
P_{trend}				0.29				0.15		0.18		0.39		0.77

Abbreviations: 95%CI, 95% confidence interval; cigs, cigarettes; ETS, environmental tobacco smoke; OR, odds ratio; Ref, reference category.
[a]Logistic regression models conditioned on matching variables (date of birth, sex, residence area of the child).
[b]Logistic regression model adjusted by age class and maternal educational level.
[c]Logistic regression model adjusted by age class and maternal educational level.
[d]Logistic regression model adjusted by duration of breastfeeding and paternal educational level.
[e]Logistic regression model adjusted by age class, maternal and paternal educational level.
[f]Logistic regression model adjusted sex, age class, residence area, birth order, birth weight, duration of breastfeeding, maternal and paternal age at child birth, maternal and paternal educational level, birth year of the mother, and parental occupational exposure to benzene (inverse probability weighting).

Risk of acute non–lymphocytic leukemia
Interaction between paternal smoking and maternal age

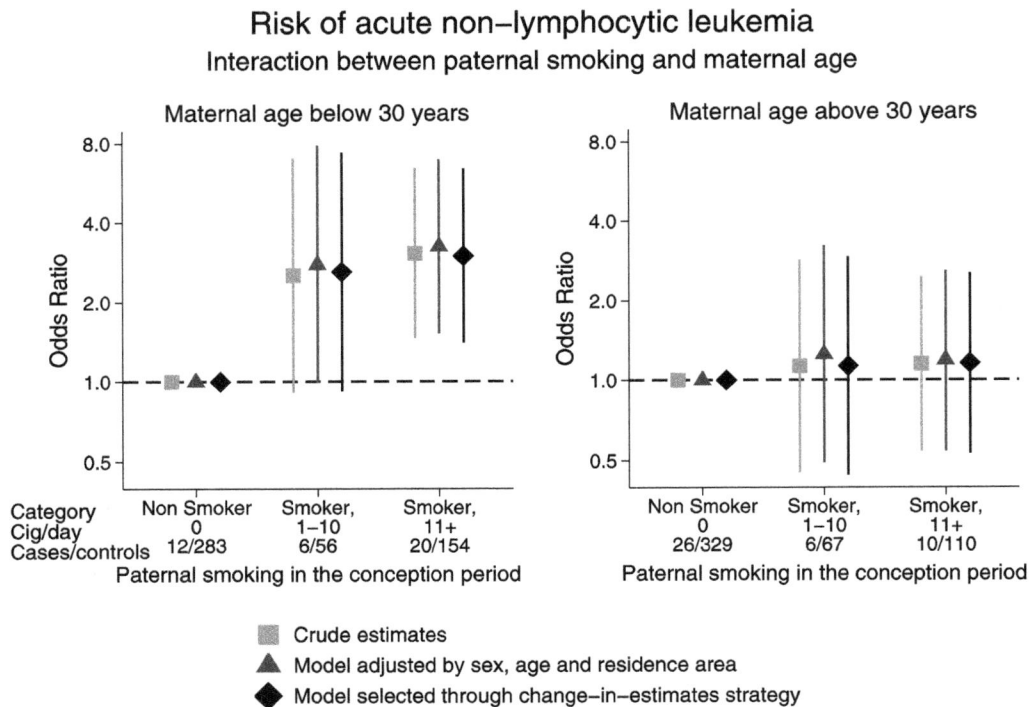

Figure 1. Association Between Paternal Smoking Status During the Period of Conception and Risk of Childhood Acute Non-Lymphocytic Leukemia, According to Maternal Age at Delivery. The SETIL Study, Italy, 1998–2003.

more than 10 cigarettes/day during the first trimester of pregnancy.

Results for maternal exposure to second-hand smoke suggest a possible association with AnLL: to the best of our knowledge, this finding is the first supporting this association [23,24] which makes us cautious in interpreting this apparent association as causal since we consider the self-assessment of second-hand smoke to be a measure prone to misclassification and recall bias. In fact, the presence of a raised risk only for maternal exposure to ETS and not for maternal active smoking is difficult to explain from a biological point of view. Furthermore, evidence suggesting a strong recall bias for maternal exposure to ETS emerged from a former study of ALL performed data from the SETIL study [13].

In most past studies on exposure of children to second-hand smoke and risk of AnLL authors used parental smoking status after pregnancy as a proxy of exposure, and most findings were negative. [25] In the SETIL study, a quantification of child exposure was attempted with direct questions in the questionnaire, but we failed to find any sign of an association between second-hand smoke and AnLL risk.

Strengths and limitations

One strength of this study is the population based design: the identification of incident cases in participating Regions proved to be very accurate [12] and information on exposures was collected by trained interviewers.

Conversely, several limitations should be considered: the response rate of controls was 0.71 and we cannot exclude a selection bias. Recall bias is always a concern when investigating self-reported exposures. Nevertheless, a Swedish study highlighted that retrospective recall of pregnancy smoking is fairly stable over time. [26] Also, interviewed subjects and interviewers were

unaware of the hypothesis investigated in the present report since studying the association between smoking and childhood ALL was not one of the main purposes of the SETIL study; furthermore, the sections aimed at collecting information on smoking were only a small part of the entire questionnaire. On the balance, we do not believe that recall bias is a serious limitation for the study of parental active smoking; on the contrary, recall bias could affect the study of ETS. As the SETIL study was not primarily designed to study the effect of tobacco smoking, misclassification of exposure could be an issue, particularly for ETS exposure.

In the present analysis we were unable to consider the effect of residential and domestic exposure to benzene, possible confounders of the relationship between exposure to cigarette smoke and risk of childhood AnLL.

We decided to break the matching in order to avoid loss of cases and expand the control group. Therefore, we should consider a possible bias due to the use of unconditional logistic regression in analysis that involved both matched and unmatched controls, with respect to AnLL cases. Of note, estimates from conditional logistic regression models (matched analysis) were consistent with the results from unmatched analysis.

The use of a propensity score or inverse probability weighting in case-control studies has been reported to be more problematic than in cohort studies, since estimates might be affected by an artefactual effect modification and residual confounding [27]. To assess whether this sort of bias might influence our estimates a supplemental set of analyses where covariates were selected based on the change-in-estimates method was performed. It is noteworthy to observe that figures from the two sets of analyses were consistent.

Conclusions

Our study supports the hypothesis that paternal smoking is associated with the risk of childhood AnLL; we also found signs of a possible effect modification due to maternal age at delivery that should be considered in future investigations. We found weak evidence of a possible effect of maternal exposure to second-hand smoke on the risk of childhood AnLL. This finding has to be consider with a degree of caution since recall bias is likely. No evidence at all emerged in our analysis for maternal smoking and exposure of the child to second-hand smoke; these results are broadly in line with knowledge from previous researches, but we should underline that the power of our study to detect an association for these exposures was low.

Supporting Information

Table S1 Studies on Paternal Tobacco Smoking and Risk of Childhood Acute non-Lymphocytic Leukemia.

Appendix S1 Smoking questionnaire.

Acknowledgments

The members of the SETIL Study Group (Principal Investigator: Prof. Corrado Magnani, email: magnani@med.unipmn.it) are:

Aricò Maurizio, AOU Meyer, Firenze, Italia;

Assennato Giorgio, ARPA Puglia, Bari, Italy;

Bernini Gabriella, Dipartimento di Oncoematologia, Azienda Ospedaliera Universitaria Meyer, Firenze, Italy (retired);

Biddau Pierfranco, Ospedale Microcitemico, Cagliari, Italia;

Bisanti Luigi, ASL di Milano, Milano, Italia;

Bochicchio Francesco, Istituto Superiore di Sanità, Roma, Italia;

Bocchini Vittorio, Istituto Nazionale per la Ricerca sul Cancro, Genova, Italia;

Cannizzaro Santina, Lega Italiana per la Lotta contro i Tumori Onlus, Ragusa, Italia;

Casotto Veronica, IRCCS Burlo Garofolo, Trieste, Italia;

Celentano Egidio, ARSAN - Agenzia Regionale Sanitaria della Campania, Napoli, Italia;

Chiavarini Manuela, Dipartimento di Specialità Medico Chirurgiche e Sanità Pubblica – Sezione di Sanità Pubblica, Facoltà di Medicina e Chirurgia, Università degli Studi di Perugia, Perugia, Italia;

Cocco Pierluigi, Università di Cagliari, Cagliari, Italia;

Cuttini Marina, Ospedale Pediatrico Bambino Gesù, Roma, Italia;

de Nichilo Gigliola, SPESAL, Barletta, Italia;

De Salvo Gian Luigi, Istituto Oncologico Veneto IRCCS, Padova, Italia;

Forastiere Francesco, Department of Epidemiology, Regional Health Authority - Lazio Region, Rome, Italy;

Gafà Lorenzo, Lega Italiana per la Lotta contro i Tumori Onlus, Ragusa Ibla, Italia;

Galassi Claudia, AOU S.Giovanni Battista e CPO Piemonte, Torino, Italia;

Greco Alessandra, Istituto Oncologico Veneto—IRCCS Padova, Padova, Italia;

Guarino Erni, Istituto Nazionale Tumori, Napoli, Italia

Haupt Riccardo, Istituto Giannina Gaslini, Genova, Italia;

Lagorio Susanna, National Institute of Health, Rome, Italia;

Locatelli Franco, Università di Pavia, Pavia, Italia;

Luzzatto Lia Lidia, ASL 1, Torino, Italy;

Kirchmayer Ursula, Dipartimento Epidemiologia Regione Lazio, Roma, Italia;

Masera Giuseppe, Università Milano Bicocca, Monza, Italia;

Massaglia Pia, Neuropsichiatria Infantile, Torino, Italia;

Merlo Domenico Franco, IRCCS Azienda Ospedaliera Universitaria San Martino- IST Istituto Nazionale per Minelli Liliana, Università degli Studi di Perugia, Perugia, Italia;

Monetti Daniele, Istituto Oncologico Veneto IRCCS, Padova, Italia;

Mosciatti Paola, Università di Camerino, Camerino, Italia;

la Ricerca sul Cancro, Genova, Italia;

Michelozzi Paola, Department of Epidemiology, Regional Health Authority – Lazio – Region, Rome, Italy;

Nuccetelli Cristina, Istituto Superiore di Sanità, Roma, Italia;

Pannelli Franco, Università di Camerino, Dipartimento di Medicina Sperimentale e di Sanità Pubblica, Camerino, Italy;

Pession Andrea, University of Bologna, Bologna, Italia;

Polichetti Alessandro, National Institute of Health, Roma, Italia;

Poggi Vincenzo, A.O.R.N. Santobono – Pausilipon, Napoli, Italia;

Pulsoni Alessandro, La Sapienza, Università di Roma, Roma, Italia;

Sampietro Giuseppe, ASL Città di Milano, Milano, Italia;

Schilirò Gino, Università di Catania, Catania, Italia;

Risica Serena, Istituto Superiore di Sanità, Roma, Italia;

Rizzari Carmelo, A.O. San Gerardo, Fondazione MBBM, Monza, Italia;

Targhetta Roberto, Servizio di Oncoematologia Pediatrica, Ospedale Microcitemico, Cagliari, Italia;

Torregrossa Maria Valeria, Università degli Studi di Palermo; Palermo, Italia;

Valenti Rosaria Maria, Università degli Studi di Palermo, Palermo, Italia;

Varotto Stefania, Dipartimento di Pediatria, Università di Padova, Italia;

Zambon Paola, Registro Tumori del Veneto, Università di Padova, Padova, Italia;

Andrea Farioli's work on this paper was supported by the Master's Degree in Epidemiology, University of Turin.

A special thank to Ms. Victoria Franzinetti for her careful revision of the text.

The SETIL study was financially supported by research grants received by AIRC (Italian Association on Research on Cancer), MIUR (Ministry for Instruction, University and Research, PRIN Program), Ministry of Health (Ricerca Sanitaria Finalizzata Program), Ministry of Labour and Welfare, Associazione Neuroblastoma, Piemonte Region (Ricerca Sanitaria Finalizzata Regione Piemonte Program), Liguria Region, ONLUS Comitato per la vita "Daniele Chianelli"- Associazione per la Ricerca e la Cura delle Leucemie, Linfomi e Tumori di Adulti e Bambini, (Perugia).

Author Contributions

Conceived and designed the experiments: SM LM AS RR CM. Performed the experiments: AF PL AB AR. Analyzed the data: AF SM PL CM. Contributed reagents/materials/analysis tools: AB AR AS. Wrote the paper: AF SM CM.

References

1. Pui CH (2006) Childhood Leukemia. 2nd ed. Cambridge University Press: New York.
2. Greaves MF, Alexander FE (1993) An infectious etiology for common acute lymphoblastic leukemia in childhood? Leukemia 7: 349–360.
3. Belson M, Kingsley B, Holmes A (2007) Risk factors for acute leukemia in children: a review. Environ Health Perspect 115: 138–145.
4. Eden T (2010) Aetiology of childhood leukaemia. Cancer Treat Rev 36: 286–297, doi: 10.1016/j.ctrv.2010.02.004
5. Greaves M (2006) Infection, immune responses and the aetiology of childhood leukaemia. Nat Rev Cancer 6: 193–203, doi: 10.1038/nrc1816
6. Schnatter AR, Rosamilia K, Wojcik NC (2005) Review of the literature on benzene exposure and leukemia subtypes. Chem Biol Interact 153–154: 9–21, doi: 10.1016/j.cbi.2005.03.039
7. WHO-IARC (2009) IARC Monographs on the Evaluation of Carcinogenic Risks to Humans. Volume 100. A Review of Human Carcinogens. Part E: Personal Habits and Indoor Combustions. Lyon: WHO Press.
8. Milne E, Greenop KR, Scott RJ, Bailey HD, Attia J, et al. (2012) Parental prenatal smoking and risk of childhood acute lymphoblastic leukemia. Am J Epidemiol 175: 43–53, doi: 10.1093/aje/kwr275

9. Chang JS (2009) Parental smoking and childhood leukemia. Methods Mol Biol 472: 10–37, doi: 10.1007/978-1-60327-492-0_5

10. Miligi L, Benvenuti A, Mattioli S, Salvan A, Tozzi GA, et al. (2013) Risk of childhood leukaemia and non-Hodgkin's lymphoma after parental occupational exposure to solvents and other agents: the SETIL Study. Occup Environ Med 70: 648–655, doi: 10.1136/oemed-2012-100951

11. Badaloni C, Ranucci A, Cesaroni G, Zanini G, Vienneau D, et al. (2013) Air pollution and childhood leukaemia: a nationwide case-control study in Italy. Occup Environ Med 70: 876–883, doi: 10.1136/oemed-2013-101604

12. AIRTUM Working Group (2008) Italian cancer figures-report 2008. 1. Childhood cancer. (In Italian) Epidemiol Prev 32: 1, 5–13, 16–35.

13. Farioli A, Legittimo P, Mattioli S, Miligi L, Benvenuti A el al. (2014) Tobacco smoke and risk of childhood acute lymphoblastic leukemia: findings from the SETIL case-control study. Cancer Causes Control, doi:10.1007/s10552-014-0371-9

14. Metayer C, Milne E, Clavel J, Infante-Rivard C, Petridou E, et al. (2013) The Childhood Leukemia International Consortium. Cancer Epidemiol 37: 336–47.

15. Cochran WG (1954) Some methods for strengthening the common $\chi 2$ tests. Biometrics 10: 417–451.

16. Robins JM, Hernán MA, Brumback B (2000) Marginal structural models and causal inference in epidemiology. Epidemiology 11: 550–560.

17. Tchernis R, Horvitz-Lennon M, Normand SL (2005) On the use of discrete choice models for causal inference. Stat Med 24: 2197–2212, doi: 10.1002/sim.2095

18. Hernan MA, Brumback BA, Robins JM (2000) Marginal Structural Models to Estimate the Causal Effect of Zidovudine on the Survival of HIV-Positive Men. Epidemiology 11: 561–570.

19. Maldonado G, Greenland S (1993) Simulation study of confounder-selection strategies. Am J Epidemiol 138: 923–36.

20. Lee KM, Ward MH, Han S, Ahn HS, Kang HJ, et al. (2009) Paternal smoking, genetic polymorphisms in CYP1A1 and childhood leukemia risk. Leuk Res 33: 250–258, doi: 10.1016/j.leukres.2008.06.031

21. Greaves M (2005) In utero origins of childhood leukaemia. Early Hum Dev 81: 123–129, doi: 10.1016/j.earlhumdev.2004.10.004

22. Ménézo YJ (2006) Paternal and maternal factors in preimplantation embryogenesis: interaction with the biochemical environment. Reprod Biomed Online 12: 616–621, doi:10.1016/S1472-6483(10)61188-1

23. Trédaniel J, Boffetta P, Little J, Saracci R, Hirsch A (1994) Exposure to passive smoking during pregnancy and childhood, and cancer risk: the epidemiological evidence. Paediatr Perinat Epidemiol 8: 233–255, doi: 10.1111/j.1365-3016.1994.tb00455.x

24. Sasco AJ, Vainio H (1999) From in utero and childhood exposure to parental smoking to childhood cancer: a possible link and the need for action. Hum Exp Toxicol 18: 192–201, doi: 10.1191/096032799678839905

25. Boffetta P, Trédaniel J, Greco A (2000) Risk of childhood cancer and adult lung cancer after childhood exposure to passive smoke: A meta-analysis. Environ Health Perspect 108: 73–82.

26. Post A, Gilljam H, Bremberg S, Galanti MR (2008) Maternal smoking during pregnancy: a comparison between concurrent and retrospective self-reports. Paediatr Perinat Epidemiol 22: 155–161, doi: 10.1111/j.1365-3016.2007.00917.x

27. Månsson R, Joffe MM, Sun W, Hennessy S (2007) On the estimation and use of propensity scores in case-control and case-cohort studies. Am J Epidemiol 166: 332–9.

4

Developing Item Banks for Measuring Pediatric Generic Health-Related Quality of Life: An Application of the International Classification of Functioning, Disability and Health for Children and Youth and Item Response Theory

Pranav K. Gandhi[1], Lindsay A. Thompson[2], Sanjeev Y. Tuli[2], Dennis A. Revicki[3], Elizabeth Shenkman[4,5], I-Chan Huang[4,5]*

1 Department of Pharmacy Practice, School of Pharmacy, South College, Knoxville, TN, United States of America, 2 Department of Pediatrics, College of Medicine, University of Florida, Gainesville, FL, United States of America, 3 Outcomes Research, Evidera, Bethesda, MD, United States of America, 4 Department of Health Outcomes and Policy, College of Medicine, University of Florida, Gainesville, FL, United States of America, 5 Department of Epidemiology and Cancer Control, St. Jude Children's Research Hospital, Memphis, TN, United States of America

Abstract

The purpose of this study was to develop item banks by linking items from three pediatric health-related quality of life (HRQoL) instruments using a mixed methodology. Secondary data were collected from 469 parents of children aged 8-16 years. The International Classification of Functioning, Disability and Health-Children and Youth (ICF-CY) served as a framework to compare the concepts of items from three HRQoL instruments. The structural validity of the individual domains was examined using confirmatory factor analyses. Samejima's Graded Response Model was used to calibrate items from different instruments. The known-groups validity of each domain was examined using the status of children with special health care needs (CSHCN). Concepts represented by the items in the three instruments were linked to 24 different second-level categories of the ICF-CY. Eight item banks representing eight unidimensional domains were created based on the linkage of the concepts measured by the items of the three instruments to the ICF-CY. The HRQoL results of CSHCN in seven out of eight domains (except personality) were significantly lower compared with children without special health care needs ($p < 0.05$). This study demonstrates a useful approach to compare the item concepts from the three instruments and to generate item banks for a pediatric population.

Editor: Jacobus van Wouwe, TNO Quality of Life, Netherlands

Funding: This study is supported by a grant from the National Institutes of Health U01 AR052181 (LAT, EAS, ICH). The funder had no role in study design, data collection and analysis, decision to publish, or preparation of the manuscript.

Competing Interests: The authors have declared that no competing interests exist.

* Email: I-Chan.Huang@StJude.org

Introduction

Over the past decade, pediatric research has shifted its attention from advancing treatments and survival rates for children with various diseases and disorders to improving their functional status and health-related quality of life (HRQoL). In parallel to this paradigm shift, the World Health Organization (WHO) elaborated the concept of health by emphasizing its components and determinants, which include body functions, body structures, activities and participation, and environmental and personal factors [1,2]. The use of this bio-psycho-social model helps us understand the psychological, social, and environmental determinants of health outcomes, especially in children and adolescents with various diseases, at different developmental stages and who are often under-served [3–5].

Several generic- and disease-specific HRQoL instruments have been developed for use in pediatric populations. The commonly used generic HRQoL instruments are the Child Health and Illness Profile (CHIP) [6], the Child Health Questionnaire (CHQ) [7], the KIDSCREEN-52 [8], the KINDL-R [9], and the Pediatric Quality of Life Inventory (PedsQL) [10]. Ideally, pediatric HRQoL instruments should be brief in content, related to the child's age and developmental stage, and demonstrate good measurement properties such as reliability, validity, and responsiveness [11]. In addition, good generic instruments should be able to assess the HRQoL in children with varying health conditions and across different languages and cultures [12,13]. Using a large sample of children enrolled in the Medicaid program, our previous study based on the classical test theory (CTT) method suggested that none of the existing pediatric HRQoL instruments (the CHIP, KIDSCREEN, KINDL-R, or PedsQL) was superior to any other in the different psychometric properties [14,15]. Although the CTT has often been applied to compare or develop new HRQoL instruments, the use of the CTT alone may neglect item-level information, which might bias the conclusions in comparative effectiveness research and clinical applications [16]. Using qualitative methodologies to compare the heterogeneity of item content, followed by advanced quantitative methodologies (e.g., item response theory; IRT) [16,17] to quantify the measurement properties of individual items for the design of appropriate pediatric instruments, is important [4,18].

The International Classification of Functioning, Disability and Health for Children and Youth (ICF-CY) taxonomy represents an international classification system for pediatric health and disability. The ICF-CY has been used in research and clinical practice to understand the components and determinants of pediatric health outcomes and to help design HRQoL instruments [19]. The ICF-CY can also serve as a framework to compare the contents of items in existing HRQoL instruments, thus providing evidence of content validity [5,20,21]. Although researchers have used the ICF-CY to investigate the contents of items in pediatric HRQoL instruments [4,5,22–24], few studies have used the ICF-CY to conduct head-to-head comparisons among items from different pediatric HRQoL instruments combined with quantitative methods to validate these items and generate item banks for use in pediatric settings [25].

Designing and administering HRQOL items in children must account for several pediatric issues related to age, neurocognitive development, and special health care needs. Although there is a consensus that children as young as 8 years old are able to and should self-report their HRQoL [26,27], the use of parent-proxy reports remains important, especially when the children are mentally disabled, too young, or too sick to self-report [26,28,29]. Parent-proxy reports of a child's HRQoL is of particular importance for children enrolled in public insurance programs such as Medicaid [30] because the parents are responsible for evaluating their child's health outcomes and making decisions for health services. Children from low-income families and those enrolled in Medicaid have a greater likelihood of a poorer HRQoL related to multiple chronic conditions than children of high-income families and those in private health insurance programs [31].

The main purpose of this study was to use a mixed qualitative and quantitative methodology to develop initial items banks on the basis of three most frequently used pediatric legacy HRQoL instruments (KIDSCREEN-52, KINDL-R, and PedsQL). The KIDSCREEN-52 and KINDL-R are among the most widely used pediatric generic HRQoL instruments in Europe, whereas the PedsQL is the most popular generic instrument in the United States. These three instruments capture the common aspects of HRQoL including physical, psychological and social domains, and are suitable for children and adolescents. Our first objective was to apply the ICF-CY framework to compare the contents of items from three pediatric legacy instruments and map these items into the domains suggested by the ICF-CY. The second objective was to apply IRT methodology to develop item banks using items mapped to the same HRQoL domain represented by the ICF-CY. The advantage of the IRT is that it can calibrate items from different instruments on the same metric by capturing comparable underlying constructs of HRQoL. The developed item banks were further validated using the Children with Special Health Care Needs (CSHCNs) Screener [32].

Methods

Study sample, inclusion and exclusion criteria, and data collection

The secondary data were analyzed using a 2009 survey comprising parents who had children aged 2–17 years old who

were enrolled in Florida's Medicaid program. Only families with 12 months of continuous enrollment in Medicaid were considered eligible for this study. Eligible families were sent a primer letter followed by a phone call for recruitment (n = 5,789). Families with disconnected and non-working numbers were excluded (n = 2,783). A total of 908 parents among the remaining 3,006 eligible participants completed the telephone interview (response rate 30.2%: 908/3006) by trained interviewers using a structured questionnaire including three legacy instruments (KIDSCREEN-52, KINDL-R, and PedsQL) and demographic information. Age-appropriate versions of the instruments were administered to each child and adolescent (Table 1). The present study analyzed the data of 469 surveys that were collected from the parents of children aged 8–16 years to allow for the comparison of all items across the three instruments.

The University of Florida's Institutional Review Board approved the study protocol. This study is part of the Quality Assurance project of the Florida Health Department for public insurance programs, and the survey was conducted via telephone. Per the University's IRB, we obtained a waiver for collecting written informed consent. Instead, we collected verbal agreement from all study participants over the phone when they were enrolled.

Survey instruments

The three pediatric legacy instruments, the KIDSCREEN-52, KINDL-R, and PedsQL, were chosen for the present study and are given in Table 1. Additionally, the parent participants answered the CSHCN Screener [32] for the analysis of the known-groups validity of the item banks. The domains and total scores were transformed into a 0–100 point scale (100 = best HRQoL and 0 = worst HRQoL). The characteristics of the three HRQoL instruments and the CSHCN Screener are described as follows:

The KIDSCREEN-52 is the most commonly administered pediatric HRQoL instrument in Europe [8,33]. The instrument contains 10 domains (52 items) including physical well-being (5 items), psychological well-being (6 items), moods and emotions (7 items), self-perception (5 items), autonomy (5 items), parent relationship and home life (6 items), social support and peers (6 items), social acceptance and bullying (3 items), school environment (6 items), and financial resources (3 items).

The KINDL-R was developed to assess HRQoL in healthy, chronically ill, and acutely ill children [9]. The Kid/Kiddo KINDL was especially designed for older children and adolescents between 8 and 16 years of age. Each version has 6 domains with 4 items per domain. The domains include physical well-being, psychological well-being, self-esteem, family functioning, friends, and school functioning.

The PedsQL 4.0 was developed to assess the WHO's core concept of health (physical, mental, and social functioning) plus school functioning [10]. This instrument contains 23 items measuring the problems associated with performing daily functions. The four domains include physical functioning (8 items), emotional functioning (5 items), social functioning (5 items), and school functioning (5 items).

CSHCN are defined as having a chronic condition (physical, developmental, behavioral, or emotional) and requiring health-related services and/or medication. The CSHCN Screener consists of five questions to evaluate the presence and duration of health conditions captured by three domains (dependency on prescription medications, service use above routine levels, and functional limitations). If a parent responds "yes" to a health consequence item, two follow-up items are asked to determine if

Table 1. Descriptions of the three pediatric health-related quality of life (HRQoL) instruments used in this study.

	KIDSCREEN-52	KINDL-R	PedsQL
Number of items	52	24	23
Number of subscales/domains	10	6	4
Age ranges suggested by the original instrument	8–18 years old	Kiddy KINDL: 4–7	Toddler: 2–4
		Kid KINDL: 8–12	Young child: 5–7
		Kiddo KINDL: 13–16	Child: 8–12
			Teen: 13–18
Age range used in this study	8–16 years old	8–16 years old	8–16 years old
Item scoring	5-point Likert scale	5-point Likert scale	5-point Likert scale
	Items scored so higher scores indicate better HRQoL	All items scored so that higher scores indicate better HRQoL	All items reverse scored so higher scores indicate better HRQoL

the consequence is due to a medical or health condition. Both follow-up items must be answered "yes" to qualify the child as a CSHCN for that domain.

Mapping, linking, and validation methodology

The ICF-CY framework. This study used the ICF-CY as a framework to link the items from the three pediatric HRQoL instruments. The ICF-CY includes four major components, and each has its respective classification codes and categories. The four components are 'body functions', represented as code letter b; 'body structure', represented as code letter s; 'activities and participation', represented as code letter d; and 'environmental factors', represented as code letter e. The numeric codes following these letters represent the chapter number (one digit), the second level (two digits), and the third and fourth levels (one digit each). The letters with the suffix of numeric codes are termed as categories. In this study, the items from the three HRQoL instruments were linked to the second-level categories of the ICF-CY [18], and these categories were used to form the domains of HRQoL and the item banks. The specific steps to map, link, and calibrate the items from the three instruments and to develop and validate the item banks are described as follows:

Step 1: Mapping items from the three pediatric HRQoL instruments using the ICF-CY framework. The rules suggested by Cieza et al. [18] were used to link the meaningful concepts of the items in the three HRQoL instruments to the ICF-CY. Prior to linking the items, the meaningful concepts of individual items were extracted by two authors using a data extraction form (see below). Per Cieza et al. [18], when the concept from each item of the three HRQoL instruments could not be linked with a specific ICF-CY category, the item was identified as 'not definable (nd)' [18]. For example, the KINDL item of 'my child worried about his/her future' was assigned 'nd' because it could not be represented by any specific ICF-CY category. Additionally, the abbreviation 'nc' (not covered) was used when the ICF-CY classification did not include a specific concept of the item [18].

In addition to the rules of Cieza et al. [18], other rules for item linkage were applied in this study. If an item from the three HRQoL instruments was linked to more than one category of the ICF-CY, multiple categories were reported for that particular item. However, to create different item banks with each measuring a unidimensional concept of HRQoL, we chose the most relevant ICF-CY category to represent the content of each individual item.

In line with the rules of Cieza et al. [18], the linking procedure was conducted independently by two authors (PG and ICH). To resolve any disagreements, a third rater was consulted, and a final decision based on a consensus among the three raters was made. Items that were linked from different instruments and placed in the same ICF-CY category are supposed to measure the same underlying construct of HRQoL. Subsequently, specific domains were created for these items that capture the same underlying constructs, and individual item banks were developed to represent the specific domains of HRQoL.

Step 2: Psychometric analysis using IRT. Confirmatory factor analyses (CFA) were used to test the structural validity of the individual domains. Specifically, CFA was used to test unidimensionality and local independence, which are two basic assumptions of IRT analysis. For the unidimensionality of individual domains, various fit indices were used to assess the structural validity, including the goodness-of-fit index χ^2 (a non-significant chi-square indicates a good model fit) and the root mean square error of approximation (RMSEA) (a value below 0.08 indicates a good model fit, and values below 0.05 indicate a close fit) [34]. Items with acceptable magnitudes of factor loading on the corresponding domains ($\lambda > 0.4$; $p < 0.05$) were considered to be appropriate for the IRT application. Non-significant items and items with a lower factor loading ($\lambda < 0.4$; $p > 0.05$) were removed from the analysis. For local independence, residual correlations of paired items from the same domains were investigated, and one of the paired items with a high residual covariance (>10.0) was considered for removal because both items might measure similar content.

Following the CFA, we used Samejima's Graded Response Model (GRM), a unidimensional IRT model for items with categorical response categories, to test and calibrate item parameter estimates and to calculate domain scores for specific HRQoL domains that were identified in the previous step. We examined different measurement properties to further remove some items from the item banks, including item thresholds and discrimination as well as item and test information functioning (IIF/TIF). Items with discrimination values>1.0, higher or lower threshold values (i.e., able to measure easiest or most challenging underlying HRQoL, respectively), and a higher IIF were considered for retention. Additionally, standardized local dependence (LD) χ^2 statistics were examined to test local independence between paired items in a specific domain [35]. Items that failed to satisfy more than one of the criteria described above were deleted from the item banks. Various fit indices were adopted to assess the

Table 2. Demographic characteristics (N = 469).

Characteristics	N (%) or mean (SD)
Child age, years	11.96 (2.55)
Parent age, years	41.46 (11.73)
Child gender, %	
Male	221 (47.1)
Female	248 (52.9)
Child race/ethnicity, %	
White	208 (44.3)
Black	143 (30.5)
Hispanic	53 (11.3)
Other	62 (13.2)
Refused	3 (0.6)
Parent race/ethnicity, %	
White	233 (49.7)
Black	140 (29.9)
Hispanic	51 (10.9)
Other	43 (9.2)
Refused	2 (0.4)
Parent education, %	
Less than HS	112 (23.9)
GED/HS degree	183 (39.0)
Vocational/some college/AA Degree	133 (28.4)
College graduate	30 (6.4)
Graduate degree	8 (1.7)
Marital status, %	
Married	187 (39.9)
Single	134 (28.6)
Other	143 (30.49)
Family income, %	
<$9,999	132 (28.2)
$10,000–$19,999	153 (32.6)
$20,000+	156 (33.3)
Refused	28 (6.0)

SD: standard deviation.

appropriateness of individual domains, including marginal reliability estimates (≥ 0.60 as acceptable), the M_2 statistic [36,37], and RMSEA (<0.08 as a good model fit for unidimensionality and <0.05 as a close fit).

Step 3: Validation analysis using the known-groups approach. The CSHCN Screener [32] was used to investigate the known-groups validity of item banks measuring different domains of pediatric HRQoL. Known-groups validity was demonstrated when the mean HRQoL domain scores derived from the item banks were able to better discriminate among the clinically meaningful groups (i.e., CSHCN versus children without special health care needs). For each individual, the underlying HRQoL domain scores were estimated using an expected a posteriori estimation (EAP) based on the Bayesian statistical principle. Bivariate relationships were examined using an independent t-test to compare the mean difference in the underlying HRQoL domain scores between the two groups. Additional analyses comparing the underlying HRQoL scores between the

two groups were conducted with adjustments for the children's age and gender and for the parent's race and education. Cohen's effect size (ES; Cohen's d) estimates were reported to indicate the magnitude of difference in the domain scores between CSHCN and children without special health care needs divided by the smaller value of the standard deviation (SD). Cohen's d values of <0.2, 0.2–0.49, 0.5–0.79, and >0.8 were regarded as a negligible, small, moderate, and large ES, respectively [38].

LISREL 8.8 was used to perform CFA [39], the Item Response Theory for Patient-Reported Outcomes (IRTPRO) v2.1 [40] was used for the IRT analysis, and the SAS 9.1 software [41] was used for the remaining analyses.

Results

Description of sample

Table 2 shows the characteristics of 469 parents of children aged 8–16 years. The average ages were 11.96 years old

Table 3. Specific items and their linkage to ICF-CY second-level categories for the development of item banks.

Domain	Item	Item question	ICF-CY category
Personality	Kindl11	My child felt pleased with him-/herself	b126 Temperament and personality functions
	Kindl20	My child felt different from other children	b126 Temperament and personality functions
	Kdscrn10	Has your child felt cheerful?	b126 Temperament and personality functions
	Kdscrn12	Has your child felt that he/she does everything badly?	b126 Temperament and personality functions
	Kdscrn19	Has your child been happy with the way he/she is?	b126 Temperament and personality functions
	Kdscrn43	Has your child been able to rely on his/her friends?	b126 Temperament and personality functions
Emotional function	Pedsql13	Worrying about what will happen to him/her	b152 Emotional functions
	Kindl5	My child had fun and laughed a lot	b152 Emotional functions
	Kindl8	My child felt scared or unsure of her/him-self	b152 Emotional functions
	Kdscrn6	Has your child felt that life was enjoyable?	b152 Emotional functions
	Kdscrn13	Has your child felt sad?	b152 Emotional functions
	Kdscrn14	Has your child felt so bad that he/she didn't want to do anything?	b152 Emotional functions
	Kdscrn15	Has your child felt that everything in his/her life goes wrong?	b152 Emotional functions
	Kdscrn16	Has your child felt fed up?	b152 Emotional functions
	Kdscrn17	Has your child felt lonely?	b152 Emotional functions
	Kdscrn18	Has your child felt under pressure?	b152 Emotional functions
	Kdscrn20	Has your child been happy with his/her clothes?	b152 Emotional functions
	Kdscrn31	Has your child been happy at home?	b152 Emotional functions
	Kdscrn44	Has your child been happy at school?	b152 Emotional functions
	Kdscrn50	Has your child been afraid of other girls and boys?	b152 Emotional functions
Mobility	Pedsql4	Lifting something heavy?	d430 Lifting and carrying objects
	Pedsql1	Walking more than one block?	d450 Walking
	Kdscrn2	Has your child felt physically well and fit?	d455 Moving around
	Pedsql2	Running?	d455 Moving around
Energy	Pedsql8	Low energy level?	b130 Energy and drive functions
	Kindl3	My child was tired and worn-out	b130 Energy and drive functions
	Kindl6	My child didn't feel much like doing anything	b130 Energy and drive functions
	Kdscrn5	Has your child felt full of energy?	b130 Energy and drive functions
	Pedsql12	Trouble sleeping?	b134 Sleep functions
Social function	Kindl19	My child got along well with his/her friends	d750 Informal social relationships
	Kdscrn27	Has your child had enough time to meet friends?	d750 Informal social relationships
	Kdscrn38	Has your child spent time with his/her friends?	d750 Informal social relationships
	Kdscrn40	Has your child had fun with his/her friends?	d750 Informal social relationships
	Kdscrn41	Has your child and his/her friends helped each other?	d750 Informal social relationships
	Kdscrn51	Have other girls and boys made fun of your child?	d750 Informal social relationships
Task accomplishment	Pedsql22	Missing school because of not feeling well?	d230 Carrying out daily routine
	Pedsql5	Taking a bath or shower by him or herself?	d510 Washing oneself
	Pedsql6	Doing chores around the house?	d640 Doing housework
	Pedsql3	Participating in sports activity or exercise?	d920 Recreation and leisure
Family function	Kindl13	My child got on well with us as parents	d760 Family relationships
	Kdscrn29	Has your child felt understood by his/her parents?	d760 Family relationships
	Kdscrn30	Has your child felt loved by his/her friends?	d760 Family relationships
	Kdscrn33	Has your child felt that his/her parent(s) treated him/her fairly?	d760 Family relationships
	Kdscrn34	Has your child been able to talk to his/her parent(s) when he/she wanted to?	d760 Family relationships
School function	Pedsql21	Keeping up with schoolwork?	d820 School education
	Kindl22	My child enjoyed the school lessons	d820 School education
	Kdscrn45	Has your child gotten on well at school?	d820 School education
	Kdscrn49	Has your child gotten along well with his/her teachers?	d820 School education
	Kindl17	My child played with friends	d880 Engagement in play

Table 3. Cont.

Domain	Item	Item question	ICF-CY category
	Pedsql17	Not being able to do things that other children/teens his or her age can do?	nd
	Pedsql18a	Keeping up with other teens	nd
	Kindl23	My child worried about his/her future	nd
	Kindl1	My child felt ill	nc
	Kindl14	My child felt fine at home	nc
	Kdscrn1	In general, how would your child rate his/her health?	nc

Kdscrn: KIDSCREEN-52; Kindl: KINDL-R; Pedsql: PedsQL; nd: not definable; nc: not covered.
All Kindl items start with "During the past week...."; All Kdscrn items start with "Please try to remember your child's experiences over the last month..."; and all Pedsql items start with "How much of a problem has your child/teen had with...".

(SD = 2.55) for the children and 41.46 years old (SD = 11.73) for the parents. A plurality of the parents were white (49.7%), and the majority had received at least a high school diploma or equivalent degree (75.5%). A third (33.3%) of the families had an income of $20,000 or above.

Step 1: Mapping items from the three pediatric HRQoL instruments using the ICF-CY framework. Table 3 displays an overview regarding the mapping of the concepts of specific items to the second-level categories of the ICF-CY. The concepts represented by the items were linked to 24 different second-level ICF-CY categories, including nine categories in the body functions component, 13 categories in the activities and participation component, and two categories in the environmental factor component. None of the items from the three HRQoL instruments were assigned to the body structures component, and three items each were not definable or not covered.

Meaningful concepts in items from the KIDSCREEN-52, KINDL-R, and PedsQL were almost equally represented by the body functions categories: six, four, and five second-level categories, respectively. In contrast, meaningful concepts of items from the PedsQL were greatly represented by the activities and participation categories: 10 second-level categories for the PedsQL compared with six and five second-level categories for KINDL-R and KIDSCREEN-52, respectively. The environmental factor component was not well represented by any of the three instruments as only one item each from the KIDSCREEN-52 and PedsQL was linked to a single category of the environmental factor component.

Appendix S1 shows the detailed mapping results between the concepts of individual items from the three instruments and the specific codes for the ICF-CY's body functions, activity and participation, and environmental factor components. This specifically informs how each item is represented by the ICF-CY components and categories. A higher representation for the items from the HRQoL instrument to a specific ICF-CY category suggests that the same concept was captured by potentially redundant items from this specific instrument. Items from the three instruments that were linked to the same ICF-CY category represented the same underlying construct, and a specific domain comprising items measuring this construct was created. As a result, 10 initial HRQoL domains were created based on the criterion of all the items in that domain that potentially measured the same underlying construct and had a minimum of four items per domain, including personality, emotion, mobility, energy, social function, task accomplishment, family function, school function, cognition, and experience of self (Table 3 and Appendix S2). However, two of the ten domains (cognition and experience of self)

were not considered further as they contained only a few items measuring those domains. Three of the six items measuring the experience of self domain were deleted because they had factor loadings <0.4 (see Step 2 below and Appendix S2). The remaining three items were considered too few to measure the experience of self. Four out of the five items from the cognition domain were assigned to different ICF-CY categories (b140, b144, b160, and b164), suggesting that these items might not measure the same underlying construct (Appendix S2).

Step 2: Psychometric analysis using IRT. CFA was performed to test the structural validity of the individual HRQoL domains with the goal of retaining items to meet the assumptions of unidimensionality and local independence to conduct the IRT analysis (Table 3 and Appendix S2). In the CFA, items that were significantly associated with the corresponding domains with factor loadings ($\lambda > 0.4$; $p < 0.05$) and residual covariance (<10.0) were considered for retention (Table 3). As a result, a total of six items were deleted due to either a low factor loading (<0.4) or a high residual covariance (>10.0), including one item in the mobility domain, three items in the social function domain, and two items in the task accomplishment domain (Appendix S2).

Item parameter estimates from the GRM for eight specific HRQoL domains are presented in Table 4. Items that did not satisfy one of the criteria explained in the Methods section were excluded from the analysis (Appendix S2). For example, item 23 of the PedsQL (name: Pedsql23) was deleted because of a poor item fit and a high correlation (>10.0) with item 22 from the PedsQL (name: Pedsql22). A total of 21 items were deleted across different domains due to poor item fit, high correlation, and/or poor discrimination value (Appendix S2). Overall, we did not consider 50 items to be assigned to any of the eight domains, leaving 49 items in the eight item banks that measure eight HRQoL domains (Table 3, Table 4, and Appendix S2). After deleting specific items across different domains, the RMSEA values for all eight domains suggested a good model fit (<0.08), and the marginal reliability of the eight domains ranged from 0.63–0.87. The majority of the threshold parameters (representing item difficulty) corresponding to the response categories of each item in a specific domain had negative values, suggesting that the majority of items captured lower levels of underlying HRQoL (Table 4).

Step 3: Validation analysis using known-groups approach. Table 5 shows known-groups validity related to CSHCN for the eight specific domains. Overall, the eight domains were able to distinguish the underlying HRQoL between children with and without special health care needs. Bivariate analyses suggested that the HRQoL domain scores for seven domains (with the exception of personality) in the CSHCN were significantly

Table 4. Item parameter estimates using item response theory for individual HRQoL domains.

Domain	Item	Discrimination parameter	Location parameters (standard error)				Chi-square	Probability
		a (se)	b_1 (se)	b_2 (se)	b_3 (se)	b_4 (se)		
Personality trait	Kindl11	1.72 (0.19)	−2.7 (0.25)	−2.22 (0.19)	−0.97 (0.1)	0.17 (0.08)	40.34	0.21
	Kindl20	1.28 (0.16)	−3.0 (0.34)	−2.27 (0.24)	−0.81 (0.11)	−0.32 (0.09)	46.35	0.20
	Kdscrn10	1.83 (0.20)	−3.79 (0.49)	−2.98 (0.29)	−1.1 (0.1)	0.44 (0.08)	44.09	0.02
	Kdscrn12	1.35 (0.16)	−3.3 (0.36)	−2.7 (0.27)	−0.86 (0.11)	0.05 (0.09)	58.39	0.01
	Kdscrn19	2.23 (0.26)	−2.61 (0.23)	−2.36 (0.19)	−1.11 (0.09)	0.01 (0.07)	37.92	0.12
	Kdscrn43	0.82 (0.12)	−3.82 (0.55)	−2.95 (0.42)	0.23 (0.13)	1.90 (0.28)	52.01	0.06
	$M_2 = 978.80$, df (234), $p = 0.0001$, RMSEA = 0.08; Marginal reliability: 0.76							
Emotion	Pedsql13	1.45 (0.15)	−3.06 (0.30)	−2.57 (0.24)	−1.00 (0.11)	−0.33 (0.09)	84.59	0.05
	Kindl5	1.51 (0.15)	−3.45 (0.36)	−2.73 (0.25)	−1.26 (0.12)	−0.20 (0.08)	101.17	0.0007
	Kindl8	1.59 (0.19)	−4.15 (0.57)	−2.82 (0.28)	−1.66 (0.15)	−0.96 (0.10)	58.54	0.10
	Kdscrn6	1.91 (0.17)	−2.58 (0.21)	−1.97 (0.15)	−1.09 (0.09)	0.24 (0.08)	72.26	0.20
	Kdscrn13	1.56 (0.15)	−3.95 (0.47)	−2.95 (0.27)	0.02 (0.08)	1.06 (0.12)	52.32	0.24
	Kdscrn14	2.06 (0.20)	−2.95 (0.27)	−2.56 (0.21)	−0.76 (0.08)	−0.14 (0.07)	59.13	0.18
	Kdscrn15	2.15 (0.20)	−2.66 (0.22)	−2.20 (0.16)	−0.88 (0.08)	−0.26 (0.07)	49.54	0.65
	Kdscrn16	2.07 (0.19)	−2.45 (0.19)	−2.12 (0.16)	−0.68 (0.08)	−0.06 (0.07)	54.66	0.53
	Kdscrn17	2.55 (0.26)	−2.48 (0.19)	−2.26 (0.16)	−0.74 (0.07)	−0.20 (0.07)	63.67	0.05
	Kdscrn18	1.82 (0.17)	−3.19 (0.31)	−2.34 (0.19)	−0.37 (0.08)	0.16 (0.08)	60.68	0.28
	Kdscrn20	1.13 (0.13)	−4.05 (0.49)	−3.34 (0.37)	−1.55 (0.17)	−0.28 (0.10)	79.29	0.09
	Kdscrn31	1.58 (0.16)	−4.17 (0.55)	−3.44 (0.36)	−1.80 (0.15)	−0.19 (0.08)	62.62	0.05
	Kdscrn44	1.28 (0.13)	−3.07 (0.30)	−2.01 (0.19)	−0.70 (0.10)	0.79 (0.12)	107.46	0.007
	Kdscrn50	1.10 (0.14)	−4.29 (0.55)	−3.63 (0.43)	−1.22 (0.15)	−0.53 (0.11)	68.40	0.17
	$M_2 = 3926.04$, df (1442), $p = 0.0001$, RMSEA = 0.06; Marginal reliability: 0.87							
Mobility	Pedsql4	1.98 (0.25)	−2.21 (0.20)	−1.99 (0.17)	−0.92 (0.09)	−0.56 (0.08)	53.36	0.008
	Pedsql1	3.35 (0.59)	−2.06 (0.16)	−1.58 (0.12)	−1.17 (0.09)	−0.87 (0.07)	40.03	0.13
	Kdscrn2	0.82 (0.13)	−3.09 (0.45)	−2.41 (0.35)	−1.07 (0.19)	0.97 (0.19)	34.25	0.51
	Pedsql2	3.70 (0.64)	−1.70 (0.13)	−1.48 (0.11)	−0.96 (0.08)	−0.62 (0.07)	42.39	0.02
	$M_2 = 351.01$, df (92), $p = 0.0001$, RMSEA = 0.08; Marginal reliability: 0.63							
Energy	Pedsql8	2.53 (0.45)	−2.46 (0.24)	−1.97 (0.18)	−0.76 (0.09)	−0.28 (0.07)	36.96	0.18
	Kindl3	1.31 (0.18)	−3.60 (0.45)	−2.83 (0.32)	−1.03 (0.13)	−0.29 (0.09)	35.89	0.25
	Kindl6	1.39 (0.19)	−3.19 (0.36)	−2.52 (0.27)	−0.98 (0.12)	−0.19 (0.09)	66.14	0.002
	Kdscrn5	1.24 (0.16)	−3.84 (0.48)	−3.18 (0.37)	−1.42 (0.17)	0.09 (0.09)	38.88	0.13
	Pedsql12	1.26 (0.17)	−3.40 (0.41)	−2.62 (0.30)	−1.28 (0.16)	−0.62 (0.11)	46.59	0.06
	$M_2 = 497.42$, df (155), $p = 0.0001$, RMSEA = 0.07; Marginal reliability: 0.69							
Social function	Kindl19	1.46 (0.16)	−3.45 (0.36)	−2.85 (0.27)	−1.26 (0.13)	−0.00 (0.09)	48.23	0.03

Table 4. Cont.

Domain	Item	Discrimination parameter	Location parameters (standard error)				Chi-square	Probability
	Kdscrn27	1.54 (0.18)	-4.30 (0.58)	-3.83 (0.45)	-1.46 (0.14)	-0.48 (0.09)	37.05	0.06
	Kdscrn38	1.58 (0.16)	-3.17 (0.30)	-2.54 (0.22)	-0.42 (0.09)	0.72 (0.10)	48.05	0.03
	Kdscrn40	3.36 (0.43)	-2.91 (0.26)	-2.56 (0.20)	-1.06 (0.08)	-0.23 (0.06)	49.94	0.0004
	Kdscrn41	2.84 (0.33)	-2.83 (0.24)	-2.47 (0.19)	-0.60 (0.07)	0.08 (0.07)	35.30	0.05
	Kdscrn51	0.90 (0.12)	-4.19 (0.56)	-3.06 (0.39)	-0.23 (0.12)	0.49 (0.13)	76.11	0.0002

M_2 = 833.87, df (234), p = 0.0001, RMSEA = 0.07; Marginal reliability: 0.79

Domain	Item	Discrimination parameter	Location parameters (standard error)				Chi-square	Probability
Task accomplishment	Pedsql22	0.74 (0.13)	-5.19 (0.90)	-4.19 (0.71)	-1.30 (0.24)	0.19 (0.15)	55.68	0.006
	Pedsql5	3.86 (1.22)	-1.40 (0.13)	-1.29 (0.12)	-1.02 (0.10)	-0.94 (0.09)	29.16	0.21
	Pedsql6	2.25 (0.32)	-1.68 (0.14)	-1.50 (0.13)	-0.45 (0.08)	-0.14 (0.07)	28.20	0.51
	Pedsql3	1.49 (0.21)	-2.32 (0.25)	-2.06 (0.22)	-1.21 (0.14)	-0.67 (0.10)	44.38	0.13

M_2 = 235.41, df (92), p = 0.0001, RMSEA = 0.06; Marginal reliability: 0.64

Domain	Item	Discrimination parameter	Location parameters (standard error)				Chi-square	Probability
Family function	Kindl13	1.15 (0.15)	-3.31 (0.40)	-2.78 (0.32)	-1.45 (0.18)	-0.01 (0.10)	73.88	0.0001
	Kdscrn29	1.97 (0.22)	-2.27 (0.19)	-1.69 (0.14)	-0.65 (0.08)	0.53 (0.09)	99.67	0.0001
	Kdscrn30	2.59 (0.39)	-2.66 (0.25)	-2.15 (0.18)	-1.61 (0.13)	-0.64 (0.07)	67.24	0.0001
	Kdscrn33	1.48 (0.17)	-2.55 (0.25)	-2.27 (0.22)	-0.92 (0.11)	0.26 (0.09)	43.82	0.06
	Kdscrn34	1.61 (0.23)	-3.29 (0.39)	-3.11 (0.35)	-1.87 (0.19)	-0.92 (0.10)	29.10	0.26

M_2 = 492.80, df (155), p = 0.0001, RMSEA = 0.07; Marginal reliability: 0.73

Domain	Item	Discrimination parameter	Location parameters (standard error)				Chi-square	Probability
School function	Pedsql21	0.98 (0.13)	-2.18 (0.27)	-1.87 (0.23)	0.00 (0.11)	0.67 (0.14)	79.56	0.0001
	Kindl22	1.91 (0.22)	-2.05 (0.18)	-1.47 (0.13)	-0.31 (0.08)	0.52 (0.09)	61.34	0.004
	Kdscrn45	2.02 (0.25)	-2.44 (0.22)	-1.57 (0.13)	-0.70 (0.08)	0.36 (0.08)	50.90	0.03
	Kdscrn49	2.00 (0.25)	-2.74 (0.26)	-2.41 (0.22)	-1.05 (0.11)	-0.02 (0.07)	49.73	0.005
	Kindl17	0.57 (0.11)	-5.69 (1.10)	-4.23 (0.80)	-0.98 (0.24)	1.46 (0.32)	41.84	0.052

M_2 = 610.77, df (155), p = 0.0001, RMSEA = 0.08; Marginal reliability: 0.74

RMSEA: root mean square error of approximation.

Table 5. Known-groups validity for individual domain scores among children with special health care needs (CSCHN) compared with children without special health care needs.

Domains	CSCHN	Children without special health care needs	Difference (effect size) Bivariate analysis	Difference (effect size) Multivariate analysis[#]
Personality	0.069 (0.879)	−0.049 (0.862)	−0.118 (−0.137)	−0.124 (0.142)
Emotional function	−0.337 (0.942)	0.226 (0.863)	0.562 (0.651)***	0.570 (0.609)***
Mobility	−0.245 (0.892)	0.167 (0.714)	0.415 (0.581)***	0.472 (0.581)***
Energy	−0.282 (0.901)	0.189 (0.726)	0.471 (0.649)***	0.488 (0.587)***
Social function	−0.213 (0.901)	0.143 (0.863)	0.356 (0.413)***	0.361 (0.402)***
Task accomplishment	−0.202 (0.780)	0.136 (0.804)	0.338 (0.423)***	0.379 (0.466)***
Family function	−0.157 (0.860)	0.106 (0.834)	0.263 (0.315)**	0.216 (0.255)**
School function	−0.293 (0.882)	0.196 (0.774)	0.489 (0.632)***	0.499 (0.587)***

** $p<0.01$.
*** $p<0.001$.
[#] Controlling for child's age and gender and parent's race and education.

lower than those in the children without special health care needs ($p<0.05$). The magnitude of ES was larger for domains of emotional function (ES = 0.65), energy (ES = 0.65), and school function (ES = 0.63) compared with the other domains (ES = 0.32 to 0.58; excluding the personality domain). Similar findings were replicated after adjusting for covariates (children's age and gender and parent's race and education).

Discussion

This study shows that the contents of items from the three pediatric HRQoL legacy instruments were well represented by the ICF-CY categories. Specifically, compared with the KIDSCREEN-52 and KINDL, the PedsQL was found to better represent the activity and participation components of the ICF-CY. The KINDL-R and PedsQL corresponded less with respect to the environmental factors, which is consistent with a previous study that linked items of these instruments to the ICF-CY categories [5]. However, we only linked one item in the KIDSCREEN-52 to a single category of the environmental factor component, which contrasts with the results of a previous study showing that 24% of the items in the KIDSCREEN-52 were able to link to six different categories in the environmental factor component [5]. This discrepancy might have arisen because the latter study linked each item to more than one concept, resulting in the total number of concepts exceeding the number of items in the instrument. However, because our purpose was to develop different item banks with each capturing a unidimensional concept of HRQoL, we chose the most relevant ICF-CY category to represent the content of an individual item. Since our selection criteria for linkage methodology was different from the previous studies [4,5,22–24], our findings do not allow for recommending which pediatric HRQOL instrument should be chosen. Instead, we argue that different pediatric HRQOL instruments contain items of different measurement properties and the inclusion of various items from different instruments will strengthen item banks with robust measurement properties.

This study uses the rules recommended by Cieza et al. [18] to link items from the three pediatric HRQoL instruments to the specific ICF-CY categories. Consequently, eight specific unidimensional domains emerged, which provides a foundation for developing item banks to measure pediatric HRQoL. CFA were used to test for structural validity, and IRT was used to calibrate

items from different instruments on the same metric and to calculate domain scores for individuals. Items were deleted from the item banks if they were not represented by the appropriate ICF-CY categories or if they demonstrated poor performance on the basis of psychometric properties. This combined use of qualitative and quantitative approaches allowed for the concomitant establishment of the content validity of individual domains and the confirmation of content validity using IRT. This strategy directly led to robust item banks that measure unidimensional HRQoL constructs. We identified several items represented by the same ICF-CY category, indicating an overlap in the concepts across different pediatric HRQoL instruments. Our linkage also identified some items that were not included in the item banks as the ICF-CY unfortunately does not represent meaningful concepts for these items. Future studies might replicate our approach to explore the potential similarities or discrepancies in these findings and expand our item banks based on the ICF-CY framework to link existing items from other pediatric HRQoL instruments or to add novel items.

The linking process was conducted based on a parent-proxy report rather than on a child self-report. The use of a parent versus a child version of the instruments might not result in discrepant item mapping results because the contents in the child and parent versions are almost the same. However, data collected from a parent-proxy versus a child self-report might lead to different quantitative results in terms of construct validity and item parameters because parents and children possess different perceptions with regard to interpreting and answering pediatric HRQoL items [42]. A greater discrepancy between proxy- and self-reports has been found in the more abstract domains (e.g., emotional functioning) compared with the less abstract domains (e.g., physical functioning) [43].

We found that the mean underlying HRQoL scores for seven of the eight domains (except personality) were significantly lower ($p<0.05$) in the CSHCN compared to the children without special health care needs in the bivariate and multivariate analyses (Table 5). These findings suggest a high level capacity to discriminate and differentiate CSHCN with respect to different emotional (emotional function and social function) and activity and participation (mobility, energy, task accomplishment, family function, and school function) domains compared with children without special health care needs. The ES for the underlying

HRQoL scores was the highest for the emotional function domain, followed by the energy domain. This finding echoes our previous study suggesting that CSHCN require more physical, developmental, and emotional support than children without special health care needs [44]. Not surprisingly, children with and without special health care needs had similar personality domain scores because personality is a trait that is less likely to be related to different levels of special health care needs.

The linkage of ICF-CY categories to the concepts measured by the items in the three pediatric HRQoL instruments helped with the development of the item banks, which in turn assists clinicians in using the measurement tools to evaluate the comparative effectiveness of different interventions [3,45]. However, there is limited evidence of the ability of HRQoL tools to measure the impact of environmental and personal factors on a child's health status. The ICF-CY framework provides an important foundation for creating the unidimensional item banks. Through the ICF-CY framework we were able to identify items from different pediatric HRQoL instruments that specifically capture life experiences, activities and participation appropriate for the child's age and developmental stage. The broader perspective embedded in the ICF-CY framework provides a valuable opportunity to develop measures to capture factors influencing physical and emotional functioning and activity and participation, further facilitating the ability of researchers and clinicians to design appropriate interventions targeting these modifiable factors [3].

The ICF framework was primarily developed to measure disability, functional status, and social participation rather than quality of life [46]. The components of the ICF are more objective (e.g., ability to perform specific functioning) than subjective (e.g., satisfaction with health). In this regard, the linkage exercise using the ICF-CY framework might not have distinguishable concepts for some items that measure specific pediatric HRQoL. The concepts for some categories in the ICF-CY are general and thus susceptible to a broader description of the meaningful concepts for the items. For example, the ICF-CY body function category b152 (emotional functions) can be explained by several aspects regarding emotions such as sadness, laughter, and fear. In turn, this general nature resulted in linking a specific ICF-CY category to several items from the pediatric HRQoL instruments.

Several limitations should be noted when interpreting the findings of this study. First, the generalizability of the findings is limited due to the use of a Medicaid population from Florida. Second, the linkage was conducted based on the perspective of the investigators and did not include the perspectives of the parents and children themselves. Indeed, investigators, parents and children may interpret the meaning of items differently [47]. With an emphasis on a patient-centeredness approach, future studies might consider engaging parents and children as stakeholders alongside researchers in the item mapping process to strengthen the content validity and develop a robust methodology for the synergy of findings from different stakeholders. Third, the CSHCN status reported by parents was used for evaluating the known-groups validity. This information may result in varying outcomes compared with the use of categorical approaches, such as disease diagnoses. Finally, the survey response rate (30.2%) was lower than that of previous studies (usually 60%) focusing on Medicaid pediatric populations [48–50]. However, responders and nonresponders did not differ significantly on children's age and sex ($p > 0.05$). The lower response rate is in part due to the inclusion of a lengthy survey (approximately 50 minutes per survey) that precludes subjects from the study participation. Although the lower response rate may threaten the generalizability of our findings, this population is important to assess because they were below 100% of the federal poverty level and possess greater risk of poor health status due to poor socioeconomic circumstances.

Conclusions

The ICF-CY serves as a useful framework to compare the concepts of items from the three pediatric HRQoL legacy instruments and to generate item banks for a pediatric population. This study provides useful insights regarding the content coverage of items from three instruments represented by the ICF-CY framework. This study has implications for researchers to refine pediatric HRQoL instruments and for clinicians to use these instruments in clinical practice.

Acknowledgments

The authors thank Katie Zidonik-Eddelton, MPH, for determining patient eligibility and coordinating data collection and Kelly Kenzik, PhD, for resolving discrepancies in the item mapping process conducted by the two primary raters (PG and ICH).

Author Contributions

Conceived and designed the experiments: PKG ICH. Performed the experiments: EAS ICH. Analyzed the data: PKG ICH. Wrote the paper: PKG LAT SYT DAR EAS ICH. Data collection: EAS ICH. Result interpretation: PKG LAT SYT DAR EAS ICH.

References

1. World Health Organization (2001) International Classification of Functioning, Disability and Health: ICF. Geneva: WHO.
2. World Health Organization. International classification of functioning, disability and health - version for children and youth (2007) Geneva: WHO Library Cataloguing-in-Publication Data.
3. Fava L, Muehlan H, Bullinger M (2009) Linking the DISABKIDS modules for health-related quality of life assessment with the International Classification of Functioning, Disability and Health (ICF). Disabil Rehabil 31: 1943–54.
4. Fayed N, Cieza A, Bickenbach J (2012) Illustrating child-specific linking issues using the Child Health Questionnaire. Am J Phys Med Rehabil 91(suppl): S189–S198.
5. Petersson C, Simeonsson RJ, Enskar K, Huus K (2013) Comparing children's self-report instruments for health-related quality of life using the International Classification of Functioning, Disability and Health for Children and Youth (ICF-CY). Health Qual Life Outcomes 11: 75.
6. Starfield B, Riley AW, Green BF, Ensminger ME, Ryan SA, et al. (1995) The adolescent child health and illness profile: A population-based measure of health. Med Care 33: 553–566.
7. Landgraf JM, Abetz L, Ware JE (1996) Child Health Questionnaire (CHQ): A user's manual. The Health Institute New England Medical: Boston, MA.
8. Ravens-Sieberer U, Gosch A, Rajmil L, Erhart M, Bruil J, et al. (2005) KIDSCREEN-52 quality-of-life measure for children and adolescents. Expert Rev Pharmacoecon Outcomes Res 5: 353–364.
9. Ravens-Sieberer U, Bullinger M (1998) Assessing health-related quality of life in chronically ill children with the german KINDL: First psychometric and content analytical results. Qual Life Res 7: 399–407.
10. Varni JW, Seid M, Rode CA (1999) The PedsQL™: Measurement model for the pediatric quality of life inventory. Med Care 37: 126–139.
11. Varni JW, Burwinkle TM, Lane MM (2005) Health-related quality of life measurement in pediatric clinical practice: An appraisal and precept for future research and application. Health Qual Life Outcomes 3: 34.

12. De Civita M, Regier D, Alamgir AH, Anis AH, Fitzgerald MJ, et al. (2005) Evaluating health-related quality-of-life studies in paediatric populations: Some conceptual, methodological and developmental considerations and recent applications. Pharmacoeconomics 23: 659–685.

13. Waters E, Davis E, Ronen GM, Rosenbaum P, Livingston M, et al. (2009) Quality of life instruments for children and adolescents with neurodisabilities: How to choose the appropriate instrument. Dev Med Child Neurol 51: 660–669.

14. Kenzik KM, Huang I-C, Tuli SY, Nackashi JA, Revicki D, et al. (2011) Head-to-head comparison of four legacy pediatric health-related quality of life instruments: a study on parent proxy-report. Qual Life Res (Suppl 1): 98.

15. Kenzik KM, Tuli SY, Revicki D, Shenkman EA, Huang I-C (2014) Comparison of 4 pediatric health-related quality of life instruments: a study on a Medicaid population. Med Dec Making 34(5): 590–602.

16. Hays RD, Morales LS, Reise SP (2000) Item response theory and health outcomes measurement in the 21st century. Med Care 38(9 Suppl): II28–42.

17. Hambleton RK, Jones RW (1993) Comparison of classical test theory and item response theory and their applications to test development. Educ Meas Issues Pract 12: 38–47.

18. Cieza A, Geyh S, Chatterji S, Kostanjsek N, Ustun B, et al. (2005) ICF linking rules: an update based on lessons learned. J Rehabil Med 37(4): 212–218.

19. The World Health Organization's (WHO) International Classification of Functioning, Disability and Health, Children and Youth (ICF-CY). ICF-CY Developmental Code Sets (2014). Available: http://www.icf-cydevelopmentalcodesets.com/. Accessed 2014 April 8.

20. Cieza A, Stucki G (2005) Content comparison of health-related quality of life (HRQOL) instruments based on the international classification of functioning, disability and health (ICF). Qual Life Res 14: 1225–1237.

21. Geyh S, Cieza A, Kollerits B, Grimby G, Stucki G (2007) Content comparison of health-related quality of life measures used in stroke based on the international classification of functioning, disability and health (ICF): a systematic review. Qual Life Res 16: 833–851.

22. Bendixen RM, Senesac C, Lott DJ, Vandenborne K (2012) Participation and quality of life in children with Duchenne muscular dystrophy using the International Classification of Functioning, Disability, and Health. Health Qual Life Outcomes 10: 43.

23. Krasuska M, Riva S, Fava L, von Mackensen S, Bullinger M (2012) Linking quality-of-life measures using the International Classification of Functioning, Disability and Health and the International Classification of Functioning, Disability and Health-Children and Youth Version in chronic health conditions: the example of young people with hemophilia. Am J Phys Med Rehabil 91(13 Suppl 1): S74–S83.

24. Riva S, Bullinger M, Amann E, von Mackensen S (2010) Content comparison of haemophilia specific patient-rated outcome measures with the International classification of functioning, disability and health (ICF, ICF-CY). Health Qual Life Outcomes 8: 139.

25. Lee AM (2011) Using the ICF-CY to organize characteristics of children's functioning. Disabil Rehabil 33(7): 605–16.

26. Riley AW (2004) Evidence that school-age children can self-report on their health. Ambul Pediatr 4: 371–376.

27. U.S. Department of Health and Human Services FDA Center for Drug Evaluation and Research; U.S. Department of Health and Human Services FDA Center for Biologics Evaluation and Research; U.S. Department of Health and Human Services FDA Center for Devices and Radiological Health (2006) Guidance for industry: patient-reported outcome measures: use in medical product development to support labeling claims: draft guidance. Health Qual Life Outcomes 4: 79.

28. Varni JW, Limbers CA, Burwinkle TM (2007) Parent proxy-report of their children's health-related quality of life: an analysis of 13,878 parents' reliability and validity across age subgroups using the PedsQL 4.0 Generic Core Scales. Health Qual Life Outcomes 5: 2.

29. Ingerski LM, Janicke DM, Silverstein JH (2007) Brief report: quality of life in overweight youth-the role of multiple informants and perceived social support. J Pediatr Psychol 32: 869–874.

30. Solans M, Pane S, Estrada M, Serra-Sutton V, Berra S, et al. (2008) Health-related quality of life measurement in children and adolescents: A systematic review of generic and disease-specific instruments. Value Health 11: 742–764.

31. Todd J, Armon C, Griggs A, Poole S, Berman S (2006) Increased rates of morbidity, mortality, and charges for hospitalized children with public or no health insurance as compared with children with private insurance in Colorado and the United States. Pediatrics 118: 577–585.

32. Bethell CD, Read D, Stein REK, Blumberg SJ, Wells N, et al. (2002) Identifying children with special health care needs: Development and evaluation of a short screening instrument. Ambul Pediatr 2: 38–48.

33. The KIDSCREEN Group Europe (2006) The KIDSCREEN questionnaires: Quality of life questionnaires for children and adolescents handbook. Pabst Science Publishers: Lengerich, Germany.

34. Brown TA (2006) Confirmatory factor analysis for applied research. The Guilford Press: New York: London.

35. Chen W-H, Thissen D (1997) Local dependence indices for item pairs using item response theory. J Educ Behav Stat 22: 265–289.

36. Maydeu-Olivares A, Joe H (2006) Limited information goodness-of-fit testing in multidimensional contingency tables. Psychometrika 71: 713–732.

37. Maydeu-Olivares A, Joe H (2005) Limited and full information estimation and testing in 2nd contingency tables: A unified framework. J Am Stat Assoc 100: 1009–1020.

38. Cohen J (1988) Statistical power analysis for the behavioral sciences. L. Erlbaum Associates: Hillsdale, NJ.

39. Jöreskog K, Sörbom D (1993) LISREL 8. Lincolnwood, Il: Scientific Software International, Inc.

40. Cai L, du Toit SHC, Thissen D (2011) IRTPRO: Computer software. Chicago: SSI International.

41. SAS Institute (2004) SAS users guide, version 9.1. Cary, NC; SAS institute, Inc.

42. Huang I-C, Shenkman EA, Leite W, Knapp CA, Thompson LA, et al. (2009) Agreement was not found in adolescent's quality of life rated by parents and adolescents. J Clin Epidemiol 62 (3): 337–346.

43. Theunissen NC, Vogel TG, Koopman HM, Verrips GH, Zwinderman KA, et al. (1998) The proxy problem: child report versus parent report in health related quality of life measure. Qual Life Res 7: 387–397.

44. Huang I-C, Leite WL, Shearer P, Seid M, Revicki DA, et al. (2011) Differential item functioning in quality of life measure between children with and without special health-care needs. Value Health 14 (6): 872–83.

45. Rosenbaum P, Stewart D (2004) The World Health Organization International Classification of Functioning, Disability, and Health: A model to guide clinical thinking, practice and research in the field of cerebral palsy. Seminars Ped Neurology 11: 5–10.

46. Valderas JM, Alonso J (2008) Patient reported outcome measures: a model-based classification system for research and clinical practice. Qual Life Res 17: 1125–1135.

47. Davis E, Nicolas C, Waters E, Cook K, Gibbs L, et al. (2007) Parent-proxy and child self-reported health-related quality of life: using qualitative methods to explain the discordance. Qual Life Res 16: 863–71.

48. Huang IC, Shenkman EA, Leite W, Knapp CA, Thompson LA, et al. (2009) Agreement was not found in adolescents' quality of life rated by parents and adolescents. J Clin Epidemiol 62(3): 337–46.

49. Huang IC, Thompson LA, Chi YY, Knapp CA, Revicki DA, et al. (2009) The linkage between pediatric quality of life and health conditions: establishing clinically meaningful cutoff scores for the PedsQL. Value Health 12(5): 773–81.

50. Huang IC, Wen PS, Revicki DA, Shenkman EA (2011) Quality of Life Measurement for Children with Life-Threatening Conditions: Limitations and a New Framework. Child Indic Res 4(1): 145–160.

5

Asthma Trajectories in Early Childhood: Identifying Modifiable Factors

Lidia Panico[1]*, **Beth Stuart**[2], **Mel Bartley**[3], **Yvonne Kelly**[3]

1 Institut National d'Etudes Démographiques, Paris, France, **2** Faculty of Medicine, University of Southampton, Southampton, United Kingdom, **3** International Centre for Lifecourse Studies, Department for Epidemiology and Population Health, University College London, London, United Kingdom

Abstract

Background: There are conflicting views as to whether childhood wheezing represents several discreet entities or a single but variable disease. Classification has centered on phenotypes often derived using subjective criteria, small samples, and/or with little data for young children. This is particularly problematic as asthmatic features appear to be entrenched by age 6/7. In this paper we aim to: identify longitudinal trajectories of wheeze and other atopic symptoms in early childhood; characterize the resulting trajectories by the socio-economic background of children; and identify potentially modifiable processes in infancy correlated with these trajectories.

Data and Methods: The Millennium Cohort Study is a large, representative birth cohort of British children born in 2000–2002. Our analytical sample includes 11,632 children with data on key variables (wheeze in the last year; ever hay-fever and/or eczema) reported by the main carers at age 3, 5 and 7 using a validated tool, the International Study of Asthma and Allergies in Childhood module. We employ longitudinal Latent Class Analysis, a clustering methodology which identifies classes underlying the observed population heterogeneity.

Results: Our model distinguished four latent trajectories: a trajectory with both low levels of wheeze and other atopic symptoms (54% of the sample); a trajectory with low levels of wheeze but high prevalence of other atopic symptoms (29%); a trajectory with high prevalence of both wheeze and other atopic symptoms (9%); and a trajectory with high levels of wheeze but low levels of other atopic symptoms (8%). These groups differed in terms of socio-economic markers and potential intervenable factors, including household damp and breastfeeding initiation.

Conclusion: Using data-driven techniques, we derived four trajectories of asthmatic symptoms in early childhood in a large, population based sample. These groups differ in terms of their socio-economic profiles. We identified correlated intervenable pathways in infancy, including household damp and breastfeeding initiation.

Editor: Kimon Divaris, UNC School of Dentistry, University of North Carolina-Chapel Hill, United States of America

Funding: The Millennium Cohort Study is funded by the Economic and Social Research Council (ESRC), UK. This work was partly funded by the ESRC International Centre for Lifecourse Studies in Society and Health (RES-596-28-0001). The funders had no role in study design, data collection and analysis, decision to publish, or preparation of the manuscript.

Competing Interests: The authors have declared that no competing interests exist.

* Email: lidia.panico@ined.fr

Introduction

In developed countries, both the incidence and the prevalence of asthma has increased dramatically in the last few decades [1,2]. Asthma and wheezing illnesses are common in childhood, with about 1 in 5 British children reporting recent wheezing symptoms [3,4] and a similar proportion reporting a doctor diagnosis of asthma [5]. Asthma is a heterogeneous disease with different clinical expressions and there is a conflicting view as to whether associated symptoms in childhood represent several discreet entities or a single but variable disease. Current classifications, such as those based on the Tucson Children's Respiratory Health Study of early transient, late onset and persistent wheeze [6], have become popular as a basis for academic research and are also increasingly used in clinical settings [7].

Studying asthma trajectories in childhood is important because different patterns of asthma expressed during childhood are important predictors of future outcomes [8], and because asthma trajectories appear to entrench early, possibly before age 6/7 [9]. Therefore, detecting early predictors of later childhood respiratory health may be important to identify interventions to potentially alter the course of the disease. However, little data is available for very young children, and therefore most studies investigating asthma phenotypes start with school aged children. Furthermore, many studies have been carried out in clinical rather than population-based samples and have relied on subjective classifications by researchers. This may explain why it has been difficult to replicate asthma groupings across studies, a key step to determine whether these groupings constitute "real" discrete phenotypes.

While studies have focused on describing clinical features, few studies have explicitly tested differences in socio-economic characteristics between asthma groupings. However, such analyses can help better understand the causation of asthma. Furthermore, when thinking about potential interventions, most studies have considered various aspects of clinical treatments, there has been less exploring potential intervenable factors in the child's environment, such as household damp and parental smoking, that could be of interest to public policy. Therefore, this paper aims to identify longitudinal trajectories of wheeze and other atopic symptoms, starting in early childhood, using a large, nationally representative sample of British children; we then describe the socio-economic profiles of these different groups of children, and we aim to identify potentially modifiable processes in infancy correlated with these different trajectories.

In this paper we propose to use a prospective birth cohort, the British Millennium Cohort Study (MCS), which follows over 19,000 children at regular intervals from 9 months after birth. As a large multi-purpose study, the MCS does not have the scope to make clinical measurements. However, the MCS does include a validated instrument to measure asthma and wheezing symptoms, the International Study of Asthma and Allergies in Childhood module, as well as detailed information on the socio-economic background and the home environment. Such variables are often measured out as "confounders" in asthma research. Therefore, this study does not aim to add to the already rich literature on the clinical features of asthma phenotypes. Instead, using a large, population-based sample, we aim to identify and characterize groups of children according to their reported symptoms in early childhood using data driven clustering methodologies, and, crucially, to identify early environmental and potentially intervenable influences on later respiratory health.

Context

The importance of early childhood for the genesis of asthma

Deficits in lung function, bronchial hyper-responsiveness, and structural airway remodeling are key features of asthma, and they appear to be established during the pre-school years in most individuals [9]. For example, the population-based Melbourne Asthma Study, which followed 401 children from age 7 in 1964 [8], found that no significant loss of pulmonary function occurred after ages 7–10, even in individuals with a severe disease at age 35. More recently, data from a New Zealand cohort of about 1000 children followed from age 9 also showed that lower levels of lung function in patients with persistent asthma were already evident by the start of the study with no further deterioration after that age [10]. The Tucson Children's Respiratory Study, a cohort of 1,246 newborns born between 1980 and 1984, showed that, for children with persistent wheezing symptoms, lung function deficits were not related to poorer lung function shortly after birth, but such deficits were already evident by age 6 and probably irreversible by age 9 [6]. This highlights the importance of the early years for the emergence and the entrenchment of life-long asthma trajectories.

Associations with socio-economic characteristics and intevenable factors

Although the association of lung function and other clinical outcomes with asthma phenotypes are well documented, the variation in environmental risk factors across asthma groups has been less explored. We know that there is a cross sectional association between socio-economic position and current asthma or lung function in adults [11–14], and a smaller body of work has

found similar associations in childhood [15–17]. How these associations vary across longitudinal measures of asthma has been less explicitly explored as such factors are often considered as confounders in that particular literature.

On the other hand, we know that there are strong associations between asthma and a number of potentially modifiable factors such as exposure to smoking. Such exposures are also often controlled out as "confounders" [18]. Exceptions include studies that have shown that the "transient early phenotype" (children who wheeze in early childhood whose symptoms resolve by school age) appears to be linked to prematurity, having siblings, attending group care settings, maternal smoking during pregnancy and post-natal exposure to smoke [19–23]. Daycare attendance appears to increase the risk of early wheeze but protect against older childhood wheezing [23,24].

Classifications derivation

Asthma classifications are useful both for research and to assist in clinical diagnosis. While the classifications derived in the literature have provided useful descriptions, they have been difficult to replicate across datasets, a key to establish whether the suggested categorizations are indeed true disease phenotypes. Currently, there is a wide range of concepts among clinicians [25] and no phenotype model appears to be more valid than others [26], with perhaps the exception of the "early transient wheeze" group which has been identified by different studies [27]. Some of these problems may exist because models do not allow multiple features or complex group definitions. Furthermore, the samples used (clinical or community populations) may be problematic. Small sample sizes may compound the problem.

Classifications are often subjective, using criteria suggested by clinicians or researchers, such as physiological characteristics (atopy, severity, age at onset, chronic airflow obstruction), triggers (exercise, allergens, irritants, viral infection) or their time course (transient, early onset, late onset, persistent). Classic categorizations derived in this manner include the Tucson Children's Respiratory Study's groupings. Martinez and colleagues [6] proposed a four category phenotype: non-wheezers, transient wheezers (at least one wheezing symptom before age 3, no wheezing at 6 years), late onset wheezers (no wheeze until age 3, wheezing at 6 years), and persistent wheeze (wheezed in the first 3 years of life, wheezing at age 6). The last group is sometime split into non-atopic persistent wheezers and atopic persistent wheezers [22,28]. Using data from the New Zealand cohort, Sears and colleagues (2003) proposed six longitudinal wheezing phenotypes: persistent wheeze, relapse (wheeze stopped then recurred), in remission, intermittent wheezing, transient wheezing, and wheezing never reported.

This subjective approach produces easily understood classifications, which can be easily applied in both research and clinical practice. However, rather than allow the researcher to subjectively determine the classifications, it is possible to use data-driven techniques to explore whether homogeneous subgroups exist within the study population. These techniques have recently been explored in the context of childhood asthma trajectories by two papers using a sample from the Avon Longitudinal Study of Parents and Children (ALSPAC), a community based sample of children born in Avon, a British county. Henderson and colleagues (2008) used a longitudinal LCA model applied to reports of wheezing from 5,760 children at several time points between ages 1 and 8 and identified 5 wheezing groups: never/infrequent wheeze (75%), intermediate onset wheeze (3%), persistent wheeze (3.5%), transient early wheeze (17%), and late onset wheeze (2%). The same model was tested on the Dutch PIAMA (Prevention and

Incidence of Asthma and Mite Allergy) study [29]. Based on a sample of about 2,800 children, similar classifications were derived. However, both studies were relatively small and not nationally representative. As far as we are aware, no study has been able to use a large, nationally representative sample to derive asthma trajectories.

Research Aims

We have three main research aims that structure our analyses: (1) to identify longitudinal trajectories of wheeze and atopic symptoms in early childhood using longitudinal latent class analysis in a large, nationally representative birth cohort; (2) to characterize the resulting trajectories according to the socio-economic background of children and their households at 9 months of age; and (3) to use multinomial regression techniques to identify modifiable processes at 9 months correlated with these trajectories, taking into account socio-economic profiles.

Data and Methods

The Millennium Cohort Study

The Millennium Cohort Study (MCS) is a nationally representative birth cohort study of infants born in the UK from September 2000 to January 2002. The survey design, recruitment process and fieldwork have been described in detail elsewhere [30]. Briefly, 18553 households agreed to participate in the initial survey, an overall response rate of 68%. Households were identified through the Department of Work and Pensions Child Benefit system, and selected on the basis of where the family was resident shortly after the time of birth. Uptake of Child Benefit is almost universal (98%). The sample has a probability design and is clustered at the electoral ward level, with disadvantaged residential areas and areas with a high proportion of ethnic minority population being over represented.

We use data from the first wave of data collection carried out when the child was about 9 months of age to characterize the socio-economic profiles of the households and identify potentially intervenable factors. For classification purposes, we use data from the second, third and fourth wave of interviews, carried out through home visits when the cohort member was aged approximately 3, 5 and 7 years, respectively. Data was collected through home interviews with the main carer, usually the mother. The overall sample size for wave 2 was 15 307, 15 246 at wave 3, and 14 043 at wave 4. This analysis is based on 11,632 cases with complete data on questions on recent wheeze, and ever eczema and ever hayfever at ages 3, 5 and 7.

Variables employed

At ages 3, 5 and 7, the ISAAC (International Study of Asthma and Allergies in Childhood) core questionnaire for asthma was included in the interview with the main carer. ISAAC is a widely used and validated instrument to measure childhood asthma and wheezing illnesses and includes questions on the occurrence of asthma and wheezing symptoms [31] (see Annex S1). For the latent class analysis, we use the question on recent wheeze (reported as whether the child wheezed in the last year) at ages 3, 5 and 7. The second key variable used is a proxy for atopy, namely other atopic symptoms. Studies often ignore the distinction between atopic and non-atopic asthma even though these phenotypes are likely to have distinct causal mechanisms [32]. As atopy cannot be measured objectively in the MCS, we rely on two questions on other atopic symptoms (hayfever and eczema), as reported by the parent. Questions asked to the main carer at ages

3, 5 and 7 on whether the child ever had eczema and whether the child ever had hay fever, adapted from the ISAAC module, are used. In this proxy therefore atopic simply means the absence of eczema and/or hay fever, and may include some asymptomatic children who are atopic (by skin test or IgE levels). Cases with complete information at all waves on these key variables were retained (n = 11,632).

A number of markers for socio-economic background were considered. We used a forward selection exercise, a data-driven model building approach, to reduce the number of variables included in the model. Under this approach, variables are added to the model one at a time and tested for inclusion. The most significant variables are retained in the model, as long as its p-value is below a pre-set level. It is customary to set p-values above the conventional .05 level because of the exploratory nature of this method. The exercise begins with the variable that appears to be most significant in initial analyses, and continue adding variables until none of remaining variables are "significant" when added to the model. Following this exercise, we retained three socio-economic variables which were significant at the level p = 0.20: parental income, parental education, and a persistent poverty indicator. This allowed us to keep the model relatively simple while maximising its predictive power.

The first two variables are based on the first interview with the main carer, carried out when the child was about 9 months old. Annual parental income is modelled as a log-transformed measure; and parental education is operationalised by the highest educational qualification for either resident parents (no educational qualifications; only overseas qualifications; qualifications equivalent to an NVQ1, NVQ2, NVQ3, NVQ4 and NVQ5). The National Vocational Qualifications (NVQs) is a system of competence-based education and training that aims to recognize individual levels of competence. The framework indicates the "equivalence" of both vocational and academic qualifications, and reflects the level of skills acquired. As an indicator, an NVQ5 is equivalent to a graduate degree; an NVQ3 is equivalent to two A-levels, a high-school qualification. A persistent poverty indicator, which captures the frequency the household was classed as poor over the 4 waves of data collection (from 9 months to 7 years of age), was calculated using data from those waves. Households were classed as poor if their equivalised income was 60% below the mean income for that wave. Equivalised income takes into account household composition and was calculated using the McClements equivalence scale [33].

To explore potentially intervenable processes, a number of variables were selected, measured at the 9 month interview. All variables are binary (yes/no) unless otherwise indicated. Over-crowding was defined as having more than one individual per room, excluding the bathroom and kitchen; damp in the home is measured on a five point scale ranging from no problems with damp to severe damp problems (modelled as a continuous variable); exposure to tobacco smoke was defined as whether either resident parental figure smokes; any smoking during pregnancy by the mother is also included; breastfeeding initiation, irrespective of duration, was included. A number of potential confounders linked to an increased risk of asthma and wheezing symptoms were included in the analytical models: the child's gender; whether the child weighed less than 2500 grams at birth; and the number of co-resident siblings in infancy (modelled as a continuous variable).

Statistical analysis

For classification purposes, we use longitudinal Latent Class Analysis (LLCA), a data driven approach to derive categories.

Using the sequences of responses at each wave for each child, LLCA identifies groups that share similar longitudinal response patterns. It assumes that the population is composed of subsets (latent classes), each having distinctive distributions of the key variables [34]. The LLCA model estimates two sets of parameters: the conditional response probabilities and the latent class prevalences. The conditional response probabilities give the probability of observing a particular response pattern within the group. So, for example, the probability that an individual in latent class 1 will respond "Yes" at age 3 to "Has your child wheezed in the last year?". The latent class prevalence gives the proportion of children in each latent class.

In order to choose the appropriate number of latent classes, the model was repeatedly fitted with the number of latent classes increasing step-wise from 1 to 6. The calculations were carried out in LEM, a statistical package designed specifically for categorical data analysis, including latent class models, with parameters estimated using maximum likelihood criterion, computed using the Expectation-maximization (EM) algorithm [35]. There is no single statistical test to determine the correct number of latent classes [36]. Selecting the best model requires a consideration both of the substantive interpretation of the output and the statistical measures of model fit. We assessed model fit using a range of measures: the Bayesian Information Criteria (BIC), the dissimilarity index, the likelihood ratio chi-squared test statistic, and the percentage of classification error based on modal assignment [37,38].

The model allocates individuals to the latent class for which they have the highest probability, called modal allocation. Sensitivity analyses were carried out using a random allocation, which classified differently cases were individuals have similar probabilities of belonging to two different classes. These analyses confirmed the substantive findings presented below.

To evaluate the distribution of the latent classes with respect to key covariates we use multinomial logistic regression carried out in Stata 11 [39]. These models produce Relative Risk Ratios (RRRs) which estimate the relative risk of a child belonging to a given class compared to the reference class, which is always the largest group. We first assessed the relative importance of each intervenable factor (household damp, breastfeeding initiation, parental smoke, and overcrowding) individually, taking into account a number of socio-economic markers and confounding factors. We then test a full model, which includes all intervenable factors alongside the full set of socio-economic and control variables. Survey weights are applied to all cross tabulations and regression analyses. This allows correcting for cohort members having unequal probabilities of selection in the study due to the stratified and clustered sample design, as well as to take account of attrition between data collection waves and unit non-response [40,41].

Results

Descriptive sample characteristics

Weighted analyses showed that, by age 7, 15.1% of children reported ever having had asthma and 25.8% had ever wheezed. 42.9% reported ever having eczema or hay fever (see Table 1). Reports of recent wheeze were higher in early childhood (at age 3, 18.5% of children had wheezed in the previous 12 months) than in the primary school years (at age 7, 11.4% of children reported wheezing in the previous 12 months). The rest of the results section is structured around the three main aims of this paper: (1) to identify longitudinal latent trajectories of wheeze and other atopic symptoms; (2) to characterize the resulting trajectories by a number of household socio-economic variables measured in infancy; and (3) to identify modifiable processes in infancy which may be correlated with these trajectories, taking into account differing socio-economic profiles.

Aim 1: Latent trajectories identification

For this aim, we use our key variables (wheeze, and the atopy proxy, namely other atopic symptoms) to derive latent trajectories of symptoms. We tested a number of models with different number of classes, Table 2 gives the measures of model fit that we used to select the solution with the optimal number of classes. The four class solution was chosen as the best fit as it had the lowest BIC value, a dissimilarity index below 0.05, a significant p-value on the chi-squared LRT and an acceptable level of potential classification error (9% of children).

Table 3 shows the categorizations produced by the four class model. The four identified latent trajectories of wheeze and other atopic symptoms from age 3 to 7 emerging from this model are also shown on Figures 1 and 2. They can be summarized as follows:

- Trajectory 1: a trajectory with both low levels of wheeze and other atopic symptoms (54% of children): this category is characterized by low levels of all symptoms. Children in this group who do wheeze are least likely to report severe or limiting symptoms (results available upon request).

- Trajectory 2: a trajectory with low levels of wheeze and high prevalence of other atopic symptoms (29% of children): this category has low levels of wheeze at all ages, however this group is characterized by high levels of eczema and/or hayfever, with about 85% of the sample reporting eczema or hay fever by age 7.

- Trajectory 3: a trajectory with a high prevalence of both wheeze and other atopic symptoms (9% of children): the "classic" asthmatic group, this category has the highest levels of wheeze (81% of the sample reported recent wheeze at age 5) and the highest proportion of children reporting eczema and/or hayfever, peaking at about 93% by age 7. Children in this group report the most severe wheezing symptoms and the most limitations due to wheeze.

- Trajectory 4: a trajectory with high levels of wheeze but low levels of other atopic symptoms (8% of children): this group had relatively high levels of wheeze, although both overall levels and severity of symptoms are below that of trajectory 3. Only about 20% of the sample reported eczema or hay fever by age 7 in this group.

Aim 2: The socio-economic characteristics of the latent trajectories of wheeze and other atopic symptoms

Next, we describe the socio-economic characteristics of the four identified latent trajectories. Table 4 shows the characteristics of the groups in terms of their socio-economic profiles at the first wave of data available, when the children were aged about 9 months. Across a number of indicators, including parental income and education, trajectory 2 (low wheeze, high levels of other atopic symptoms) appears to be the most advantaged group, slightly more so than largest group, trajectory 1 (both low wheeze and other atopic symptoms). Trajectory 4 (high wheeze, low levels of other atopic symptoms) appears to be disproportionately disadvantaged. These differences extend to other early markers of well-being (see the second panel of Table 4): trajectory 2 was on average least likely to be born at a low birthweight, while trajectory 4 appeared to have the highest risk of being low weight at birth. Interestingly,

Table 1. Prevalence of asthma and wheezing symptoms at ages 3, 5 & 7.

	Age 3 %	Age 5 %	Age 7 %
Ever had asthma	11.5	13.7	15.1
Ever had wheeze	29.3	28.4	25.8
Wheezed in last year	18.5	15.0	11.4
Ever had eczema and/or hay fever	37.8	40.1	42.9
Total sample size	11,632		

Weighted percentages.

if we compare each group with high levels of wheeze with its low-wheeze counterpart (i.e. trajectory 2 versus trajectory 3), it appears that the most advantaged of the two groups have the lower levels of wheeze.

The third panel of Table 4 shows that when looking at characteristics normally associated with atopy such as gender and sibship size, the groups perform as expected: the two groups reporting high levels of eczema and/or hayfever are more likely to include boys than the groups with low levels of these symptoms, and are more likely not to have older siblings. There was however no clear associations with being exposed to group care at a young age.

Aim 3: Identifying intervenable factors

The final phase of analyses consisted of identifying potentially intervenable predictors, taking account of the differing socio-economic profiles and a number of control factors such as sex and sibship size. Table 5 shows the multinomial logistic regressions for the relative risk of being in a given trajectory compared to being in the largest trajectory. The results suggest that, once their more deprived socio-economic background is accounted for, the children in trajectory 4 were more likely to have been exposed to household damp at 9 months of age, and were less likely to have been breastfed. In the fully adjusted model, when all potentially intervenable factors are included, breastfeeding initiation and household damp remain significant. Both groups reporting high levels of eczema and/or hayfever (trajectories 2 and 3) were more likely to be exposed to household damp at 9 months in the fully adjusted model.

Discussion

In this work, we use parental reports of wheeze, eczema and hayfever at age 3, 5 and 7 from a large birth cohort representative of British children born in 2000–2001. We identify four latent trajectories of symptoms, and quantified their associations with a number of factors in infancy that could form a basis for intervention. We employed longitudinal Latent Class Analysis to derive categories in a data-driven manner based on the heterogeneity of our sample.

Our model distinguished four classes of children: (1) a trajectory with both low levels of wheeze and other atopic symptoms, into which over half our population is classed; (2) a trajectory with low levels of wheeze and the highest prevalence of other atopic symptoms, which included nearly a third of the population; (3) a trajectory with the highest prevalence of wheeze, and higher than average levels of other atopic symptoms, which comprised 9% of our sample; and (4) a trajectory with high levels of wheeze but low levels of other atopic symptoms, which included 8% of our population.

While a non-atopic high-wheeze group was identified in previous literature [42,43], our identified trajectories differ from previously reported patterns of early childhood wheezing. Notably, they contrast with previous classifications that focus on early versus late onset of wheezing symptoms as one of the most important distinction. This dichotomy did not appear in our findings. Our results also challenge the current model that early wheezing is normally not associated with atopy, while late wheeze is associated with atopic symptoms. Such categorizations did not emerge from our data.

The main aim of this paper was to characterize the resulting latent trajectories according to the child's socio-economic back-

Table 2. Measures of model fit, Longitudinal Latent Class model of wheeze and other atopic symptoms.

Number of latent classes	BIC	Dissimilarity index	Likelihood ratio chi-squared test statistic	Percentage classification error based on modal class assignment
1	76455.00	0.4476	N/A	N/A
2	65549.56	0.1459	<0.0001	3.68%
3	63768.25	0.0644	<0.0001	5.86%
4	63029.01	0.0158	<0.0001	9.02%
5	63064.27	0.0138	<0.0001	19.60%
6	63118.96	0.0106	0.1462	59.42%

Table 3. Conditional response probabilities for the key model variables (recent wheeze, and other atopic symptoms) by latent trajectories (1).

	Trajectory 1	Trajectory 2	Trajectory 3	Trajectory 4
Recent wheeze, age 3	0.0913	0.1358	0.6279	0.5190
Recent wheeze, age 5	0.0195	0.0385	0.8088	0.6968
Recent wheeze, age 7	0.0176	0.0583	0.6231	0.3958
Ever eczema and/or hayfever, age 3	0.0868	0.7611	0.8427	0.1432
Ever eczema and/or hayfever, age 5	0.0461	0.8821	0.9480	0.1592
Ever eczema and/or hayfever, age 7	0.0949	0.8564	0.9356	0.1986
% of total sample (sample size)	54% (6,275)	29% (3,393)	9% (1,043)	8% (921)

(1) Trajectory 1: low levels of wheeze and low levels of other atopic symptoms; Trajectory 2: low levels of wheeze and high prevalence of other atopic symptoms; Trajectory 3: high levels of wheeze and high levels of other atopic symptoms; Trajectory 4: high levels of wheeze and low levels of other atopic symptoms.

ground and to identify potentially intervenable factors in children's early environment. We found that the four groups were different in terms of a number of socio-economic markers. The group with low levels of wheeze but the highest levels of eczema and/or hayfever appeared to be the most advantaged in terms of parental incomes and educational qualifications, showing a slightly more advantaged profile than all other groups. The two groups with high levels of wheeze were less advantaged. The group with high levels of wheeze but low levels of other atopic symptoms appeared to be the most disadvantaged, showing the lowest incomes and fewest parental educational qualifications. Taking into account these differing socio-economic backgrounds, we looked at a number of potential modifiable factors. In fully adjusted models, the two groups with high levels of eczema and/or hayfever were more likely to have lived in damp homes in infancy than the largest group. The trajectory reporting high levels of wheeze but low levels of other atopic symptoms appeared to be less likely to have been breastfed and more likely to be living in damp homes at 9 months of age, even when taking account of its already disadvantaged socio-economic profile.

Taussig and colleagues (2003) suggested that non-atopic wheezers are probably more likely to develop acute airway obstruction in relation to viral infection because they have an alteration in the control of airway tone that determines this increased risk. Our results could lend support to this hypothesis: trajectory 4 (high wheeze, low levels of other atopic symptoms) appeared to be a disadvantaged group exposed to a number of potential risk factors in infancy, including living in damp homes and not being breastfed. Furthermore, Taussig et al. (2003) concluded that perhaps, for children with atopic symptoms, early (before age 3) allergic sensitization may be an important risk factor for more severe disease. In our results, the risk of living in a damp home at 9 months (which may be linked to allergic sensitization through inhaled mould spores) was highest in two groups with high levels of eczema and/or hayfever.

Strengths and limitations

The present work enjoys a number of characteristics which increase the robustness of our results. Historically, studies have attempted to classify asthma in an attempt to categorize a complex

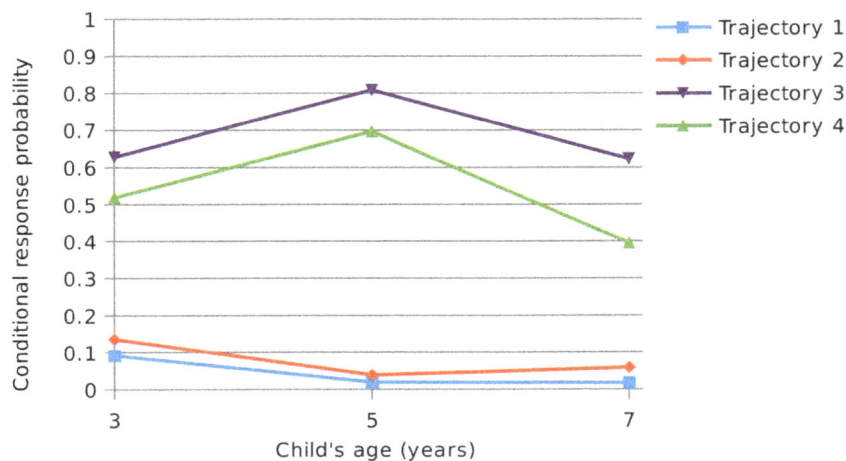

Figure 1. Conditional response probabilities of reporting wheeze in the last 12 months, ages 3 to 7. Trajectory 1: low levels of wheeze and low levels of other atopic symptoms; Trajectory 2: low levels of wheeze and high prevalence of other atopic symptoms; Trajectory 3: high levels of wheeze and high levels of other atopic symptoms; Trajectory 4 high levels of wheeze and low levels of other atopic symptoms.

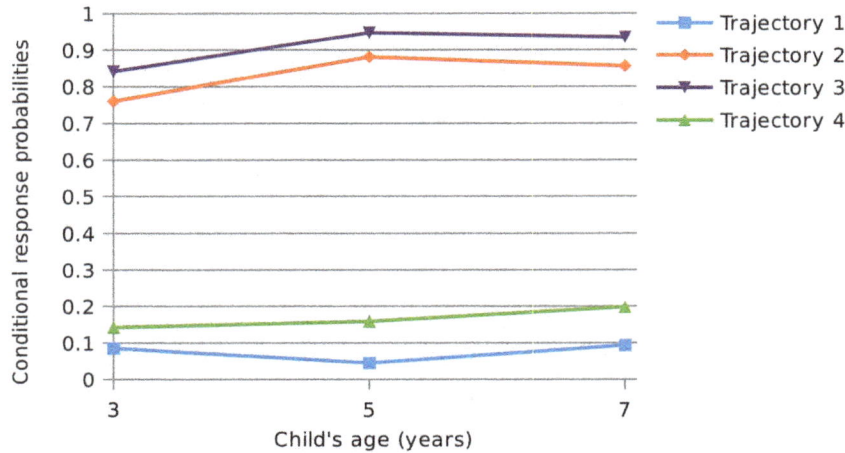

Figure 2. Conditional response probabilities of reporting ever eczema and/or ever hayfever, ages 3 to 7. Trajectory 1: low levels of wheeze and low levels of other atopic symptoms; Trajectory 2: low levels of wheeze and high prevalence of other atopic symptoms; Trajectory 3: high levels of wheeze and high levels of other atopic symptoms; Trajectory 4 high levels of wheeze and low levels of other atopic symptoms.

disease into discrete, clinically useful subsets. In this study, groupings were derived from the observed population heterogeneity using a clustering technique, longitudinal LCA, which requires a relatively small number of subjective choices. LCA clustering is not rigid as each individual is assigned different probabilities of belonging to various classes. This soft form of classification is similar to clinical situations, where patients often present symptoms common to more than one condition. In the present study, the majority of children could be clearly assigned to one class, but for a minority (9%), there remained some ambiguity about the class they were assigned to. Sensitivity analyses using a different classification for these ambiguous cases indicate that the results presented here are robust to this issue.

The second major strength comes from our use of a large, nationally representative and prospective birth cohort study. Our analytical sample included 11,652 children; as a result, each identified trajectory was based on a sample of at least 1,000 children. A second strength of this data is that children are observed from early ages, when the development of lung function, lung responsiveness and atopy is likely to occur. Third, the rich data available in the Millennium Cohort Study means that, rather than just identify trajectories of asthma, we can also attempt to describe them in terms of their socio-economic background, and find early predictors of these trajectories. Significantly, we use data on potentially modifiable factors collected when the child was 9 months old, before diagnoses and treatments of asthma (and, for many children, before even the onset of symptoms) has begun. Therefore, parental report of, for example, problems with damp in the home, might be less likely to be coloured by the child's later symptoms and diagnosis. And we identify predictors when policy intervention could have most impact, as symptoms are just beginning to develop and before the disease is fully entrenched.

Given the nature of the MCS, which tracks a very large number of children and is a multi-disciplinary study, lung function or objective measures of atopy (such as measured by skin prick test or IgE) were not available. Therefore, all outcomes were self-reported, although based on a validated tool. Self-report of

symptoms by parents is a widely accepted method in epidemiological studies and reliably reflects the incidence of asthmatic symptoms in young children; furthermore, in preschool children a diagnosis of asthma is often based on symptoms rather clinical measurements. Objective tests, including spirometry or bronchial hyperresponsiveness, are difficult to perform in young children, and especially so within a large cohort of a general population. Furthermore, data on wheeze before 3 years of age was not available.

Wheeze is however a difficult symptom for parents to describe and report. Studies show that parents can have very different perceptions of what wheeze sounds like [44]. While parental-reported wheezing in early life is imprecise [45] and correlates poorly with objective observations [46], previous work found strong correlations between wheezing classifications as derived by parent-reports of wheeze and physician diagnosed asthma at about 7 years [47]. Furthermore, the data used here was collected using the ISAAC module, a widely used and validated questionnaire.

Other atopic symptoms used in our study, such as eczema and hayfever, are also based on parental report. Although symptoms such as eczema have been used as proxy for atopy in previous studies of young children [48,49], not all children presenting these symptoms are atopic, and some asymptomatic children may be atopic (as identified for example by a skin test or IgE levels). Therefore, some degree of outcome misclassification may be present. However, the prevalence of symptoms in this population-based study was comparable with prevalence rates in equivalent British populations, and we observed consistent associations of our proxy for atopic symptoms with a number of classic variables associated with atopy, such as the child's sex, and the number of older siblings living in the household.

A further limitation to consider is that, as most longitudinal studies, loss to follow-up was greater in children from more socially deprived backgrounds. Given known associations of social deprivation with early childhood wheezing (Baker and Henderson, 1999), it is likely that children excluded because of missing data had higher rates of wheezing than those included in our analyses.

Table 4. Socio-economic variables and exposure variables, by latent trajectories (1).

		Trajectory 1	Trajectory 2	Trajectory 3	Trajectory 4
Socio-economic variables					
Parental income, 9 months	Don't know	6.1	6.2	6.6	5.8
	Under 10 400 pounds	14.7	13.1	19.4	20.0
	10 400–20 800	27.8	28.5	30.4	32.4
	20 800–31 200	24.5	22.7	21.2	18.0
	31 200–52 000	19.1	20.8	16.3	18.3
	52 000 and over	7.7	8.6	6.1	5.5
	p-value	<0.001			
	Mean income, pounds	26 608	27 792	24 205	23 570
Highest parental education, 9 months	None of these	5.5	3.7	5.1	8.3
	Overseas quals only	1.2	1.0	1.7	1.7
	NVQ 1	4.3	3.8	5.0	7.5
	NVQ 2	22.8	21.5	24.9	23.9
	NVQ 3	16.7	15.6	14.3	17.3
	NVQ 4	41.3	45.7	42.1	35.1
	NVQ 5	8.2	8.7	7.0	6.3
	p-value	<0.001			
Persistent poverty indicator, 9 months to 7 years	Never poor	64.7	67.3	58.4	54.7
	Poor at one wave	12.9	14.2	13.2	16.2
	Poor at two waves	7.0	6.6	8.7	9.3
	Poor at three waves	7.1	5.3	9.6	8.7
	Always poor	8.3	6.6	10.0	11.0
	p-value	<0.001			
Exposures					
Overcrowding	% overcrowded home	10.9	7.5	9.6	12.4
Either parent smokes	% parental smoke	41.6	39.9	44.3	48.8
Damp home	Yes	11.8	14.7	14.7	16.1
Breastfeeding initiated	Yes	71.1	74.2	69.7	64.2
Confounders					
Gender	Male	48.1	49.7	62.1	56.3
	p-value	<0.001			
Low birthweight	% low birthweight	6.7	5.0	7.7	9.8
	p-value	0.002			
Formal group care	% formal group care	6.5	6.6	6.9	4.7
	p-value	0.0501			

Weighted percentages.
(1) Trajectory 1: low levels of wheeze and low levels of other atopic symptoms; Trajectory 2: low levels of wheeze and high prevalence of other atopic symptoms; Trajectory 3: high levels of wheeze and high levels of other atopic symptoms; Trajectory 4: high levels of wheeze and low levels of other atopic symptoms.

As more symptomatic children may not have been included in our analytical sample, it is likely that our estimates are an under representations of the true effects.

Finally, our analytical technique, longitudinal LCA, shares the limitations of other clustering techniques. First, even though researchers use a number of statistical fit criteria as a guide, the problem of determining the number of classes has not been completely resolved. Second, some a priori decisions have to be made, notably about which variables to include in the model. This does introduce a degree of subjectivity to the model. Third, as the term "latent class" implies, these are not directly observed clusters but groups constructed on the basis of the pattern of responses over a fixed number of observation periods. These methods therefore do not predict the natural history of symptoms in an individual, nor produce overall population prevalences, instead trajectories are derived by assigning each child a probability of membership based on their overall symptom history.

Table 5. Multinomial logistic regression of intervenable factors by latent trajectories (1).

	Model 1	Model 2	Model 3	Model 4	Model 5	Model 6
	RRR	RRR	RRR	RRR	RRR	RRR
Trajectory 1	— reference class —					
Trajectory 2						
Breastfeeding initiation	0.94					0.92
Parental smoke, 9 months		0.98				0.99
Smoke during pregnancy			0.96			0.95
Damp, 9 months				1.31*		1.35*
Overcrowd, 9 months					0.95	.94
Log income, 9 months	.86	.86*	.87	.87	.86*	.89
No educational quals	.68	.68	.70	.69	.68	.70
Overseas ed quals only	.91	.91	.92	.89	.91	.91
NVQ 1	.84	.85	.84	.83	.85	.82
NVQ 2	.76*	.76*	.76	.75*	.76*	.75*
NVQ 4	1.11	1.10	1.10	1.10	1.10	1.11
NVQ 5	1.00	0.99	0.98	0.99	1.00	0.98
Poor at one wave	1.10	1.11	1.13	1.10	1.10	1.12
Poor at two waves	1.31	1.33	1.31	1.38	1.33	1.27
Poor at three waves	1.52*	1.53*	1.58*	1.51*	1.53*	1.57*
Always poor	1.35	1.37	1.43	1.32	1.37	1.40
Gender	.54***	.54***	.54***	.54***	.54***	.54***
Low birth weight	.94	.94	.94	.93	.94	.93
Co-resident siblings	.84**	.84**	.84**	.84**	.84**	.84**
Trajectory 3						
Breastfeeding initiation	1.04					1.03
Parental smoke, 9 months		0.98				1.02
Smoke during pregnancy			0.91			.89
Damp, 9 months				1.25*		1.26*
Overcrowd, 9 months					0.91	.88
Income, 9 months	0.97	0.97	0.97	0.98	0.97	0.98
No educational quals	.88	.87	.88	.87	0.87	.88
Overseas ed quals only	.82	.82	.86	.82	0.82	.82
NVQ 1	1.07	1.06	1.06	1.06	1.07	1.06
NVQ 2	0.91	0.92	0.90	0.92	0.92	0.90
NVQ 4	1.10	1.10	1.09	1.10	1.10	1.08
NVQ 5	0.99	1.00	0.99	1.01	1.01	0.98
Poor at one wave	1.10	1.11	1.13	1.10	1.11	1.13
Poor at two waves	.96	.96	.98	.94	.96	.96
Poor at three waves	.79	.80	.82	.78	.80	.81
Always poor	.88	.88	.92	.86	.89	.91
Gender	.96	.96	.96	.96	.96	.96
Low birth weight	1.33*	1.33*	1.31*	1.33*	1.33*	1.30*
Co-resident siblings	.84***	.84***	.84***	.84***	.85***	.85***
Trajectory 4						
Breastfeeding initiation	.79*					.78*
Parental smoke, 9 months		1.17				1.10
Smoke during pregnancy			1.22			1.36
Damp, 9 months				1.38*		1.36*
Overcrowd, 9 months					1.34	1.32
Income, 9 months	.90	.89	.90	.90	.89	.92
No educational quals	1.33	1.38	1.33	1.38	1.37	1.27

Table 5. Cont.

	Model 1	Model 2	Model 3	Model 4	Model 5	Model 6
	RRR	RRR	RRR	RRR	RRR	RRR
Overseas ed quals only	1.18	1.16	0.95	1.13	1.13	0.94
NVQ 1	1.58*	1.62*	1.56*	1.60*	1.62*	1.49*
NVQ 2	1.02	1.02	1.02	1.00	1.01	1.03
NVQ 4	.93	.91	.92	.89	0.89	.97
NVQ 5	.96	.94	.94	.90	0.92	1.02
Poor at one wave	1.26	1.26	1.28	1.26	1.26	1.26
Poor at two waves	1.24	1.23	1.22	1.21	1.24	1.14
Poor at three waves	1.02	1.00	0.99	1.01	1.01	0.96
Always poor	1.01	0.99	0.97	0.99	0.98	0.90
Gender	.74**	.74**	.77**	.75**	.75**	.75**
Low birth weight	.75	.76	.73	.75	.76	.74
Co-resident siblings	1.03	1.05	1.04	1.04	1.02	1.00

Weighted Relative Risk Ratios.
*** p<0,001** p <0,01 *p<0,05.
(1) Trajectory 1: low levels of wheeze and low levels of other atopic symptoms; Trajectory 2: low levels of wheeze and high prevalence of other atopic symptoms; Trajectory 3: high levels of wheeze and high levels of other atopic symptoms; Trajectory 4: high levels of wheeze and low levels of other atopic symptoms.

Conclusions

In summary, we use a nationally-representative sample of young British children with longitudinal, prospective information on wheeze and other atopic symptoms and apply latent class techniques to derive trajectories of symptoms over the first seven years of life in a relatively objective and data-driven manner. Four latent trajectories of wheeze and atopy symptoms measured at age 3, 5 and 7 were derived. The rich data set used allowed characterization of the socio-economic profiles of these groups, and studying the association between these latent trajectories to a number of potentially intervenable factors in infancy, before trajectories have entrenched. Exposure to household damp at 9 months, and for a particularly socio-economically disadvantaged group of children with high levels of wheeze, breastfeeding initiation, appeared to be potentially important modifiable factors to focus on.

Acknowledgments

We thank the Millennium Cohort Study families for their time and cooperation, as well as the MCS team at the Institute of Education. We are grateful to two anonymous reviewers for their helpful comments, and to Dr John Armitage for expert technical assistance.

Author Contributions

Analyzed the data: LP BS. Wrote the paper: LP BS. Conceived and designed analyses: LP BS MB YK.

References

1. Kuehni CE, Davis A, Brooke AM, Silverman M (2001) Are all wheezing disorders in very young (preschool) children increasing in prevalence? The Lancet 357: 1821–1825.
2. Burr ML, Wat D, Evans C, Dunstan FD, Doull IJ (2006) Asthma prevalence in 1973, 1988 and 2003. Thorax 61: 296–299.
3. Pearce N, Aït-Khaled N, Beasley R, Mallol J, Keil U, et al. (2007) Worldwide trends in the prevalence of asthma symptoms: phase III of the International Study of Asthma and Allergies in Childhood (ISAAC). Thorax 62: 758–766.
4. Panico L, Bartley M, Marmot M, Nazroo JY, Sacker A, et al. (2007) Ethnic variation in childhood asthma and wheezing illnesses: findings from the Millennium Cohort Study. International journal of epidemiology 36: 1093–1102.
5. Fuller E (2006) Children's health. Health Survey for England 2004: The health of minority ethnic groups. Leeds: The Information Centre.
6. Martinez FD, Wright AL, Taussig LM, Holberg CJ, Halonen M, et al. (1995) Asthma and wheezing in the first six years of life. New England Journal of Medicine 332: 133–138.
7. Pedersen SE, Hurd SS, Lemanske Jr RF, Becker A, Zar HJ, et al. (2011) Global strategy for the diagnosis and management of asthma in children 5 years and younger. Pediatric pulmonology 46: 1–17.
8. Oswald H, Phelan PD, Lanigan A, Hibbert M, Carlin JB, et al. (1998) Childhood asthma and lung function in mid-adult life. Pediatric pulmonology 23: 14–20.
9. Martinez FD (2009) The origins of asthma and chronic obstructive pulmonary disease in early life. Proceedings of the American Thoracic Society 6: 272–277.
10. Sears MR, Greene JM, Willan AR, Wiecek EM, Taylor DR, et al. (2003) A longitudinal, population-based, cohort study of childhood asthma followed to adulthood. New England Journal of Medicine 349: 1414–1422.
11. Shiue I (2013) Associated social factors of prevalent asthma in adults and the very old in the UK. Allergy 68: 392–396.
12. Hedlund U, Eriksson K, Rönmark E (2006) Socio-economic status is related to incidence of asthma and respiratory symptoms in adults. European Respiratory Journal 28: 303–410.
13. Hegewald MJ, Crapo RO (2007) Socioeconomic status and lung function. CHEST Journal 132: 1608–1614.
14. Kanervisto M, Vasankari T, Laitinen T, Heliövaara M, Jousilahti P, et al. (2011) Low socioeconomic status is associated with chronic obstructive airway diseases. Respiratory medicine 105: 1140–1146.
15. Almqvist C, Pershagen G, Wickman M (2005) Low socioeconomic status as a risk factor for asthma, rhinitis and sensitization at 4 years in a birth cohort. Clinical & Experimental Allergy 35: 612–618.
16. Kozyrskyj AL, Kendall GE, Jacoby P, Sly PD, Zubrick SR (2010) Association between socioeconomic status and the development of asthma: analyses of income trajectories. American journal of public health 100: 540.
17. Williams DR, Sternthal M, Wright RJ (2009) Social determinants: taking the social context of asthma seriously. Pediatrics 123: S174–S184.

18. Moore WC, Meyers DA, Wenzel SE, Teague WG, Li H, et al. (2010) Identification of asthma phenotypes using cluster analysis in the Severe Asthma Research Program. American journal of respiratory and critical care medicine 181: 315–323.

19. Ball TM, Castro-Rodriguez JA, Griffith KA, Holberg CJ, Martinez FD, et al. (2000) Siblings, day-care attendance, and the risk of asthma and wheezing during childhood. New England Journal of Medicine 343: 538–543.

20. Søyseth V, Kongerud J, Boe J (1995) Postnatal maternal smoking increases the prevalence of asthma but not of bronchial hyperresponsiveness or atopy in their children. CHEST Journal 107: 389–394.

21. Speer C, Silverman M (1998) Issues relating to children born prematurely. The European respiratory journal Supplement 27: 13s.

22. Stein RT, Holberg CJ, Sherrill D, Wright AL, Morgan WJ, et al. (1999) Influence of Parental Smoking on Respiratory Symptoms during the First Decade of Life The Tucson Children's Respiratory Study. American journal of epidemiology 149: 1030–1037.

23. Midodzi WK, Rowe BH, Majaesic CM, Saunders LD, Senthilselvan A (2008) Predictors for wheezing phenotypes in the first decade of life. Respirology 13: 537–545.

24. Rusconi F, Galassi C, Bellasio M, Piffer S, Lombardi E, et al. (2005) [Risk factors in the pre-, perinatal and early life (first year) for wheezing in young children]. Epidemiologia e prevenzione 29: 47.

25. Spycher BD, Silverman M, Barben J, Eber E, Guinand S, et al. (2009) A disease model for wheezing disorders in preschool children based on clinicians' perceptions. PloS one 4: e8533.

26. Spycher BD, Silverman M, Kuehni C (2010) Phenotypes of childhood asthma: are they real? Clinical & Experimental Allergy 40: 1130–1141.

27. von Mutius E (2011) Trajectories of childhood wheeze. Journal of Allergy and Clinical Immunology 127: 1513–1514.

28. Martinez FD (2002) Development of wheezing disorders and asthma in preschool children. Pediatrics 109: 362–367.

29. Savenije OE, Granell R, Caudri D, Koppelman GH, Smit HA, et al. (2011) Comparison of childhood wheezing phenotypes in 2 birth cohorts: ALSPAC and PIAMA. Journal of Allergy and Clinical Immunology 127: 1505–1512. e1514.

30. Dex S, Joshi H (2005) Children of the 21st century: from birth to nine months: The Policy Press.

31. Asher MI, Keil U, Anderson HR, Beasley R, Crane J, et al. (1995) International Study of Asthma and Allergies in Childhood (ISAAC): rationale and methods. Eur Respir J 8: 483–491.

32. Strina A, Barreto ML, Cooper PJ, Rodrigues LC (2014) Risk factors for non-atopic asthma/wheeze in children and adolescents: a systematic review. Emerging Themes in Epidemiology 11: 5.

33. McClements LD (1977) Equivalence scales for children. Journal of Public Economics 8: 191–210.

34. McLachlan G, Peel D (2000) Finite mixture models: Wiley-Interscience.

35. Vermunt JK (1997) LEM: A general program for the analysis of categorical data. Department of Methodology and Statistics, Tilburg University.

36. Storr CL, Zhou H, Liang K-Y, Anthony JC (2004) Empirically derived latent classes of tobacco dependence syndromes observed in recent-onset tobacco smokers: Epidemiological evidence from a national probability sample survey. Nicotine and Tobacco Research 6: 533–545.

37. Magidson J, Vermunt JK (2004) Latent class models. In: Kaplan D, editor. The Sage handbook of quantitative methodology for the social sciences. Thousand Oaks, CA: Sage. pp. 175–198.

38. Biemer PP (2010) Latent class analysis of survey error. Hoboken, New Jersey: John Wiley & Sons.

39. StataCorp (2009) Stata: release 11: StataCorp LP.

40. Plewis I (2007) Non-response in a birth cohort study: the case of the Millennium Cohort Study. International Journal of Social Research Methodology 10: 325–334.

41. Plewis I (2007) The Millennium Cohort Study: technical report on sampling. London: Centre for Longitudinal Study, Institute of Education.

42. Taussig LM, Wright AL, Holberg CJ, Halonen M, Morgan WJ, et al. (2003) Tucson children's respiratory study: 1980 to present. Journal of Allergy and Clinical Immunology 111: 661–675.

43. Spycher BD, Silverman M, Brooke AM, Minder CE, Kuehni CE (2008) Distinguishing phenotypes of childhood wheeze and cough using latent class analysis. European Respiratory Journal 31: 974–981.

44. Cane R, Pao C, McKenzie S (2001) Understanding childhood asthma in focus groups: perspectives from mothers of different ethnic backgrounds. BMC family practice 2: 4.

45. Elphick H, Sherlock P, Foxall G, Simpson E, Shiell N, et al. (2001) Survey of respiratory sounds in infants. Archives of disease in childhood 84: 35–39.

46. Elphick H, Ritson S, Rodgers H, Everard M (2000) When a" wheeze" is not a wheeze: acoustic analysis of breath sounds in infants. European Respiratory Journal 16: 593–597.

47. Henderson J, Granell R, Heron J, Sherriff A, Simpson A, et al. (2008) Associations of wheezing phenotypes in the first 6 years of life with atopy, lung function and airway responsiveness in mid-childhood. Thorax 63: 974–980.

48. Font-Ribera L, Kogevinas M, Zock J-P, Nieuwenhuijsen MJ, Heederik D, et al. (2009) Swimming pool attendance and risk of asthma and allergic symptoms in children. European Respiratory Journal 34: 1304–1310.

49. Leermakers E, Sonnenschein-van der Voort A, Heppe D, De Jongste J, Moll H, et al. (2013) Maternal fish consumption during pregnancy and risks of wheezing and eczema in childhood: The Generation R Study. European journal of clinical nutrition 67: 353–359.

6

"Nothing Special, Everything Is *Maamuli*": Socio-Cultural and Family Practices Influencing the Perinatal Period in Urban India

Shanti Raman[1]*, Krishnamachari Srinivasan[2], Anura Kurpad[3], Husna Razee[4], Jan Ritchie[4]

1 Department of Community Paediatrics, South Western Sydney Local Health District, Liverpool Hospital, Liverpool, New South Wales, Australia, 2 Department of Psychiatry, St John's Medical College, Bangalore, India, 3 Department of Physiology, St John's Medical College, Bangalore, India, 4 School of Public Health & Community Medicine, University of New South Wales, Sydney, New South Wales, Australia

Abstract

Background: Globally, India contributes the largest share in sheer numbers to the burden of maternal and infant under-nutrition, morbidity and mortality. A major gap in our knowledge is how socio-cultural practices and beliefs influence the perinatal period and thus perinatal outcomes, particularly in the rapidly growing urban setting.

Methods and Findings: Using data from a qualitative study in urban south India, including in-depth interviews with 36 women who had recently been through childbirth as well as observations of family life and clinic encounters, we explored the territory of familial, cultural and traditional practices and beliefs influencing women and their families through pregnancy, childbirth and infancy. We found that while there were some similarities in cultural practices to those described before in studies from low resource village settings, there are changing practices and ideas. Fertility concerns dominate women's experience of married life; notions of gender preference and ideal family size are changing rapidly in response to the urban context; however inter-generational family pressures are still considerable. While a rich repertoire of cultural practices persists throughout the perinatal continuum, their existence is normalised and even underplayed. In terms of diet and nutrition, traditional messages including notions of 'hot' and 'cold' foods, are stronger than health messages; however breastfeeding is the cultural norm and the practice of delayed breastfeeding appears to be disappearing in this urban setting. Marriage, pregnancy and childbirth are so much part of the norm for women, that there is little expectation of individual choice in any of these major life events.

Conclusions: A greater understanding is needed of the dynamic factors shaping the perinatal period in urban India, including an acknowledgment of the health promoting as well as potentially harmful cultural practices and the critical role of the family. This will help plan culturally appropriate integrated perinatal health care.

Editor: Ignacio Correa-Velez, Queensland University of Technology, Australia

Funding: The authors have no funding or support to report.

Competing Interests: The authors have declared that no competing interests exist.

* Email: shanti.raman@sswahs.nsw.gov.au

Introduction

Health conditions affecting the perinatal period still account for a major contribution to disease burden in sub-Saharan Africa and South Asia despite the significant global shift in disease burden towards non-communicable diseases [1,2], making the perinatal period i.e. pregnancy, childbirth and infancy, a key period for health intervention. Of this global burden of maternal and neonatal deaths, India contributes the largest share [3–6]. India also contributes the largest share in terms of sheer numbers, of maternal and infant under-nutrition, starting with low birth weight infants [7]. Public health approaches to maternal and newborn health over the last decade have emphasized the need for access to services, chiefly skilled attendance and emergency obstetric care, but have paid comparatively less attention to improving family and

community practices [8]. A major gap in our knowledge on how to improve perinatal outcomes, is how family and community practices influence maternal/child health care-seeking behaviours [9]. Given India's significant contribution to global maternal and infant mortality, a focus on this country is integral to any successful global effort [10].

Over the past two decades there has been considerable interest in understanding the socio-cultural milieu of pregnancy and childbirth in low-and middle-income countries so that interventions can be culturally appropriate and have a greater chance of success. The majority of the research has centred on 'traditional' or cultural care practices around birth and delivery and the newborn period; and much of it is based on rural populations [11–13]. There has been understandable emphasis in the research on potentially harmful traditional practices, particularly in settings such as in rural South Asia and sub-Saharan Africa, where home deliveries are common. We know from recent research in rural India that unhygienic cord cutting, delayed breastfeeding and early bathing [14], and a combination of traditional and modern practices rooted in the concept of inducing heat to facilitate labour, continue to take place [12]. There has also been robust research aimed at describing early infant nutrition, particularly cultural approaches to breastfeeding initiation and duration [15–18].

Less understood and described and, we would argue no less important, are the socio-cultural milieu and practices across the whole of the perinatal continuum and in the urban setting. Darmstadt et al. [19] reviewed the literature of antenatal, intra-partum, and postpartum care practices for mothers and newborns in Bangladeshi communities and found a dearth of information. Studies of newborn care practices in the slums of Dhaka [20], and Karachi [21], have found that these were similar to those in rural areas of the South Asia region, including lack of exclusive breastfeeding, bathing the baby soon after birth and applying substances to the umbilical cord. During the 1990s, the MotherCare Project conducted qualitative research to determine the major barriers and facilitators of iron supplementation programs for pregnant women in eight developing countries; beliefs against consuming medications during pregnancy, and fears that taking too much iron may cause too much blood or a big baby, making delivery more difficult were common [22]. In summary, research has been more focused on the potentially dangerous cultural practices during pregnancy, childbirth and newborn period, and less interested in the health promoting aspects of cultural practices.

In 2003 a prospective birth cohort study was commenced at St John's Medical College (SJMC) Hospital, Bangalore, India, to explore the association of maternal health and nutrition with pregnancy and child health outcomes. Several salient reports and results have already emerged out of this cohort study [23,24]; in keeping with international research findings, the single most important factor in determining birth weight and hence infant outcomes in this cohort was maternal education level [25]. We situated our qualitative study within this cohort to elicit psychosocial and cultural factors that influence the perinatal period, for mother and infant dyads in urban India. In particular we wanted to explore how 'cultural' practices and beliefs influenced women's pregnancy and childbirth experiences, their pregnancy and family planning choices, their self-care including nutrition through the perinatal continuum.

Empirical Setting, Methods and Data

This paper draws on ethnographic work carried out in greater metropolitan Bangalore, (now Bengaluru), a contemporary urban landscape in India which includes large areas that were until recently considered villages (rural), but have become incorporated into the city. Our previous paper focused on sources of support available to mother-infant dyads [26], we have also reported on the challenges of accessing healthcare in the perinatal period [27]. In this paper we report specifically on the role cultural ideas, beliefs and practices play in influencing the perinatal period in the urban setting.

SJMC Hospital is a 1200-bed tertiary healthcare service in Bangalore, which draws patients of diverse socioeconomic status, from urban slums to high-income residential areas. For the in-depth interviews, we identified women from the cohort who had been through pregnancy and childbirth within the last two years. We used maximum variation sampling [28], to ensure a mix of

social and cultural groups (i.e. language and religion) from within three education levels from the cohort. These included women with low education levels (primary school-Group 1), women with medium education levels (completed high school-Group 2) and women with high education levels (tertiary education – Group 3). Prior to commencing the interviews, an interview guide was formulated based on a literature review including topics such as home environment, sources of support, pregnancy and childbirth expectations including gender preference, choice and control over reproduction, cultural practices, dietary practices and self-care. Participants were initially contacted by telephone to locate them, as most addresses were incomplete or wrong; the mobile phone proving the most useful method of reaching even the most unreachable. None of the women refused to participate; some were unable to be located due to change in mobile phone number. Participants were interviewed by female researchers (the first author and research assistant) in the location of their choice; most often it was their home, sometimes it was their mother's house, or their in-laws' house, occasionally it was their workplace. While the interview subjects were recent mothers, due to the ethnographic approach taken and the reality of conducting qualitative research in India, often the extended family or even friendship network participated. Interviews were continued till a saturation of themes was reached. Each in-depth interview lasted between 1.5 hours to two hours.

Ethnographic observations were carried out during fieldwork by the first author between August 2008 to January 2009 and in December 2010 in Bangalore. Observations were carried out during formal and informal encounters in family homes or workplaces and while interacting with the extended family and friendship network of the participants or during maternal and child antenatal and postnatal healthcare visits in SJMC and a government health centre. The ethnographic approach was influenced strongly by active listening [29], and used a range of methodologies as described by Fitzgerald including observation, participation, formal and informal interviewing and critical self-reflection [30].

Audio taped interviews were transcribed (from the language of interview to English) as soon as possible following the interview either by the first author or the research assistant (RA) and verified by each other. Observation notes were recorded as field notes in a journal and reflective observations entered in Microsoft Word. The transcripts were open-coded manually and re-categorised by the first author and the RA [28]. One other member of the research team in Bangalore independently read all the transcripts and cross-coded the interviews to ensure data integrity Data were analysed using thematic analysis and constant comparative techniques [31]. Overall analysis was iterative, being guided by the principles of grounded theory and phenomenology and incorporating critical reflexivity [32].

Ethics statement

Ethics clearance was obtained from the Institutional Ethical Review Board of the St John's Medical College and Hospital prior to commencing the fieldwork. Informed consent was read and translated to the language of choice by the first author or RA; all participants provided written consent through a signature or initials in English or in Kannada.

Results

In all, in-depth interviews were carried out with 36 women, 13 in group one, 12 in group two, 11 in group three. Table 1 summarises characteristics of those interviewed. The results of the

Table 1. Characteristics of participants, perinatal socio-cultural study, Bangalore.

	Group 1 Low education	Group 2 Medium education	Group 3 Tertiary education
Number	13	12	11
Languages spoken	6	5	5
Maternal age (mean)	23 years	24 years	26 years
Baby birth weight (mean)	2.6 kg	2.7 kg	3.1 kg
Infant outcomes	1 death, 1 disability, 2 stunted	1 stunted, 1 mild disability	Good overall

analysis and interpretation of the qualitative data are presented as key themes identified with respect to the research question: how do cultural practices and beliefs impact on the perinatal continuum for maternal-infant dyads in Bangalore? The following themes emerged:

1. Pregnancy related expectations and experiences

- **Fertility concerns**
- **Gender preference**
- **Desire for small family**
- **Reproductive choice**

2. Traditional cultural practices
3. Dietary practices through perinatal period

Pregnancy related expectations and experiences

I was very "tense" because I did not get pregnant: Fertility concerns. An overwhelming concern for many women, who were asked about their pregnancy, was around demonstrating their fertility early, following marriage. This cut across education levels, religious and cultural affiliations. Many women when asked about details about pregnancy would recount their problems with 'falling pregnant' first. As 27 year old Priya (names have been changed throughout to preserve anonymity) who worked as a teacher recounted, "I was very tense [English word used] because I did not get pregnant." Priya and her husband had been trying to get pregnant for two years ever since she got married, "after the [fertility] treatment and many tests" the couple were successful in their quest. Thirty year old Sumathi, related with some distress the hazardous journey that fertility and reproductive services had been for her. Sumathi and her husband had lost their first son in a tragic drowning accident in their village. After some difficulty, the couple had a girl. Following this, the extended family said "get another baby". Although her husband was happy with one child, family pressure prevailed. "I have had lots of investigations and ultrasounds, *tumbane* (too much) problem." The couple had spent a lot of money and waited seven years for another successful pregnancy. After five miscarriages in as many years, Sumathi finally had a successful pregnancy; she related that her doctor had said "we have tried our best; the rest is up to God."

Very often the question about whether the pregnancy was planned would be interpreted as a query regarding family planning or contraception use. Invariably women would offer up their accounts of their fertility concerns. As 20 year old Shashi with limited high school education said,

I thought of having three years [*family*] planning. But my in-laws started acting differently towards me as I was not pregnant. Due to their forcing I got pregnant so soon (i.e. within three months).

Only girls look after their families: Gender preference. Contrary to our expectations most women asked about gender preference in their pregnancy expressed a strong desire for a girl, especially if it was the first pregnancy. None of the women we spoke to admitted to any knowledge during the pregnancy of the expected gender of the baby. As typified by Ganga, a working woman with low education levels, who at 31 years was one of the oldest women in the cohort, said:

We both wanted girl child only. Only girls look after their families, boys are a waste. Girls understand family issues better, that is why we like girls. I want only one girl, and I want to give her a good education.

Women, as well as their husbands if they were around, reflected a preference for girls. Some women acknowledged that their families, more importantly their mothers-in-law, expected a boy. As 20 year old Shashi said, "for my in-laws' sake I was expecting for boy.... but I preferred girl only. I am very happy with a girl now."

While all women denied any ultrasound-assisted gender identification prenatally, many women spoke of having 'abortions'. Sometimes this term related to spontaneous miscarriages, other times it was specifically used to denote medical terminations of pregnancy. Twenty year old Shobha who had eloped to have a 'love marriage' and had suffered from financial stresses in the past said, "Actually I had two abortions between first and second child. This time we were happy about pregnancy, both husband and I wanted a girl."

Women who expressed a preference for a boy were in a minority and usually had strong family pressure bearing down on them. The two women who had a strong preference for a boy were both Muslim, and already had two girls each. As Shabnam (29 years old, educated, teacher) said:

I really, really wanted a boy after two girls. I had a lot of health problems associated with pregnancy, in the past. I was told **not** to become pregnant (emphatic hand gestures), by doctors and all. But so much I was praying for a boy.

Shabnam also admitted that even her husband had suggested she go for an abortion, given her past health problems. However her mother supported her throughout this pregnancy saying, "I have prayed for you, this time it will be different, you *will* have a boy." Only one other young mother Kala, a 22 year old with little education expressed a desire for a boy with this pregnancy, she also already had two daughters. Her mother, who often spoke in her stead, said, "we thought if it is a boy, she can go for family planning [*referring to tubal ligation*], but now [*meaning the next pregnancy*] she will try for a boy."

We are not planning for another one: Desire for small, healthy family. Another strong sentiment expressed, often unsolicited was for a small, healthy family. Many families were living in cramped one room dwellings. The emphasis seemed to be on making sure that the family unit was able to provide adequately for and bring up optimally, a finite number of children. Only three women we spoke to were even contemplating having more than two children. A surprising minority expressed a preference for having only one child; this view was expressed by Hindus and Christians across class divides, but never by Muslim women. "We just wanted a healthy baby", was oft repeated, the emphasis being on 'healthy'. As 26 year old Anita (Christian, poorly educated), who already had one boy said, "We are not planning for another one; because in our family all are telling us, next will be a boy only." Ganga who had expressed strong views about the benefits of having girls, was preparing to have her "family planning operation." Educated and well off Sumithra at 25 years of age and with one daughter said, "No, one is enough, I feel tired to look after this child only." Women often said, "I feel one child is enough, but my husband wants another."

We did some planning for two years: Reproductive choice. We did not specifically probe about whether women had control over their fertility or reproductive choice. Various questions and observations were analysed to gather information about women's choice in fertility and reproduction. Choice and control over reproduction was linked to choice of marriage partner and ability to make choices regarding fertility. For example, Shobha who had primary school education only and came from a poor rural family had defied tradition to marry a man from her village across caste lines. The couple were isolated from both their families of origin. Despite her young age, at 21 years, Shobha had decided, "I am not having any more pregnancies; I will get operated on soon". Twenty-four year old Pooja, who had also had a love marriage, and insisted that they had planned the pregnancy, when asked when she actually got pregnant replied happily, "After one month of my marriage I got pregnant." Twenty-eight year old Grace, Catholic with tertiary education also admitted to a 'love marriage'. Grace worked as a marriage counsellor; she followed birth spacing and Billings method for contraception, "as I give advice on such things only in my counselling."

Love marriages were an exception; most of the women we interviewed had arranged marriages. At least half of the women particularly from the less educated groups originally hailed from villages in South India and endogamy was widely practised (cross-cousin and maternal uncle marriages common). Mumtaz, who was poorly educated, yet was extremely confident in the social sphere, said she and her husband did "some (family) planning for two years" prior to the first successful pregnancy at 25 years. About half the women in the less educated groups said they had some choice and control over their reproduction and fertility, women usually referred to this as 'planning' (English term used). Mostly women said that they did some planning for two years, rarely longer than that. Among highly educated women, more of them said they had some measure of control over their planning. However those that had the least say in their marriage choice likewise had little choice or control over their fertility. Twenty-two year old Sameena (Muslim) got married "within one week after

finishing my exams" and admitted, "We didn't have any planning, after two months of my marriage I got pregnant."

Nothing special. Everything is "maamuli" only: Traditional (cultural) practices. Most women in their first pregnancy described having a religious or cultural ritual in the third trimester to celebrate the mother and the pregnancy; this was celebrated by Hindus, Muslims and Christians in some manner. However the question of whether women did anything special during their pregnancy was often responded to with, "nothing special, everything is *maamuli* (ordinary) only"; suggesting that pregnancy and birthing rituals and other practices were commonplace and were nothing out of the ordinary. The South Indian term for the special ritual in pregnancy is *Seemantha* or *Vallécāpu*, and is celebrated during a woman's first pregnancy, in preparation for her first delivery; it is a rite of passage into motherhood. In many cases the ritual is performed in the woman's in-laws' house, but the bulk of expenses are expected to be borne by her own natal kin. It is commonly performed as a ritual celebrating fertility and the mother, various emic symbols are used as presents and offerings to the mother-to-be including bangles, coconuts and special saris. It is customary for the pregnant woman to return to her own mother's house following the ritual and remain with her mother for the customary six weeks or three months post-delivery. Despite the expectations of following this script, in reality the *Seemantha* or equivalent ceremony was celebrated in a range of ways in Bangalore. For example, Savitha who had an early pregnancy miscarriage previously was being specially cared for at her own parents' (natal) home. This lasted from mid pregnancy through to almost 9 months post baby's birth. "Yes, here they arranged *seemantha* for me, my husband's family bought everything here (to her natal home) and they did the ceremony." Twenty-four year old Pooja and her husband, came from Northeastern India and had no family in Bangalore. Pooja admitted to missing her mother and her natal family very much through her pregnancy. However, neighbours in this crowded and dilapidated housing complex had taken on family responsibility for Pooja and her husband, despite being from different cultural and language backgrounds. The husband gratefully described, "Our neighbours arranged function in the next building. I got a priest to do *puja* (religious ritual); rest all they did." Mumtaz, 25 year old Muslim woman with primary school education, said "We had a seven month function (using English word) here (at husband's place)."

Many women talked of missing the ceremony if it wasn't performed. Shobha who was isolated from her natal family "because I did love marriage", said regretfully, "We did *Seemantha* for the first pregnancy, but nothing special this time. I did not go to mother's place even; I feel my mother does not have much love for me." Sometimes the ritual was avoided because of medical complications, "We did nothing special cultural, mainly followed medical advice, as this was a very precious pregnancy." Sometimes it was due to family tension or financial tensions. As with 20 year old Shashi who related that her parents requested her in-laws, "shall we arrange a function?" but was told that they (in-laws) "didn't have time for all those things." This was a family with major in-law tensions; exacerbated by the fact that the couple's marriage was endogamous (related).

Specific cultural practices for the infant were also commonly performed, but unless specifically asked about, not mentioned. A range of naming ceremonies or specific religious ceremonies was carried out in early infancy, depending on cultural group. As 23 year old Mary said, "For the baby, he was baptized and we did 'holy communion'; we also recently went to Velankanni temple and offered baby's hair as thanksgiving." Most infants wore charms, talismans (*rakshé* or *tabiz*), or religious icons around their waists or necks, many also had beauty spots (black mark) on the face to ward off the evil eye.

Cool foods and 'heaty' foods: Dietary practices in pregnancy and postnatally. Women and their families had strongly held cultural views about food and nutrition. While all the women were part of the larger cohort study and were being asked questions about their diet and provided dietary advice in pregnancy; they most often spoke about cool foods and heaty foods and the effect these had on their pregnancy. Anita a 25 year old woman with little education said, that the "doctor told me eat whatever you want, but avoid 'heaty' food." She also said that many of her family and friends had suggested that she "avoid cool food" and "have heat food" instead. Others were equally adamant that they must avoid 'heaty' foods. Thirty-two year old Ganga who had a high school education level and strongly held views said, "Doctor suggested me to take lot of spinach, fruits, fish; but I was avoiding *musumbi* [sweet lime] as it causes cold effect on me. I was avoiding papaya, as it is 'heaty.'" Most women had some idea about whether their body type was 'heaty' or 'cool'. Radhika, who was well educated and even worked for a health firm in the past, said "I used to avoid papaya, because mine is a 'heat' body. Whenever I ate papaya, the next day only I used to get urine problems." None of the women admitted to restricting their diet to have a small baby or facilitate easy delivery. Some women spoke about special foods that were made for them usually by their mothers, during pregnancy and also for the immediate post-natal period; the nutritional content was never mentioned. *Nāti aushadi* or folk medicine was also mentioned, as part of the diet particularly to combat nausea in pregnancy. All the women as part of the cohort were given iron and calcium supplements throughout pregnancy and the early postnatal period, most women said they took these tablets. However when they described their diets, it was mostly about the fit between the foods and their body type rather than the nutritional content. Twenty-five year old Mumtaz (Muslim, poorly educated), was the only one who specifically mentioned taking rest in pregnancy and also being supported by the family to take rest. Her desire was to have a 'fair child', "everyone told me to eat two apples daily and half litre of milk, I did that daily; that's why I have such a beautiful, fair baby (laughing)!".

Breastfeeding was universally practised, all had initiated breastfeeding early. When asked specifically about breastfeeding initiation, the usual response was "soon after delivery". Apart from one woman, who did say she needed some help and support from her mother with establishing breastfeeding, there were none who reported problems. Baby massages with application of oil was also common. Another universally common practice was ensuring clean water for the infant, usually "I boil water for baby". Even where families had difficulties accessing adequate water supply, they would ensure that any water used to feed or cook for the infant was boiled. Complementary feeds for the infant were usually traditional foods, slightly modified according to the age of the child, but not by cultural group. "Morning we are giving rusk, *dosa* or *idli* (rice and lentil based local food), also we are giving him almonds, *ragi* (local millet) malt." This description of complementary feeding was repeated many times and by women from all cultural groups.

Discussion

This qualitative study explores the socio-cultural factors that shape the perinatal period in urban India today. Public health researchers and policymakers are increasingly acknowledging the need to understand pregnancy and childbirth beyond morbidity and mortality statistics [10,33]. More than two decades ago Cleland and van Ginneken suggested that the intervening role of cultural beliefs and domestic practices may be very important in the explanation of the maternal education-perinatal mortality relationship [34]. We found that while there were many similarities in cultural practices and beliefs in South Asian anthropological studies [35–39], there are changing practices and ideas that deserve documenting and recognising. We found in our study that fertility concerns dominate women's experience of married life; that notions of ideal family size and gender preference are changing rapidly in response to the urban context; that while a rich repertoire of cultural practices persist throughout the perinatal continuum their existence is normalised and even underplayed; and that in terms of diet and nutrition traditional messages are stronger than health messages. Marriage, pregnancy and child-birth are so much part of the norm for women that there is little expectation of individual choice in any of these major life events. The family unit, including extended family, exerts a critical influence throughout the perinatal period, as noted previously [26].

There has been acknowledgement that infertility is an important public health issue [40,41]; the International Conference on Population and Development Programme of Action stating that reproductive health services should include the prevention and appropriate treatment of infertility [42]. Yet this common problem has received little attention from health policy makers in India. While the World Health Organization recommends the epidemiological definition of infertility, which is the inability to conceive within two years of exposure to pregnancy [43], we found that women in our study felt pressured to demonstrate their fertility soon after they got married, and if that did not occur concerns about infertility dominated family life. We found that the language used to probe about planning for pregnancy was loosely interpreted or misinterpreted, such that the term 'planning' has to be understood within its socio-cultural context. Any exploration of pregnancy therefore has to acknowledge the important role of infertility in reproductive health concerns. Indeed, infertility and fertility exist in a dialectical relationship of contrast, such that understanding one leads to a much greater understanding of the other [44]. Much has been written about infertility and its consequences for couples in Africa [45–47]; in south Asia the stigma associated with infertility can be seen as a "social response to the breakdown of a conceptual bind that conjoins the sacrament of marriage to the task of producing offspring" [48]. In Hindu families, the very notion of auspiciousness is linked to female fertility [49] across all cultural groups, however infertility is largely blamed on the woman and thought to be due to evil spirits or physiological defects in the woman [50].

The deep-rooted culturally determined beliefs of son preference in Asia are well documented. Much has been written about female foeticide, infanticide, abandonment, out-adoption, under-reporting of female births, and selective neglect of girls leading to higher death rates in South Asia in particular [51]. There are 44 million missing women in India; the sex ratio in second children if the first is a girl is even lower; strongly suggesting sex selective abortions after antenatal sex determination [52]. Given this publicly available knowledge, hearing the very real and current desire of women in Bangalore to have female children was surprising. Equally surprising was the oft repeated desire for 'small family' size, even a one child family. This suggests that change is occurring in socio-cultural norms and quite rapidly in certain urban settings. There is growing evidence in China that son preference is on the decline, but a recent study in both rural and urban China revealed that while son preference has weakened considerably in this generation, it has by no means disappeared [53]. Kodzi et al. [54], found the desire to stop childbearing in Ghana is influenced by reproductive life stage; events; perceptions of personal health; the household's economic welfare; and the overall subjective cost of children. Cost of living concerns were definitely a factor in influencing the desire for small family size; however there was a strongly expressed love and appreciation of the girl child, which has not been documented before to our knowledge. The sociocultural roots of son preference even for non-resident Indians is extremely strong; in our study similarly, women were particularly pressurised to have sons by female in-laws and husbands [55]. This raises the whole question of how much if any reproductive "choice" women do have. We found that there was an ambivalence with which women regarded their own experience of reproductive choice; this began with the lack of choice or control over their marriage and extended through to their 'planning', family planning or pregnancy planning. The small minority of women who had had love marriages in our study had the greatest choice in planning their families, as exemplified by the young woman who became pregnant a month after her 'love' marriage and proudly proclaimed that she had done "planning".

The tendency for rural South Indian women to prefer smaller babies and the relationship of this preference to dietary behaviour and quantity of food consumed during pregnancy have been well described by Nichter and Nichter [39]. We found that traditional, cultural messages about food and diet, including bewildering notions of hot and cold foods versus body habitus which have been well described, still hold meaning and relevance [56]. However curtailing diet consumed in order to have a small baby was never mentioned; the nutritional content of the food was also not a preoccupation for our mothers. A recent qualitative study of pregnant women in Mumbai similarly found that despite the knowledge that the best solution for anaemia in pregnancy was a nutritious diet, respondents did not consume appropriate diets, nor provide details of dietary regimens that would help improve iron content [57]. Breastfeeding, indeed prolonged breastfeeding, was universally practiced; other studies from this region have confirmed that prolonged breastfeeding is the norm and complementary feeding commences around four months [58]. Interestingly the 'drink boiled water' message, especially for baby, had translated into practice; this is clearly a change in behaviour over practices from decades ago [59]. Delayed breastfeeding, the early feeding of substitutes such as honey and *ghutti* to the newborn, which have been described in other studies from rural and urban settings [21,60], appears to be changing in this urban setting. Cultural and religious practices from pregnancy through to the first year of life clearly have meaning, even though they were normalised (*maamuli*) and diverse in nature. Rodrigues' study from Goa found that the failure to observe rituals and dietary practices associated with childbirth, such as the use of special diets and body massages with oil, was associated with perinatal depression [61]. Similarly women in our study who did not have a pregnancy ceremony, or were deprived of a culturally sanctioned celebration for whatever reason were unhappy.

These findings should be interpreted with certain limitations in mind. Although our study provides in-depth qualitative insight into cultural practices and beliefs throughout the perinatal period in Bangalore, it cannot be generalised beyond the urban South Indian population. Urban populations are by nature fluid and dynamic, the particular mix of cultural groups that reside in urban South India may not be similar to urban populations elsewhere.

We did not specifically interview husbands, however the nature of doing field-based qualitative research in India means that the interview is with more than just the woman so that often family or friends participate, with husbands and fathers-in-law regularly attending the interviews.

In conclusion, in the great melting pot of metropolitan Bangalore, traditional and cultural practices and beliefs do strongly influence the perinatal continuum, but they are morphing and moulding according to the socio-environmental context. Kesterton and Cleland [14], from their qualitative study of birthing practices in rural Karnataka also found that movement away from traditional practices is already taking place, particularly amongst the more educated and better off. We would argue that the sometimes accusatory gaze with which 'traditional' practices in pregnancy and childbirth have been described, needs to be re-positioned to encompass the health and wellbeing-enhancing practices that continue to play a role for today's mothers. There also needs to be an acknowledgement that culture is dynamic and that change is a constant. Clearly some health messages are getting through such as the need to have clean water and early attachment to the breast, while others are not. We know from research in India that community-based intervention, targeted at certain high-risk newborn-care practices, can lead to substantial behavioural modification and reduction in neonatal mortality [62]; however not all domestic behaviours change easily as our study illustrates. Further research is required to elucidate the nexus between receipt of health information and desired behaviour change. We would suggest that ethnographic research, which is multi-methodology research par excellence [30], should be given more importance both in understanding the socio-cultural contexts and in helping shape public health interventions.

We call for a greater understanding of the dynamic factors influencing and shaping the perinatal period in urban India. This includes acknowledging the critical importance of the family both in supporting and in disrupting perinatal wellbeing. It also includes acknowledging the health promoting as well as potentially harmful perinatal practices and beliefs, to result in better targeting of culturally appropriate public health interventions throughout the perinatal continuum. Behaviour change interventions to improve maternal and newborn health need to address potentially harmful practices through appropriate training of healthcare providers, changing their perceptions and attitudes, and arming them with the skills to promote positive, culturally sanctioned behaviour. Beyond merely targeting 'practices', healthcare providers also need to understand the socio-cultural contexts which influence beliefs and practices. This can only be achieved by involving the extended family and community in the perinatal journey.

Acknowledgments

We gratefully acknowledge the invaluable support and help provided by Dr Sumithra Mutthayya and members of the Nutrition Research team from St John's Research Institute, St John's Medical College, Bangalore. The first author is particularly grateful to all the women and families who so freely gave their time to this research.

Author Contributions

Conceived and designed the experiments: SR KS AK. Performed the experiments: SR. Analyzed the data: SR KS HR JR. Contributed reagents/materials/analysis tools: SR KS AK. Contributed to the writing of the manuscript: SR HR JR KS.

References

1. Lopez AD, Mathers CD, Ezzati M, Jamison DT, Murray CJL (2006) Global and regional burden of disease and risk factors, 2001: systematic analysis of population health data. Lancet 367: 1747–1757.
2. Murray CJL, Vos T, Lozano R, Naghavi M, Flaxman AD, et al. (2012) Disability-adjusted life years (DALYs) for 291 diseases and injuries in 21 regions, 1990–2010: a systematic analysis for the Global Burden of Disease Study 2010. The Lancet 380: 2197–2223.
3. Lawn J, Cousens S, Zupan J (2005) 4 million neonatal deaths: When? Where? Why? Lancet 365: 891–900.
4. Ministry of Health and Family Welfare (2008) 2005–2006 National Family Health Survey (NFHS-3). National Fact Sheet- India, Provisional Data. In: Ministry of Health and Family Welfare GoI, editor. New Delhi.
5. Oestergaard MZ, Inoue M, Yoshida S, Mahanani WR, Gore FM, et al. (2011) Neonatal Mortality Levels for 193 Countries in 2009 with Trends since 1990: A Systematic Analysis of Progress, Projections, and Priorities. PLoS Med 8: e1001080.
6. Kassebaum NJ, Bertozzi-Villa A, Coggeshall MS, Shackelford KA, Steiner C, et al. (2014) Global, regional, and national levels and causes of maternal mortality during 1990?2013: a systematic analysis for the Global Burden of Disease Study 2013. The Lancet.
7. Gragnolati M, Shekar M, Gupta MD, Bredenkamp C, Lee Y-K (2005) India's Undernourished Children: A Call for Reform and Action. Washington DC: The World Bank.
8. Campbell O, Graham W, group oboTLs (2006) Strategies for reducing maternal mortality: getting on with what works. Lancet 368: 1284–1299.
9. Bhutta ZA, Darmstadt GL, Hasan BS, Haws RA (2005) Community-based interventions for improving perinatal and neonatal health outcomes in developing countries: a review of the evidence. Pediatrics 115: 519–617.
10. Bhutta ZA, Chopra M, Axelson H, Berman P, Boerma T, et al. (2010) Countdown to 2015 decade report (2000–10): taking stock of maternal, newborn, and child survival. The Lancet 375: 2032–2044.
11. Maimbolwa MC, Yamba B, Diwan V, Ransjö-Arvidson A-B (2003) Cultural childbirth practices and beliefs in Zambia. Journal of Advanced Nursing 43: 263–274.
12. Iyengar SD, Iyengar K, Martines JC, Dashora K, Deora KK (2008) Childbirth practices in rural Rajasthan, India: implications for neonatal health and survival. J Perinatol 28: S23–S30.
13. Callaghan-Koru J, Seifu A, Tholandi M, de Graft-Johnson J, Daniel E, et al. (2013) Newborn care practices at home and in health facilities in 4 regions of Ethiopia. BMC Pediatrics 13: 198.
14. Kesterton AJ, Cleland J (2009) Neonatal care in rural Karnataka: healthy and harmful practices, the potential for change. BMC Pregnancy and Childbirth 9: 13.
15. Aborigo RA, Moyer C, Rominski S, Adongo P, Williams J, et al. (2012) Infant nutrition in the first seven days of life in rural northern Ghana. BMC Pregnancy and Childbirth 12: 76.
16. Kimani-Murage EW, Madise NJ, Fotso JC, Kyobutungi C, Mutua MK, et al. (2011) Patterns and determinants of breastfeeding and complementary feeding practices in urban informal settlements, Nairobi Kenya. BMC Public Health 11: 396.
17. Holder K (2011) Birthing support and breastfeeding initiation in Somaliland: experiences at the Edna Adan Maternity Hospital in Hargeisa, Somaliland. East African Journal of Public Health 8: 38–41.
18. Lee H, Durham J, Booth J, Sychareun V (2013) A qualitative study on the breastfeeding experiences of first-time mothers in Vientiane, Lao PDR. BMC Pregnancy and Childbirth 13: 223.
19. Darmstadt GL, Syed U, Patel Z, Kabir N (2006) Review of Domiciliary Newborn-care Practices in Bangladesh. The Journal of Health, Population and Nutrition 24: 380–393.
20. Moran A, Choudhury N, Uz Zaman Khan N, Ahsan Karar Z, Wahed T, et al. (2009) Newborn care practices among slum dwellers in Dhaka, Bangladesh: a quantitative and qualitative exploratory study. BMC Pregnancy and Childbirth 9: 54.
21. Fikree FF, Ali TS, Durocher JM, Rahbar MH (2005) Newborn care practices in low socioeconomic settlements of Karachi, Pakistan. Social Science & Medicine 60: 911–921.
22. Galloway R, Dusch E, Elder L, Achadi E, Grajeda R, et al. (2002) Women's perceptions of iron deficiency and anemia prevention and control in eight developing countries. Social Science & Medicine 55: 529–544.
23. Dwarkanath P, Muthayya S, Vaz M, Thomas T, Mhaskar A, et al. (2007) The relationship between maternal physical activity during pregnancy and birth weight. Asia Pac J Clin Nutr 16: 704–710.
24. Muthayya S, Dwarkanath P, Mhaskar M, Mhaskar P, Thomas A, et al. (2006) The relationship of neonatal serum vitamin B12 status with birth weight. Asia Pac J Clin Nutr 15: 538–543.
25. Thomas T, Dwarkanath P, Muthayya S, Vaz M, Kurpad AV (2009) Raising the minimum education of the girl child in India may lead to improvement in birth outcomes. Bangalore, India: St. John's Research Institute, St. John National Academy of Health Sciences.
26. Raman S, Srinivasan K, Kurpad A, Dwarkanath P, Ritchie J, et al. (2014) 'My Mother… My Sisters… and My Friends': Sources of maternal support in the perinatal period in urban India. Midwifery 30: 130–137.
27. Raman S (2014) Faith, trust and the perinatal healthcare maze in urban India. Health, Culture and Society 6: 73–84.
28. Grbich C (2003) Qualitative Research in Health: An introduction. London: Sage Publications. 312 p.
29. Forsey MG (2010) Ethnography as participant listening. Ethnography 11 558–572.
30. Fitzgerald M (1997) Ethnography. In: Higgs J, editor. Qualitative research: Discourse on methodologies. Sydney: Hamden Press and The Centre for Professional Education Advancement, University of Sydney. 48–60.
31. Braun V, Clarke V (2006) Using thematic analysis in psychology. Qualitative Research in Psychology 3: 77–101.
32. Green J, Thorogood N (2009) Qualitative methods for health research. Second edition. London: Sage Publications. 304 p.
33. Bhutta ZA, Lassi ZS (2010) Empowering communities for maternal and newborn health. The Lancet 375: 1142–1144.
34. Cleland JG, van Ginneken JK (1988) Maternal education and child survival in developing countries: The search for pathways of influence. Social Science & Medicine 27: 1357–1368.
35. Gideon H (1962) A baby is born in the Punjab. American Anthropologist 64: 1220–1234.
36. Blanchet T (1984) Women, pollution and marginality: meanings and rituals of birth in rural Bangladesh: Dhaka: University Press.
37. Ram K (1994) Medical management and giving birth: Responses of coastal women in Tamil Nadu. Reproductive Health Matters 2: 20–26.
38. Rozario S (1998) The dai and the doctor: discourses on women's reproductive health in rural Bangladesh In: Ram K, Jolly M, editors. Maternities and Modernities: Colonial and Postcolonial Experiences in Asia and the Pacific. Cambridge: Cambridge University Press 144–176.
39. Nichter M, Nichter M (1983) The ethnophysiology and folk dietetics of pregnancy: A case study from South India. Human Organization 42: 235–246.
40. Inhorn MC (2009) Right to assisted reproductive technology: Overcoming infertility in low-resource countries. International Journal of Gynecology & Obstetrics 106: 172–174.
41. Nachtigall RD (2006) International disparities in access to infertility services. Fertility and Sterility 85: 871–875.
42. ICPD. International Conference on Population and Development - ICPD - Programme of Action. In: UNFPA, editor (1994) Cairo. United Nations Population Fund.
43. WHO (1987) Infections, pregnancies, and infertility: perspectives on prevention. Fertility and Sterility 47: 964–968.
44. Inhorn MC (1994) Interpreting infertility: Medical anthropological perspectives: Introduction. Social Science & Medicine 39: 459–461.
45. Feldman-Savelsberg P (1994) Plundered kitchens and empty wombs: Fear of infertility in the Cameroonian Grassfields. Social Science & Medicine 39: 463–474.
46. Hollos M, Larsen U (2008) Motherhood in sub-Saharan Africa: The social consequences of infertility in an urban population in northern Tanzania. Culture, Health & Sexuality 10: 159–173.
47. Tabong PT-N, Adongo PB (2013) Understanding the social meaning of infertility and childbearing: A qualitative study of the perception of childbearing and childlessness in northern Ghana. PLoS ONE 8: e54429.
48. Bharadwaj A (2003) Why adoption is not an option in India: the visibility of infertility, the secrecy of donor insemination, and other cultural complexities. Social Science & Medicine 56: 1867–1880.
49. Neff DL (1994) The social construction of infertility: The case of the matrilineal Nāyars in South India. Social Science & Medicine 39: 475–485.
50. Papreen N, Sharma A, Sabin K, Begum L, Ahsan SK, et al. (2000) Living with infertility: Experiences among urban slum populations in Bangladesh. Reproductive Health Matters 8: 33–44.
51. Bandyopadhyay M (2003) Missing girls and son preference in rural India: looking beyond popular myth. Health Care for Women International 24: 910–926.
52. Sahni M, Verma N, Narula D, Varghese RM, Sreenivas V, et al. (2008) Missing girls in India: Infanticide, feticide and made-to-order pregnancies? Insights from hospital-based sex-ratio-at-birth over the last century. PLoS ONE 3.
53. Chi Z, Dong ZX, Lei WX, Jun ZW, Lu L, et al. (2013) Changing Gender Preference in China Today: Implications for the Sex Ratio. Indian Journal of Gender Studies 20: 51–68.
54. Kodzi IA, Johnson DR, Casterline JB (2012) To have or not to have another child: Life cycle, health and cost considerations of Ghanaian women. Social Science & Medicine 74: 966–972.
55. Puri S, Adams V, Ivey S, Nachtigall RD (2011) "There is such a thing as too many daughters, but not too many sons": A qualitative study of son preference and fetal sex selection among Indian immigrants in the United States. Social Science & Medicine 72: 1169–1176.
56. Nichter M (1987) Cultural dimensions of hot, cold and sema in Sinhalese health culture Soc Sci Med 25: 377–387.

57. Chatterjee N, Fernandes G (2013) "This is normal during pregnancy" A qualitative study of anaemia-related perceptions and practices among pregnant women in Mumbai, India. Midwifery.

58. Veena SR, Krishnaveni GV, Srinivasan K, Wills AK, Hill JC, et al. (2010) Infant feeding practice and childhood cognitive performance in South India. Archives of Disease in Childhood 95: 347–354.

59. Nichter M (1985) Drink boiled water: A cultural analysis of a health education message. Social Science & Medicine 21: 667–669.

60. Barnett S, Azad K, Barua S, Mridha M, Abrar M, et al. (2006) Maternal and newborn-care practices during pregnancy, childbirth, and the postnatal period: a comparison in three rural districts in Bangladesh. Journal of health, population, and nutrition 14: 394–402.

61. Rodrigues M, Patel V, Jaswal S, de Souza N (2003) Listening to mothers: qualitative studies on motherhood and depression from Goa, India. Social Science & Medicine 57: 1797–1806.

62. Kumar V, Mohanty S, Kumar A, Misra R, Santosham M, et al. (2008) Effect of community-based behaviour change management on neonatal mortality in Shivgarh, Uttar Pradesh, India: a cluster-randomised controlled trial. Lancet 372: 1151–1162.

7

A Systematic Review of Individual and Contextual Factors Affecting ART Initiation, Adherence, and Retention for HIV-Infected Pregnant and Postpartum Women

Ian Hodgson[1], Mary L. Plummer[2], Sarah N. Konopka[3]*, Christopher J. Colvin[4], Edna Jonas[3], Jennifer Albertini[5], Anouk Amzel[6], Karen P. Fogg[7]

1 Independent Consultant, Bingley, United Kingdom, 2 Independent Consultant, Dar es Salaam, Tanzania, 3 Center for Health Services, Management Sciences for Health, Arlington, Virginia, USA, 4 Centre for Infectious Disease Epidemiology and Research (CIDER), Division of Social and Behavioural Sciences, School of Public Health and Family Medicine, University of Cape Town, Cape Town, South Africa, 5 United States Agency for International Development (USAID)/Africa Bureau, Washington, D.C., USA, 6 USAID/Bureau for Global Health (BGH)/Office of HIV/AIDS, Washington, D.C., USA, 7 USAID/BGH/Office of Health, Infectious Diseases, and Nutrition, Washington, D.C., USA

Abstract

Background: Despite progress reducing maternal mortality, HIV-related maternal deaths remain high, accounting, for example, for up to 24 percent of all pregnancy-related deaths in sub-Saharan Africa. Antiretroviral therapy (ART) is effective in improving outcomes among HIV-infected pregnant and postpartum women, yet rates of initiation, adherence, and retention remain low. This systematic literature review synthesized evidence about individual and contextual factors affecting ART use among HIV-infected pregnant and postpartum women.

Methods: Searches were conducted for studies addressing the population (HIV-infected pregnant and postpartum women), intervention (ART), and outcomes of interest (initiation, adherence, and retention). Quantitative and qualitative studies published in English since January 2008 were included. Individual and contextual enablers and barriers to ART use were extracted and organized thematically within a framework of individual, interpersonal, community, and structural categories.

Results: Thirty-four studies were included in the review. Individual-level factors included both those within and outside a woman's awareness and control (e.g., commitment to child's health or age). Individual-level barriers included poor understanding of HIV, ART, and prevention of mother-to-child transmission, and difficulty managing practical demands of ART. At an interpersonal level, disclosure to a spouse and spousal involvement in treatment were associated with improved initiation, adherence, and retention. Fear of negative consequences was a barrier to disclosure. At a community level, stigma was a major barrier. Key structural barriers and enablers were related to health system use and engagement, including access to services and health worker attitudes.

Conclusions: To be successful, programs seeking to expand access to and continued use of ART by integrating maternal health and HIV services must identify and address the relevant barriers and enablers in their own context that are described in this review. Further research on this population, including those who drop out of or never access health services, is needed to inform effective implementation.

Editor: Marie-Louise Newell, University of Southampton, United Kingdom

Funding: This review was supported by funding from the Africa Bureau of USAID. Three coauthors on the paper are from USAID. They played a role in designing the review questions and methods, and contributed to revisions of the manuscript. They were not involved in data collection and analysis or drafting of the initial manuscript.

Competing Interests: The authors have declared that no competing interests exist.

* Email: skonopka@msh.org

Background

HIV is responsible for a large proportion of indirect maternal deaths in countries with high HIV prevalence [1–3]. New [1] analyses reveal that there is wide range in the estimated impact of HIV on pregnancy-related and maternal mortality from 24 percent of pregnancy-related deaths [4] to 6.4 percent of maternal deaths [5] in sub-Saharan Africa. Globally, estimates range from roughly 21 percent to 0.4 percent of maternal deaths [6] that are related to HIV. However, the impact of HIV on pregnancy and maternal mortality is substantial for countries with high HIV prevalence [7]. Hospital-based studies in Africa have shown relative risks of pregnancy-related death among HIV-infected women ranging from two to eight-times greater than in non-infected women [8]. There is also evidence of increased risk of direct obstetric complications, such as sepsis, among HIV-infected pregnant women [8,9].

In countries where HIV is highly prevalent, HIV infection is a leading cause of pregnancy-related deaths and has even reversed gains in reducing maternal mortality [2]. Many of these countries struggle to maintain adequate health system capacity to meet the associated service needs. Antiretroviral therapy (ART) is effective in reducing maternal mortality among HIV-infected women [10], but ART initiation, adherence, and retention in care remain problematically low in some regions, even when ART is available [11]. There is an urgent need to understand the factors affecting the uptake of this critical intervention in order to improve programming and extend the reach of services and supportive interventions to this population.

This review is one of three systematic reviews that together consider evidence around efforts to reduce mortality among HIV-infected pregnant and postpartum women. One review assesses the evidence on the effectiveness of interventions to decrease death and morbidity among HIV-infected women during pregnancy and up to one year postpartum [12]; another review examines the health system barriers and enablers to ART initiation, adherence, and retention and evidence on health system interventions that may facilitate access to maternal ART [13]. This current review synthesizes evidence on the individual and contextual barriers to and enablers of ART initiation, adherence, and retention among the same population. This systematic review was guided by the following question:

What are the individual and contextual factors affecting the initiation, adherence, and retention to ART among HIV-infected pregnant women during and following pregnancy?

Factors of interest include those individual, interpersonal, community, and structural forces which influence an HIV-infected woman's ability to initiate, adhere to, or be retained in ART care. Some health system factors identified in the other above-mentioned review are closely related to contextual factors identified in this review. We have included information on health systems factors if they capture the woman's perspectives on or experiences of health system issues.

Methodology

Review Design

We undertook a systematic review of both qualitative and quantitative evidence of individual and contextual factors that inhibit or enable access to and use of ART for HIV-infected pregnant and postpartum women. Study findings were analyzed thematically and we used a conceptual framework for data extraction and synthesis that was informed by the World Health Organization (WHO) health systems framework [14] and Supporting the Use of Research Evidence (SURE) framework [15].

Study Eligibility

Inclusion Criteria. To maximize the breadth of the study findings, we included any study that reported empirical qualitative or quantitative findings relevant to the review question. Studies from low- and middle-income countries (LMICs), as well as high-income countries, were included, as were studies conducted in community or health system settings. Due to time and resource constraints, we only included studies written in English. To maximize the relevance of the study findings to current maternal ART policy and practice, we only included studies published between January 1, 2008 and March 26, 2013.

Because this review was conducted in parallel with a separate but linked systematic review of health systems factors affecting ART initiation, adherence, and retention for pregnant and postpartum women [13], we only included studies that described health systems-related factors if these were described from the woman's perspective or experience. For example, long waiting times at health facilities are a contextual barrier from women's perspectives when they do not attend services because they do not believe they have enough time to wait. Long waiting times may also reflect broader supply-side issues within the health system, such as inefficient models of care or system-level resource constraints.

Exclusion Criteria. Studies were excluded if they focused on HIV-infected pregnant or postpartum women on ART and/or in PMTCT programs but did not identify individual or contextual barriers or enablers of ART initiation, adherence, or retention. We excluded studies that reported on relevant health systems barriers and enablers if there was no discussion of these factors from the perspective of pregnant women. We also excluded studies of broader cohorts of people with HIV (e.g., all adults on ART) if barriers and enablers specific to pregnant or postpartum women could not be distinguished in the findings.

Search Strategy and Selection Process

Search strategy. Both peer-reviewed journal articles and gray literature were searched to identify eligible studies. Peer-reviewed journal articles were searched systematically in the PubMed and Social Sciences Citation Index (SSCI) databases using variations of three key terms:

- Population of interest (i.e., pregnant women and postpartum women infected with HIV);
- Intervention of interest (i.e., ART);
- Outcomes of interest (i.e., initiation, adherence, retention).

A full search strategy for one of the database searches can be found in the Supporting Information. Gray literature was also searched on relevant conference abstract databases, multilateral and bilateral agency websites, and websites of non-governmental organizations (NGOs) conducting research or implementing programs of relevance. Articles and abstracts were excluded if they did not address the population, interventions or outcomes of interest.

Study selection. Studies were selected for review in two stages. First, three review authors independently assessed the first 100 abstracts retrieved from PubMed. Each reviewer's list of selected articles and accompanying rationale was compared with the list from the other reviewers; discrepancies were discussed and resolved. Inclusion and exclusion criteria were refined and clarified during this process. In the second step, one review author (SK) reviewed the remaining abstracts and included or excluded studies.

Quality Assessment and Data Extraction

Characterizing the evidence base. In order to assess the strength of the underlying evidence base for the review, we first developed an overview of key characteristics of the included studies by summarizing several variables, including study design, sample size and strategy, geographic region, healthcare setting, and risk of bias. We then ranked each included study as low, medium, or high with respect to overall risk of bias. Given the diversity of study designs included and the difficulty of comparing study quality assessments across widely varying study types, these rankings were based on criteria appropriate to each study design (e.g. different quality appraisal criteria were used for qualitative and quantitative studies). These rankings were further justified via short narratives. This provided an overview of the quality of the existing evidence base, as represented by the included studies. No studies were excluded on the basis of the quality assessment. Rather the quality assessment process was used to identify weaknesses in study methodologies and to guide the interpretation and assessment of study findings.

Data extraction and management. Once the study selection process was concluded, one review author (SK) extracted data from the studies using a standard template. Initial data extraction captured both the study characteristics (e.g., setting, participants, and type of ART program reviewed) as well as key findings related to factors associated with initiation, adherence, and retention of ART. A second author (IH) also reviewed the studies and extracted data relating to key individual and contextual barriers and enablers associated with initiation, adherence, and retention. Extracted findings from both authors were compared and discrepancies resolved.

Data Synthesis

The barriers and enablers identified were arranged thematically within a framework of individual, interpersonal, community, and structural categories [16]. These categories were further divided into enabling factors and barriers to ART adherence, e.g., knowledge about HIV or ART or wanting to protect one's child (individual-level enablers); domestic violence or spousal dependence (interpersonal-level barriers); stigma (community-level barrier); or health worker attitude or support group participation (structural-level enablers). This framework was reviewed by all review authors for accuracy and comprehensiveness.

The intention of the analysis process was to produce a detailed list of factors that have been reported as affecting the three ART outcomes of interest for pregnant and postpartum women, and to offer, when possible, brief explanations for how these factors might operate and in which contexts they were most salient. Given the diversity of disciplinary approaches, sociocultural contexts, study questions, and study designs in this review's included studies and the broad scope of the review question, it was not possible to develop the analysis of these factors further than a straightforward thematic analysis. The intention, therefore, is not to provide a rich explanatory model for how each of these factors might work, or to develop a global theory of barriers and enablers to maternal ART. Rather, the analysis is intended to provide policymakers and practitioners with a roadmap for how to think about, and where to look for, the factors that might shape pregnant and postpartum women's access to ART.

As a final step in the analysis process, we assessed our confidence in each of the "key review findings" by describing the strength and generalizability/transferability of the evidence supporting that finding. For each review finding, therefore, we looked back at the studies that contributed to that finding and considered: 1) how strong the underlying study design was, 2) what the risk of bias was, 3) what level of detail and/or context was provided to enable interpretation, and 4) how frequently the review finding was found across the individual studies. This approach is modeled on the CERQual approach to assessing the confidence in findings of qualitative systematic reviews [17]. We then ranked the strength of the evidence underlying each finding as high, moderate or low.

We were also interested in the generalizability or transferability–depending on whether we were considering quantitative or qualitative evidence–of the evidence with respect to public sector health services in low and middle-income countries with high HIV prevalence (where most of the global burden lies and where women and programs need the most support). The concept of 'transferability' is used in assessing qualitative research findings as a more appropriate alternative to the concept of 'generalizability' [18]. Transferability expresses the degree to which the study authors have provided contextual information and other forms of 'thick description' that allow the reader to determine to which other contexts particular findings might be transferable. For each key review finding, we therefore asked two additional questions: 5) how many of the studies supporting this finding were conducted within existing services settings, and 6) how many came from LMICs with high HIV prevalence. Here too, we ranked generalizability or transferability as high, moderate or low.

Findings on the strength and generalizability or transferability of review findings to high prevalence settings have been provided below along with a brief narrative justification for each. No studies were excluded based on the quality appraisals of the studies, but most studies used to illustrate core findings in the text were supported by strong evidence.

Results

Overview of Studies Included and ART Regimens

The results of the peer-reviewed journal article and gray literature search are summarized in the flow diagram in Figure 1. The peer-reviewed journal article search yielded 672 articles, of which 31 were included in the core review. A total of 1,487 grey literature documents were assessed, of which three were selected for inclusion in the review.

Thirty-four studies met the inclusion criteria for this review [19–52]. Table 1 provides a brief overview of the key characteristics of the included studies. A more detailed table is available in the Supporting Information that provides information on each of the studies reviewed, including each study's location, design, population size, type of ART program, and key findings related to initiation, adherence and retention during pregnancy and postpartum.

Twenty-seven of the studies were carried out in sub-Saharan Africa, one in Asia, two in Latin America, and four in Europe and the US. Sixteen studies used quantitative methods, twelve used qualitative methods and six employed both qualitative and quantitative methods. Most study participants were HIV-infected pregnant or postpartum women. Eight studies included data from interviews or focus group discussions with health care workers, community members, partners, and/or family members of HIV-infected pregnant and postpartum women.

Four studies described and evaluated interventions. These include: a study from Zambia exploring the benefits of couple counseling for initiation [32]; a study from South Africa describing the impact of text messaging on promoting positive health choices [52]; another study from South Africa describing the benefits of rapid ART initiation among pregnant women [44]; and a study from Malawi exploring the use of community health workers in promoting ART adherence [34].

There were a number of different prevention of mother-to-child transmission (PMTCT) and maternal ART regimens used in the included studies. Seven studies involved women who had initiated ART for therapeutic reasons before they enrolled in a PMTCT program. Twenty-one studies included participants not on ART who then enrolled in PMTCT programs, and examined factors

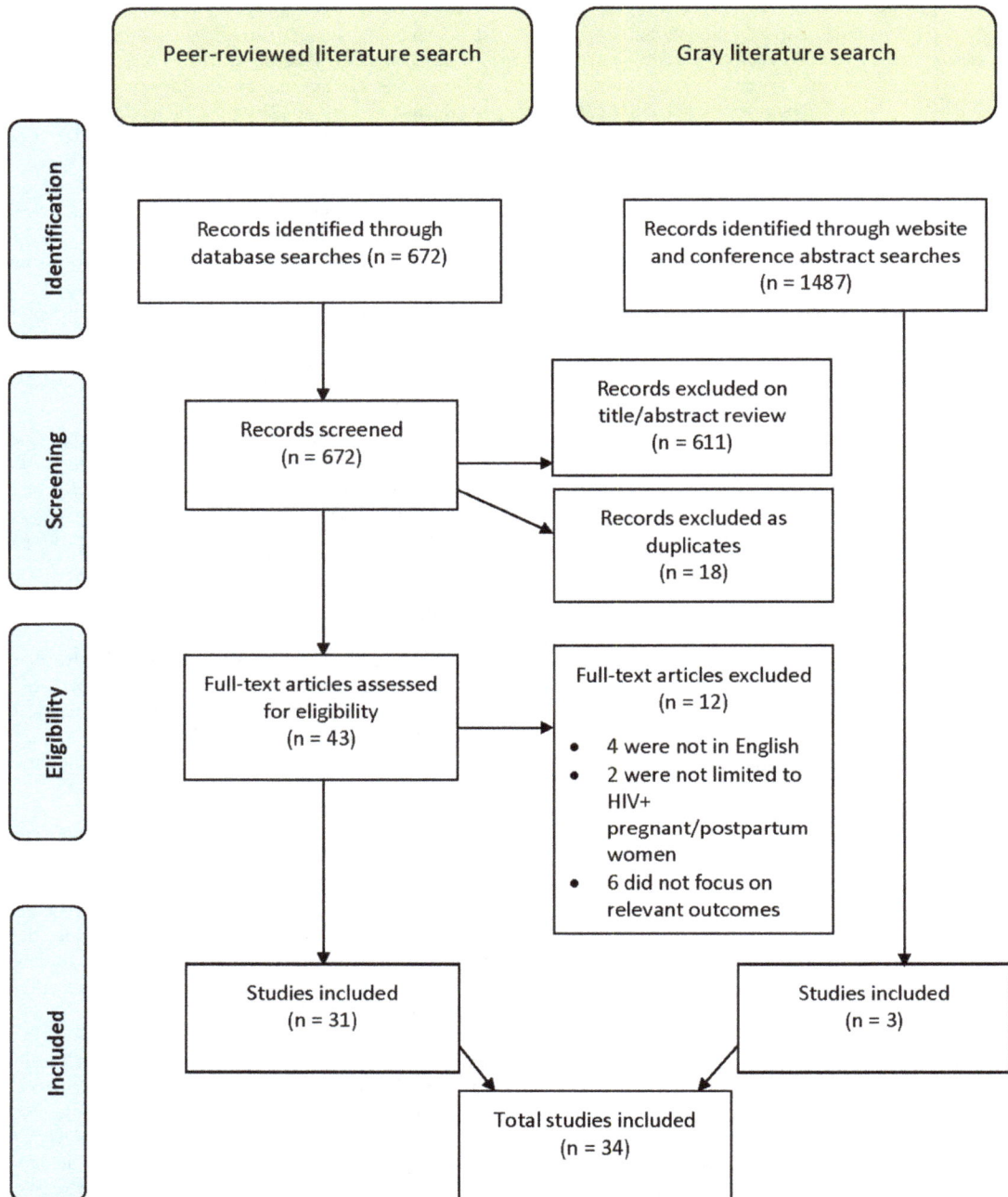

Figure 1. Flow Diagram for Study Search and Inclusion.

influencing ART initiation, adherence and/or retention during pregnancy and, depending on regimen, for a brief period thereafter. The regimens used in these studies included use of single-dose nevirapine (sdNVP), Option A, and Option B regimens (described in more detail in Table 2) [53–55].

Six studies involved women who were initiated on ART for therapeutic reasons after being enrolled in a PMTCT program. These women were eligible to initiate ART because of their advanced clinical disease and/or high CD4 count. All of the reviewed studies preceded the introduction of Option B+ (where all pregnant HIV-infected women are initiated/supported on lifelong ART regardless of WHO clinical stage and/or CD4

count). Thus, no reviewed studies examined ART initiation, adherence, or retention within an Option B+ program.

The one-time nature of the sdNVP-based PMTCT regimen means that it has only limited comparability to situations in which a woman might begin long-term or life-long ART during pregnancy. Papers reporting on sdNVP-based programs were excluded from the review unless they addressed barriers and enablers relevant to initiation, adherence or retention from the woman's point of view; seven such sdNVP-focused studies were included.

Table 1. Summary of Key Characteristics of Included Studies.

Characteristics	Number of studies
Regions	
Sub-Saharan Africa	27
Asia	1
Latin America	2
Europe/North America	4
Middle East	0
Geographic Setting	
Rural	6
Urban	12
Both	11
Unclear	5
HIV Prevalence Rates	
Low (0–5%)	9
Moderate (5–15%)	11
High (15% or higher)	14
Study Designs	
Quantitative methods	16
Qualitative methods	12
Mixed methods	6
Explicit Intervention Tested	
Yes	4
No	30

Overview of Barriers and Enablers Identified

Individual and contextual factors influencing ART initiation, adherence, and retention for pregnant and postpartum women were identified through qualitative participant reports, study author observations and interpretations, and quantitative measures of association reported in the studies. Data were extracted from both the findings sections of study reports as well as 'second-order' author interpretations of findings [56] in the discussion sections of papers.

Key barriers and enablers to ART initiation, adherence, and retention identified in the studies were categorized thematically within individual, interpersonal, community, and structural levels of influence. This approach to organising and understanding the factors shaping health practices, processes and outcomes is typically defined as the 'socio-ecological' approach [57–59]. While the findings have been divided into these four different levels of analysis, they are of course not all independent, and in fact many factors identified at one level may interact with other factors within and between levels (e.g., fear of stigma at the individual level and norms around non-disclosure at the community level).

An overview of the key identified factors is presented in Table 3. This table summarizes enablers and barriers separately, by the relevant outcome of interest. A more comprehensive table is available in the Supporting Information that provides the same information in more detail, showing the hierarchy of main themes and subcategories, and, for each finding, which studies contributed to the finding. The assessment of our confidence in these findings is provided in Table 4.

The findings extracted from the studies were identified with respect to which outcomes they related to (initiation, adherence, or retention), which region of the world they came from, the socioeconomic status of study participants, and whether they were from low or high prevalence settings. We used these characteristics to develop 'sub-groups' of the various findings, searching for example, for whether or not there were distinct variations in the barriers and enablers identified by region, or by type of outcome. In Table 3, and in the narrative findings below, we distinguish which specific findings applied to each of the three outcomes. We also make consistent reference in the narrative to the countries and world region(s) that contributed to particular findings.

Making further generalizations about patterns of findings within these sub-groups has been difficult, however, for several reasons. One is that the body of studies that contributed the most to the review findings are the studies that came from high-prevalence settings in Eastern and Southern Africa. A second challenge has been the fact that in most cases, findings are only supported by one, two, or three studies, making comparisons along various axes of region, prevalence, or outcome difficult. Finally, many of the studies provide little detailed context on the study setting and implementation process of the programs under review. Absent such context, it is difficult to develop confident explanations about how context (e.g. HIV prevalence or the SES of participants or the wealth of a particular country) might affect the finding in more precise ways.

Individual factors

Individual-level enablers and barriers to pregnant or postpartum women's ART initiation, adherence, and retention include those within a woman's awareness and control (e.g., commitment to a child's health), and those that may be outside of her awareness or control (e.g., where she lives or her level of knowledge about HIV, ART, or PMTCT).

Socio-demographic attributes. Age was associated with ART initiation, adherence and retention in several of the included studies, albeit in contrasting ways. Two studies, one from Tanzania and one from the US, found that younger women were less likely than older women to engage with the health system and/or adhere to ART [25,35]. In contrast, a multi-country study of long-term ART in Latin America found that non-adherence increased by six percent with each one-year increase in age. The study's authors posited that these findings might relate to the higher demands on older women living with HIV, particularly those with children under 18 [37].

Education was also noted as an important factor. Two studies from Kenya and one from the US found that women's education level was positively associated with ART adherence [20,21,36]. Ayuo et al. [20], in their Kenyan study of pregnant women initiating ART, reported that each additional year in school increased the likelihood of reporting perfect adherence by 10.6 percent. Similarly, a study in Rwanda found that women with lower education levels were less likely to participate in an sdNVP program. The study's authors posited that higher education levels contributed to better health literacy, which in turn promoted sdNVP program initiation and adherence [26].

Finally, two studies in Kenya found that rural residency was a barrier to ART initiation and adherence. In the first study, women enrolled in HIV care at a rural clinic were more likely to be lost to follow-up than women enrolled in similar care in a district hospital [20]. In the second study, a qualitative narrative analysis, HIV-infected pregnant women in rural settings were less likely to disclose their HIV status than urban women. The authors argued that these women, in striving to keep their status a secret, were more likely to miss clinic appointments, resulting in poor ART adherence [48].

Table 2. Antiretroviral medication regimens in included studies.

Regimen	Purpose: PMTCT Prophylaxis*	Purpose: Treatment for the Mother	Notes
Single-dose nevirapine (sdNVP)	One intrapartum dose taken at the beginning of a woman's labor	N/A	Introduced in 2000, this regimen is no longer recommended by WHO unless as part of combination PMTCT (Option A)
Option A	**For pregnant women living with HIV with CD4>350**	**For pregnant women with CD4 cells <350 or clinical Stage 3–4 disease**	
	(a) Antepartum: Antenatal zidovudine (AZT) twice daily starting as early as 14 weeks gestation	Triple antiretroviral medications (ARVs) often combined within a single pill (a "fixed dose combination") that is taken twice daily, starting as soon as diagnosed and continued for life	
	(b) Intrapartum: at onset of labor, sdNVP and AZT every 3 hours and lamivudine (3TC) every 12 hours until delivery		
	(c) Postpartum: twice daily AZT/3TC for 7 days		
Option B	Triple ARVs starting as early as 14 weeks gestation and continued intrapartum and through childbirth if not breastfeeding or until 1 week after cessation of breastfeeding	Triple ARVs starting as soon as diagnosed, continued for life	Under WHO's 2010 PMTCT ARV guidance, countries have the option to choose between two prophylaxis regimens for pregnant women living with HIV: Option A and Option B.
Option B+	Triple ARVs starting as soon as diagnosed, continued for life	Triple ARVs starting as soon as diagnosed, continued for life	Option B+ was conceived and implemented in Malawi in 2011. In April 2012, WHO released a programmatic update in which it urged countries to consider Option B and B+

*PMTCT prophylaxis refers to the use of ARV drugs solely for the purpose of reducing the risk of vertical transmission when a woman is not on standard ART for therapeutic reasons.

Knowledge of HIV, ART, PMTCT and the Health Services. In three studies in Uganda, South Africa, and Tanzania, a lack of knowledge about health services and/or ART was associated with poor ART adherence [41] or retention [27,50]. Similarly, three other studies in Kenya, Ghana, and South Africa found that sufficient knowledge of PMTCT facilitated ART initiation, adherence and/or retention during and after pregnancy [22,36,47]. For example, the Ghana study found that many study participants had a high level of essential HIV knowledge (e.g., routes of transmission; the role of ARVs in prolonging life), but that women with inadequate knowledge of PMTCT and ART were significantly more likely to be lost to follow-up [22].

Fears and Aspirations Related to HIV, ART and Motherhood. Several studies identified women's fears as barriers to ART initiation and/or adherence. For example, fear of losing a job or fear of being HIV-infected contributed to inaction and/or denial about one's HIV status. Some studies found that women feared HIV testing or the ARVs themselves, including a South African sdNVP study [47] and studies on ART in Tanzania and Malawi [23,50]. Two South African studies found women's unwillingness to commit to lifelong treatment as a barrier to ART initiation [43,47]. Furthermore, two studies from the US and Australia found that women feared ART would have a negative impact on their children [39,40].

The review of literature also found that women's desire to protect her health and her children's health could positively influence ART initiation, adherence, and retention. In a Nigerian study, an active desire to remain healthy and/or to protect one's child was an enabler of ART initiation and adherence [28]. A desire to protect one's children also motivated ART adherence

among women in a US study [40] and ART initiation among women in two South African studies [43,47].

Women's concerns about maintaining their status within their families sometimes led them to keep their HIV infection a secret, creating a barrier to initiation, adherence and retention. Some women in a Kenyan study felt that disclosure of their HIV status would undermine their roles as mothers and homemakers. This non-disclosure made ART initiation and adherence particularly challenging for the women during pregnancy, when elder women in their families make decisions about their health care [48]. Another Kenyan study found that women were reluctant to attend clinics for ART services because their visibility during long waiting times could reveal their HIV status and, in turn, enhance their risk of being stigmatized and perceived as incapable mothers [19].

Challenges to the Practical Demands of Treatment. Individuals experienced a wide variety of barriers to the day-to-day practical requirements of treatment adherence. These included difficulty remembering to take medication, misplacing medications, travel away from home, scheduling conflicts with work, and lack of regular access to food or water. Forgetting to take medication was reported in six studies, including an sdNVP study in Rwanda [26], and pregnancy and postpartum ART studies in Latin America, Nigeria, South Africa, and Tanzania [28,35,37,41]. Research in Zimbabwe found that being away from home and/or misplacing medicines impeded women's ART adherence [38], and similarly, a study in South Africa found that being away from home created a barrier when treatment was required [41].

Women also reported that scheduling challenges (e.g., due to work commitments) affected both adherence and retention,

Table 3. Summary of ART Enabler and Barrier Findings, by Level and Outcome of Interest.

Level	Initiation — Enabler	Initiation — Barrier	Adherence — Enabler	Adherence — Barrier	Retention — Enabler	Retention — Barrier
Individual	• Knowledge of PMTCT and referral process (higher) • Desire to protect child • Education level (higher)	• Age (lower) • Knowledge of PMTCT (lower) • Denial of HIV • Fear of job loss • Reluctance to start lifelong treatment • Forgetting medication • Scheduling problems • Feeling too healthy	• Age (higher) • Education level (higher) • Sufficient knowledge of PMTCT • Desire to remain healthy • Desire to protect child	• Age (lower) • Education level (lower) • Rural residency • HIV denial • Concern ART will harm child • Conflict with role as homemaker • Misplacing medication • Forgetting medication • Away from home • Lack of food/water/income • Religion • Use of drugs/alcohol	• Sufficient knowledge of PMTCT • Access to cell phone (text reminders/appointments) • Religion	• Poor knowledge of ART • HIV denial • Scheduling problems • Religion
Interpersonal	• Partner involved in care	• Dependence on or permission needed from partner • Non-disclosure to partner • Partner not involved in care • No support from family	• Disclosure to partner • Partner involved in care • Family support	• Dependence on or permission needed from partner • Fear of domestic violence after disclosure • No family support • Relatives 'stealing' ART pills	• Disclosure to partner • Partner not involved in care	• Dependence on or permission needed from partner • Fear of domestic violence after disclosure
Community		• Actual or anticipated stigma	• Disclosure without stigma	• Actual or anticipated stigma		• Actual or anticipated stigma
Structural	• Support group participation • Treatment support or counseling • Encouragement from a traditional birth attendant	• Low attendance at ANC • Negative health worker attitudes • Long queues at health center • Transportation problems	• Receiving other treatment (e.g., for tuberculosis) or vitamin supplements • Enrolment in ART pre-delivery	• Actual or anticipated breach of confidentiality in health center • Payment problems • Negative health worker attitudes • Long queues at health center • Medications not dispensed correctly • Transportation problems	• First pregnancy registration • Community health worker involvement • Successful completion of PMTCT pre-delivery • Enrolment in ART pre-delivery	• Late disengagement (within 30 days of delivery) • Low or late attendance at ANC • Negative health worker attitudes • Actual or anticipated breach of confidentiality • Long queues at health center • Transportation problems

Table 4. Strength of Evidence and Generalizability/Transferability of Key Review Findings to High Prevalence Contexts.

Level of Influence	Key Review Finding	Strength of Evidence Summary	Generalizability/Transferability Summary
Individual	1a) Socio-demographic factors (i.e., age, educational level, residency) can influence ART initiation, adherence, and retention.	**High** Eight papers reported a range of socio-demographic factors. Age and educational level were most widely reported as specific findings in papers with strong quantitative designs, specifically that older women, or those achieving a higher level of education, were more likely to adhere. Residency was reported in two papers – one quantitative (women in central hospitals were less likely to disengage than women in smaller and more remote hospitals), and one qualitative/descriptive, focusing on challenges in rural communities around maternal roles.	**Moderate** This finding was reported across a range of contexts, and is generalizable, although issues around maternal role may be context-based.
	1b) Level of knowledge about health services, ART, and/or PMTCT can affect ART initiation, adherence, and retention.	**Moderate** Six papers reported on the association between knowledge (of health services, or ART) and adherence. Mixed method and quantitative designs reported higher levels of knowledge correlating with adherence. One qualitative study based on focus group discussions and one paper derived from a conference abstract confirmed the other studies' findings. Knowledge of the referral process was only cited as an enabler in one mixed method paper.	**High** This finding was reported across a range of contexts, with no anomalies, and is likely to apply broadly, although evidence for knowledge of the referral process requires further exploration.
	1c) Women's fears and perceptions of treatment, and the desire to maintain their roles and status within families, can affect ART initiation, adherence, and retention.	**Moderate** Eleven papers reported on these issues. Qualitative and mixed method studies with strong designs reported that a woman's role in the family may conflict with her needs as a patient. A desire to protect children from HIV was reported in qualitative studies and one quantitative study, although the latter was only a second order interpretation.	**Moderate** Evidence relating to these factors was internally consistent within the review, although it did include second order interpretations. The particular forms these factors take are likely to be context-based.
	1d) Factors in a woman's daily life can affect ART initiation, adherence, and retention.	**High** Challenges managing the practical demands of ART were reported in 12 quantitative or mixed method papers, and included day-to-day demands or (in one mixed method paper) lack of access to water and/or food. Scheduling problems, or being away from home, were frequently reported barriers to adherence. All findings were of first order interpretation.	**Moderate** Evidence relating to these factors was internally consistent within the review, although the particular forms these factors take are likely to be context-based.
	1e) Beliefs (e.g., religious beliefs, feeling healthy, and having a positive outlook) can affect ART initiation, adherence, and retention.	**Moderate** Seven papers reported that individual beliefs affected initiation, adherence, and retention. The finding about feeling too well to attend HIV services was only a second order interpretation in one quantitative paper and a report by one respondent in a qualitative study. Feeling 'happy' was significant in one quantitative study. The positive role of religion was a strong finding in two papers, though one (quantitative) was a second order interpretation. Advice to use traditional medicines instead of ART was only cited as a barrier in only one mixed method study, but it was a core finding.	**Moderate** Evidence was reported across a range of contexts, confirming the relevance of the broad finding, but specific examples are likely to be context-dependent.
	1f) Behavioral factors can be key barriers to ART initiation, adherence, and retention.	**High** Behavioral factors influencing ART initiation, adherence, and retention were reported in eight papers. Three quantitative papers with strong designs reported use of alcohol or illegal drugs as barriers to adherence. Four quantitative studies, and one mixed method study, reported evidence that forgetting, or misplacing, medication was a barrier to adherence.	**High** This finding was reported across a wide range of contexts; the two essential components can be generalized.
Interpersonal	2a) Relationships with partners can have a substantial influence on ART initiation, adherence, and retention.	**High** This finding was reported across 14 studies, with quantitative and qualitative designs. Five of the papers also reported on issues around gender dynamics and six of the papers reported on the benefits of disclosure to a partner to adherence. One quantitative paper reported a significant and contrary finding that not disclosing HIV status to a partner enabled adherence, but this was not reported elsewhere.	**High** This broad finding was reported across a wide range of contexts, arguing for a high validity. The one finding that non-disclosure to a partner enabled adherence highlights how the nature of interpersonal influence may vary by context.

Table 4. Cont.

Level of Influence	Key Review Finding	Strength of Evidence Summary	Generalizability/Transferability Summary
	2b) Relationships within the family affect ART initiation, adherence, and retention.	**Moderate** This finding was reported in three qualitative papers and a mixed method study. Designs were robust and the evidence was descriptive in all four studies.	**Low** This finding was reported in a small number of largely descriptive papers.
Community	3) Stigma within a community can be a significant barrier to ART initiation, adherence, and retention.	**High** This finding was reported in 15 papers, almost all of which were based on qualitative studies. Data on stigma as a barrier typically came in the form of participant self-report. One quantitative study described self-disclosure as an enabler of access to HIV care and adherence to ART.	**High** This finding was reported across a wide range of contexts, especially studies in which women identified barriers to initiating, adhering to, or remaining on treatment.
Structural	4a) Higher participation in recommended health services leads to increased likelihood of ART initiation, adherence, and retention.	**Moderate** This was a core finding in six quantitative papers. Delivery in a health center was found to be an enabler in two studies, although one was derived from a conference abstract with limited detail. Two papers reported an association between ART adherence and receiving treatment (e.g., tuberculosis treatment or multivitamins) for other conditions.	**Moderate** This finding was reported across a range of contexts.
	4b) Logistical problems around access to services can be barriers to ART initiation, adherence, and retention.	**Moderate** Seven papers with a range of designs (i.e., four qualitative, two mixed method, and one quantitative) reported this finding. Transportation problems were described descriptively in four well-designed studies, and cost was reported as a limited finding in one quantitative study. Long queues at health facilities were report as barriers to initiation, adherence, and retention in four papers of differing methods.	**Moderate** This finding was reported across a range of contexts and designs. The finding is generalizable, though specific factors may be context-dependent.
	4c) Interactions with health workers are valued, and affect the quality of access, and likelihood of ART initiation, adherence, and retention.	**High** Seven studies reported that health worker attitudes influenced whether women initiated and adhered to ART. Qualitative studies with strong designs reported that women's perspective of beneficial interactions encouraging adherence. One quantitative paper proposed a second order interpretation that adherence is due to nurses taking opportunities to engage more effectively with patients. Positive interactions with doctors and traditional birth attendants were noted as enablers of ART initiation, adherence, and retention in two strong qualitative papers.	**Moderate** This finding was reported qualitatively across a range of contexts, suggesting strong context validity, and reasonable generalizability.

specifically for registration or ART visits in Nigeria and Zimbabwe and for support group meetings in South Africa [28,42,52]. Three studies in Kenya, Tanzania, and South Africa identified lack of food, water, or income as barriers to ART adherence; women were less likely to adhere to their medications when food was unavailable, because taking ART on an empty stomach often caused negative side effects [19,35,41].

Two studies in Africa, on the other hand, found that ART adherence among women was facilitated by the use of mobile phones and/or enrolment in a postnatal care program. Women in a South African study said they forgot to take ART medication because their phones were turned off, which the authors interpreted to mean that the women were using their phones for personal organization [41]. In Uganda, women were three times more likely to attend a six-week postnatal care appointment if they had provided a phone contact. The study's authors posited that such women were more open to being contacted by health personnel than women who did not provide a phone contact, and also might be more likely to accept entry into the medical care system and/or to have a good socioeconomic status that empowered them to make informed decisions [44].

Religious Beliefs. Religion was found to influence adherence and retention in three studies. In a quantitative study in Uganda, being Christian was found to be a predictor (through correlation) for ART adherence among women over 25 years of age [44]. Another quantitative study in Zimbabwe found that belonging to a religion that promoted the use of traditional herbs during pregnancy (i.e., not biomedical care) reduced visits to antenatal care (ANC) clinics and/or use of sdNVP [38]. Similarly, a mixed-method study from Ghana found that the use of alternative medicines and/or participation in overnight prayer camps contributed to ART interruption and loss to follow-up [22].

Alcohol and Substance Abuse. Alcohol and/or illicit drug use were barriers to ART adherence during and after pregnancy in two U.S. studies [21,25], and a multi-country Latin American study found tobacco use was negatively associated with adherence [37]. No studies from sub-Saharan Africa included these factors in their data.

Interpersonal Factors

Interpersonal barriers and enablers are those influenced by both the woman and other individuals in her life, such as her partner or family members. The review found that a woman's relationships within her immediate family could profoundly influence her ART initiation, adherence and retention. The degree of the impact of these factors often depended on the extent to which she had disclosed her status and the extent to which family members who knew her status supported her. Interpersonal findings specific to women's partners or spouses are discussed below, followed by findings related to other family members.

Spouse or partner. Eighteen studies highlighted the role and impact of a spouse/partner on ART initiation, adherence, and/or retention. This was one of the most widely reported findings across the reviewed studies. Studies in Rwanda, Uganda, and Malawi found that women often felt a need for their partners' permission to initiate, adhere to, and be retained in ART care [26,27,45]. In a rural Tanzanian study, women reported being dependent on their partners for transportation to health facilities, so consistent participation in an ART program was difficult if they had not disclosed their status [35]. Similarly, in Uganda, non-disclosure of HIV status to a partner was the second most commonly cited barrier to enrolling in a PMTCT program [27].

Many of these women explained that economic dependence on their husbands and/or fear of domestic violence inhibited them from disclosing their status [27]. Domestic violence - actual or anticipated - was also reported as a barrier to disclosure and ART adherence in a South African study [41].

Other studies in France, Kenya, South Africa, and Tanzania also found that non-disclosure of HIV infection to a spouse was a barrier to ART initiation and retention [29,30,47,50]. Three of these studies were qualitative and provided detailed insight into women's relationships with their husbands, and the influence of those relationships on ART interventions. For example, in the South African study, some women specifically asked to delay their ART enrolment because they needed more time (e.g., a week or a month) to disclose their HIV status to their partners [47]. Two quantitative studies in Zimbabwe and South Africa found strong associations between a woman disclosing her HIV status to a partner and taking sdNVP, as recommended, at the start of labor [38,46].

Several studies assessed the impact of a partner's involvement in a woman's HIV care. Partner involvement was indicated by factors such as knowledge that the woman had been referred to HIV treatment, accompanying her to health appointments, or participating in couples counselling. In Kenya and Zambia, studies identified partner involvement as an enabler of ART initiation. Similarly, in South Africa, partner involvement was identified as an enabler of ART adherence [32,36,46]. Findings for this factor in relation to retention were inconsistent in Malawi, however, where one study found lack of male involvement as a barrier to ART retention [23], and another found it as an enabler [34].

Family. Family members were cited as either important facilitating or inhibiting influences by different studies. A family's embrace of community norms around stigma (discussed in more detail below as a key community-level factor), and the consequent pressure to maintain role and status within families can lead women to keep HIV infection a secret, creating a barrier to ART initiation and adherence. This relates to the barrier created when decision making about the pregnant woman's health/health care is made by an elder female family member, as seen in a Kenyan study [48]. Another study from Malawi found that grandmothers strongly influenced pregnant women's choice of delivery, provider and location options (e.g., a traditional birth attendant at home)

[45]. This lack of autonomous maternal decision-making capacity appeared to restrict HIV-infected women's ability to adhere to ART and PMTCT protocols. Only one study reported broader family support as an enabler of adherence during pregnancy, by helping women more with domestic tasks at home and allowing them time to attend appointments [60].

Community Factors. This section addresses barriers and enablers of pregnant and postpartum women's ART initiation, adherence and retention at the community level. These factors relate to a woman's broader social network and context. Stigma and disclosure are the two critical community-level factors that appeared most frequently in the studies described below.

Stigma. Like spousal disclosure and support at the interpersonal level, stigma was one of the most widely reported influences on women's ART initiation, adherence and retention at the community level. In some cases, women's direct experience of stigma were barriers to successful ART outcomes, while in others, fear of anticipated stigma was a barrier for women who had not disclosed their HIV status publicly. Seven qualitative studies, two mixed-methods studies, and two quantitative studies reported stigma as a barrier.

Studies in Uganda, Malawi (two), South Africa, and Tanzania found that HIV-related stigma was a barrier to women's ART initiation and retention, or their use of sdNVP. Some women in these studies reported not initiating treatment because they feared others would learn of their HIV infection and blame or stigmatize them; some also feared their husbands would divorce them [23,45,49,50,61].

Similarly, other studies in Malawi, South Africa (three), Nigeria, Uganda, and Kenya reported that stigma inhibited ART adherence and, in one case, retention. Many women who had not disclosed their HIV status publicly feared there was insufficient confidentiality within health facilities; this fear contributed to women missing appointments and not participating in broader HIV services, such as patient support groups [24,28,41,43,44,48,52].

Disclosure. Studies in Zimbabwe and South Africa identified positive experiences with disclosure as enablers of ART adherence during pregnancy [38,46]. Specifically, women in the Zimbabwe study reported that disclosure to someone other than their spouse had been beneficial to their adherence [38]. The South African study similarly found that disclosure not resulting in stigmatization was positively associated with maternal ART adherence. A third study from Kenya found that having ART clinics separate from main hospital buildings reduced clinic attendance and ART adherence; women were concerned their HIV infection would be disclosed publicly by their attendance at the HIV-only sites [60].

Structural factors. Structural influences on a woman's ART initiation, adherence and retention are those within her broader environment (beyond the local community/social context) that are beyond her control and agency (e.g., organizational, economic, legal, and policy factors). The main structural barriers and enablers identified in this review relate to health system usage, access, and engagement. The studied reviewed rarely made mention of broader other barriers such as economic marginalization, gender norms or the legal and policy context. Most reference to these factors were made in relation to issues of health care access and use.

Access to health services. Difficulty obtaining or paying for transport to facilities was a barrier in studies from Uganda, Tanzania, Malawi, and South Africa [27,35,45,47,50]. No studies specifically highlighted the costs of services as a barrier to ART initiation, adherence or retention. However, authors of a Kenyan study speculated that the cost of HIV service registration may have contributed to some women not attending services or being lost to follow-up [29], while authors of a Nigerian study posited that the free nature of services was an enabler of adherence [28]. Additionally, several studies identified long queues and wait times as barriers to ART initiation, adherence, and retention in Kenya, Malawi, and Uganda, and Zimbabwe [24,27,42,60].

Use of health services. Several studies found that the more women participated in recommended health services, the more likely they were to initiate, adhere to and be retained in ART care. For example, studies in Tanzania and Kenya found that low antenatal care (ANC) attendance (i.e., less than three visits) was associated with lower rates of ART initiation and retention [29,50]. Interestingly, women who were pregnant for the first time were more likely to register at an HIV clinic than women who had been pregnant before–the authors speculated this might be because women tended to be more anxious about their own and the fetus' health during their first pregnancy [29]. In a Kenyan study, women who disengaged from HIV services in the 30 days before delivery (i.e. late disengagement) were more likely to be lost to follow up postpartum when compared to women who stayed until delivery [20].

Delivery at a health facility was associated with ART initiation in studies in Kenya and Rwanda [26,36]. The Rwandan study found that women delivering in health centers were more likely to have had two or more ANC visits, and to have received sdNVP at the onset of labor [26]. Although this study focused on sdNVP use, it was included in this review because it is indicative of the enabling effect of prior interaction with the health system. In the Kenyan study, women receiving treatment for other conditions (e.g., tuberculosis) were less likely to disengage from ART services, and those receiving PMTCT were more likely to register at an HIV clinic and to be retained in long-term HIV care [20].

Health worker attitudes. Eight studies reported that health workers' attitudes influenced women's initiation and adherence to ART. Studies in Brazil, Kenya, Malawi and South Africa found that negative health worker attitudes were barriers to ART initiation [29,31,33,49]. Studies from Australia, Malawi, Uganda, and South Africa found that negative attitudes were a barrier to both adherence and retention during and/or after pregnancy [27,39,45,47,49]. In these studies, negative provider attitudes were exemplified by health workers in Uganda who reportedly were uninterested or too busy to interact with women or provide them with medication [27], and by health workers in Malawi who reportedly shouted at women attending HIV services [45]. Studies in Kenya and Malawi found that women's concern that health workers would not maintain confidentiality also inhibited adherence or retention [24,60].

Positive, non-judgmental attitudes from health workers – described in a Brazilian study as "warmth" – were found to be an enabler for ART adherence [31]. A Malawian study found that traditional birth attendants (TBAs) were preferred over health workers because they were more accessible and positive towards women, underscoring the importance of ensuring respectful care in antenatal, maternity, postnatal and HIV services [45].

Discussion

Overview of Findings and Programmatic Implications

This review identified a range of individual, interpersonal, community, and structural factors that inhibit or facilitate HIV-infected pregnant and postpartum women's ART initiation and adherence. Only four of the 34 included studies described or evaluated an intervention. Thus, we are not able to make evidence-based recommendations for specific interventions to improve HIV-infected women's access to and use of prenatal and postpartum ART. However, the review's descriptive findings suggest broad areas of intervention needs for this population, and these are discussed below in the context of the general literature on ART adherence barriers, facilitators, and interventions.

Individual level factors. This review found that many studies reported barriers to ART initiation, adherence, and retention that were related to poor understanding of HIV, ART, and PMTCT. For example, some women believed they did not need to initiate ART because they felt too healthy or feared ART would harm the fetus. Other studies identified poor knowledge about how PMTCT worked as both a barrier to ART initiation and adherence as well as retention in care postpartum. These findings may be especially important going forward with the growing roll-out of Option B+, as increasing numbers of healthy-feeling women are initiated on ART [62].

This review did not set out to assess women's knowledge of HIV, ART and PMTCT and can therefore make no general findings about these levels of knowledge. The review can provide indirect evidence, however, that gaps in knowledge about HIV, ART and PMTCT continue to act as barriers to critical health services and highlight the need for improving the provision of information within and outside of health services. While it is disappointing that poor understanding of HIV still persists, this finding indicates a promising way forward, in that improving knowledge is generally considered one of the simplest and most straight-forward behavior change interventions [63].

Other common individual-level problems were forgetting to take ART, misplacing it, or not having access to it when traveling. Our findings indicate the women would benefit from support in developing routines and approaches for self-monitoring and remembering to take their medication. Such interventions should use locally available and culturally appropriate systems, such as intensive counseling within health facilities or strengthening community-based support systems (e.g., maximizing the discreet and convenient potential of mobile-phone text reminders or supporting home-based care providers who remind women to take and renew their medications and accompany them to appointments, as needed) [64–67]. The discipline, commitment, and coordination required for ART adherence over an extended period should not be underestimated.

Interpersonal level factors. Many studies reported on the crucial influence of husbands or partners, both positive and negative. Disclosure of HIV infection to a spouse and spousal involvement in a woman's treatment were both associated with improved initiation, adherence, and retention. However, multiple studies also reported that women were reluctant to disclose their HIV status to partners because they feared significant negative consequences. Importantly, it is not possible to know the direction of cause and effect in these findings. It is possible that women who choose to disclose to their partners already have positive and supportive relationships, in comparison to women who do not disclose, and that these positive relationships in themselves promote ART initiation, adherence, and retention. Alternatively, for some women, the process of disclosure itself (regardless of relationship quality) may be a critical factor in promoting ART initiation and/or adherence.

In either case, these findings highlight the importance of ART programs that focus on the continuum of care for women, acknowledge the role these relationships may have in ART initiation, adherence, and retention, and incorporate interventions that take into account the relevance of women's primary relationships. Maternal ART program staff can provide counseling for women who have not yet disclosed their status to their partners, communication skills exercises, couple counseling to help them to disclose, or practical strategies for ART adherence if they are unwilling or unable to disclose to their partners. Very few of the interventions identified in this review addressed the role of power and interpersonal relationships, reflecting a broader tendency among individual-level HIV interventions to focus on knowledge and planning skills [68].

Community level factors. At the community level, this review found the experience of stigma, or the fear of stigma, to be a substantial barrier to ART initiation, adherence and retention among pregnant and postpartum women. Other reviews have also found stigma to have a significant influence on ART initiation and adherence [69]. Basic misunderstandings about HIV and AIDS persist in much of the world; for example, UNAIDS' *2010 Global Report on the AIDS Epidemic* found that, in 15 of the 25 countries with the highest HIV prevalence rates, less than half of young people could answer five basic questions about HIV correctly [70]. Misunderstandings about the effectiveness and value of ART and PMTCT may contribute to community-level stigmatization of women who are discovered to be HIV-infected because they participate in ART programs. These findings highlight the need for intensive interventions focused on raising knowledge and awareness about the effectiveness and value of ART and PMTCT, and the harmful effects of stigma [71,72].

Structural level factors. This review's findings underscore the importance of HIV services providing intensive, targeted support tailored to the unique needs and circumstances of HIV-infected women during pregnancy. For effective ART initiation, adherence, and retention, women may need in-depth orientation and counseling sessions to ensure they fully comprehend the importance of ART, to help them through the process of disclosing their status to husbands/partners/families, and to strategize about how they can reliably take their medication [73,74].

HIV services ideally should be integrated with other maternal and child health services to maximize efficiency for the client, service delivery, and confidentiality (e.g., one-stop ANC and ART appointments). Integrated services would also support confidentiality and reduce fear of stigma among women who have not yet disclosed their status. Regardless of the specific program design of the maternal, child, and HIV health services in a particular context, however, this review also highlighted the critical role that health worker attitudes played in encouraging–or more often discouraging–access to and use of HIV services.

Are the pregnancy and postpartum periods unique?

Many of our findings related to ART initiation, adherence, and retention for HIV-infected pregnant and postpartum women are similar to those reported for people living with HIV (PLHIV) more broadly, including enablers such as social support [64,65] and barriers such as fear of disclosure and stigma, lack of knowledge about HIV and ART, or difficulty obtaining transportation to facilities [74,75]. In fact, the most urgent findings from this review–the continuing influence of stigma at both interpersonal and community levels, the surprising persistence in knowledge gaps, and the ongoing missteps and missed opportunities in the HIV-related health services–reflect long-standing challenges in ART programming for adults more generally.

A question arising from this recognition, however, is how individual and contextual barriers and enablers for pregnant and postpartum women might differ in important ways from those of the general population of PLHIV. While we did not directly compare findings between pregnant and non-pregnant women with HIV, the review suggests that some enablers may have a stronger influence on pregnant and postpartum women. For

example, pregnant women are more likely than others to visit health facilities regularly, which, under ideal circumstances, would promote ART initiation, adherence, and retention and relatively prompt care for other conditions. A recent assessment of the beneficial effect of pregnancy on presentation for HIV care found that non-pregnant women were twice as likely to present late when compared to pregnant women [76]. The studies in this review also identified ways in which pregnant women may receive special support from partners and other family members who assist them in domestic and other work activities. Concern for the health of the fetus may also facilitate or inhibit adherence to ART.

Some barriers to ART initiation, adherence, and retention may also be intensified for pregnant or postpartum women. Women in multiple studies reviewed reported increased demands or responsibilities due to their pregnancy, caring for an infant, and/or physical conditions post-delivery as barriers to adherence or retention in care [19,42,45,47]. Many women maintain their usual responsibilities with little assistance while pregnant. Pregnancy can be physically demanding and tiring, and there may be additional commitments to maintain, including regular health care appointments at distant facilities. This highlights a particular concern for pregnant women who only learn of their HIV infection when screened during pregnancy, and are then initiated on ART. These women must quickly adjust to being pregnant, being HIV-infected, and to a daily treatment regimen they will need to follow for the rest of their lives. Each of these changes may tax a woman emotionally and physically, and may be further exacerbated during the postpartum period, when she is both recovering from the delivery as well as breastfeeding and caring for an infant day and night. All of these conditions help suggest why barriers to ART initiation, adherence, and retention, common to many PLHIV, may become more pronounced for some women during pregnancy and postpartum.

Review limitations

The strengths of this review's design included its inclusive search strategy that ensured wide coverage, dual inclusion and data extraction, and iterative analysis. Limitations in the review design included its rapid pace, which prevented more exhaustive searches of the gray literature and inclusion of studies in languages other than English.

Given the diversity of the evidence base with respect to settings, ART/PMTCT program types and protocols, and study questions and designs, we have not been able to transform or interpret the data beyond the descriptive, thematic analysis presented above.

The diversity of evidence included here is a strength in terms of the richness it provides, but generalizability and transferability across contexts was limited by a range of factors. First, there was great variance in how adherence was defined and measured across the reviewed studies, limiting our ability to synthesize findings across studies (see Supporting Information for a table summarizing the outcome measures used in the included studies). Second, studies differed greatly in the range of ART regimens they evaluated, which also limited our ability to integrate and interpret findings, particularly since some ART barriers and enablers may be particular to specific regimens.

Third, many studies did not clearly distinguish between individual and contextual factors influencing ART initiation, adherence, and retention *during* pregnancy from those influencing *postpartum* ART adherence, a time when conditions for women are likely to be very different. Finally, many identified barriers and enablers may be regionally or culturally specific. While this may in general limit the transferability of the findings outside of sub-Saharan Africa–and in particular high-prevalence regions within

Southern Africa–it does potentially increase their transferability with this region, and possibly to regions with similar levels of HIV prevalence and health system challenges. A further threat to transferability of the contextually specific findings, however, is the fact that few of the articles provided rich enough detail to know when particular findings might be transferable to similar contexts.

Research agenda

This review has revealed several gaps in the existing evidence base, gaps that collectively point to what we argue should be key parts of the research agenda going forward. Perhaps the most important gap, and a critical focus of future research, is the women who do not appear in these studies–those who did not make it to antenatal care or HIV testing, or who dropped out along the maternal ART cascade. Much of the research we reviewed is focused on health systems issues and women's engagement with these systems. Consequently, we know a great deal more about who stayed in care and why than about those who never attended entered the system or who dropped out early [77]. None of the included studies examined the barriers that women who do not enter into care experience in accessing maternity services and initiating ART during pregnancy or postpartum. We need a great deal more research–and programming–aimed at understanding and supporting such women. Loss-to-follow-up is particularly likely to happen postpartum [40], which suggests this is an area that also needs increased attention as Option B+ is scaled up.

There is also limited examination of health beliefs in the literature. Alternative treatment-seeking, particularly for traditional medicine, is widely practiced in many countries with high HIV prevalence [78], but these choices were minimally addressed within the reviewed studies. This likely reflects the number of studies that took place within the health system, and highlights the need for community-based research focused on how alternative health-seeking behaviors may intersect with ART initiation, adherence, and retention among pregnant and postpartum women. Similarly, our understanding of how interpersonal and community-level factors operate would benefit from more research examining the impact of HIV and treatment on women's aspirations and expectations, their roles and status within families, and the broader social dynamics in relation to pregnancy and HIV.

Finally, this review highlighted a critical methodological gap and area for future improvement–the need for meaningful, standardized ART adherence and retention performance indicators within programs and research. Measuring ART adherence and retention is critical for PLHIV care and treatment and broader efforts to minimize ART resistance, but collecting valid data on these outcomes is not straightforward. Adherence measures based on dispensing and appointment-keeping data are increasingly being implemented within health systems [79], but measures which assess adherence behaviors more broadly among PLHIV vary widely. There are also important questions to answer, however, with respect to how valid adherence measures for pregnant and postpartum women may differ from standard appointment-based measures in the short-term, given pregnant women's unique schedule of contact with the health system during pregnancy and postpartum. Finally, very few of the studies measured adherence or retention measures in the long-term and provided little guidance on how and why women may cycle through periods of better and worse adherence or even drop in and out of care episodically. Our understanding of pregnant and postpartum women's access to and use of ART would benefit greatly from research that used consistent, standardized, and appropriate measures of adherence and retention that had a longitudinal component.

Conclusion

The potential of antiretroviral therapy to prevent avoidable maternal deaths among HIV-infected women is great. The success of this strategy, however, will depend on careful consideration of the barriers and enablers to pregnant and postpartum women's access to and use of ART. Managing these barriers and enhancing known enablers will require the development of respectful and locally acceptable HIV and ANC service delivery models that are responsive to women's needs and perspectives, and support them as they enter and move through the maternal ART cascade. It will also require better understanding the ways women's lives outside of the clinic affect their chances of entering into, and staying adherent to and retained in care.

This review of individual and contextual factors, along with the two companion reviews which assess the evidence on the effectiveness of interventions to decrease death and morbidity among HIV-infected pregnant and postpartum women [12] and examine the health system barriers and enablers to ART initiation, adherence, and retention among this group [13], point to strategies that may be effective in expanding the reach of ART. Translating this evidence into practice is critical for keeping pregnant women and mothers alive and preventing new HIV infections among their children as we endeavor to achieve the global goals of an AIDS-Free generation and ending preventable child and maternal deaths.

Acknowledgments

We would like to thank Thomas Finkbeiner, Katharina Hermann, John Chalker, Sara Holtz, Erik Schouten and Manana Gagua for their input into earlier versions of this review as part of their work on the team developing three systematic reviews on HIV and maternal mortality. We would also like to thank Sylvia Alford, Allisyn Moran, and Marta Levitt at the United States Agency for International Development (USAID) for their input into earlier drafts and during the review process. This publication was produced for USAID by the African Strategies for Health Project at Management Sciences for Health with support from the USAID/Africa Bureau. The authors' views expressed in this publication do not necessarily reflect the views of the United States Agency for International Development or the United States Government.

Author Contributions

Conceived and designed the experiments: IH MLP SNK CJC EJ JA AA KF. Analyzed the data: IH SNK CJC. Contributed reagents/materials/analysis tools: IH MLP SNK CJC EJ. Wrote the paper: IH MLP CJC SNK. Conducted the search and screening/inclusion process: SNK. Conducted the data extraction: SNK IH CJC. Contributed to the revision process: IH MLP SNK CJC EJ JA AA KF.

References

1. Abdool-Karim Q, Abouzahr C, Dehne K, Mangiaterra V, Moodley J, et al. (2010) HIV and maternal mortality: turning the tide. Lancet 375: 1948–1949.

2. Hogan MC, Foreman KJ, Naghavi M, Ahn SY, Wang M, et al. (2010) Maternal mortality for 181 countries, 1980–2008: a systematic analysis of progress towards Millennium Development Goal 5. Lancet 375: 1609–1623.

3. WHO UNICEF, UNFPA, World Bank (2010) Trends in Maternal Mortality: 1990 to 2008. Geneva: World Health Organisation.

4. Zaba B, Calvert C, Marston M, Isingo R, Nakiyingi-Miiro J, et al. (2013) Effect of HIV infection on pregnancy-related mortality in sub-Saharan Africa: secondary analyses of pooled community-based data from the network for Analysing Longitudinal Population-based HIV/AIDS data on Africa (ALPHA). Lancet 381: 1763–1771.

5. Say L, Chou D, Gemmill A, Tuncalp O, Moller AB, et al. (2014) Global causes of maternal death: a WHO systematic analysis. Lancet Glob Health 2: e323–333.

6. Lozano R, Wang H, Foreman KJ, Rajaratnam JK, Naghavi M, et al. (2011) Progress towards Millennium Development Goals 4 and 5 on maternal and child mortality: an updated systematic analysis. Lancet 378: 1139–1165.

7. WHO UNICEF, UNFPA, World Bank, United Nations Population Division (2014) Trends in Maternal Mortality: 1990 to 2013. Geneva, Switzerland: World Health Organisation.

8. Calvert C, Ronsmans C (2013) The contribution of HIV to pregnancy-related mortality: a systematic review and meta-analysis. Aids.

9. McIntyre J (2003) Mothers infected with HIV: Reducing maternal death and disability during pregnancy. British Medical Bulletin 67: 127–135.

10. Liotta G, Mancinelli S, Nielsen-Saines K, Gennaro E, Scarcella P, et al. (2013) Reduction of maternal mortality with highly active antiretroviral therapy in a large cohort of HIV-infected pregnant women in Malawi and Mozambique. PLoS One 8: e71653.

11. Hoffman RM, Black V, Technau K, van der Merwe KJ, Currier J, et al. (2010) Effects of highly active antiretroviral therapy duration and regimen on risk for mother-to-child transmission of HIV in Johannesburg, South Africa. J Acquir Immune Defic Syndr 54: 35–41.

12. Thetard R, Holtz S, Gagua M, Jonas E, Albertini J (2014) A Systematic Review of Interventions to Reduce Mortality among HIV-Infected Pregnant and Postpartum Women. Submitted for publication.

13. Colvin C, Konopka S, Chalker J, Jonas E, Albertini J (in press) A Systematic Review of Health System Barriers and Enablers for Antiretroviral Therapy (ART) for HIV-Infected Pregnant and Postpartum Women. PLoS ONE.

14. WHO (2007) Everybody's Business: Strengthening Health Systems to Improve Health Outcomes. Geneva: World Health Organization.

15. SURE Collaboration (2011) Identifying and addressing barriers to implementing policy options. Version 2.1. Geneva: World Health Organization.

16. Coates TJ, Richter L, Caceres C (2008) Behavioural strategies to reduce HIV transmission: how to make them work better. Lancet 372: 669–684.

17. Lewin S, Glenton C, Noyes J, Hendry M, Rashidian A (2013) CerQual approach: Assessing how much certainty to place in findings from qualitative evidence syntheses. 21st Cochrane Colloquium. Quebec, Canada.

18. Lincoln YS, Guba EG (1985) Naturalistic inquiry. Beverly Hills, Calif.: Sage Publications. 416 p.

19. Awiti Ujiji O, Ekström AM, Ilako F, Indalo D, Wamalwa D, et al. (2011) 'Keeping healthy in the backseat': How motherhood interrupted HIV treatment in recently delivered women in Kenya. African Journal of AIDS Research 10: 157–163.

20. Ayuo P, Musick B, Liu H, Braitstein P, Nyandiko W, et al. (2013) Frequency and factors associated with adherence to and completion of combination antiretroviral therapy for prevention of mother to child transmission in western Kenya. J Int AIDS Soc 16: 17994.

21. Bardeguez AD, Lindsey JC, Shannon M, Tuomala RE, Cohn SE, et al. (2008) Adherence to Antiretrovirals Among US Women During and After Pregnancy. JAIDS Journal of Acquired Immune Deficiency Syndromes 48: 408–417 410.1097/QAI.1090b1013e31817bbe31880.

22. Boateng D, Kwapong GD, Agyei-Baffour P (2013) Knowledge, perception about antiretroviral therapy (ART) and prevention of mother-to-child-transmission (PMTCT) and adherence to ART among HIV positive women in the Ashanti Region, Ghana: a cross-sectional study. BMC Womens Health 13: 8.

23. Bwirire LD, Fitzgerald M, Zachariah R, Chikafa V, Massaquoi M, et al. (2008) Reasons for loss to follow-up among mothers registered in a prevention-of-mother-to-child transmission program in rural Malawi. Transactions of the Royal Society of Tropical Medicine and Hygiene 102: 1195–1200.

24. Chinkonde JR, Sundby J, Martinson F (2009) The prevention of mother-to-child HIV transmission programme in Lilongwe, Malawi: why do so many women drop out. Reprod Health Matters 17: 143–151.

25. Cohn SE, Umbleja T, Mrus J, Bardeguez AD, Andersen JW, et al. (2008) Prior illicit drug use and missed prenatal vitamins predict nonadherence to antiretroviral therapy in pregnancy: adherence analysis A5084. Aids Patient Care and Stds 22: 29–40.

26. Delvaux T, Elul B, Ndagije F, Munyana E, Roberfroid D, et al. (2009) Determinants of Nonadherence to a Single-Dose Nevirapine Regimen for the Prevention of Mother-to-Child HIV Transmission in Rwanda. JAIDS Journal of

Acquired Immune Deficiency Syndromes 50: 223–230 210.1097/QAI.1090-b1013e31819001a31819003.

27. Duff P, Kipp W, Wild TC, Rubaale T, Okech-Ojony J (2010) Barriers to accessing highly active antiretroviral therapy by HIV-positive women attending an antenatal clinic in a regional hospital in western Uganda. J Int AIDS Soc 13: 37.

28. Ekama SO, Herbertson EC, Addeh EJ, Gab-Okafor CV, Onwujekwe DI, et al. (2012) Pattern and Determinants of Antiretroviral Drug Adherence among Nigerian Pregnant Women. Journal Of Pregnancy 2012: 851810–851810.

29. Ferguson L, Lewis J, Grant AD, Watson-Jones D, Vusha S, et al. (2012) Patient Attrition Between Diagnosis With HIV in Pregnancy-Related Services and Long-Term HIV Care and Treatment Services in Kenya: A Retrospective Study. Jaids-Journal of Acquired Immune Deficiency Syndromes 60: E90-E97.

30. Jasseron C, Mandelbrot L, Dollfus C, Trocmé N, Tubiana R, et al. (2013) Non-Disclosure of a Pregnant Woman's HIV Status to Her Partner is Associated with Non-Optimal Prevention of Mother-to-Child Transmission. Aids and Behavior 17: 488–497.

31. Jerome JS, Galvao MTG, Lindau ST (2011) Brazilian mothers with HIV: experiences with diagnosis and treatment in a human rights based health care system. Aids Care-Psychological and Socio-Medical Aspects of Aids/Hiv 24: 491–495.

32. Kanjipite W, Nikisi J, Chilila M, Shasulwe H, Banda J, et al. (2012) Couple counseling increases antiretroviral (ARV) uptake by pregnant women: a case report in Zambia Defense Force health facilities. Journal of the International AIDS Society 2012, 15 (Suppl 3) 15: 132.

33. Kasenga F (2010) Making it happen: prevention of mother to child transmission of HIV in rural Malawi. Glob Health Action 3.

34. Kim MH, Ahmed S, Buck WC, Preidis GA, Hosseinipour MC, et al. (2012) The Tingathe programme: a pilot intervention using community health workers to create a continuum of care in the prevention of mother to child transmission of HIV (PMTCT) cascade of services in Malawi. J Int AIDS Soc 15 Suppl 2: 17389.

35. Kirsten I, Sewangi J, Kunz A, Dugange F, Ziske J, et al. (2011) Adherence to Combination Prophylaxis for Prevention of Mother-to-Child-Transmission of HIV in Tanzania. PLoS ONE 6: e21020.

36. Kohler P, Okanda J, Kinuthia J, Olilo G, Odhiambo F, et al. (2012) Social and structural barriers to uptake of PMTCT in Nyanza province, Kenya - a community-based survey. Journal of the International AIDS Society 15: 131.

37. Kreitchmann R, Harris DR, Kakehasi F, Haberer JE, Cahn P, et al. (2012) Antiretroviral adherence during pregnancy and postpartum in Latin America. AIDS Patient Care STDS 26: 486–495.

38. Kuonza L, Tshuma C, Shambira G, Tshimanga M (2010) Non-adherence to the single dose nevirapine regimen for the prevention of mother-to-child transmission of HIV in Bindura town, Zimbabwe: a cross-sectional analytic study. BMC Public Health 10: 218.

39. McDonald K, Kirkman M (2011) HIV-positive women in Australia explain their use and non-use of antiretroviral therapy in preventing mother-to-child transmission. Aids Care-Psychological and Socio-Medical Aspects of Aids/Hiv 23: 578–584.

40. Mellins CA, Chu C, Malee K, Allison S, Smith R, et al. (2008) Adherence to antiretroviral treatment among pregnant and postpartum HIV-infected women. Aids Care-Psychological and Socio-Medical Aspects of Aids/Hiv 20: 958–968.

41. Mepham S, Zondi Z, Mbuyazi A, Mkhwanazi N, Newell ML (2011) Challenges in PMTCT antiretroviral adherence in northern KwaZulu-Natal, South Africa. Aids Care-Psychological and Socio-Medical Aspects of Aids/Hiv 23: 741–747.

42. Muchedzi A, Chandisarewa W, Keatinge J, Stranix-Chibanda L, Woelk G, et al. (2010) Factors associated with access to HIV care and treatment in a prevention of mother to child transmission programme in urban Zimbabwe. J Int AIDS Soc 13: 38.

43. Myer L, Zulliger R, Black S, Pienaar D, Bekker LG (2012) Pilot programme for the rapid initiation of antiretroviral therapy in pregnancy in Cape Town, South Africa. Aids Care-Psychological and Socio-Medical Aspects of Aids/Hiv 24: 986–992.

44. Nassali M, Nakanjako D, Kyabayinze D, Beyeza J, Okoth A, et al. (2009) Access to HIV/AIDS care for mothers and children in sub-Saharan Africa: adherence to the postnatal PMTCT program. Aids Care-Psychological and Socio-Medical Aspects of Aids/Hiv 21: 1124–1131.

45. O'Gorman DA, Nyirenda LJ, Theobald SJ (2010) Prevention of mother-to-child transmission of HIV infection: views and perceptions about swallowing nevirapine in rural Lilongwe, Malawi. BMC Public Health 10: 354.

46. Peltzer K, Sikwane E, Majaja M (2011) Factors associated with short-course antiretroviral prophylaxis (dual therapy) adherence for PMTCT in Nkangala district, South Africa. Acta Paediatrica 100: 1253–1257.

47. Stinson K, Myer L (2012) Barriers to initiating antiretroviral therapy during pregnancy: a qualitative study of women attending services in Cape Town, South Africa. Ajar-African Journal of Aids Research 11: 65–73.

48. Ujiji OA, Ekström AM, Ilako F, Indalo D, Wamalwa D, et al. (2011) Reasoning and deciding PMTCT-adherence during pregnancy among women living with HIV in Kenya. Culture, health & sexuality 13: 829–840.

49. Varga C, Brookes H (2008) Factors influencing teen mothers' enrollment and participation in prevention of mother-to-child HIV transmission services in Limpopo Province, South Africa. Qual Health Res 18: 786–802.

50. Watson-Jones D, Balira R, Ross DA, Weiss HA, Mabey D (2012) Missed opportunities: poor linkage into ongoing care for HIV-positive pregnant women in Mwanza, Tanzania. PLoS One 7: e40091.

51. Aziz SA, Mubiru D, Rose N (2011) Acceptability of short-course AZT prevention regimen by HIV-infected pregnant women: Should VCT in the antenatal setting be modified? Sex Transm Infect 87: A356.

52. Dean AL, Makin JD, Kydd AS, Biriotti M, Forsyth BW (2012) A pilot study using interactive SMS support groups to prevent mother-to-child HIV transmission in South Africa. J Telemed Telecare 18: 399–403.

53. WHO (2010) Antiretroviral drugs for treating pregnant women and preventing HIV infection in infants: towards universal access. Geneva, Switzerland: WHO.

54. WHO (2012) Programmatic Update: Use of Antiretroviral Drugs for Treating Pregnant Women and Preventing HIV Infection in Infants. Geneva, Switzerland: WHO.

55. UNICEF (2012) Options B and B+: Key Considerations for Countries to Implement an Equity-Focused Approach. Geneva, Switzerland: UNICEF.

56. Schutz A (1962) Collected papers, Volume 1. The Hague: Martinus Nijhoff.

57. McLeroy KR, Bibeau D, Steckler A, Glanz K (1988) An ecological perspective on health promotion programs. Health Educ Q 15: 351–377.

58. Sword W (1999) A socio-ecological approach to understanding barriers to prenatal care for women of low income. J Adv Nurs 29: 1170–1177.

59. Richard L, Gauvin L, Raine K (2011) Ecological models revisited: their uses and evolution in health promotion over two decades. Annu Rev Public Health 32: 307–326.

60. Awiti Ujiji O (2011) Reasoning and deciding PMTCT-adherence during pregnancy among women living with HIV in Kenya. Culture, health & sexuality 13: 829–840.

61. Duff P, Kipp W, Wild TC, Rubaale T, Okech-Ojony J (2010) Barriers to accessing highly active antiretroviral therapy by HIV-positive women attending an antenatal clinic in a regional hospital in western Uganda. J Int AIDS Soc. England. 37.

62. Coutsoudis A, Goga A, Desmond C, Barron P, Black V, et al. (2013) Is Option B+ the best choice? Lancet 381: 269–271.

63. Bandura A (2004) Health promotion by social cognitive means. Health Educ Behav 31: 143–164.

64. Barnighausen T, Chaiyachati K, Chimbindi N, Peoples A, Haberer J, et al. (2011) Interventions to increase antiretroviral adherence in sub-Saharan Africa: a systematic review of evaluation studies. Lancet Infectious Diseases 11: 942–951.

65. Kenya S, Chida N, Symes S, Shor-Posner G (2011) Can community health workers improve adherence to highly active antiretroviral therapy in the USA? A review of the literature. Hiv Medicine 12: 525–534.

66. Pellowski JA, Kalichman SC (2012) Recent advances (2011–2012) in technology-delivered interventions for people living with HIV. Curr HIV/AIDS Rep 9: 326–334.

67. Wise J, Operario D (2008) Use of electronic reminder devices to improve adherence to antiretroviral therapy: a systematic review. AIDS Patient Care STDS 22: 495–504.

68. Burton J, Darbes LA, Operario D (2010) Couples-focused behavioral interventions for prevention of HIV: systematic review of the state of evidence. Aids and Behavior 14: 1–10.

69. Turan JM, Hatcher AH, Medema-Wijnveen J, Onono M, Miller S, et al. (2012) The role of HIV-related stigma in utilization of skilled childbirth services in rural Kenya: a prospective mixed-methods study. PLoS Med 9: e1001295.

70. UNAIDS (2010) UNAIDS Report on the Global AIDS Epidemic. Geneva: UNAIDS.

71. Sengupta S, Banks B, Jonas D, Miles MS, Smith GC (2011) HIV interventions to reduce HIV/AIDS stigma: a systematic review. Aids and Behavior 15: 1075–1087.

72. Skevington SM, Sovetkina EC, Gillison FB (2013) A systematic review to quantitatively evaluate 'Stepping Stones': a participatory community-based HIV/AIDS prevention intervention. Aids and Behavior 17: 1025–1039.

73. Finocchario-Kessler S, Catley D, Thomson D, Bradley-Ewing A, Berkley-Patton J, et al. (2012) Patient communication tools to enhance ART adherence counseling in low and high resource settings. Patient Educ Couns 89: 163–170.

74. Higa DH, Marks G, Crepaz N, Liau A, Lyles CM (2012) Interventions to improve retention in HIV primary care: a systematic review of U.S. studies. Curr HIV/AIDS Rep 9: 313–325.

75. Rosen S, Ketlhapile M (2010) Cost of using a patient tracer to reduce loss to follow-up and ascertain patient status in a large antiretroviral therapy program in Johannesburg, South Africa. Tropical Medicine & International Health 15 Suppl 1: 98–104.

76. Dourado I, MacCarthy S, Lima C, Veras M, Kerr L, et al. (2014) What's pregnancy got to do with it? Late presentation to HIV/AIDS services in Northeastern Brazil. AIDS Care epub ahead of print.

77. Moodley J, Pattinson RC, Baxter C, Sibeko S, Abdool Karim Q (2011) Strengthening HIV services for pregnant women: an opportunity to reduce maternal mortality rates in Southern Africa/sub-Saharan Africa. BJOG 118: 219–225.

78. Peltzer K (2009) Utilization and practice of traditional/complementary/alternative medicine (TM/CAM) in South Africa. Afr J Tradit Complement Altern Med 6: 175–185.

79. Chalker J, Wagner A, Tomson G, Laing R, Johnson K, et al. (2010) Urgent need for coordination in adopting standardized antiretroviral adherence performance indicators. J Acquir Immune Defic Syndr 53: 159–161.

8

Missed Opportunities for Early Access to Care of HIV-Infected Infants in Burkina Faso

Malik Coulibaly[1]*, Nicolas Meda[1,2], Caroline Yonaba[3], Sylvie Ouedraogo[4], Malika Congo[5], Mamoudou Barry[6], Elisabeth Thio[1], Issa Siribié[1], Fla Koueta[4], Diarra Ye[4], Ludovic Kam[3], Stéphane Blanche[7], Phillipe Van De Perre[8], Valériane Leroy[9], for the MONOD Study Group ANRS 12206[¶]

1 Projet MONOD ANRS 12206, Centre de Recherche Internationale pour la Santé, Site ANRS Burkina, Université de Ouagadougou, Ouagadougou, Burkina Faso, 2 Centre Muraz, Bobo Dioulasso, Burkina Faso, 3 Service de Pédiatrie, CHU Yalgado Ouédraogo, Ouagadougou, Burkina Faso, 4 Service de Pédiatrie Médicale, CHU Charles de Gaulle, Ouagadougou, Burkina Faso, 5 Laboratoire de Bactériologie - Virologie CHU Yalgado Ouédraogo, Ouagadougou, Burkina Faso, 6 Service de laboratoire, CHU Charles de Gaulle, Ouagadougou, Burkina Faso, 7 Groupe hospitalier Necker- Enfants malades, Paris, France, 8 Inserm U1058, Université Montpellier 1, Montpellier, France, 9 Inserm, U897, Institut de Santé Publique, Epidémiologie et Développement (ISPED), Université de Bordeaux, Bordeaux, France

Abstract

Objective: The World Health Organization (WHO) has recommended a universal antiretroviral therapy (ART) for all HIV-infected children before the age of two since 2010, but this implies an early identification of these infants. We described the Prevention of Mother-to-Child HIV Transmission (PMTCT) cascade, the staffing and the quality of infrastructures in pediatric HIV care facilities, in Ouagadougou, Burkina Faso.

Methods: We conducted a cross-sectional survey in 2011 in all health care facilities involved in PMTCT and pediatric HIV care in Ouagadougou. We assessed them according to their coverage in pediatric HIV care and WHO standards, through a desk review of medical registers and a semi-structured questionnaire administered to health-care workers (HCW).

Results: In 2011, there was no offer of care in primary health care facilities for HIV-infected children in Ouagadougou. Six district hospitals and two university hospitals provided pediatric HIV care. Among the 67 592 pregnant women attending antenatal clinics in 2011, 85.9% were tested for HIV. The prevalence of HIV was 1.8% (95% Confidence Interval: 1.7%–1.9%). Among the 1 064 HIV-infected pregnant women attending antenatal clinics, 41.4% received a mother-to-child HIV transmission prevention intervention. Among the HIV-exposed infants, 313 (29.4%) had an early infant HIV test, and 306 (97.8%) of these infants tested received their result within a four-month period. Among the 40 children initially tested HIV-infected, 33 (82.5%) were referred to a health care facility, 3 (9.0%) were false positive, and 27 (90.0%) were initiated on ART. Although health care facilities were adequately supplied with HIV drugs, they were hindered by operational challenges such as shortage of infrastructures, laboratory reagents, and trained HCW.

Conclusions: The PMTCT cascade revealed bottle necks in PMTCT intervention and HIV early infant diagnosis. The staffing in HIV care and quality of health care infrastructures were also insufficient in 2011 in Ouagadougou.

Editor: Julian W. Tang, Alberta Provincial Laboratory for Public Health/University of Alberta, Canada

Funding: The study was supported in part by the MONOD ANRS 12206 project granted by the European and Developing Countries Clinical Trial Partnership (EDCTP), the CRP-santé in Luxembourg and the French ANRS-Inserm. Dr. Malik Coulibaly is a fellow PhD candidate of the Doctoral School of Society, Politics and Public Health, Bordeaux, France funded by the MONOD consortium. The content of this publication is solely the responsibility of the authors and does not necessarily represent the official views of any of the institutions mentioned above. The funders had no role in study design, data collection and analysis, decision to publish, or preparation of the manuscript.

Competing Interests: The authors have declared that no competing interests exist.

* Email: coulmalik@yahoo.fr

¶ Membership of the MONOD Study Group ANRS 12206 is provided in Appendix S1.

Introduction

Despite the efficacy of Prevention of Mother-To-Child- HIV Transmission (PMTCT), Human Immunodeficiency Virus (HIV) pediatric infection still occurs in Africa because of the lack of operational access to this intervention. Without any intervention, mortality of HIV infected children can reach up to 35% before the first birthday and up to 52% before the second birthday [1,2], and the untreated survivors would need substantial care [3]. However early antiretroviral treatment routinely started before 12 weeks of age significantly increases infant survival by 76%, reduces morbidity and enhances immunological benefits [4,5,6,7]. The 2010 World Health Organization (WHO) revised guidelines recommend early antiretroviral treatment in all HIV infected children less than two years of age, regardless of their immune status [8]. These guidelines also recommend a routine Early Infant Diagnosis (EID) from six-weeks of age of all HIV-exposed children. EID requires sophisticated technology before 18 months of age because of the persistence of maternal antibodies in infants [9]. In addition, the uptake at each step in the EID cascade highlights that even with the highest reported level of uptake, nearly half of HIV-infected infants may not successfully complete the cumulative cascade [10]. In sub-Saharan Africa, HIV-exposed infants continue to suffer from insufficient access to EID and antiretroviral therapy. In 2010, a survey was conducted in Burkina Faso, Ghana and Côte d'Ivoire, to identify the major challenges regarding HIV prophylaxis for children in West Africa [11]. The results of this survey indicated that only a small proportion of HIV-exposed newborns received antiretroviral prophylaxis. Scaling-up management of early pediatric HIV infection remains challenging in West African countries in 2011. But there is a need to increase the PMTCT coverage and to trace the children born in the setting of the PMTCT programs [12]. It is crucial to identify the barriers at the national level. Burkina Faso is a West-African developing country where HIV prevalence was about 1.0% in 2010 [13]. HIV EID in children born to HIV-infected mothers is organized in cascade from the district health care facilities, towards district hospital laboratories, to the university hospital laboratories. There are few data on the full PMTCT cascade coverage and postnatal services in regard to infants born to HIV-infected mothers. Problems are related to resource management, and lack of assessment of sites.

We described the access to pediatric HIV diagnosis and care in Ouagadougou, the capital of Burkina Faso. We also assessed the health care facilities regarding the conformance of staff and infrastructures with WHO standards for the care of HIV infected infants in Ouagadougou in 2010–2011.

Methods

Access to HIV care for infants in Burkina Faso

Burkina Faso is administratively divided into 13 regions, 45 provinces and 351 rural and urban municipalities. In 2011, the public health system was organized around four types of hospitals: district, confessional, regional, and university hospitals. Besides the public health facilities, Burkina Faso had also a large number of private health care facilities and traditional healers [14].

The "big" Ouagadougou equated the Center region with a population of 2 136 582 inhabitants in 2011, of whom 39.7% were children less than 15 years of age [14]. The Center region was the most populous and urbanized of the 13 administrative regions of Burkina Faso, with a land area of 2 869 square kilometers [15]. We identified in this region two university hospitals, five district hospitals, one confessional hospital, eight hospitals without surgical units, and 81 primary health care facilities [16]. According to the 2010 health and demographic survey, the HIV prevalence in Ouagadougou was estimated at 2.1% (95% CI: 1.5–2.7) in 2010 [13].

PMTCT services are integrated in the national health system. All pregnant women who come for antenatal care in a health care facility are expected to be counseled for HIV testing. In case of consent, HIV screening is performed on-site using rapid HIV antibody tests, with a simultaneous HIV result delivery. The pregnant women who attend antenatal consultation with a documented positive result are also tested for the sake control, unless that they are already treated with antiretroviral drugs. In any case, there were included in the PMTCT cascade.

In Burkina Faso, the option A of PMTCT was still recommended in 2011 and HIV-infected pregnant women were eligible to antiretroviral treatment on the basis of CD4 count. Pregnant women with more than 350 cells/mm^3 CD4 count were prescribed zidovudine at 28 weeks gestation in antepartum. In intrapartum, at onset of labor, a single dose of nevirapine and the first dose of zidovudine/lamivudine were given. In postpartum, a

daily zidovudine/lamivudine was given for seven days. Whenever the pregnant women's CD4 count was inferior or equal to 350 cells/mm^3 a triple antiretroviral therapy was started as soon as diagnosed, and continued for life. Infants received a daily nevirapine dose from birth up to one week after the complete cessation of breastfeeding. When mothers were not breastfeeding or were on antiretroviral drugs, infants were given *a* daily nevirapine dose up to six weeks of age. Infant breastfeeding was the most recommended feeding option.

After delivery, HIV-infected mothers and their children were advised to go to the nearest health care facility for a postnatal visit and an EID preformed since six weeks of age. This EID was based on a first deoxyribonucleic acid polymerase chain reaction (DNA PCR) test on a Dried Blood Spot (DBS) and was scheduled once a month. The DBS were sent for processing by the corresponding district hospital to one of the three laboratories in Ouagadougou region (the university hospital Yalgado Ouédraogo, the university hospital Charles de Gaulle, and the Saint Camille hospital). All HIV tests results were sent back to the health care facilities via the corresponding district hospitals. In case of a first positive DBS result, a second DNA PCR test is performed on a blood sample to confirm HIV infection [17].

Context and study design

The study was conducted in the implementation phase of the MONOD ANRS 12206 clinical trial (ClinicalTrial.gov registry n°NCT01127204), which was approved by the national ethics committee and the Burkina Faso Ministry of Health. The study was conducted in the capital of the country (Ouagadougou). Health professionals who were interviewed and parents of children who were enrolled for treatment provided a clear written consent. The ethics committee approved the consent procedure. The informed consent was waived for the use of aggregate register data.

The ANRS 12206 MONOD trial is a randomized controlled trial whose aim is to assess a simplified once daily antiretroviral treatment in virologically suppressed HIV infected children initially treated with a triple therapy containing lopinavir/ritonavir before the age of two (Appendix S1).

We undertook a cross-sectional survey from January 2011 to January 2012, to evaluate the performance of PMTCT cascade, and the conformance of infrastructures and staff in health care facilities with pediatric HIV services in Ouagadougou.

Study site and population

We included all the health care facilities providing PMTCT services, infant HIV diagnosis and antiretroviral treatments in Ouagadougou. We first used their 2011 aggregate data to document the PMTCT cascade. Then, in each health care facility, we interviewed all the heads of the various services: health districts, health care facilities, PMTCT services, laboratories, pharmacies, pediatric services, statistics and epidemiology surveillance division, and human resource services.

Data collection

We used 2010 and 2011 Ministry of Health statistical yearbook, as the reference figures [14,16]. We designed a semi-structured questionnaire with three sections according to the staff targeted: pediatric, laboratory and pharmacy services. Two medical epidemiologists, one midwife and one sociologist carried out the desk review and interviewed the selected health professionals. The questionnaire reviewed variables related to PMTCT statistics (cascade of HIV care from antenatal services to EID of HIV-exposed children at six weeks of age and antiretroviral treatment care for HIV-infected children), infrastructures, laboratory reagents, essential drug management and health professionals staffing (doctors, nurses, pharmacists, and laboratory technicians). The staff interviews helped to check registers and identify difficulties faced in providing early HIV infant diagnosis and treatment, and possible solutions.

In 2011, there were 103 health care facilities providing PMTCT services in Ouagadougou and we collected data from all of them. In each health care facility, there was a statistics manager who was in charge of collecting data monthly in a register provided by the Ministry of Health. Pregnant women received for antenatal consultation were recorded in a register that was later used by the statistics manager. A report was then sent to the district head of statistics and epidemiology surveillance division, who compiled the different health care facility reports with Excel software. In our study, we monthly recorded data in term of aggregate number of the different variables related to the PMTCT cascade, from the health care facility registers as well as the district registers, for comparison. In case of discrepancies, we monitored the data recording process to correct the errors. Finally, we were able to document individual data for the HIV-infected children diagnosed and transferred to HIV pediatric care for antiretroviral treatment in the MONOD trial.

For drug management, we checked the registers where the drug management was recorded to determine the availability of drugs and stock-outs. We checked the availability of antiretroviral drugs needed for the national guideline treatment: zidovudine or stavudine or abacavir, lamivudine or emtricitabine, nevirapine or efavirenz, and lopinavir/ritonavir. For opportunistic infection treatment and prophylaxis, we checked the availability of the following drugs: cotrimoxazole, nistatine, miconazole, amphotericine B, ciprofloxacine, ceftriaxone, acyclovir, and anti-tuberculosis drugs.

Finally, we checked the laboratory reagent management and availability with the responsible of laboratories in the corresponding registers.

To document the PMTCT cascade, we used the Ministry of Health method to estimate the expected number of pregnancies, based on the expected number of births multiplied by 1.10 [14]. The expected number of births is equal to the number of women of childbearing age multiplied by the corrected fertility rate of the Center region, equal to 0.1247. The logic of multiplying the expected number of births by 1.10 to obtain the number of expected pregnancies comes from a study of Sedgh et al. who found that 10% of pregnancies end in abortions in Western Africa [18].

Essential infrastructure requirement for health care centers

In 2008, WHO published an operational manual for HIV high prevalence resource constraint settings, to assess health care facilities serving HIV infected people [19].

The WHO defines health care facility's space, design, power supply, water, hygiene and sanitation, and equipment requirements to be able to deliver quality HIV prevention, care and treatment services. We assessed health care facilities using the following WHO criteria: space, privacy and confidentiality, infection control (tuberculosis infection and HIV infection), safe water supply and hygiene (sanitation, hand washing and other hygiene practices, waste management, latrine/toilet, and cleaning), communications, power, and fire safety. The standards require using color-coded waste containers and fire extinguishers. Space requirement is at least 9 m^2 for consultation room, 2.25 m^2 for counseling room, 9 m^2 for laboratory specimen analysis room, and 9 m^2 for pharmacy room [19].

We checked the space available in pediatric consultation ward, laboratory, and pharmacy rooms. This criteria was classified as conform if the available space was superior or equal to that required by the WHO standards. We also checked other qualitative criteria such as the availability of power supply, infection control and the respect of privacy and confidentiality by health professionals. The conformance was good if all the criteria were met. For laboratory tests, we assessed the capacity for performing the required tests in hospitals, without neither shortages of laboratory reagents nor failure of medical devices.

Finally, the conformance was good if antiretroviral drugs and drugs for opportunistic infection treatment and prophylaxis were available to treat HIV infected children with a regimen recommended by the national guidelines.

Statistical analysis

The prevalence of HIV infected pregnant women was calculated by dividing the number of HIV infected pregnant women by the total number of pregnant women screened for HIV infection. The 95% confidence intervals were determined according to the following formula: $(P - Z_{1-\frac{\alpha}{2}}\sqrt{\frac{P(1-P)}{n}} + \frac{1}{2n},$ $P + Z_{1-\frac{\alpha}{2}}\sqrt{\frac{P(1-P)}{n}} + \frac{1}{2n})$ [20] where p = prevalence, n = sample size. We described the coverage of pediatric HIV services and the flow from HIV-exposed children to access to ART, of HIV-infected children. The cascade of care was compiled on Microsoft Excel software using proportions. All the proportions of the PMTCT cascade were calculated by dividing the total number of favorable cases by the number of eligible cases with their 95% confidence intervals according to the formula previously mentioned.

Results

From the 103 health care facilities providing PMTCT services in Ouagadougou in 2011, 127 health professionals were interviewed: 7 (5.5%) pediatricians, 5 (3.9%) general practitioners, 10 (7.9%) pharmacists, 5 (3.9%) nurse-epidemiologists, 75 (59.1%) nurses, 7 (5.5%) midwives, 9 (7.1%) pharmacist assistants, 5 (3.9%) laboratory technicians, 2 (1.6%) biologists, and 2 (1.6%) human resource managers.

Staffing in pediatric HIV health services

In 2010, there was no HIV treatment for HIV-infected children in primary health care facilities in Ouagadougou. All pediatric HIV care was provided by the six district hospitals, and two university hospitals. In these hospitals, a total of 225 health professionals were directly involved in pediatric HIV infection care, and among them 40% worked in the two university hospitals (Table 1). Overall, 10.7% were pediatricians, 4.4% general practitioners, 19.1% nurses, 5.8% counselors, 8.9% pharmacists, and 29.8% laboratory technicians. Six of the eight hospitals had at least one pediatrician.

In 2010, the total population of children less than 15 years old in the whole region was estimated at 811 115 [16]. With an HIV prevalence of 0.26% in children less than 15 years old [11], we estimated the number of HIV infected children less than 15 to be about 2 109 (811 115×0.26%) in Ouagadougou. With 24 pediatricians in this area (10.7% of the overall staff dedicated to pediatric HIV care), one pediatrician was responsible for 33 797 (811 115/24) children less than 15 years age of whom 88 (2 109/24) were HIV infected.

Table 1. Staff involved in HIV pediatric care per health district or university hospitals, and qualification, in Ouagadougou, in 2010.

	Pediatricians	General practitioners	Pharmacists	Laboratory technicians	Psychologist/ counselors	Nurses	Others	Total
District hospitals	8	9	6	38	6	30	36	133
Mean per hospital	1.6	1.8	1.2	7.6	1.2	6	7.2	26.6
University hospital	16	1	14	29	7	13	12	92
Mean per hospital	8	0.5	7	14.5	3.5	6.5	6	46

Others: pharmacy assistants and laboratory assistants.

When evaluating the conformance of health staff requirements of the WHO standards in the health district hospitals [19], the staff is overall insufficient: general practitioners are less than 1/10 000, and pharmacists are less than 1/20 000 in all the five health districts of Ouagadougou. We had more than 1/4000 nurses in four health districts. Overall, both physician and pharmacist staff were scarce.

PMTCT cascade

In 2011, out of the 76 935 expected pregnancies in the Center region, 67 592 attended at least one antenatal consultation (87.8%). Among the pregnant women attending antenatal consultation, 58 036 accepted to be HIV-tested (85.9%) and the HIV prevalence was 1.8% (95% CI: 1.7%–1.9%). Furthermore, 441 out of the 1 064 HIV-infected pregnant women (41.4%) benefitted from a PMTCT intervention (option A). Then, only 313 (29.4%) HIV-exposed infants (0–18 months) had an HIV virologic test on a DBS, and 306 (97.8%) among these infants tested received their results, usually within a month, but sometimes within a four-month period. Still among the infants tested, 40 children were initially identified as HIV-infected, and 33 (82.5%) out the infants tested, were referred to the MONOD study sites before the age of two for an HIV test confirmation using a deoxyribonucleic acid polymerase chain reaction (DNA PCR). With three children identified as false positive (9%) and 30 (91%) confirmed to be HIV-infected, the HIV prevalence was estimated to be 9.6% (95% CI: 6.3%–12.9%). Finally, 27 children (90.0%) were enrolled in the MONOD ANRS 12206 trial and treated with a triple lopinavir/ritonavir based therapy (Table 2). Their median age at diagnosis was 13 months [IQR: 7–19].

Seven children (17.5%) were not referred for HIV care. One of them died before his laboratory result was released. The six remaining did not come back for their laboratory results and we were not able to contact them because of missing telephone numbers or addresses in the health care facility registers.

Among the six (18.2%) children who were referred to MONOD clinical sites, but were not enrolled in the trial to start an antiretroviral therapy, two died before being able to initiate treatment because of their advanced stage of HIV disease. One was lost to-follow-up after his father refusal to consent for treatment, and three were finally controlled as HIV-negative and not eligible for antiretroviral treatment.

Infrastructures

The conformance of infrastructures was globally gauged "not conform" because of two criteria: safe waste management and fire safety. Indeed, none of the health care facilities had either segregate color-coded waste containers or fire extinguishers.

Essential laboratory tests and apparatus

The availability of essential laboratory tests was checked in health care facilities (Table 3). The lack of some of the laboratory tests was associated to either a failure/lack of the corresponding laboratory apparatus or a reagent shortage. The table 4 displays the reasons for the laboratory non conformance. In addition, lack of apparatus maintenance has been underlined in all the health care facilities.

Essential drugs

The availability of essential antiretroviral drugs was quite good in 2010, and the conformance was judged to be good in spite of few shortages which did not affect the treatment of HIV-infected patient according to national guidelines. A shortage of seven days

Table 2. The PMTCT cascade until HIV pediatric care in Ouagadougou, 2011.

Designation	Number	Percentage (%)	Confidence Interval 95%
Pregnant women expected	76 935	100%	-
Pregnant women attending antenatal consultation	67 592	87.8 (100%)	[87.6–88.0]
Pregnant women having been counseled for HIV testing	60 156	89.0	[88.8–89.2]
Pregnant women having been HIV-tested	58 036	85.9 (100%) (96.5% of the counseled women)	[85.6–86.1]
HIV-infected pregnant women	1 064	1.8 (100%)	[1.7–1.9]
Pregnant women exposed to PMTCT intervention	441	41.4	[38.4–44.4]
HIV-exposed infants having been HIV-tested using DBS	313	29.4 (100%)	[26.6–32.2]
DBS tests results returned	306	97.8	[96.0–99.6]
Infants identified as HIV-infected on the first DBS test (100%)	40	12.8	[8.9–16.6]
HIV-infected infants referred to pediatric care	33	82.5	[71.9–95.5]
Infants confirmed as HIV-infected on the second test (DNA PCR on blood sample)	30	9.6 (100%)	[6.3–12.9]
HIV-infected infants initiated on antiretroviral therapy	27	90.0	[79.2–100.0]

100% is the reference number.
DNA PCR = deoxyribonucleic acid polymerase chain reaction.
DBS = dried blood spot.

was observed for lopinavir/ritonavir, lamivudine and abacavir in Charles de Gaulle university hospital in 2010. In addition, Bogodogo district hospital noticed a shortage of 30 days for the combination lamivudine + nevirapine + stavudine (triomune junior). The drugs for opportunistic infections were available and conform to WHO standards, but they were not free of charge for HIV-infected patients in 2010, except anti-tuberculosis drugs and cotrimoxazole.

Discussion

This cross-sectional survey assessed for the first time the staff, the infrastructures and the PMTCT cascade from prenatal PMTCT up to pediatric HIV care, in all health care facilities providing pediatric HIV care services in Ouagadougou. We documented that only 40% of HIV-infected women received a PMTCT intervention and less than a third of HIV-exposed children were tested during the postnatal period. Moreover, it provides a description of the health care system in this country, useful to understand some of the weaknesses of the system when it comes to the issue of EID in all HIV exposed children, and their access to antiretroviral therapy.

There are several drawbacks in our observations. Firstly, the incompleteness of the data collected may be the source of information bias in this study. Our study method was partially

based on desk review, where we checked the statistics in the available registers. Unfortunately, we could not get all the information related to our objectives. For instance, it had not been possible to routinely determine the duration of laboratory reagent shortage. Secondly, we were not able to really link one-to-one the PMTCT with the postnatal data, and we assumed that each HIV-pregnant woman was supposed to give one alive pregnancy outcome, without taking into account multiple pregnancy outcomes or stillbirth. Furthermore, some of the infants tested in 2011, had their mothers attend their first antenatal consultation in the preceding years, and some of the pregnant women tracked in 2011 will give birth in 2012 as well, resulting in a kind of compensation allowing the PMTCT and EID coverage estimates. Consequently, we feel that these figures were accurate enough to understand the overall patient flow throughout the health care system services. Thirdly, the conformance of health care services was determined with respect to the WHO standards, ideally suitable for district hospitals [19]. These standards might not be suitable when applied to university hospitals, where a higher standard of care is expected. Lastly, in terms of representativeness, our results showed a similar proportion of antenatal consultations among pregnant women in Ouagadougou, compared to the rest of the country (88%) [14]. As a matter of fact, Ouagadougou had a greater number of private health facilities compared to the rest of the country [14], and their statistics were

Table 3. Conformance of Ouagadougou hospitals according to WHO standards, in 2010.

WHO criteria of conformance	District hospital	University hospital
	N = 6	N = 2
	# conform/N	# conform/N
Infrastructure		
Room space >9 m^2	6/6	2/2
Power (electricity) available	6/6	2/2
Tap water available	6/6	2/2
Tuberculosis infection control (ventilated waiting rooms, cough control, good patient flow)	6/6	2/2
HIV infection control (injection safety, appropriate use and disposal of sharps, personal protective equipment for staff, post exposure prophylaxis available)	6/6	2/2
Waste management (3 color-containers available)	0/6	0/2
Privacy of patient's test protected	6/6	2/2
Communication (land line available)	6/6	2/2
Fire extinguisher available	0/6	0/2
Conclusion	**Not conform**	**Not conform**
Laboratory test available		
Rapid HIV antibody test	4/6	2/2
DBS	6/6	2/2
CD4 count	1/6	1/2
Hemoglobin determination	5/6	2/2
Serum alanin aminotransferase	4/6	2/2
Serum creatinin & blood urea nitrogen	4/6	2/2
Bilirubin determination	4/6	2/2
Lactic acid	5/6	2/2
Blood sugar	4/6	2/2
Tuberculosis diagnostics	6/6	2/2
Pregnancy test	6/6	2/2
Urine dipstick for sugar and protein	6/6	2/2
Conclusion	**Not conform**	**Not conform**
Drugs available		
Antiretroviral drugs	6/6	2/2
Opportunistic infection drugs	6/6	2/2
Conclusion	**Conform**	**Conform**
Staff		
One general practitioner for 10 000	0/6	Not applicable*
One pharmacist for 20 000	0/6	Not applicable*
One nurse for 4 000	4/6	Not applicable*
Conclusion	**Not conform**	**Not applicable**

*The university hospitals are located in the center region, but patients are referred from the whole country.

not included in our figures. As a result, the number of antenatal consultations was lower than that was really carried out in Ouagadougou. However, in our study, we considered all pregnant women who were on PMTCT antiretroviral protocol with the hypothesis that their children would be referred to the public system if they were found to be HIV-infected.

Our study helped to identify major challenges facing EID and antiretroviral treatment access for children in Burkina Faso. A survey conducted in Burkina Faso, Ghana and Côte d'Ivoire, from January 2010 to February 2011 had already reported the lack of access to child PMTCT prophylaxis [11]. Our results confirm that in the urban setting of Ouagadougou. The level of missed opportunities was so high that it was difficult to cover sufficiently with PMTCT intervention, the mother-infant couple, estimated at 59%, as well as to offer EID to all HIV-exposed children, reaching 71%. We also conclude that these missed opportunities should be greater at the national level considering the fact that the health

Table 4. Reasons for Ouagadougou laboratory non conformance in 2010.

Laboratory tests non available	District hospitals N = 6		University hospitals N = 2	
	Lack or apparatus failure	Reagent shortage	Lack or apparatus failure	Reagent shortage
Rapid HIV antibody test	Non applicable	2	Non applicable	0
CD4 count	5	5	1	0
Hemoglobin determination	1	0	0	0
Serum alanin aminotransferase	1	1	0	0
Serum creatinin & blood urea nitrogen	1	1	0	0
Bilirubin determination	1	1	0	0
Lactic acid	1	0	0	0
Blood sugar	1	1	0	0

care system would be more complex and thus weaker at the rural level in comparison to the urban one.

Some factors could explain these missed opportunities and could be separately addressed. Firstly, the low awareness of HIV prevention and care services in the community could explain the non-attendance of EID services or the rejection of these services by families. In Burkina Faso, only 20.1% of the population attended the secondary school in 2008/2009 [21] and therefore we think that substantial efforts should be developed to make them aware of the benefit of PMTCT services. In addition, men should also be targeted in education, because they are likely to be reluctant to carrying out HIV screening, and they can greatly support their wives in using PMTCT services [22,23].

Secondly, we highlighted the lack of adequate quantitative and qualitative health care workers (HCW) to cover the needs. At the six-week postnatal visit for instance, due to the fact that nurses were not all trained to perform DBS, the DBS could only be performed one day in a month. Mothers who would like have their infant HIV-tested could only return on this unique day, leading to a high attrition rate because of the inadequate offer of this simple service.

Thirdly, the inaccessibility to EID services is also related to the health system organization, as the current DBS sample circuit and transportation is too complicated and should be simplified. Indeed, the need to go through each district hospital while the final laboratory test is performed in each university laboratory hospital should be considered. It would be more efficient to perform the DBS directly in the health care facilities, to limit the lost to follow-up rate. In the neighboring country of Côte d'Ivoire, we had a similar problem of low coverage rate of EID, favored by the civil war, with only 24% of the HIV exposed children early diagnosed in 2010 [24]. In comparison, a study carried out in 2008, showed that DNA polymerase chain reaction testing in routine was 35.2% for children hospitalized in Malawi, but their age was not specified [25].

Similarly, the low PMTCT intervention coverage is related to problems in the health service organization. When a pregnant woman attends antenatal consultation in a health care facility, she is counseled and screened for HIV with a rapid HIV antibody test. In case of HIV infection, she is referred to the referent district hospital in order to carry out the other tests such as CD4 count, before visiting a doctor who would prescribe an option A

antiretroviral treatment, mainly based on nevirapine. Then, she is later sent back in the former health care facility, to pursue her antenatal follow-up. Although not documented, we assume that some pregnant women could not reach the district hospitals, thus increasing the number of lost to follow-up. This could explain why a lot of pregnant women attend antenatal consultation but do not benefit from PMTCT intervention, when they are HIV-infected.

Fourthly, there are also laboratory related challenges, with the need to offer routine services while the HIV-prevalence is still low, leading to frequent laboratory reagent shortages. Thairu et al. also confirmed our results about maintenance and reagent stock management, in their study in Burkina Faso and Zimbabwe [26]. A frequently-cited barrier to expansion of EID programs is the cost of the required laboratory assays.

Thus, substantial sequential barriers explain the low PMTCT and EID complete cascade coverage, and the lack of personnel and infrastructure requirements. A review reported that even with the highest reported levels of uptake, nearly half of HIV-infected infants may not complete the cascade successfully [10].

Additionally, we raise the overall problem of the EID strategy performances. In settings with low HIV prevalence or well performing PMTCT program, vertical transmission rates may be as low as 2% at six weeks and the positive predictive value of a single test will be approximately 50%, meaning that only half of infants who are tested positive are truly infected [27,28]. For this reason, a confirmatory test is essential, especially in the context of a low HIV prevalence country such as Burkina Faso. Indeed, in our study, the high rate of false positive DBS (9%) highly affects the positive predictive value of the national HIV screening strategy. Acknowledging this, the test confirmation is a priority and laboratories should implement reliable quality control system and constantly work on maintaining high quality standards of EID.

Antiretroviral access for HIV-infected children looked good in our study when compared to the estimates of the Ethiopian study, where only 8.4% of positive babies had access to antiretroviral treatment [29]. But, it is important to point out the contribution of the Monod trial implementation in our results, which set up a network whose aim was to improve the coverage of pediatric antiretroviral therapy beyond the EID.

A shortage of some antiretroviral drugs was observed in two health care facilities for several days, as a result of delays in reporting. In effect, antiretroviral drugs are provided by the Ministry of Health division for HIV/AIDS (Comité Ministériel de Lutte contre le Sida), and they required periodic reports, before delivery. Hence, a delay in providing a report will ultimately end in a delay in drug supply.

Moreover, while all antiretroviral drugs were free of charge in Burkina Faso in 2010, the opportunistic infection drugs are charged to families. It has already been reported that having to pay for HIV treatment and laboratory tests, increases the risk of lost to follow-up [30].

When analyzing the conformance of health centers with respect to the PMTCT cascade, we can point out that the infrastructure requirements are almost met, and that the absence of fire extinguishers and segregate color-codes waste containers, did not affect antenatal consultation rate which is quite good in a developing country setting such as this. However, the non conformance to laboratory test requirements explained why we observed an attrition of the cascade at the number of children tested for HIV infection. The conformance of pharmacies was found to be good and consequently two-third of HIV infected children were treated. The missed opportunity for treatment was related to communication and pregnant women HIV testing circuit problem.

Globally, the causes of non conformance at the district and university hospitals are almost similar because they are public centers (except Saint Camille hospital), run by the Ministry of Health. The causes could be a lack of resources, or a mismanagement of the available resources.

The problem could be alleviated by improving the communication process between the peripheral health services and the national procurement system. The community awareness should also be improved and contextualized to the socio-cultural needs of the region.

Moreover, training in a large scale on DBS practicing and in HIV care among HCW would be useful and promote task shifting activities [31,32,33]. Finally, characteristics of the health care facilities could be determinant in improving the pediatric HIV care in Africa as reported in the HEART project [34]: characteristics associated with favorable children enrolment in care are nutritional support, linkages with associations of people living with HIV, access to EID and integration of PMTCT services. Applying the South African strategies to improve antiretroviral treatment in the province of KwaZulu-Natal could be beneficial. In addition to training all the staff in contact with mothers and children, they carried out campaigns aimed at increasing HIV testing during immunization and clinics, routinely testing of HIV in children with tuberculosis and malnutrition, and

systematically testing for HIV, all children admitted at hospital [35]. However, in Burkina Faso, as the HIV prevalence is lower than that of South Africa, it would be more efficient to start the systematic HIV diagnosis by screening first the children with rapid HIV antibody tests. Expanding these characteristics to improve pediatric HIV treatment in Burkina Faso, warrants further evaluation for improving the scaling up of pediatric HIV care. Finally, as it was reported in South Africa, it is possible to improve the identification of HIV-infected children and ensure a prompt start on ART when needed with relatively simple measures, limited staffing and budgets [35].

Despite an overall good access to prenatal services in Ouagadougou in 2011, there are still many missed opportunities for both the prevention of mother-to-child transmission and the early access to diagnosis and antiretroviral therapy for HIV-infected children before two years of life. The government should look forward to improving the awareness and education among the population, training health care workers for HIV diagnosis and care, facilitating the access to EID and making health care facilities more attractive to families. In addition, the DBS circuit should be simplified to avoid lost to follow-up. Early access to EID and to antiretroviral therapy will require political willingness and leadership to address these health system barriers in Burkina Faso.

Acknowledgments

We acknowledge the Head of Ministry of Health division for AIDS (Comité Ministériel de Lutte contre le Sida), in Burkina Faso, Dr Marie-Joseph Sanou, the regional Director of Health, Dr Amédée Prosper Djiguemdé and all heads of health care facilities in Ouagadougou and their staff for their contribution to data collection. We are grateful to the French GIP ESTHER for its assistance to HIV infected children in Burkina Faso. We would like to give special thanks to Pr Louis Rachid Salmi for his helpful suggestion on using WHO standards.

Author Contributions

Conceived and designed the experiments: M. Coulibaly NM VL PV SB DY LK CY SO MB IS ET M. Congo. Performed the experiments: M. Coulibaly IS ET. Analyzed the data: M. Coulibaly IS VL. Contributed reagents/materials/analysis tools: CY M. Congo MB NM VL PV. Wrote the paper: M. Coulibaly VL SB PV NM FK. Edit the manuscript: VL SB PV ET MB LK CY SO IS DY FK M. Congo.

References

1. Newell ML, Brahmbhatt H, Ghys PD (2004) Child mortality and HIV infection in Africa: a review. AIDS 18 Suppl 2: S27–34.
2. Newell ML, Coovadia H, Cortina-Borja M, Rollins N, Gaillard P, et al. (2004) Mortality of infected and uninfected infants born to HIV-infected mothers in Africa: a pooled analysis. Lancet 364: 1236–1243.
3. Desmonde S, Coffie P, Aka E, Amani-Bosse C, Messou E, et al. (2011) Severe morbidity and mortality in untreated HIV-infected children in a paediatric care programme in Abidjan, Cote d'Ivoire, 2004–2009. BMC Infect Dis 11: 182.
4. Goetghebuer T, Le Chenadec J, Haelterman E, Galli L, Dollfus C, et al. (2012) Short- and long-term immunological and virological outcome in HIV-infected infants according to the age at antiretroviral treatment initiation. Clin Infect Dis 54: 878–881.
5. Prendergast AJ, Penazzato M, Cotton M, Musoke P, Mulenga V, et al. (2012) Treatment of young children with HIV infection: using evidence to inform policymakers. PLoS Med 9: e1001273.
6. Prendergast A, Mphatswe W, Tudor-Williams G, Rakgotho M, Pillay V, et al. (2008) Early virological suppression with three-class antiretroviral therapy in HIV-infected African infants. AIDS 22: 1333–1343.

7. Violari A, Cotton MF, Gibb DM, Babiker AG, Steyn J, et al. (2008) Early antiretroviral therapy and mortality among HIV-infected infants. N Engl J Med 359: 2233–2244.
8. WHO (2010) Antiretroviral therapy for HIV infection in infants and children: Towards universal access. Recommendations for a public health approach. 2010 revision.
9. Nielsen K, Bryson YJ (2000) Diagnosis of HIV infection in children. Pediatr Clin North Am 47: 39–63.
10. Ciaranello AL, Park JE, Ramirez-Avila L, Freedberg KA, Walensky RP, et al. (2011) Early infant HIV-1 diagnosis programs in resource-limited settings: opportunities for improved outcomes and more cost-effective interventions. BMC Med 9: 59.
11. Tchidjou HK, Maria Martino A, Goli LP, Diop Ly M, Zekeng L, et al. (2012) Paediatric HIV infection in Western Africa: the long way to the standard of care. J Trop Pediatr 58: 451–456.
12. Ndondoki C, Brou H, Timite-Konan M, Oga M, Amani-Bosse C, et al. (2013) Universal HIV screening at postnatal points of care: which public health approach for early infant diagnosis in Cote d'Ivoire? PLoS One 8: e67996.

13. Ministère de l'Economie et des Finances Burkina Faso (2011) Enquête Démographique et de Santé et à indicateurs Multiples (EDSBF-MICS IV) 2010. Ouagadougou, Burkina Faso. 50 p. Available: www.measuredhs.com/pubs/pdf/PR9/PR9.pdf. Accessed 2012 September 12.

14. Ministère de la Santé Burkina Faso (2012) Annuaire statistique 2011. Ouagadougou, Burkina Faso. 244 p. Available: http://www.sante.gov.bf/phocadownload/Annuaire_statistique_2011.pdf. Accessed 2013 May 27.

15. Institut National de la Statistique et de la Démographie Burkina Faso (2011) La région du centre en chiffres. Ouagadougou, Burkina Faso. 7 p. Available: http://www.insd.bf/n/contenu/statistiques_regions/regions_en_chiffres_en_2011/reg_chif_c_2011.pdf. Accessed 2014 August 4.

16. Ministère de la Santé Burkina Faso (2011) Annaire statistique 2010. Ouagadougou, Burkina Faso. 204p. Availaible: http://www.sante.gov.bf/phocadownload/Publications_statistiques/Annuaire/annuaire_statistique_sante_2010.pdf. Accessed: 2014 October 5.

17. Ministère de la Santé Comité Ministériel de Lutte contre le SIDA Burkina Faso (2008) Normes et protocoles de prise en charge médicale des personnes vivant avec le VIH au Burkina Faso. Ouagadougou.

18. Sedgh G, Henshaw S, Singh S, Ahman E, Shah IH (2007) Induced abortion: estimated rates and trends worldwide. Lancet 370: 1338–1345.

19. WHO (2008) Operations Manual for Delivery of HIV Prevention, Care and Treatment at Primary Health Centres in High-Prevalence, Resource-Constrained Settings. Geneva, Switzerland. 392 p.

20. Forthofer RN, Lee ES, Hernandez M (2007) Biostatistics: A guide to Design, Analysis, and Discovery: Elsevier. 502 p.

21. Institut National de la Statistique et de la Démographie Burkina Faso (2013) Tableau 05.34: Evolution du taux brut de scolarisation de l'ensemble du secondaire (en %). Ouagadougou, Burkina Faso. Available: http://www.insd.bf/n/contenu/tableaux/T0534.htm. Accessed 2013 May 27.

22. Desgrees-Du-Lou A, Brou H, Djohan G, Becquet R, Ekouevi DK, et al. (2009) Beneficial effects of offering prenatal HIV counselling and testing on developing a HIV preventive attitude among couples. Abidjan, 2002–2005. AIDS Behav 13: 348–355.

23. Brou H, Djohan G, Becquet R, Allou G, Ekouevi DK, et al. (2008) Sexual prevention of HIV within the couple after prenatal HIV-testing in West Africa. AIDS Care 20: 413–418.

24. Folquet-Amonissani M, Dainguy M. E, Amani-Bossé C, Elian-Kouakou J, Méa-Assandé V, et al. Early infant diagnosis and access to pediatric HIV care: barriers and challenges in Abidjan, Ivory Coast in 2011; 2012; Washington DC, USA.

25. Van Rompaey S, Kimfuta J, Kimbondo P, Monn C, Buve A (2011) Operational assessment of access to ART in rural Africa: the example of Kisantu in Democratic Republic of the Congo. AIDS Care 23: 686–693.

26. Thairu L, Katzenstein D, Israelski D (2011) Operational challenges in delivering CD4 diagnostics in sub-Saharan Africa. AIDS Care 23: 814–821.

27. WHO (2010) WHO recommendations on the diagnosis of HIV infection in infants and children. Geneva, Switzerland. 64 p.

28. WHO (2014) March 2014 supplement to the 2013 consolidated guidelines on the use of antiretroviral drugs for treating and preventing HIV infection recommendations for a public health approch. Geneva, Swetzerland. 128 p.

29. Nigatu T, Woldegebriel Y (2011) Analysis of the prevention of mother-to-child transmission (PMTCT) service utilization in Ethiopia: 2006–2010. Reprod Health 8: 6.

30. Leroy V, Malateste K, Rabie H, Lumbiganon P, Ayaya S, et al. (2013) Outcomes of antiretroviral therapy in children in Asia and Africa: a comparative analysis of the IeDEA pediatric multiregional collaboration. J Acquir Immune Defic Syndr 62: 208–219.

31. Zachariah R, Ford N, Philips M, Lynch S, Massaquoi M, et al. (2009) Task shifting in HIV/AIDS: opportunities, challenges and proposed actions for sub-Saharan Africa. Trans R Soc Trop Med Hyg 103: 549–558.

32. Creek T, Tanuri A, Smith M, Seipone K, Smit M, et al. (2008) Early diagnosis of human immunodeficiency virus in infants using polymerase chain reaction on dried blood spots in Botswana's national program for prevention of mother-to-child transmission. Pediatr Infect Dis J 27: 22–26.

33. Oga MA, Ndondoki C, Brou H, Salmon A, Bosse-Amani C, et al. (2011) Attitudes and practices of health care workers toward routine HIV testing of infants in Cote d'Ivoire: the PEDI-TEST ANRS 12165 Project. J Acquir Immune Defic Syndr 57 Suppl 1: S16–21.

34. Adjorlolo-Johnson G, Wahl Uheling A, Ramachandran S, Strasser S, Kouakou J, et al. (2013) Scaling up pediatric HIV care and treatment in Africa: clinical site characteristics associated with favorable service utilization. J Acquir Immune Defic Syndr 62: e7–e13.

35. Bland RM, Ndirangu J, Newell ML (2013) Maximising opportunities for increased antiretroviral treatment in children in an existing HIV programme in rural South Africa. BMJ 346: f550.

9

Safety and Effectiveness of Combination Antiretroviral Therapy during the First Year of Treatment in HIV-1 Infected Rwandan Children: A Prospective Study

Philippe R. Mutwa[1,2]*, Kimberly R. Boer[2,6], Brenda Asiimwe-Kateera[2], Diane Tuyishimire[7], Narcisse Muganga[1], Joep M. A. Lange[2], Janneke van de Wijgert[2,3,4], Anita Asiimwe[8], Peter Reiss[2], Sibyl P. M. Geelen[2,5]

1 Kigali University Teaching Hospital, Department of Pediatrics, Kigali, Rwanda, **2** Department of Global Health and Amsterdam Institute for Global Health and Development, Academic Medical Center, Amsterdam, The Netherlands, **3** Institute of Infection and Global Health, University of Liverpool, Liverpool, United of Kingdom, **4** Rinda Ubuzima, Kigali, Rwanda, **5** Wilhelmina Children's Hospital, University Medical Centre Utrecht, Utrecht, The Netherlands, **6** Biomedical Research, Epidemiology Unit, Royal Tropical Institute, Amsterdam, The Netherlands, **7** Outpatients Clinic, Treatment and Research on HIV/AIDS Centre, Kigali, Rwanda, **8** Ministry of Health of Rwanda. Kigali, Rwanda

Abstract

Background: With increased availability of paediatric combination antiretroviral therapy (cART) in resource limited settings, cART outcomes and factors associated with outcomes should be assessed.

Methods: HIV-infected children <15 years of age, initiating cART in Kigali, Rwanda, were followed for 18 months. Prospective clinical and laboratory assessments included weight-for-age (WAZ) and height-for-age (HAZ) z-scores, complete blood cell count, liver transaminases, creatinine and lipid profiles, CD4 T-cell count/percent, and plasma HIV-1 RNA concentration. Clinical success was defined as WAZ and WAZ >−2, immunological success as CD4 cells ≥500/mm^3 and ≥25% for respectively children over 5 years and under 5 years, and virological success as a plasma HIV-1 RNA concentration <40 copies/mL.

Results: Between March 2008 and December 2009, 123 HIV-infected children were included. The median (interquartile (IQR) age at cART initiation was 7.4 (3.2, 11.5) years; 40% were <5 years and 54% were female. Mean (95% confidence interval (95%CI)) HAZ and WAZ at baseline were −2.01 (−2.23, −1.80) and −1.73 (−1.95, −1.50) respectively and rose to −1.75 (−1.98, −1.51) and −1.17 (−1.38, −0.96) after 12 months of cART. The median (IQR) CD4 T-cell values for children <5 and ≥5 years of age were 20% (13, 28) and 337 (236, 484) cells/mm^3 respectively, and increased to 36% (28, 41) and 620 (375, 880) cells/mm^3. After 12 months of cART, 24% of children had a detectable viral load, including 16% with virological failure (HIV-RNA>1000 c/mL). Older age at cART initiation, poor adherence, and exposure to antiretrovirals around birth were associated with virological failure. A third (33%) of children had side effects (by self-report or clinical assessment), but only 9% experienced a severe side effect requiring a cART regimen change.

Conclusions: cART in Rwandan HIV-infected children was successful but success might be improved further by initiating cART as early as possible, optimizing adherence and optimizing management of side effects.

Editor: Rashida A. Ferrand, London School of Hygiene and Tropical Medicine, United Kingdom

Funding: This work was funded by Infectious Diseases Network for Treatment and Research in Africa. An African-Dutch partnership programme, funded by The Netherlands-African partnership for Capacity development and Clinical interventions against Poverty-related diseases (NACCAP). The funders had no role in study design, data collection and analysis, decision to publish, or preparation of the manuscript.

Competing Interests: The authors have declared that no competing interests exist.

* Email: mutwaph@gmail.com

Introduction

There is strong evidence that combination antiretroviral therapy (cART) reduces morbidity and mortality, promotes normal growth and development, and improves quality of life in children infected by HIV [1,2,3,4,5,6]. However, cART effectiveness depends on durable suppression of viral replication. Ongoing HIV replication leads to chronic inflammation, and when cART is not used appropriately this can lead to HIV drug resistance and treatment failure, which limits future treatment options [7,8]. Data

from low and middle-income countries (LMIC) have demonstrated good cART effectiveness and tolerability in most children, but some children remain underweight and stunted or do not improve their CD4 T-cell count or viral load after several years of treatment [9,10,11]. Advanced disease at cART initiation was found to be associated with poor outcomes [9,12,13,14], indicating that earlier treatment may improve effectiveness of cART. Initiation of cART in children is guided by pediatric clinical staging and age-dependent CD4 values.

In Rwanda the national ART guidelines were recently revised to promote an earlier start of cART in children and adolescents, and a roll out of pediatric care and treatment centers throughout the country was achieved [15]. As a result, the number of HIV-infected children on cART in Rwanda has rapidly increased from 468 in 2005 to an estimated 8,032 in 2013 [16]. The main objectives of this study were to prospectively document responses to cART in the first year of treatment in a cohort of HIV-infected Rwandan children, and to determine the incidence and severity of side effects of cART.

Methods

Ethical considerations

The Rwanda National Ethics Committee (RNEC) and the Medical Ethics Review Committee of the University Medical Center of Utrecht, the Netherlands, approved the study protocol. In accordance with the RNEC guidelines written informed consent was obtained from primary caregivers of all children. In addition, verbal assent was obtained from children between 7 and 12 years of age, and written assent from children age 12 or older. The Rwandan national guidelines for disclosure to children recommend to inform children at 7 years of age of their HIV status.

Study design, population and period

In this longitudinal prospective cohort study, HIV-infected cART-naïve children below 15 years of age who initiated cART between March 2008 and December 2009 were followed by the study team for a minimum of 9 and a maximum of 18 months. Study participation ended after 18 months of follow-up or in September 2010, when funding for the study ended. All children continued to be followed in routine HIV care at a public clinic after their study participation ended. The study was conducted at the Treatment and Research AIDS Center (TRACplus) Outpatient Clinic in Kigali, Rwanda. During the study period, the TRACplus clinic was providing HIV care and treatment to 686 HIV-infected children. Among these children, 444 (65%) were already on cART before the study period, 174 became eligible for treatment. With the strategy to scale up pediatric treatment services, 51 children were transferred to clinics closer to their homes, hence they were not enrolled for the study. One hundred and twenty three (18%) children were enrolled. These children were usually referred from Kigali University Teaching Hospital (which is adjacent to the TRACplus clinic), nearby district hospitals, or health centers providing Prevention of Mother to Child HIV Transmission (PMTCT) services; a few children were diagnosed at the TRACplus facility itself. All children below the age of 15 years who initiated cART at the TRACplus clinic during the study period were given the opportunity to enroll in the study.

cART guidelines and regimens

At the time of study initiation, the 2007 Rwandan ART guidelines (based on the 2006 WHO ART guidelines) were operational, which recommended cART initiation in children and adolescents less than 15 years of age if they were classified as WHO pediatric clinical stage III or IV, or had a severe immunodeficiency based on age-dependent CD4 values: CD4 $<1500/mm^3$ or $<25\%$ if ≤ 11 months; $<750/mm^3$ or $<20\%$ if 12–35 months; $<15\%$ or $<350/mm^3$ if 36–59 months; and $<350/mm^3$ if ≥ 5 years of age [17,18]. Children enrolled in the study received cART, cotrimoxazole prophylaxis, and free medication for all acute illnesses during the length of the study. They were initiated on a first-line cART regimen consisting of two

nucleoside reverse transcriptase inhibitors (NRTIs) and a non-nucleoside reverse transcriptase inhibitor (NNRTI). A cART regimen was defined as nevirapine-based, efavirenz-based or protease-inhibitor (PI)-based. The Rwandan ART guidelines were revised in 2009, and from then onwards, children known to have been exposed to nevirapine in the context of PMTCT were initiated on a first-line regimen with two NRTIs and a protease inhibitor (PI) [19]. For the purposes of this study, a treatment switch was defined as modifying the regimen to another regimen, within the first-line (including modification from one NRTI to another) or from first-line to second-line. Children would typically switch from a nevirapine-containing regimen to an efavirenz-containing regimen if side effects occurred due to nevirapine, or if they developed tuberculosis. A treatment switch from one NRTI to another NRTI could be due to national ART guidelines changes, side effects, or stock outs. A modification from a first line (NNRTI-containing) regimen to a second line (PI-containing) regimen was indicated in case of virological failure.

Clinic procedures

By the time a child and caregiver were approached for study participation, the decision to start cART had already been taken by a committee of clinicians and social workers as per routine clinic procedures. Children who subsequently also consented to study participation initiated cART at study enrollment. At this enrollment visit, primary caregivers and children were counseled and interviewed by study staff. The face-to-face interviews included questions about socio-demographics (including orphan status and guardianship), HIV infection history, and variables deemed of importance in the context of cART adherence (see below). In accordance with the national ART guidelines, a clinical assessment was conducted at enrollment and at 2, 4, 8 and 12 weeks after enrollment, and subsequently every three months if the child was clinically doing well, until a maximum of 18 months of follow up was reached or the end of the study (whichever came earlier). Children had additional visits to the clinic in case of unforeseen problems (e.g. infections, or presumed adverse effects of cART). The study was conducted within the public health sector; clinic visits combined routine follow-up procedures and additional study-related procedures such as close laboratory monitoring including CD4 and viral load as well as treatment adverse effect assessment. The study was designed in such a way that no extra visits were needed for the sake of the study. For the study a reimbursement of transport fees was given to the parents per visit for the equivalent of 5 USD. The assessment included a physical examination with measurement of height and weight, pediatric WHO clinical staging, clinical symptoms, and targeted evaluations of side-effects using a standardized checklist. A general physical exam was also conducted and clinician findings were recorded on a standardized CRF covering each body system. In addition to the clinical and laboratory evaluations targeting side effects (see below), side effects were also assessed by standardized face-to-face interview at each study visit. In addition, participants were asked if they had any other symptoms that had not yet been covered in the interview.

Laboratory testing

All laboratory tests were performed at the National Reference Laboratory (NRL) in Kigali, Rwanda. Blood was drawn by venipuncture: a complete blood cell count and liver transaminases [Alanine Amino Transferase (AST) and Aspartate Amino Transferase (AST)] were determined by Cobas Integra 400 plus (Roche Diagnostics, Indianapolis IN, USA) at enrollment and at 1, 3, 6, 12, and 18 months follow-up. CD4 T-cell counts and percentages were determined at enrollment and at 3, 6, 12 and 18 months follow-up by flow-cytometric measurement using a FACS Calibur (Becton Dickinson, San Jose, CA, USA). Plasma HIV-1 RNA concentration (Roche Cobas AmpliPrep/Cobas TaqMan HIV-1, Roche Molecular Systems, France, with a lower limit of detection of 40 copies/mL), creatinine (Cobas Integra 400 plus, Roche Diagnostics, Indianapolis IN, USA) and a lipid profile (low-density lipoprotein. high-density lipoprotein and triglycerides, Human Humastar 180, Human GmbH, Wiesbaden Germany) were determined at enrollment and at months 6, 12 and 18. Children with virological failure (see definition below) and children with plasma HIV-RNA concentrations between 40 and 1000 copies/ mL were scheduled for additional HIV-1 RNA testing within 6 months.

Adherence assessments

Caregivers and children, if age appropriate, received adherence counseling before enrollment and then at each follow-up visit. Caregivers were requested to return all medication containers and any unused medications at the next scheduled visit. For adherence monitoring, the caregivers were asked questions by face-to-face interviewing using a structured questionnaire; adherence assessment was conducted at every clinic and pharmacy follow-up visit.

They were asked how many doses of the prescribed medication the child had missed during the previous 30 days and at what time points this occurred, and reasons for non-adherence, both child-related (e.g. refusal, spitting, or vomiting) or caregiver-related (e.g. forgetting). They were also asked questions about the socio-economic status of the household (level of caregivers' education, household income), and distance to the clinic. Children were categorized as non-adherent if having taken less than 95% of the prescribed medication in the last 30 days. In addition, study nurses and pharmacy staff counted pills dispensed and returned unused, assuming that all other pills were used.

Statistical analysis

All statistical analyses were performed using STATA Version 12 (Copyright 1984–2007 StataCorp TX USA). All statistical analyses were assessed for statistical significance at the $p<0.05$ level. Descriptive statistics are presented as proportions for categorical data and means with standard deviations (SD) and medians with IQR for parametric and non-parametric continuous data, respectively.

Study endpoints. The primary objective of this study was to determine the proportion of children achieving good clinical, immunological, and virological outcomes in the first year of cART as well as predictors of these outcomes. Good clinical outcome was defined as weight-for-age (WAZ) or height-for-age (HAZ)≥ -2 z-score. WAZ and HAZ were calculated using Epinfo version 3.5.1 (Centers for Disease Control and Prevention, Atlanta, GA). Immunological success was defined as achievement of CD4 cells $\geq 500/mm^3$ for children above 5 years of age and a CD4 percentage $\geq 25\%$ for children under 5 years of age. Virological success was defined as an HIV-1 RNA concentration <40 copies/ mL per study time point. Children were categorized as WHO clinical stage I–IV throughout the study according to the WHO pediatric clinical classification system [18].

A secondary objective of the study was to document the occurrence and severity of side effects at any time point as well as predictors of the occurrence of side effects. Self-reported side effects and clinical findings were categorized into 5 main groups: gastro-intestinal, neurological, skin/mucosal, respiratory, and other. The severity of each side effect was assessed using the US National Institute of Allergy and Infectious Diseases Division of AIDS Table for Grading the Severity of Adult and Pediatric Adverse Events (DAIDS-AE) [20]. Grade 1 (mild) was defined as symptoms causing no or minimal interference with usual social and functional activities; grade 2 (moderate) as symptoms causing greater than minimal interference with usual social and functional activities; grade 3 (severe) as symptoms causing inability to perform usual social and functional activities; and grade 4 (potentially life-threatening) as symptoms causing inability to perform basic self-care functions or medical or operative intervention indicated to prevent permanent impairment, persistent disability, or death. Side effects were classified as transient if they were recorded at one or multiple time-points but eventually disappeared without any changes to cART regimen and without treatment of the side effects. They were classified as persistent when they required cART regimen changes or treatment of the side effect. Children were considered to have severe anemia if hemoglobin was <7.5 g/dl, and severe liver abnormality if ALT and/or AST was >5 times the normal values.

Another secondary objective of the study was to assess adherence over time and predictors of adherence. Children were categorized as poorly adherent if they had taken less than 95% of the prescribed medication, based on either self-report or pill counts, or if the caregiver had missed a scheduled pharmacy appointments for ≥ 2 consecutive days, as only a 15- or 30-day supply of medication was provided at each clinic visit. Adherence assessment was conducted at every visit and was measured for the last 30 days preceding the clinic visit.

Statistical modeling. Due to repeated measurements of the outcome, generalizing estimating equation (GEE) models were used to determine outcome changes over time, assuming an exchangeable correlation, (where the correlation is the same for all outcomes within a subject; which is best suited for longitudinal studies in which the same subjects are followed over time). The associations between outcomes and different explanatory variables were evaluated using bivariable GEE models (due to sample size limitations, only one explanatory factor was added at a time). In the WAZ and HAZ models, these explanatory variables included age group, CD4 count, gender, PMTCT exposure and adherence at visits 3, 6 and 9. In the models with positive immunological response as the outcome, children of all ages were combined into one model by combining percentages $\geq 25\%$ for children below 5 years and absolute CD4 T-cell counts ≥ 500 cell/mm^3 for children older than 5 years of age as positive outcomes. Explanatory variables included age group, CD4 count, WHO stage, gender, PMTCT exposure and adherence during the previous 3 or 6 months. In the models with virological success as the outcome, the same explanatory variables were tested as in the immunological success models, but also distance to the TRACplus clinic, orphan status, caregiver education, viral load at initiation and history of treatment switches. Furthermore, adherence over the last 6 months was used (instead of the last 3 months in all other models) because viral load was only measured once every 6 months. In the models with adherence over time as the outcome, explanatory variables included cART regimen, gender, caregiver's educational level, orphan status, and distance to the TRACplus clinic. The proportions of children with side effects were calculated per time point. From the literature, the most relevant predictors associated with side effects were considered gender and age [21]. Using Kaplan–Meier survival analysis, gender and age were analyzed for all side effects jointly and for each group separately.

Results

Baseline characteristics

One hundred and twenty three children were enrolled in the study (figure 1). The median (IQR) age at cART initiation was 7.4 years (3.2, 11.5); 40% of children were below 5 years of age and 54% were female (Table 1). Twenty-five (20%) children were diagnosed with HIV during PMTCT follow-up services, 58 (47%) children when they presented with clinical symptoms, and 40 (33%) children after their parents or siblings were diagnosed with HIV or were suspected to have died of HIV-related diseases. More than a quarter of the children (26%) were orphaned and cared for by other family members or living in an orphanage.

More children were stunted than underweight, with a mean (SD) HAZ and WAZ of -2.01 (1.2) and -1.73 (1.3), respectively. The median (IQR) CD4 T-cell values for children <5 years and $\geq$ 5 years of age were 20 (13, 28) percent and 337 (236, 484) cells/mm^3 respectively. The median (IQR) plasma HIV-1 RNA concentration was 283,000 copies/mL (59,800, 1,100,000) for children less than 5 years of age and 90,600 copies/mL (12,800, 268,000) for those $\geq$5 years. The initial cART regimens are described in Table 1.

Study follow-up and clinical outcomes

Due to termination of funding in September 2010, not all children could be followed for 18 months; 116 children had been followed for 9 months; 104 for 12 months and 72 children for 18 months. The longitudinal analysis includes all data up to 12 months. One child (14 years old) presenting with WHO clinical stage 4 and a CD4 T-cell count of 2 cells/mm^3 died one month after cART initiation. He developed high fever, respiratory distress and increased lymphadenopathy, and the presumed cause of death was immune reconstitution inflammatory syndrome (IRIS). Two children were diagnosed with tuberculosis (one after 1 month on cART and the second child after 4 months of cART); no other children developed opportunistic infections during follow-up. One child was lost to follow-up, and one child moved and was transferred to another treatment center. At the time of the current analysis 98% of children were alive.

Table 2 summarizes anthropometric and biological parameters over time. Mean WAZ (GEE odds ratio (OR): 1.05 (95% confidence interval (CI): 1.03, 1.06; p-value <0.001)) and HAZ (GEE OR: 1.02 (95% CI: 1.01, 1.03; p-value <0.001)) improved significantly during the 12 months. At 12 months of follow-up, the proportion of children who were underweight had decreased from 42% to 20% (GEE OR: 0.90 (95% CI: 0.87, 0.94; p-value <0.001)) and the proportion of children who were stunted decreased from 51% to 41% (GEE OR: 0.96 (95% CI: 0.95, 0.99; p-value<0.001)). The median (range) ALT and AST concentrations at baseline were 19.5 (15.0, 25.0) and 39.0 (29.0,

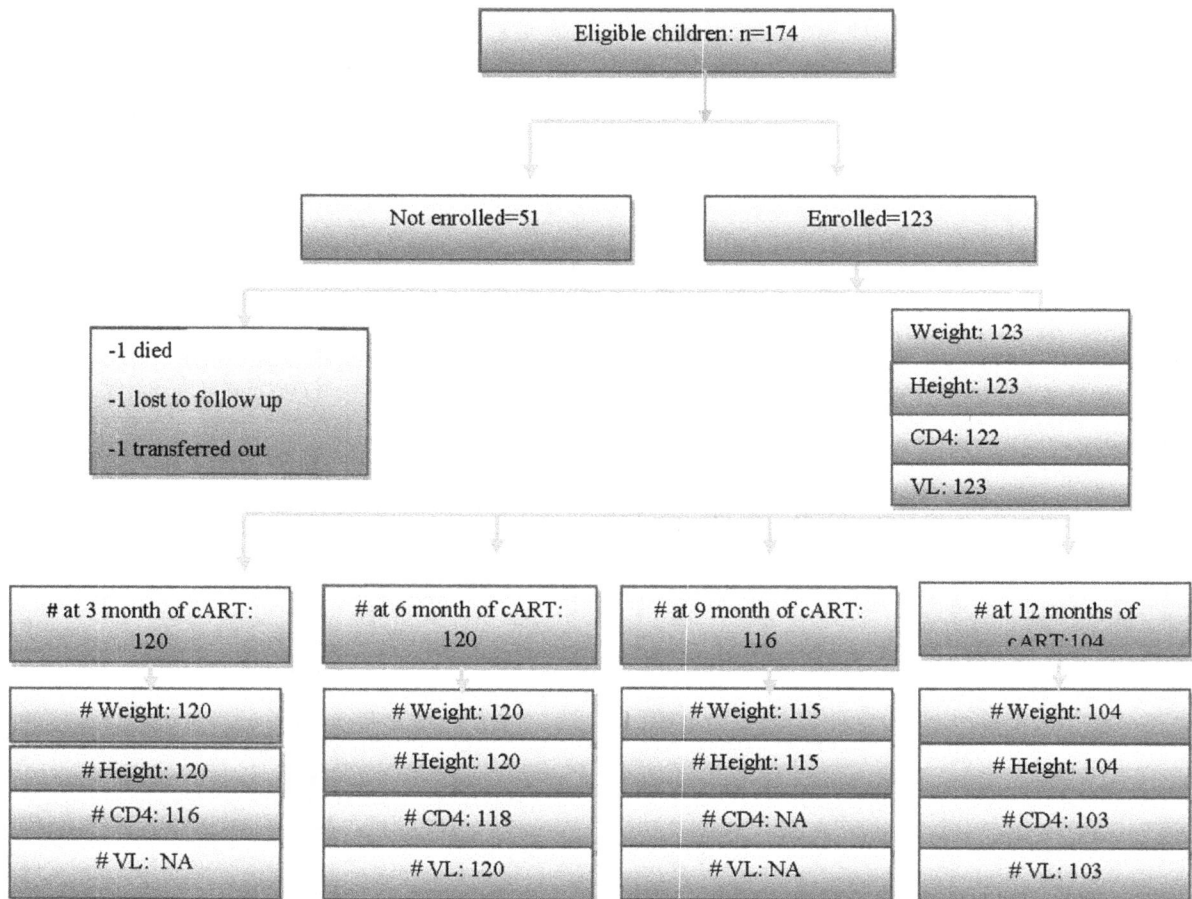

Figure 1. Flowchart summarizing the number of children at each stage of the study.

Table 1. Baseline characteristics at cART initiation (n = 123).

	<5 years (n = 49)	≥5 years (n = 74)	N
DEMOGRAPHIC AND SOCIAL			
Median (IQR) age, years	2.5(1.8–3.5)	11.0(9.0–13.4)	123
Female n (%)	28(57)	39(53)	123
Perinatal infection n (%)	49(100)	74(100)	123
Children exposed to PMTCT, n (%)	15(33)	10(15)	110
Parent status n (%)*			123
Both parents alive	28(57)	34(46)	
Only mother alive	7(14)	12(16)	
Only father alive	4(8)	6(8)	
Both parents died	10(20)	22(30)	
Guardians/caregivers n (%)			123
Both parents	19(39)	20(27)	
Mother only	15(31)	25(34)	
Father only	2(4)	3(4)	
Other family member	11(23)	23(31)	
Other	2(4)	3(4)	
Caregiver's educational status n (%)**			123
No education/few years primary school	17(34.7)	28(37.85)	
At least primary school completed	32(65.3)	46(62.2)	
Distance from healthcare center n (%)***			123
Living in Kigali	39(79.6)	16(21.6)	
Living outside of Kigali	10(20.4)	58(78.4)	
Tested and Diagnosed n (%)			123
PMTCT services	15	10	
Family member died/sick	15	25	
Symptoms	19	39	
CLINICAL			
Weight-for-age z-score			123
Mean (SD)	−2.04(1.6)	−1.49(1.1)	
z-score ≤−2 n (%)	26(53)	25(34)	
Height-for-age z-score			123
Mean (SD)	−2.5(1.4)	−1.7(0.9)	
z-score ≤−2 n (%)	34(69)	29(39)	
WHO stage, n (%)			122
Stage 1 & II	5(10.2)	18(24.7)	
Stage III & IV	44(89.8)	55(75.3)	
Tuberculosis at cART, n (%)	11(22)	19(26)	123
LABORATORY			
Immunological status at baseline			119
Median (IQR) CD4 values	20(13–28)	337/mm3(236–484)	
Children with CD4<15% or <350/mm3, n (%)	13(28)	41 (57)	
Virological status at baseline			123
Median (IQR) HIV-1 RNA copies/mL	283,000(59,800–1,100,000)	90,600(12,800–268,000)	
Biochemistry & Hematology at baseline			122
Median (IQR) ALT, UI/l	20(15–32)	19(15–25)	
Median (IQR) AST, UI/l	40(34–50)	34(29–40)	
Median (IQR) Hemoglobin, g/dL	11(10.2–11.6)	12(11.7–12.8)	
INITIAL cART REGIMEN n (%)			123
AZT/3TC/NVP	38(77.5)	46(62.2)	
ABC/3TC/NVP	1(2	2(2.7)	

Table 1. Cont.

	<5 years (n = 49)	≥5 years (n = 74)	N
D4T/3TC/NVP	2(4)	11(15.0)	
AZT/3TC/EFV	4(8)	12(16.2)	
D4T/3TC/EFV	2(4)	2(2.7)	
ABC/3TC/LPV/r	2(4)	1(1.4)	
Treatment switch	9(18.4)	12(16.2)	

*Orphan status was defined as having at least one biological parent vs. none.
**Caregiver's educational level was categorized as non-educated/few years of primary school vs. completed at least primary school.
***Distance to the clinic was defined as living in Kigali vs. outside of Kigali.

50.0) IU/mL and rose to 22.0 (15.0, 30.0) and 54.1 (29.9, 91.9) IU/mL at 12 months, respectively. The median (range) hemoglobin at cART initiation was 11.6 (11.3, 12.0) g/dL and increased to 12.3 (12.1, 12.5) at 12 months of cART.

Both age groups, above and below 5 years at cART initiation, had a significant increase in HAZ z-scores on therapy, but improvement was better in children above 5 years of age (GEE OR: 3.7 (95% CI: 1.8, 7.6)). Children who were not underweight when initiating cART were more likely to experience a significant HAZ and reduction of stunting overtime (GEE OR: 4.1 (95% CI:

1.9, 8.6)) as compared to those who were underweight (data not presented). WAZ increase was observed in both children with good and poor adherence, but the increase was slightly better in children with good adherence than children with poor adherence (GEE OR: 1.2 (95% CI: 0.9, 1.7)). Children who initiated treatment with CD4 ≥350 cells/µ/L or CD4 ≥15% had better improvement in WAZ scores compared to children who initiated treatment with CD4 below these cut offs (GEE OR: 1.9 (95% CI: 0.9, 3.8)). Children who achieved viral suppression compared to children with virological failure had significant WAZ (GEE OR:

Table 2. Changes of WAZ, HAZ, Hemoglobin, CD4 values and HIV RNA overtime.

	Baseline (n = 123)	3 Months (n = 119)	6 Months (n = 119)	12 Months (n = 104)	P-values
Nutritional status					
WAZ (mean, 95%CI*)	−1.73(−1.95,−1.50)	−1.38(−1.59,−1.17)	−1.28(−1.47,−1.08)	−1.17(−1.38,−0.96)	**<0.001**
Underweight (WAZ<−2) (n, %)	52(42)	36 (30)	31(26)	21(20)	**<0.001**
HAZ (mean, 95%CI*)	−2.01(−2.23,−1.80)	−1.93(−2.15,−1.71)	−1.82(−2.04,−1.60)	−1.75(−1.98,−1,51)	**<0.001**
Stunting (HAZ<−2) (n, %)	63(51)	57(47)	53(44)	43(41)	**0.001**
Hemoglobin (mean, 95 CI*), g/dL	11.6(11.3–12.0)	12.1(11.8–12.4)	12.2(12.0–12.4)	12.3(12.1–12.5)	**<0.001**
Immunological status					
Children ≥5 years, n = 74					
CD4 T-cells (median, IQR)	337(236–484)	500(345–675)	567(365–765)	620(375–880)	**<0.001**
CD4 T-cells <500, n (%),	57(79)	34(49)	29(40)	22(34)	**<0.001**
Children <5 years, n = 49					
CD4 T-cell % (median, IQR)	20(13–28)	29(22–36)	33(26–39)	36(28–41)	**<0.001**
CD4T-cell <25%, n (%),	30(65)	17(38)	11(24)	5(13)	**<0.001**
Virological status (HIV-RNA)					
<40 (copies/mL), n (%)	0(0)	Not determined	52(43)	79(76)	**<0.001**
>1000 copies/mL, n (%)	123(100)		46(38)	17(16)	**<0.001**

P values bold: Changes over time for all variables were statistically significant at p<0.05 using a univariate Generalized estimating equation model for categorical, normal and no normal distributed outcomes.

2.3 (95% CI: 1.6, 3.3)) and HAZ increases over time (GEE OR: 1.3 (95% CI: 1.1, 1.5)). A small percentage of children did not show any improvement in WAZ (4%) and HAZ (9%) after 12 months of cART. Out of 5 children who did not have increased WAZ, three had virological and immunological failure, and 4 had poor adherence. Out of 12 who did not have increased HAZ, 9 had virological failure, 7 had immunological failure, and 7 had poor adherence.

Immunological and virological responses

A significant increase in CD4 T- cells was observed in both children younger than 5 years of age as well as in those over 5 years of age. The median CD4 T-cell percent for younger children increased from 20% to 36% and the median CD4 T-cell count for children above 5 years increased from 337 to 620cells/mm^3 by 12 months follow-up; the proportion of children who achieved immunological success was 87% for children under 5 years and 66% for children 5 years of age and above. In bivariable models, independent predictors of immunological success included age and CD4 T-cell baseline value, with children below 5 years and those having a CD4 T-cell baseline value above 350/mm^3 showing a more robust increase in median CD4 T-cells (GEE OR: 1.9 (95% CI: 1.1, 4.1) and 7.0 (4.3, 11.6), respectively). PMTCT exposure, WHO stage at baseline, poor adherence, and socio-economic characteristics were not statistically associated with CD4 T-cell recovery in the first 12 months of cART.

The mean changes in HIV RNA plasma concentration over time are presented in Table 2. After 12 months of cART, 24% had detectable HIV RNA (>40 copies/mL), including 16% with virologic failure (>1000 copies/mL). In bivariable analyses, independent predictors of virological failure were being less than 5 years old at baseline (GEE OR: 2.6 (95% CI: 1.3, 5.2)), exposure to PMTCT (GEE OR: 3.4 (95% CI: (1.5, 7.8)), poor adherence during the first six months of treatment (GEE OR: 2.5 (95% CI: 1.3, 5.0)) and initiating cART with viral load ≥50.000 copies/mL (GEE OR: 4.6 (95% CI: 2.3, 156.2)). Other medical and social characteristics were not significantly associated with HIV RNA change over time (Table 3).

Adverse effects of treatment and treatment switches

There were 158 cumulative adverse effects reported in 52 (42%) children during the period of 12 months. The highest number was reported at month two of treatment in 40 (33%) of the children. The majority (47 out of 52) of children reported the same adverse effect at 2 or more time points; 41 children had mild and transient adverse effects which recovered without stopping treatment, 11/123 (9%) children experienced persistent side effects and/or worsening over time and underwent cART regimen changes as a result. The incidence of side-effects was higher within the first 6 months of cART initiation than thereafter (Figure 2a, 2b). The most common side effects were nausea and vomiting (14.8%), nevirapine-associated skin rash and hypersensitivity (13.2%), any grade of anemia (7%), diarrhea (6%), and dizziness and fatigue (5%) (Table 4). Eighty six percent of mild/moderate side effects improved without additional therapy.

During the follow-up period of 18 months, 21 (17%) children switched their initial cART regimen. Reasons for switching included persistent side effects (n = 11), virological failure (n = 3), tuberculosis treatment (replacement of nevirapine by efavirenz, n = 2), replacement of stavudine following a change of the Rwandan cART guidelines (n = 3), and replacement due to

stock-out issues (n = 2). The children who developed nevirapine-associated skin-related side effects and/or significant liver enzyme elevations stopped treatment and their symptoms abated after treatment cessation; they resumed treatment with an efavirenz-based regimen. In three children with significant anemia, zidovudine was replaced by abacavir or tenofovir, hemoglobin improved to ≥10 g/dl within 6 months after treatment change. Two adolescents on a stavudine-based regimen developed signs of lipoatrophy (n = 1) and lipohypertrophy (n = 1) during the second year of treatment, and switched from stavudine to tenofovir. Eighteen out of the 21 treatment modifications were from one drug to another within the first line; 3 children switched from the first line NNRTI based regimen to a second line with lopinavir/ritonavir because of virologic failure.

Adherence assessment

Adherence as estimated by self-report was high, with a median >95% at all-time points. In only 77 (11%) out of 710 scheduled visits at least one missed dose was reported by self-report. Incorrect dosage of any drug or change of time of taking medication was reported in 44 (6%) of all scheduled visits. Poor adherence on self-report was highly predictive of poor adherence on pill count (data not shown); however, good adherence by self-report was often not confirmed by pill count data. Pill count data showed that pills or scheduled visits were missed at 269 (38%) of visits. The proportion of children who were poor adherent according to pill count and recorded missed visits (adherence <95%) decreased over time, from 38% at month 3 to 20% by 12 months.

In bivariable analysis, after 6 months of cART 48% of children with good adherence had an undetectable viral load while only 34% of children with poor adherence had an undetectable viral load. The proportion of children with an undetectable viral load increased to 80% in the adherent group and to 57% in the less adherent group after 12 months of cART.

In bivariable analysis, lower caregiver educational status (GEE OR: 1.2 (95% CI: (1.1, 9.8)) and being an orphan ((GEE OR: 1.6 (95% CI): (1.2, 8.3)) were associated with lower adherence. None of the other factors, including gender, age, regimen or distance to the clinic were found to be statistically associated with adherence over time.

Discussion

The majority of children in this study showed good clinical and immunologic recovery, good adherence to cART and retention in care, as well as improved height and weight after 12 months of cART. Although the study showed overall treatment success after 12 months, HIV viral load was not fully suppressed in nearly a quarter of children, and immunologic recovery was less successful in children 5 years or older and those with more advanced HIV disease at cART initiation. Approximately one in 10 children developed severe side effects resulting in temporary cART cessation and regimen switches.

At baseline, slightly more than half of children were stunted and 40% were underweight. These proportions were higher than those reported by various recent national surveys in children regardless of HIV status, in which 27–44% of children were stunted, and up to 12% of children were underweight, depending on the area of the survey [22,23]. The lowest proportion of underweight children (6%) was found in Kigali district [22]. However, in our study, the number of children stunted and underweight after 12 months of cART was close to these survey figures. Furthermore, the overall

Table 3. Number of children with virological failure* over time.

	Month 6	Month 12	p-values**	Odds Ratio(95%%CI)
Parent status				
Both died	12(38)	6(21)	0.872	0.9(0.4–2.0)
At least one lives	34(39)	11(15)		
Caregiver's educational status				
Completed at least Primary school	17(37)	9(19)	0.678	0.6(0.3–3.1)
Non educated	30(39)	16(20)		
Distance from healthcare center				
Living in Kigali	22(40)	9(17)	0.567	0.8(0.5–2.7)
Outside of Kigali	28(41)	13(19)		
Age group				
Age ≥5 years at cART initiation	21(29)	7(11)	**0.006**	**2.6(1.3–5.2)**
Age <5 years at cART initiation	25(52)	10(25)		
Immunological status at baseline				
CD4≥15% or 350/mm3	21(34)	6(12)	0.282	1.5(0.7–2.9)
CD4<15% or <350/mm3	23(43)	10(20)		
WHO stage at baseline				
Baseline WHO I&II	8(35)	0	0.171	1.7(0.8–3.9)
Baseline WHO III&IV	37(39)	16(19)		
95% Adherence				
Adherent	26(32)	12(15)	**0.009**	**2.5(1.3–5.0)**
Non-adherent	20(53)	5(24)		
PMTCT exposure				
No-exposure	26(31)	9(12)	**0.003**	**3.4(1.5–7.9)**
Exposure	14(58)	6(38)		
Regimen switch up to 6 or 9 months				
No treatment change	40(37)	12(14)	0.337	1.6(0.6–4.3)
Treatment change	6(54)	7(49)		

*Virological failure defined as VL≥1000 copies/mL for one measurement;
**between group comparisons.
P values bold: significant difference at p<0.05.

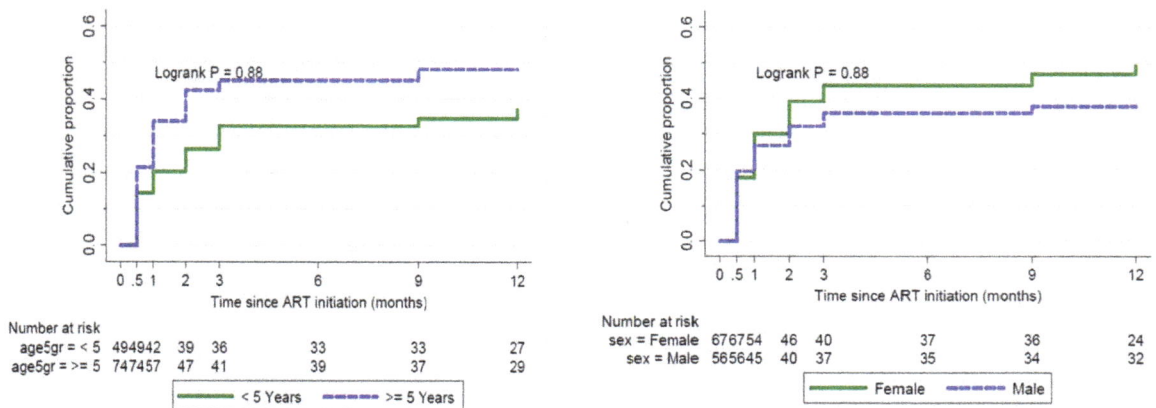

Figure 2. Cumulative of proportion of children with any side effect by sex (left) and age group (right) from baseline to 12 months of Treatment.

Table 4. Clinical and laboratory side effects.

	Day 15	Month 1	Month 2	Month 3	Month 6	Month 9	Month 12
Clinical side effects, n (%)							
Skin, mucosa and nails							
Hypersensitivity/Skin rash	16(13)	31(26)	26(21)	18(15)	6(5)	5(4)	2(2)
Nail pigmentation	-	-	-	2(2)	7(6)	9(8)	9(9)
Gastro-intestinal							
Nausea and vomiting, n (%)	21(17)	30(25)	34(28)	18(15)	4(3)	2(2)	1(1)
Diarrhea, n(%)	12(10)	13(11)	15(13)	11(9)	-	-	-
Abdominal pain, n (%)	4(3)	1(1)	2(2)	1(1)	-	-	-
Neurological							
Dizziness, n(%)	3(2)	6(5)	6(5)	6(5)	2(2)	2(2)	1(1)
Insomnia, n(%)	-	-	-	2(2)	2(2)	2(2)	1(1)
Laboratory							
Anemia (Hb<10 g/dl)	NA	NA	19(16)	6(5)	4(3)	2(2)	2(2)
Liver functions elevated (ALT), n (%)	7(6)	13(10)	8(7)	8(7)	3(3)	2(2)	-
Other*, n (%)	4(3)	2(2)	5(4)	3(2)	1(1)	-	-

*other included fatigue, anxiety and nightmares.

increase in weight among all children, and increase of height by baseline nutrition status and age are comparable to increases reported in other studies from similar resource constrained settings [9,24,25,26,27,28,29]. These findings reflect the efficacy of cART and offer reassuring evidence of its safety and tolerability in Rwandan children in which regular clinical monitoring is routine. Children who did not show any improvement in WAZ and HAZ after 12 months of treatment also showed poor ART adherence, poor immunologic recovery and virological failure.

In our study, children above 5 years of age were more likely to have impaired immunological recovery after 12 months of cART; conversely those under five were more likely to experience virologic failure. The robust immunologic recovery that we observed in young children may be partially explained by the superior ability of young infants to repopulate T lymphocytes [30,31], or by the hypothesis that later initiation of cART allows for more architectural damage to lymphatic tissues, which in turn hampers immune reconstitution [4,32]. The relationship between young age and virological failure has been documented in other studies in sub-Saharan Africa [13,33]. It is also consistent with earlier observations that infants and young children often present with high viral load and that it takes longer to fully suppress viral replication [34,35,36,37,38]. Prospective studies with longer follow-up periods should be conducted to determine whether the association between age at cART initiation and suboptimal virologic suppression is maintained after a longer period on cART. Not surprisingly, age and immune status at cART initiation were the factors most strongly associated with immunological success [9,39]. This observation emphasizes the fact that efforts should be made to diagnose and treat HIV infected children as early as possible.

The proportion of children with a detectable viral load and virological failure after 12 months of cART in this study is a serious finding that needs urgent attention. Poor adherence to cART and nevirapine exposure during PMTCT were associated with cART failure in our study as has been shown in other studies [40,41]. Previous studies confirmed that one in two infants exposed to single dose nevirapine prophylaxis develop nevirapine resistance, which in turn may expose children to more resistant viral strains and compromise therapy with NNRTI-containing regimens [42,43,44,45,46,47]. The finding that non-adherence measured by pill count was a strong predictor of virologic response reiterates the importance of adherence to cART and adherence monitoring through other means than self-report, in which patients are more likely to report high adherence [48]. Although it is obvious that adherence is paramount for achieving and maintaining viral suppression, and prevention of drug-resistance [49,50], it seems that the specific challenges regarding adherence in pediatric populations have not yet been sufficiently tackled. Issues such as drug administration in young children, adolescent behavior, socio-economic status and the dependency on the caregiver [51,52] may all play a role and are often difficult to solve. Additionally, the pharmacokinetic properties of ARVs in young children are not well known; underdosing or increased metabolism may lead to suboptimal plasma drug levels and thereby influence virologic outcomes. In an earlier study conducted in Rwanda, we observed that 14% of children using efavirenz were not adequately dosed [53], and other studies have shown similar results for other drug combinations [54,55].

The incidence of mild and moderate side effects in this study, mainly associated with nevirapine use, were similar to the findings from Uganda by Tukei [56], but were higher than what was reported by Lapphra in Thai children [57] and by Oumar in Malian children [58]. Most of the severe symptoms reported were reversed after discontinuation of the suspected drug and treatment changes to potentially less toxic medication as has been reported previously by Shubber et al [59]. The number of children with severe and/or persistent side effects leading to drug substitution was higher in our study compared to the studies mentioned previously [56,57,58]. Side effects and treatment switches may impact on treatment adherence, and potentially undermine the success of cART [60,61]. The side effects and regimen changes may have contributed to the relatively high percentage of children with treatment failure that we have seen in our study. More than half of the children without viral suppression had persistent side effects and/or regimen switches. Careful monitoring of the safety of cART remains needed, especially during the first months of cART, and we strongly support the national ART guidelines recommending PI-based regimens for all children <3 years of age [15].

This study has a number of limitations. Due to funding constraints, the sample size was relatively small; results for the present study on 123 children may not be generalizable to the larger population of children in Rwanda, given that data were only collected from children in one center in Kigali. Moreover, data for this study were collected a few years ago, current practice, validity and implication of some recommendations may be affected. However, the study presents more comprehensive information on cART outcomes in children than is available from national Rwandan HIV programs. The study highlights an important point that treatment failures are common in Rwandan children and emphasizes the importance of close virological monitoring. Another limitation is that the duration of follow-up was shorter than originally planned. This means that we were unable to assess the long term impact of cART on growth, immune and virologic responses, and long term toxicity. Studies with a longer duration of follow up are needed to inform national programs. Furthermore, we could not attribute the incidence of anemia solely to use of zidovudine as coexisting nutritional deficiencies and other chronic diseases may also have played a role [56,62,63]. Finally, we could not assess cART drug resistance in this particular study, but an earlier study in Rwanda showed that >90% of children with a viral load ≥1000 copies/mL after 12 months of cART were reported to have at least one NRTI or NNRTI's major mutations [10].

In conclusion, the importance of timely initiation of cART before profound immunodeficiency occurs in children should not be underestimated, as has been reported previously [9,11,12,13,14]. The Ministry of Health in Rwanda has recognized this and has adjusted its guidelines accordingly. Initiation of cART is now recommended for all children under 5 regardless of clinical condition and CD4 status, and for all children and adults older than 5 years with CD4 T-cells <500/mm^3. However, several challenges related to side effects, and achieving long-term adherence and virologic suppression remain. To be truly successful, pediatric HIV programs must aim to find HIV infected children before disease progression occurs, initiate cART timely, and monitor treatment success and side effects closely. Furthermore, the main causes of virologic failure should be further investigated, so that strategies for early recognition of children at high risk and appropriate interventions can be developed [64,65].

Acknowledgments

The authors would like to thank all the patients and families from Treatment and Research for AIDS Center participating in this study and the team of the INTERACT Project and the Rwandan Ministry of Health. Laboratory technicians from the National Reference Laboratory, Rwanda are kindly acknowledged for the analysis of laboratory tests that were performed for the purpose of this study.

References

1. HHS Panel on Antiretroviral Therapy and Medical Management of HIV-Infected Children (2012) Guidelines for the Use of Antiretroviral Agents in Pediatric HIV Infection. Available: http://aidsinfonihgov/contentfiles/lvguidelines/pediatricguidelinespdf Accessed September 2013
2. Mofenson LM, Brady MT, Danner SP, Dominguez KL, Hazra R, et al. (2009) Guidelines for the Prevention and Treatment of Opportunistic Infections among HIV-exposed and HIV-infected children: recommendations from CDC, the National Institutes of Health, the HIV Medicine Association of the Infectious Diseases Society of America, the Pediatric Infectious Diseases Society, and the American Academy of Pediatrics. MMWR Recomm Rep 58: 1–166.
3. Penazzato M, Crowley S, Mofenson L, Franceschetto G, Nannyonga MM, et al. (2012) Programmatic impact of the evolution of WHO pediatric antiretroviral treatment guidelines for resource-limited countries (Tukula Fenna Project, Uganda). J Acquir Immune Defic Syndr 61: 522–525.
4. Puthanakit T, Kerr S, Ananworanich J, Bunupuradah T, Boonrak P, et al. (2009) Pattern and predictors of immunologic recovery in human immunodeficiency virus-infected children receiving non-nucleoside reverse transcriptase inhibitor-based highly active antiretroviral therapy. Pediatr Infect Dis J 28: 488–492.
5. Sutcliffe CG, van Dijk JH, Munsanje B, Hamangaba F, Siniwymaanzi P, et al. (2011) Risk factors for pre-treatment mortality among HIV-infected children in rural Zambia: a cohort study. PLoS One 6: e29294.
6. Yotebieng M, Van Rie A, Moultrie H, Meyers T (2010) Six-month gain in weight, height, and CD4 predict subsequent antiretroviral treatment responses in HIV-infected South African children. AIDS 24: 139–146.
7. Clavel F, Hance AJ (2004) HIV drug resistance. N Engl J Med 350: 1023–1035.
8. Musiime V, Kaudha E, Kayiwa J, Mirembe G, Odera M, et al. (2013) Antiretroviral drug resistance profiles and response to second-line therapy among HIV type 1-infected Ugandan children. AIDS Res Hum Retroviruses 29: 449–455.
9. Musoke PM, Mudiope P, Barlow-Mosha LN, Ajuna P, Bagenda D, et al. (2010) Growth, immune and viral responses in HIV infected African children receiving highly active antiretroviral therapy: a prospective cohort study. BMC Pediatr 10: 56.
10. Mutwa PR, Boer KR, Rusine J, Muganga N, Tuyishimire D, et al. (2014) Long-term effectiveness of combination antiretroviral therapy and prevalence of HIV drug resistance in HIV-1-infected children and adolescents in Rwanda. Pediatr Infect Dis J 33: 63–69.
11. Sutcliffe CG, van Dijk JH, Munsanje B, Hamangaba F, Sinywimaanzi P, et al. (2011) Weight and height z-scores improve after initiating ART among HIV-infected children in rural Zambia: a cohort study. BMC Infect Dis 11: 98.
12. Ndumbi P, Falutz J, Pant Pai N, Tsoukas CM (2014) Delay in cART Initiation Results in Persistent Immune Dysregulation and Poor Recovery of T-Cell Phenotype Despite a Decade of Successful HIV Suppression. PLoS One 9: e94018.
13. Okomo U, Togun T, Oko F, Peterson K, Townend J, et al. (2012) Treatment outcomes among HIV-1 and HIV-2 infected children initiating antiretroviral therapy in a concentrated low prevalence setting in West Africa. BMC Pediatr 12: 95.
14. Mossdorf E, Stoeckle M, Mwaigomole EG, Chiweka E, Kibatala PL, et al. (2011) Improved antiretroviral treatment outcome in a rural African setting is associated with cART initiation at higher CD4 cell counts and better general health condition. BMC Infect Dis 11: 54.
15. Rwanda Ministry of Health (2012) National Guidelines for Comprehensive Care of People Living with HIV in Rwanda.
16. Rwanda Ministry of Health (2012) National Annual Report on HIV&AIDS July 2011–June 2012. Available: http://wwwrbcgovrw/spipphp?article503 Accessed August 2013.
17. Rwanda Ministry of Health (2007) Guide de Prise en Charge des Personnes Infectées par le VIH au Rwanda. Available: http://wwwaidstar-onecom/focus_areas/treatment/resources. Accessed July 2013.
18. World Health Organization (2006) Antiretroviral Therapy of HIV infection in Infants and Children: Towards universal access Recommendations for a public health approach. Available: http://wwwwhoint/hiv/pub/guidelines/art/en/ Accessed August 2013
19. Rwanda Ministry of Health (2009) Guidelines for the provision of comprehensive care to persons infected by HIV in Rwanda.
20. (2004) Division of AIDS Table for Grading the Severity of adult and Pediatric Adverse Events Available: http://rsctech-rescom/safetyandpharmacovigilance/gradingtablesaspx Accessed November 2013 Version 1.0.
21. Phan V, Thai S, Choun K, Lynen L, van Griensven J (2012) Incidence of treatment-limiting toxicity with stavudine-based antiretroviral therapy in Cambodia: a retrospective cohort study. PLoS One 7: e30647.
22. National Institute of Statistics of Rwanda/Ministry of Finance and Economic Planning Kigali R (2010) Rwanda Demographic and Health Survey. Available: http://wwwstatisticsgovrw/survey/demographic-and-health-survey-dhs Accessed September 2013.
23. National Institute of Statistics of Rwanda/Ministry of Finance and Economic Planning R (2012) Comprehensive Food Security and Vulnerability Analysis and Nutrition Survey Available: http://wwwstatisticsgovrw/publications/comprehensive-food-security-and-vulnerability-analysis-and-nutrition-survey-cfsva-2012 Accessed November 2013
24. Bolton-Moore C, Mubiana-Mbewe M, Cantrell RA, Chintu N, Stringer EM, et al. (2007) Clinical outcomes and CD4 cell response in children receiving antiretroviral therapy at primary health care facilities in Zambia. JAMA 298: 1888–1899.
25. Davies MA, Keiser O, Technau K, Eley B, Rabie H, et al. (2009) Outcomes of the South African National Antiretroviral Treatment Programme for children: the IeDEA Southern Africa collaboration. S Afr Med J 99: 730–737.
26. Essajee SM, Kim M, Gonzalez C, Rigaud M, Kaul A, et al. (1999) Immunologic and virologic responses to HAART in severely immunocompromised HIV-1-infected children. AIDS 13: 2523–2532.
27. Kamya MR, Mayanja-Kizza H, Kambugu A, Bakeera-Kitaka S, Semitala F, et al. (2007) Predictors of long-term viral failure among ugandan children and adults treated with antiretroviral therapy. J Acquir Immune Defic Syndr 46: 187–193.
28. Sutcliffe CG, Moss WJ (2010) Do children infected with HIV receiving HAART need to be revaccinated? Lancet Infect Dis 10: 630–642.
29. Wamalwa DC, Farquhar C, Obimbo EM, Selig S, Mbori-Ngacha DA, et al. (2007) Early response to highly active antiretroviral therapy in HIV-1-infected Kenyan children. J Acquir Immune Defic Syndr 45: 311–317.
30. Franco JM, Leon-Leal JA, Leal M, Cano-Rodriguez A, Pineda JA, et al. (2000) CD4+ and CD8+ T lymphocyte regeneration after anti-retroviral therapy in HIV-1-infected children and adult patients. Clin Exp Immunol 119: 493–498.
31. Soh CH, Oleske JM, Brady MT, Spector SA, Borkowsky W, et al. (2003) Long-term effects of protease-inhibitor-based combination therapy on CD4 T-cell recovery in HIV-1-infected children and adolescents. Lancet 362: 2045–2051.
32. Walker AS, Doerholt K, Sharland M, Gibb DM, Collaborative HIVPSSC (2004) Response to highly active antiretroviral therapy varies with age: the UK and Ireland Collaborative HIV Paediatric Study. AIDS 18: 1915–1924.
33. Wittkop L, Ngo-Giang_huong N, Team E-C-EP (2013) Prevalence and impact of transmitted drug resistance (TDR) on response to ART in children. Abstract Presented at 7th Conference on HIV Pathogenesis, treatment and Prevention.
34. van Rossum AM, Geelen SP, Hartwig NG, Wolfs TF, Weemaes CM, et al. (2002) Results of 2 years of treatment with protease-inhibitor–containing antiretroviral therapy in dutch children infected with human immunodeficiency virus type 1. Clin Infect Dis 34: 1008–1016.
35. Starr SE, Fletcher CV, Spector SA, Yong FH, Fenton T, et al. (1999) Combination therapy with efavirenz, nelfinavir, and nucleoside reverse-transcriptase inhibitors in children infected with human immunodeficiency virus type 1. Pediatric AIDS Clinical Trials Group 382 Team. N Engl J Med 341: 1874–1881.
36. Nachman SA, Stanley K, Yogev R, Pelton S, Wiznia A, et al. (2000) Nucleoside analogs plus ritonavir in stable antiretroviral therapy-experienced HIV-infected children: a randomized controlled trial. Pediatric AIDS Clinical Trials Group 338 Study Team. JAMA 283: 492–498.
37. Pelton SI, Johnson D, Chadwick E, Baldwin Z, Yogev R (1999) A one year experience: T cell responses and viral replication in children with advanced human immunodeficiency virus type 1 disease treated with combination therapy including ritonavir. Pediatr Infect Dis J 18: 650–652.
38. Palumbo PE, Kwok S, Waters S, Wesley Y, Lewis D, et al. (1995) Viral measurement by polymerase chain reaction-based assays in human immunodeficiency virus-infected infants. J Pediatr 126: 592–595.
39. Lewis J, Walker AS, Castro H, De Rossi A, Gibb DM, et al. (2012) Age and CD4 count at initiation of antiretroviral therapy in HIV-infected children: effects on long-term T-cell reconstitution. J Infect Dis 205: 548–556.
40. Teasdale CA, Abrams EJ, Coovadia A, Strehlau R, Martens L, et al. (2013) Adherence and viral suppression among infants and young children initiating protease inhibitor-based antiretroviral therapy. Pediatr Infect Dis J 32: 489–494.
41. Nachega JB, Hislop M, Nguyen H, Dowdy DW, Chaisson RE, et al. (2009) Antiretroviral therapy adherence, virologic and immunologic outcomes in

Author Contributions

Conceived and designed the experiments: PRM NM JMAL JvdW AA PR SPMG. Performed the experiments: PRM KRB NM DT. Analyzed the data: PRM KRB BAK. Contributed reagents/materials/analysis tools: PRM KRB NM JMAL JvdW BAK DT PR SPMG. Wrote the paper: PRM KRB NM JMAL JvdW AA BAK DT PR SPMG.

adolescents compared with adults in southern Africa. J Acquir Immune Defic Syndr 51: 65–71.

42. Persaud D, Bedri A, Ziemniak C, Moorthy A, Gudetta B, et al. (2011) Slower clearance of nevirapine resistant virus in infants failing extended nevirapine prophylaxis for prevention of mother-to-child HIV transmission. AIDS Res Hum Retroviruses 27: 823–829.

43. Palumbo P, Lindsey JC, Hughes MD, Cotton MF, Bobat R, et al. (2010) Antiretroviral treatment for children with peripartum nevirapine exposure. N Engl J Med 363: 1510–1520.

44. Mphatswe W, Blanckenberg N, Tudor-Williams G, Prendergast A, Thobakgale C, et al. (2007) High frequency of rapid immunological progression in African infants infected in the era of perinatal HIV prophylaxis. AIDS 21: 1253–1261.

45. Lockman S, Shapiro RL, Smeaton LM, Wester C, Thior I, et al. (2007) Response to antiretroviral therapy after a single, peripartum dose of nevirapine. N Engl J Med 356: 135–147.

46. Coovadia A, Abrams EJ, Stehlau R, Meyers T, Martens L, et al. (2010) Reuse of nevirapine in exposed HIV-infected children after protease inhibitor-based viral suppression: a randomized controlled trial. JAMA 304: 1082–1090.

47. Arrive E, Newell ML, Ekouevi DK, Chaix ML, Thiebaut R, et al. (2007) Prevalence of resistance to nevirapine in mothers and children after single-dose exposure to prevent vertical transmission of HIV-1: a meta-analysis. Int J Epidemiol 36: 1009–1021.

48. Vyankandondera J, Mitchell K, Asiimwe-Kateera B, Boer K, Mutwa P, et al. (2013) Antiretroviral therapy drug adherence in Rwanda: perspectives from patients and healthcare workers using a mixed-methods approach. AIDS Care 25: 1504–1512.

49. Mofenson LM, Cotton MF (2013) The challenges of success: adolescents with perinatal HIV infection. J Int AIDS Soc 16: 18650.

50. Mghamba FW, Minzi OM, Massawe A, Sasi P (2013) Adherence to antiretroviral therapy among HIV infected children measured by caretaker report, medication return, and drug level in Dar Es Salaam, Tanzania. BMC Pediatr 13: 95.

51. Vreeman RC, Wiehe SE, Ayaya SO, Musick BS, Nyandiko WM (2008) Association of antiretroviral and clinic adherence with orphan status among HIV-infected children in Western Kenya. J Acquir Immune Defic Syndr 49: 163–170.

52. Azmeraw D, Wasie B (2012) Factors associated with adherence to highly active antiretroviral therapy among children in two referral hospitals, northwest Ethiopia. Ethiop Med J 50: 115–124.

53. Mutwa PR, Fillekes Q, Malgaz M, Tuyishimire D, Kraats R, et al. (2012) Mid-dosing interval efavirenz plasma concentrations in HIV-1-infected children in Rwanda: treatment efficacy, tolerability, adherence, and the influence of CYP2B6 polymorphisms. J Acquir Immune Defic Syndr 60: 400–404.

54. Menson EN, Walker AS, Sharland M, Wells C, Tudor-Williams G, et al. (2006) Underdosing of antiretrovirals in UK and Irish children with HIV as an example of problems in prescribing medicines to children, 1997–2005: cohort study. BMJ 332: 1183–1187.

55. King JR, Kimberlin DW, Aldrovandi GM, Acosta EP (2002) Antiretroviral pharmacokinetics in the paediatric population: a review. Clin Pharmacokinet 41: 1115–1133.

56. Tukei VJ, Asiimwe A, Maganda A, Atugonza R, Sebuliba I, et al. (2012) Safety and tolerability of antiretroviral therapy among HIV-infected children and adolescents in Uganda. J Acquir Immune Defic Syndr 59: 274–280.

57. Lapphra K, Vanprapar N, Chearskul S, Phongsamart W, Chearskul P, et al. (2008) Efficacy and tolerability of nevirapine- versus efavirenz-containing regimens in HIV-infected Thai children. Int J Infect Dis 12: e33–38.

58. Oumar AA, Diallo K, Dembele JP, Samake L, Sidibe I, et al. (2012) Adverse drug reactions to antiretroviral therapy: prospective study in children in sikasso (mali). J Pediatr Pharmacol Ther 17: 382–388.

59. Shubber Z, Calmy A, Andrieux-Meyer I, Vitoria M, Renaud-Thery F, et al. (2013) Adverse events associated with nevirapine and efavirenz-based first-line antiretroviral therapy: a systematic review and meta-analysis. AIDS 27: 1403–1412.

60. Moh R, Danel C, Messou E, Ouassa T, Gabillard D, et al. (2007) Incidence and determinants of mortality and morbidity following early antiretroviral therapy initiation in HIV-infected adults in West Africa. AIDS 21: 2483–2491.

61. Padua CA, Cesar CC, Bonolo PF, Acurcio FA, Guimaraes MD (2006) High incidence of adverse reactions to initial antiretroviral therapy in Brazil. Braz J Med Biol Res 39: 495–505.

62. Pryce C, Pierre RB, Steel-Duncan J, Evans-Gilbert T, Palmer P, et al. (2008) Safety of antiretroviral drug therapy in Jamaican children with HIV/AIDS. West Indian Med J 57: 238–245.

63. Shah I (2006) Adverse effects of antiretroviral therapy in HIV-1 infected children. J Trop Pediatr 52: 244–248.

64. Scanlon ML, Vreeman RC (2013) Current strategies for improving access and adherence to antiretroviral therapies in resource-limited settings. HIV AIDS (Auckl) 5: 1–17.

65. Gusdal AK, Obua C, Andualem T, Wahlstrom R, Chalker J, et al. (2011) Peer counselors' role in supporting patients' adherence to ART in Ethiopia and Uganda. AIDS Care 23: 657–662.

10

Free Preconceptual Screening Examination Service in Rural Areas of Hubei Province, China in 2012

Cui-ling Li[1,9], Kai Zhao[1,9], Hui Li[2], Omar Ibrahim Farah[1], Jiao-jiao Wang[1], Rong-ze Sun[3], Hui-ping Zhang[1]*

1 Family Planning Research Institute, Tongji Medical College, Huazhong University of Science and Technology, Wuhan, Hubei, China, 2 Department of Science and Technology Service, Hubei Provincial Population and Family Planning Commission, Wuhan, Hubei, China, 3 Renmin Hospital of Wuhan University, Wuhan, Hubei, China

Abstract

Objective: This work aims to collect and summarize the outcomes on free preconceptual screening examination in rural areas of Hubei Province in 2012. Moreover, this review promotes further understanding of the status of this activity to provide the Family Planning Commission valid scientific data upon which to construct effective policies.

Methods: Couples, who complied with the family planning policy and were the residents in agricultural areas or lived in a local rural area for more than six months, were encouraged to participate in the free preconceptual screening examination service provided by the Hubei Provincial Population and Family Planning Commission. This service included 19 screening tests. All the data, including forms, manuals, and test results, were collected from 1 January 2012 to 31 December 2012 in rural areas in Hubei Province.

Results: A total of 497,860 individuals participated in the free preconceptual screening examination service, with a coverage rate of 97.1%. 4.0% and 4.8% of the participants exhibited with abnormal blood levels of ALT and creatinine, respectively; 0.36% of the participants tested positive for syphilis; 0.44% and 3.6% of the female participants tested positive for *Neisseria gonorrhoeae* and *Chlamydia trachomatis*, respectively; and 0.84% and 1.8% of the female participants tested positive for cytomegalovirus (IgM) and *Toxoplasma gondii* (IgM), respectively. After risk assessment, 59,935 participants might have high-risk of adverse pregnancy outcomes. In 2012, the prevalence of birth defects among the parturient who participated in the preconceptual screening examination service was 0.04%, while the prevalence was 0.08% among those who did not participate in the service.

Conclusion: Preconceptual screening examination service may help to address the risk factors that can lead to adverse pregnancy outcome. More studies on the relationship between preconceptual screening examination service and prevalence of birth defect or other adverse pregnancy outcomes should be conducted.

Editor: Sten H. Vermund, Vanderbilt University, United States of America

Funding: The funders had no role in study design, data collection and analysis, decision to publish, or preparation of the manuscript. This study was supported by the Foundation of Hubei Provincial Population and Family Planning Commission (grant no. JS-2011011).

Competing Interests: The authors have declared that no competing interests exist.

* Email: familyplanning2013@163.com

9 These authors contributed equally to this work.

Introduction

A birth defect is an abnormality that is present at birth, such as a missing limb, malformed heart, or Down's syndrome. Birth defects occur in approximately 6% of births worldwide each year [1]. In China, the birth defect incidence is 4% to 6% [2], and the prevalence in 2008 was 1.4% in Hubei Province [3]. In China, there are some free basic public health service for the people that are provided by the government, such as tuberculosis treatment, HIV screening and treatment, vaccinations, infectious disease monitoring, maternal and child health care, seniors health care, and health education. Women can access to the maternal and child health care service in local medical health care organizations for free [4]. However, maternal and child health care are carried out in the antepartum and postpartum period, which is consistent with the concept of primary prevention. The concept of preconception health care has been articulated for over a decade

but are yet to become part of free medical service in China. Preconception health care is a preventive strategy that helps men and women prepare for pregnancy by improving their health prior to conception, including health practices related to safeguarding fertility, preparing for pregnancy, and identifying and addressing risk factors [5–8]. Thus, preconception health care is important to improve pregnancy outcomes and birth quality.

Considering the importance of preconception health care, the National Population and Family Planning Commission officially launched the national project for the free preconceptual screening examination in China on 22 April 2010. The National Population and Family Planning Commission selected 18 provinces as the first batch of pilot provinces to carry out this national project. While there are many screening tests that are related with the pregnancy and preconception health, the National Population and Family Planning Commission set 19 items of screening tests that are provided in the preconceptual screening examination project due to they are the basic examinations and known associations with adverse pregnancy outcomes. Hubei Province is one of the 18 pilot provinces. Hubei Province is the 14th largest province with the ninth largest population in China (57,237,727 individuals, 2010) [9]. Since 22 April 2010, the Hubei Provincial Population and Family Planning Commission (HPPFPC) had employed the free preconceptual screening examination project to promote the comprehensive development of people, balanced development of the population, and healthy development of the family. Depending upon locality in rural areas, this project aimed to provide free preconceptual screening examination service for 256,274 pairs of rural couples (512,548 individuals) in Hubei Province in 2012.

The main objectives of the project included the following: to improve the quality of births, reduce the prevalence of birth defects, improve the knowledge of preconception health care among couples, enhance the consciousness and initiative of couples to participate in this project, and enhance the competence of primary service agencies to conduct the primary prevention of birth defects. Improving preconception health care can improve pregnancy outcomes by improving the overall health of men and women [10,11]. Screening by a knowledgeable professional can identify unrecognized risks to the mother and child [12]. Preconception counseling can increase men and women's knowledge and, more importantly, the likelihood that they will make any behavioral changes needed before and during pregnancy to reduce the risk of adverse pregnancy outcomes.

Many studies document the effectiveness of interventions targeted at increasing awareness of preconception folic acid supplementation. However, limited evidence links comprehensive preconception health care promotion to improve pregnancy outcomes [13–16]. In this study, data were collected and summarized to understand the status of the preconceptual screening examination work in Hubei Province. The pregnancy outcomes among the pregnant and parturient who participated in and who did not participate in the preconceptual screening examination service in 2012 were compared and analyzed. Greater understanding of these concepts will lead to better informed strategies by researchers, policy makers, and clinicians to assist men and women to optimize preconception health and reduce adverse pregnancy outcomes.

Materials and Methods

Target service population

The target population who were eligible to participate in the free preconceptual screening examination service met the following conditions:

1). Couples who complied with the family planning policy and prepared for pregnancy in 2012.

2). A couple, at least one of whom was a resident in an agricultural area or was defined as a rural resident.

3). A couple, at least one of whom was a local residence. Alternatively, none of them was a local resident, but both lived in the locale for more than six months.

Data source

A list of all eligible individuals was obtained from the Ministry of Civil Affairs and local family planning institutions. All the couples were confirmed to be married in accordance with the data of Ministry of Civil Affairs. Couples who prepared for pregnancy registered in the local family planning institutions and obtained a birth certificate before pregnancy. From 1 January 2012 to 31 December 2012, a total of 256,274 pairs of couples in rural areas of 46 pilot counties in Hubei Province met the conditions that the free preconceptual screening examination service required. All the data, including forms, manuals, test results and pregnancy follow-ups record, were collected from 1 January 2012 to 31 December 2012 in rural areas in Hubei Province.

Additional data specific to the pregnancy outcomes of 177416 pregnant and parturient who did not participate in the preconceptual screening examination service were collected from 1 January 2012 to 31 December 2012, and were obtained from the department of Obstetrics and Gynecology in the local hospitals in other 21 counties in Hubei Province.

Service content

The service provided 19 items of preconception health care screening tests, including health education on childbearing knowledge, history taking, physical examination, reproductive examination, clinical laboratory tests, risk assessment, and counseling and guidance for both male and female participants. History taking included birth history, history of diseases, family history, medication, lifestyle, diet and nutrition, and environmental risk factors. Physical examination included height, weight, blood pressure, heart rate, thyroid palpation, heart lung auscultation, palpation of liver and spleen, and limb and spinal column inspection. Reproductive examination included inspection and palpation of the external genitalia. Clinical laboratory tests included urinalysis, blood type (ABO type and Rh type), glutamin-pyruvic transaminase (ALT), hepatitis B serologic markers, creatinine, and syphilis screening.

Moreover, some were tests only for female participants, including gynecological ultrasound examination, vaginal leucorrhea exam, *Neisseria gonorrhoeae* and *Chlamydia trachomatis*, complete blood count (CBC), serum glucose, thyroid-stimulating hormone (TSH), rubella virus (IgG), cytomegalovirus (IgM and IgG), *Toxoplasma gondii* (IgM and IgG), early pregnancy follow-up, and pregnancy outcome follow-up. Early pregnancy follow-up was carried out within 12 weeks of pregnancy, and pregnancy outcome follow-up was within 6 weeks after childbirth or within 2 weeks after other terminated pregnancy. The main objective of early pregnancy follow-up was to inform precautions during pregnancy and prenatal care, and to give necessary health guidance and counseling. Pregnancy outcomes, such as normal newborn, preterm birth, low birth weight, androgyneity, birth defect, spontaneous abortion, elective abortion, abortion by labor induction, ectopic gestation, and fetal death/stillbirth were recorded in the Pregnancy Outcome Record during the pregnancy outcome follow-up. Sex, birth weight, gestational age and physical examination of the newborn were also recorded.

Service agencies

Preconceptual screening examination service were provided by the county-level family planning institutions that obtained the Practice License of the Family Planning Technical Institutions and Medical Institutions Permit.

Engaging in health education work were the health care personnel who received professional training. Engaging in history taking, physical and reproductive examination, ultrasound, clinical laboratory tests, risk assessment, and counseling and guidance were the licensed physicians or physician's assistants. The congenital anomalies and adverse pregnancy outcomes were diagnosed and recorded by the doctors working the department of Obstetrics and Gynecology.

Financial support

The elementary cost was RMB 240 ($ 39.45), including female RMB 190 ($31.24) and male RMB 50 ($8.21), per child time for the preconceptual screening examination service for every couple. Approximately 50% of the cost was supported by national finance, 30% was provided by provincial public finance, and 20% was supported by county-level public finance.

Information management

1) Information collection

Data on the free preconceptual screening examination service were collected from 1 January 2012 to 31 December 2012 in rural areas of 46 pilot counties in Hubei Province. The data on eligible couples within the jurisdiction were collected and reported by the family planning administrators in the village (community) to the township (town, street) family planning office. Data were subsequently reported to the family planning institutions at the county level. Finally, all data were collected and reported to the HPPFPC.

A Family Archive was established for each eligible couple. All documents in the Family Archive included the Information Consent Form, service record manual, tests results, risk assessment guidance document, records of early pregnancy follow-up, and pregnancy outcome follow-up. All data were encoded into a network system called "National Project of Free Preconceptual Screening Examination Service Information Management System".

2) Data quality control

At the first week of each month, the personnel working in local family planning institutions used the "National Project of Free Preconceptual Screening Examination Service Information Management System" to generate the reports and statistics, which handed over to the HPPFPC. The personnel working in HPPFPC organized spot checks once every three months to ensure the accuracy, authenticity and reliability of the data.

Ethical review

The study protocol was approved by the institutional review boards of the Tongji Medical College, Huazhong University of Science and Technology. All the participants signed the informed written consent after the personnel explained the study protocol.

Results

Number of women participating in each pregnancy-related service

From 1 January 2012 to 31 December 2012, a total of 256,274 couples (512,548 individuals) were eligible to participate in the free preconceptual screening examination service in rural areas of 49 pilot counties in Hubei, whereas 497,860 individuals participated in the service, with a coverage rate of 97.1% (497,860/512,548). According to the results of all tests, participants were divided into two groups: general population and high-risk population. Participants with one or more abnormal history, physical examination and test results that might result in a birth defect or other adverse pregnancy outcomes were grouped to the high-risk population. After the risk assessment, 59,935 participants (12.0%) were grouped to the high-risk population, among whom 40.5% were male and 59.5% were female. A total of 86,970 pregnant women participated in the early pregnancy follow-up, and 55,136 pregnant and parturient participated in the pregnancy outcome follow-up (Table 1).

Results of tests for both male and female participants

A total of 496,331, 497,359, and 490,427 participants took the history taking, physical examination, and reproductive examination, respectively, among whom 19.6%, 13.0%, and 6.6% showed abnormalities. Moreover, 4.0% of the participants exhibited an abnormal blood level of ALT, and 4.8% exhibited an abnormal blood level of creatinine. In addition, 0.36% of the participants tested positive for syphilis (Table 2).

Results of the tests only for female participants

A total of 248,385 and 247,616 female participants were tested for *Neisseria gonorrhoeae* and *Chlamydia trachomatis*, respectively, among whom 0.44% and 3.6% tested positive. Moreover, 7.7% of the female participants had abnormal serum glucose, and 6.6% exhibited abnormal blood levels of TSH. In addition, 0.84% and 1.8% of female participants tested positive for cytomegalovirus (IgM) and *Toxoplasma gondii* (IgM) tests, respectively (Table 3).

Pregnancy outcomes among the pregnant and parturient who participated in and who did not participate in preconceptual screening examination

In 2012, a total of 60,398 pregnant and parturient (including some pregnant and parturient who participated in the service in 2011 and delivered in 2012) from 46 pilot counties, who participated in the preconceptual screening examination service delivered or terminated the pregnancy; while a total of 177,416 pregnant and parturient from other 21 counties, who did not participate in the service, delivered or terminated the pregnancy. The general information of pregnancy outcomes follow-up individuals who participated or did not participate in the service were shown in Table 4, including age, minority, smoking status and education level. There was no significant difference between the pregnant and parturient who participated or did not participate in the service. The prevalence of birth defects was 0.04% among 58,928 follow-up newborns, while the prevalence was 0.08% among those whose parturient did not participate in the service (Table 5). The prevalence of spontaneous abortion, ectopic gestation, and fetal death/stillbirth among 60,398 pregnant and parturient were 1.3%, 0.07%, and 0.13%, respectively (Table 5). The prevalence of birth defects among the parturient who participated in the service was lower than that among the parturient who did not ($\chi^2 = 10.7$, $P = 0.001$). Also, the prevalence of other adverse pregnancy outcomes was lower among the pregnant and parturient who participated in the service ($\chi^2 = 1820.2$, $P < 0.001$) (Table 5).

Birth defects in different regions of Hubei Province

The areas of Hubei Province are divided into five regions, mainly according to the location and economic development, which are Wuhan City (capital city of Hubei Province), Northeast, Northwest, Southeast and Southwest in Hubei Province (Fig. 1). The number and prevalence of birth defects in every region were summarized and compared respectively. The prevalence of birth defects among the parturient who participated in the service was lower than that among the parturient who did not participate in Northwest ($\chi2 = 6.77$, $P = 0.003$) and Southwest ($\chi2 = 8.67$, $P = 0.009$) (Table 6).

Discussion

While prenatal care or maternal care and other interventions during pregnancy can address conditions that occur during pregnancy, they are not designed to address the high-risk factors

Table 1. Individuals Who Participated in the Preconception Health Care Check-up.

Individuals	Male	Percent (%)	Female	Percent (%)	In Total (per child time)
Participant	242578	48.7	255282	51.3	497860
Health Education on Childbearing knowledge	—	—	—	—	596858
High-risk Population	24273	40.5	35662	59.5	59935
Counseling and Guidance	—	—	—	—	494587
Early Pregnancy Follow-up	—	—	86970	—	86970
Pregnancy Outcome Follow-up	—	—	55136	—	55136

to adverse pregnancy outcomes before pregnancy. Interventions to reduce the adverse pregnancy outcomes or improve the birth outcomes may need to start before pregnancy. Presently, preconception health care is strongly endorsed by the researchers and clinicians [17–19]. This study provides an overview of preconceptual screening examination service in rural areas of Hubei Province in 2012. The local family planning institutes provided the free preconceptual screening examination service for 497,860 individuals in rural areas, which covered 97.1% of the eligible individuals, higher than the coverage rates in 2010 (68.0%, 65,170/95,838) and 2011 (94.8%, 186,452/196,596). In the coming years, the government still need to invest more funding in this service to increase the coverage rate and cover the individuals not only in rural areas but also in the urban areas.

HPPFPC recently released 10 recommendations to improve preconception and primary health care for women and men. These recommendations included increased public awareness of the importance of preconception health behavior and preconception care services, as well as the provision of risk assessment and educational and health promotion counseling to all women of childbearing age to reduce reproductive risks and improve pregnancy outcomes in the event of pregnancy. An increasing number of couples were made aware of the importance of preconceptual screening examination and thus participated in this project. A total of 497,860 individuals participated in the free preconceptual screening examination service in 2012, but not all couples participated in the service together. Moreover, not all eligible individuals participated in this service. The couples living in remote areas might have less willingness for and interest in

preconception health care. Thus, HPPFPC still needs to improve its service and strive to cover more couples, particularly in those remote areas. The local family planning institutes should put more effort into the propaganda of preconception health care, so that to raise the people's awareness of the importance of preconception health and people's self-consciousness to participate in this service.

After history taking, physical examination, and medical tests, the physicians would identify and assess the potential factors, including genetic, environmental, psychological, and behavioral factors, which might result in birth defects or other adverse pregnancy outcomes. For couples without risk factors, physicians would suggest that they come regularly to gain more health education and guidance. If only one partner participated in the service, physicians would suggest that the other partner participate as soon as possible. For those who had potential risk factors, physicians would inform the couple of the risk factors and potential effects on the fetus, aside from recommending further consultation, examination, referral, and treatment, while postponing childbearing if necessary. In 2012, 59,935 participants (12.04%) were grouped to the high-risk population and suggested to get further examination and treatment in hospital, which might help reduce the prevalence of adverse pregnancy outcomes. Also, preconceptual screening examination service might help to address the risk factors that could lead to adverse pregnancy outcome, so increased attention were given by the participants and physicians.

Although adequate prenatal, obstetric, and primary care services can reduce infant and maternal mortality, preconception health care refers not only to the primary prevention of maternal and perinatal morbidity and mortality, but also to a primary

Table 2. Results of Tests for both Male and Female individuals.

Individuals	Normal	Percent (%)	Abnormal	Percent (%)	In Total (per child time)
History Taking	399197	80.4	97134	19.6	496331
Physical Examination	432461	87.0	64898	13.1	497359
Reproductive Examination	458160	93.4	32267	6.6	490427
Urinalysis	463898	95.6	21234	4.4	485132
Glutamin-Pyruvic Transaminase	471441	96.0	19711	4.0	491152
Hepatitis B Serologic Markers*	452449	91.9	39713	8.1	492162
Creatinine	465701	95.2	23598	4.8	489299
Syphilis Test*	465303	99.6	1681	0.36	466984
	Ordinary Blood Type	**Percent (%)**	**Special Blood Type**	**Percent (%)**	**In Total (per child time)**
Blood Type	474360	98.3	8053	1.7	482413

*Hepatitis B Serologic Markers: includes HBs-Ag, HBs-Ab, HBe-Ag, HBe-Ab and HBc-Ab; **Syphilis Test:** *Treponema pallidum* Hemagglutination Assay.

Table 3. Results of Tests Only for Female Individuals.

Individuals	Normal	Percent(%)	Abnormal	Percent(%)	In Total (per child time)
Gynecological Ultrasound Examination	248687	96.6	8840	3.4	257527
Vaginal Leucorrhea Exam	234095	93.1	17395	6.9	251490
Serum Glucose	248737	92.3	20877	7.7	269614
Complete Blood Count	220258	79.6	56328	20.4	276586
Thyrcid-stimulating Hormone	247348	93.4	17397	6.6	264745
	Negative	**Percent(%)**	**Positive**	**Percent(%)**	**In Total**
Neisseria Gonorrheae	247304	99.6	1081	0.44	248385
Chlamydia Trochoatis	238677	96.4	8939	3.6	247616
Rubelia Virus IgG	124033	47.7	136105	52.3	260138
Cytomegalovirus IgM	254650	99.2	2150	0.84	256800
Cytomegalovirus IgG	146142	57.1	109804	42.9	255946
Toxoplasma Gondii IgM	251122	98.2	4693	1.8	255815
Toxoplasma Gondii IgG	245389	95.9	10391	4.1	255780

approach used to address various health issues [16,20]. In this study, the number of pregnant and parturient who came for the pregnancy outcome follow-up increased in 2012 compared with that in 2010 (753 pregnant and parturient) and 2011 (24778 pregnant and parturient). However, there were some loss between the pregnant and parturient who came for the early pregnancy follow-up and pregnancy outcome follow-up, as some pregnant and parturient would prefer hospitals in the urban area for the delivery or abortion, instead of local family planning institutions. The prevalence of birth defect among the parturient who participated in pregnancy follow-up was lower than that among

the parturient who did not, so was the prevalence of other adverse pregnancy outcomes. In details, the prevalence of birth defects in Northwest and Southwest in Hubei Province was lower among the parturient who participated in the service than that among the parturient who did not. However, determining whether preconceptual screening examination service can decrease the birth defect or other adverse pregnancy outcomes is difficult. Because the detailed data of every individual are not available now and the time of pregnancy follow-up is limited. Luckily, the project of preconceptual screening service have been still carried on among larger population in Hubei Province with some technological

Table 4. General Information Distribution among Pregnancy Outcomes Follow-up Individuals.

	Individuals who participated in the service		Individuals who did not participate in the service		
	(n = 58928)		(n = 166819)		
	Number	Percent (%)	Number	Percent(%)	P value
Age					
20–24	7778	13.2	22353	13.4	P>0.05
25–29	29641	50.3	84244	50.5	P>0.05
30–34	15793	26.8	44374	26.6	P>0.05
≥35	5716	9.7	15848	9.5	P>0.05
Minority					
Han	56754	96.3	160547	96.2	P>0.05
Others	2174	3.7	6272	3.8	P>0.05
Smoking Status					
Smoking	1503	2.6	4003	2.4	P>0.05
Second-hand Smoking	6417	10.9	16398	9.8	P>0.05
Education level					
Junior/Middle School	47779	81.1	136975	82.1	P>0.05
High School	10460	17.8	27759	16.6	P>0.05
College/University	689	1.2	2085	1.3	P>0.05

Table 5. Pregnancy Outcome among the Individuals who Participated/did not Participated in Preconception Health Check-up.

Pregnancy Outcome	Individuals who Participated in Check-up Service		Individuals who did not Participate in Check-up Service	
	Number	Percent (%)	Number	Percent (%)
Total Newborn	58928	97.6	166819	94.0
Normal Newborn	57779	98.1	165234	99.1
Male	30990	52.6	88138	52.8
Female	26789	45.5	77096	46.2
Prematurity	569	0.97	497	0.30
Low Birth Weight	557	0.95	954	0.57
Androgyneity	0	0.00	1	0.0006
Birth Defect *	23	0.04	134	0.08
Male	15	0.03	87	0.05
Female	8	0.01	46	0.03
Total Terminated Pregnancy #	1470	2.43	10597	5.97
Spontaneous Abortion	797	1.32	1282	0.72
Elective Abortion	350	0.58	6917	3.90
Abortion by Labor Induction	69	0.11	943	0.53
Ectopic Gestation	45	0.07	666	0.38
Fetal Death/Stillbirth	76	0.13	308	0.17
Others	133	0.22	481	0.27
In Total	60398	100.00	177416	100.00

*$\chi 2 = 10.685$, $P = 0.001$; #$\chi 2 = 1820.17$, $P < 0.0001$.

improvement. Also, analysis such as regression and correlation analysis will be done to determine the relationship between preconceptual screening examination service and prevalence of birth defect or adverse pregnancy outcomes in the future. Furthermore, the couples living in those remote areas and isolated from health care might have a higher prevalence. The number of spontaneous abortion might be under-reported, given that data were only obtained from local family planning institutions. Some pregnant with spontaneous abortion did not come for the early pregnancy follow-up, instead, they went to hospitals. The data

about spontaneous abortion of the pregnant who did not participate in this service were only reported from the department of Obstetrics and Gynecology, not including the outpatient department, where an important proportion of the abortion were carried out.

As more women than before have access to education and information, are employed, have personal income and decision making power, and delay pregnancy, many opportunities are available to inform them about the need for preconception care, risk factors leading to birth defects, and the importance of a healthy reproductive life. A good opportunity for the health of the mother and the infant to improve if for any adverse condition to be identified and addressed before pregnancy [21]. A number of lifestyle modifications and medical interventions can be of benefit to maternal and neonatal health when applied prior to conception [8,22]. These interventions include making a pregnancy plan, smoking cessation, supplementation with folic acid, cessation or moderation of alcohol intake, avoiding contact with toxic and hazardous substances, improvement of diabetic control, and maintaining healthy lifestyle and behavior [22–24]. Preconception health care is a good method for health promotion (including advice and education and screening tests) and risk assessment for every couple and should thus be implemented widely in China.

This study has a number of limitations. Firstly, not every individual participated in all the 19 screening tests for several reasons. For example, some participants might not have been aware that the service included 19 screening tests. Thus, the family planning institutes need to take some measures to ensure that participants complete the whole process. The 19 screening tests included in this service are the basic examinations that related to the pregnancy outcomes, and only RMB 240 ($ 39.45) are provided by national finance and local public finance. Tests, such

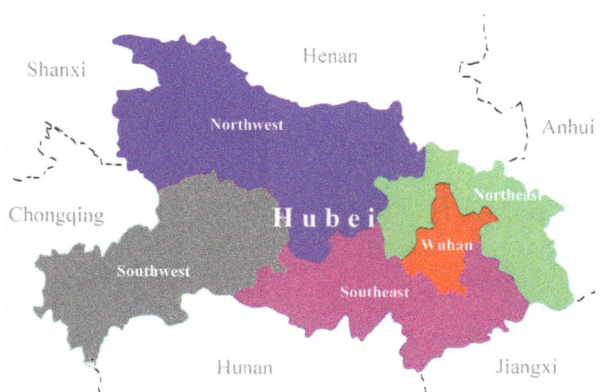

Figure 1. The map of Hubei Province, China. Wuhan, the capital city, and four regions of Hubei Province are highlighted with different colors.

Table 6. Birth defect in different regions of Hubei Province.

Regions	Individuals who participated in the service				Individuals who did not participate in the service				
	Numbers of County	Number of Newborns	Birth Defect	Percent (%)	Number of County	Number of Newborns	Number of Birth Defect	Percent (%)	P value
Wuhan	7	6400	5	0.078	2	23848	39	0.160	P=0.11
Northeast	9	13968	3	0.021	4	23155	6	0.026	P=0.94
Southeast	11	18742	9	0.048	5	19090	27	0.140	P=0.003
Northwest	9	7443	4	0.054	4	22399	43	0.190	P=0.009
Southwest	10	12375	2	0.016	6	78327	19	0.024	P=0.81
Total	46	58928	23	0.04	21	166819	134	0.08	P=0.001

as chromosome examination, Mediterranean anemia screening, and sex hormones, which are also important and known associations with adverse pregnancy outcomes, are not included in this service. Also, some other free medical service, such as HIV screening and premarital health care, are carried out in local Centers for Disease Control and Prevention (CDC) or local maternal and child health care hospital, not in the same institution. In the future, the funding invested by the government shall be increased to carry out more screening tests, and the cross-service and information exchange between different health care service institutions shall be coordinated and implemented. Secondly, this work only included physicians working in family planning institutes and does not represent the preconception care that may be provided by other primary care providers, such as obstetricians and gynecologists, midwives, and personnel working in maternal and child health-care institutes. Individuals who participated in the study may have had a higher interest in preconception health or greater concern about preconception care services, but this study could not represent all individuals. More studies in varying populations may validate the role of preconceptual screening examination service. This study did not assess the prevalence of adverse pregnancy outcomes among men who participated in the service, as we did not collect the data in this respect. Furthermore, the data generated by the "National Project of Free Preconceptual Screening Examination Service Information Management System" were not divided into male and female sections, such that the number of male and female participants in every item is unclear. Although it is important to assure the completeness of data, it is also important to report and show the data from the health management system to the readers when not all the data are publicly available. The results may has certain significance and provide a useful and meaningful suggestion to the government and concerned departments in the future.

Preconception health strategies include aspects related to awareness, knowledge, skills, motivation, opportunity, access, supportive environments, policy development, and ultimately, behavioral change [5,25]. The provision of routine health promotion before conception may encourage changes to improve health and may be an opportunity to identify risk factors, such as infection, that can be treated before pregnancy begins [6]. However, preconception health care is not widely practiced in China despite being apparently acceptable to health professionals and to women of childbearing age. In the future, the expansion of access to preconception health risk assessment and counseling at community health centers and publicly funded primary care sites should been proposed as a strategy for improving preconception health and health care for women and men. This study presented the basic data about the status of preconceptual screening examination service in rural areas of Hubei Province in 2012, which provided the National Population and Family Planning Commission a valid scientific bases upon which to construct effective policies. More detailed data and analysis shall be studied in the future to better understanding the importance of preconception health care to pregnancy outcome.

Author Contributions

Conceived and designed the experiments: HPZ. Performed the experiments: CLL KZ. Analyzed the data: HL OIF JJW. Contributed reagents/materials/analysis tools: RZS. Wrote the paper: CLL KZ HPZ.

References

1. Lobo I, Zhaurova K (2008) Birth Defects: Causes and Statistics. Nature Education 1(1).
2. Chen Z (2011) Report on Women and Children's Health Development in China. Ministry of Health, People's Republic of China 2011.
3. Tu L, Li H, Zhang H, Li X, Lin J, et al. (2012) Birth defects data from surveillance hospitals in hubei province, china, 2001-2008. Iran J Public Health 41: 20-25.
4. Li CL, Jiang T, Hu XZ, Zhao K, Yu Q, et al. (2013) Analysis of the maternal and child health care status in Suizhou City, Hubei Province, China, from 2005 to 2011. PLoS One 8: e72649.
5. Centre BSR (2009) Preconception Health: Physician Practices in Ontario. Toronto, Ontario, Canada
6. Witters I, Bogaerts A, Fryns JP (2010) Preconception care. Genet Couns 21: 169-182.
7. Dunlop AL, Jack B, Frey K (2007) National recommendations for preconception care: the essential role of the family physician. J Am Board Fam Med 20: 81-84.
8. Weisman CS, Hillemeier MM, Downs DS, Feinberg ME, Chuang CH, et al. (2011) Improving women's preconceptional health: long-term effects of the Strong Healthy Women behavior change intervention in the central Pennsylvania Women's Health Study. Womens Health Issues 21: 265-271.
9. National Bureau of Statistics of China (2010) Available: http://www.stats.gov. cn/tjsj/pcsj/rkpc/6rp/indexch.htm.
10. Johnson K, Posner SF, Biermann J, Cordero JF, Atrash HK, et al. (2006) Recommendations to improve preconception health and health care—United States. A report of the CDC/ATSDR Preconception Care Work Group and the Select Panel on Preconception Care. MMWR Recomm Rep 55: 1-23.
11. Moos MK, Dunlop AL, Jack BW, Nelson L, Coonrod DV, et al. (2008) Healthier women, healthier reproductive outcomes: recommendations for the routine care of all women of reproductive age. Am J Obstet Gynecol 199: S280-289.
12. Allaire AD, Cefalo RC (1998) Preconceptional health care model. Eur J Obstet Gynecol Reprod Biol 78: 163-168.
13. de Weerd S, Thomas CM, Cikot RJ, Steegers-Theunissen RP, de Boo TM, et al. (2002) Preconception counseling improves folate status of women planning pregnancy. Obstet Gynecol 99: 45-50.
14. Morin P, De Wals P, Noiseux M, Niyonsenga T, St-Cyr-Tribble D, et al. (2002) Pregnancy planning and folic acid supplement use: results from a survey in Quebec. Prev Med 35: 143-149.
15. de Jong-Van den Berg LT, Hernandez-Diaz S, Werler MM, Louik C, Mitchell AA (2005) Trends and predictors of folic acid awareness and periconceptional use in pregnant women. Am J Obstet Gynecol 192: 121-128.
16. Frey KA, Files JA (2006) Preconception healthcare: what women know and believe. Matern Child Health J 10: S73-77.
17. Livingood WC, Brady C, Pierce K, Atrash H, Hou T, et al. (2010) Impact of pre-conception health care: evaluation of a social determinants focused intervention. Matern Child Health J 14: 382-391.
18. Boulet SL, Johnson K, Parker C, Posner SF, Atrash H (2006) A perspective of preconception health activities in the United States. Matern Child Health J 10: S13-20.
19. Liu Y, Liu J, Ye R, Li Z (2006) Association of preconceptional health care utilization and early initiation of prenatal care. J Perinatol 26: 409-413.
20. Ebrahim SH, Lo SS, Zhuo J, Han JY, Delvoye P, et al. (2006) Models of preconception care implementation in selected countries. Matern Child Health J 10: S37-42.
21. Jack BW, Atrash H, Coonrod DV, Moos MK, O'Donnell J, et al. (2008) The clinical content of preconception care: an overview and preparation of this supplement. Am J Obstet Gynecol 199: S266-279.
22. Heyes T, Long S, Mathers N (2004) Preconception care: practice and beliefs of primary care workers. Fam Pract 21: 22-27.
23. Xaverius PK, Salas J (2013) Surveillance of preconception health indicators in behavioral risk factor surveillance system: emerging trends in the 21st century. J Womens Health (Larchmt) 22: 203-209.
24. Campbell SK, Lynch J, Esterman A, McDermott R (2012) Pre-pregnancy predictors of diabetes in pregnancy among Aboriginal and Torres Strait Islander women in North Queensland, Australia. Matern Child Health J 16: 1284-1292.
25. Dunlop AL, Logue KM, Thorne C, Badal HJ (2013) Change in women's knowledge of general and personal preconception health risks following targeted brief counseling in publicly funded primary care settings. Am J Health Promot 27: S50-57.

11

Bacterial Load of Pneumococcal Serotypes Correlates with Their Prevalence and Multiple Serotypes Is Associated with Acute Respiratory Infections among Children Less Than 5 Years of Age

Bhim Gopal Dhoubhadel[1,5], Michio Yasunami[1], Hien Anh Thi Nguyen[2], Motoi Suzuki[1], Thu Huong Vu[2], Ai Thi Thuy Nguyen[3], Duc Anh Dang[2], Lay-Myint Yoshida[4]*, Koya Ariyoshi[1,5]

1 Department of Clinical Medicine, Institute of Tropical Medicine, Nagasaki University, Nagasaki, Japan, **2** Department of Bacteriology, National Institute of Hygiene and Epidemiology, Hanoi, Vietnam, **3** Department of Microbiology, Khanh Hoa General Hospital, NhaTrang, Vietnam, **4** Department of Pediatric Infectious Diseases, Institute of Tropical Medicine, Nagasaki University, Nagasaki, Japan, **5** Graduate School of Biomedical Sciences, Nagasaki University, Nagasaki, Japan

Abstract

Background: Among pneumococcal serotypes, some serotypes are more prevalent in the nasopharynx than others; determining factors for higher prevalence remain to be fully explored. As non-vaccine serotypes have emerged after the introduction of 7-valent conjugate vaccines, study of serotype specific epidemiology is in need. When two or more serotypes co-colonize, they evolve rapidly to defend host's immune responses; however, a clear association of co-colonization with a clinical outcome is lacking.

Methods: Children less than 5 years old who were admitted to hospital due to acute respiratory infections (ARI) (n = 595) and healthy children (n = 350) were recruited. Carriage of pneumococcus was determined by culture and lytA PCR in the nasopharyngeal samples. Serotype/serogroup detection and its quantification were done by the nanofluidic real time PCR system. Spearman's correlation and logistic regression were used to examine a correlation of serotype/serogroup specific bacterial load with its prevalence and an association of co-colonization with ARI respectively.

Results: Serotype/serogroup specific bacterial load was correlated with its prevalence, both in ARI cases (Spearman's rho = 0.44, n = 186; P<0.0001) and healthy children (Spearman's rho = 0.41, n = 115; P<0.0001). The prevalence of multiple serotypes was more common in ARI cases than in healthy children (18.5% vs 7.1%; aOR 2.92, 95% CI: 1.27–6.71; P = 0.01). The dominant serotype in the co-colonization had a 2 log10 higher bacterial load than the subdominant serotype, both in ARI cases (P<0.001) and healthy children (P<0.05).

Conclusions: High bacterial load in the nasopharynx may help transmit pneumococci among hosts, and increase the chance of successful acquisition and colonization. Co-colonization of multiple serotypes of pneumococci is linked with ARI, which infers the interactions of multiple serotypes may increase their pathogenicity; however, they may compete for growth in number.

Editor: Cristina Costa, University Hospital San Giovanni Battista di Torino, Italy

Funding: BGD received scholarship from the Government of Japan, Ministry of Education, Culture, Sports, Science, and Technology for Monbukagakusho (MEXT) scholarship. The study was funded by Japan Initiative for Global Research Network on Infectious Diseases (J-GRID) and Japan Science and Technology, Japan. The funders had no role in study design, data collection and analysis, decision to publish, or preparation of the manuscript.

Competing Interests: The authors have declared that no competing interests exist.

* Email: lmyoshi@nagasaki-u.ac.jp

Introduction

Streptococcus pneumoniae (pneumococcus) is a major cause of life threatening diseases including pneumonia, sepsis and meningitis in children worldwide [1]. Pneumococcus has distinct polysaccharide capsule which characterizes its more than 90 serotypes. It colonizes in the nasopharynx, which is the precursor for pneumococcal diseases and the source for transmission among

people [2]. The emergence of non-vaccine serotypes (19A, 35B) after the introduction of 7-valent pneumococcal conjugate vaccine (PCV7) has become a concern for future epidemiology of pneumococcal diseases, and it highlights the need of serotype specific study of this common pathogen [3,4].

The prevalence of a serotype in the nasopharynx is inversely correlated with the invasiveness of the serotype [5]. Less invasive serotypes such as 6A, 6B, 19F, 23F tend to colonize more frequently and maintain the carriage for longer time; while the more invasive serotypes such as 1, 4, 5, 7F tend to colonize less frequently and maintain colonization for less duration [6,7]. The pneumococcal capsule, which is a major virulent factor, determines the serotype. It is found the thickness of the capsule positively correlates with the prevalence of the serotype/serogroup [8]. Furthermore, the capacity to grow of a serotype is correlated with its prevalence in an in vitro study [9]; however, it is unknown whether similar relationship exists in the natural niche in humans.

Co-colonization of multiple pneumococcal serotypes in the nasopharynx affects vaccine serotype replacement, carriage detection and pneumonia diagnosis [10]. Accurate determination of co-colonization and its role in pathogenesis are difficult to establish by using conventional serotyping method because of its low sensitivity and tedious laboratory work; therefore, a highly sensitive and specific molecular method is in need to detect multiple serotypes accurately and efficiently [11,12]. Although varied prevalence rates of co-colonization have been reported from different parts of the world [11–15], an epidemiological evidence of their association with a clinical outcome is lacking. Some epidemiological models have demonstrated that the serotypes compete among themselves for acquisition and persistence of colonization in the nasopharynx [16,17]; however, it is yet to be demonstrated quantitatively in humans.

In this study, we applied a highly sensitive and specific novel nanofluidic real time PCR system to identify serotypes/serogroups and quantify their bacterial load in nasopharyngeal samples of hospitalized acute respiratory infections (ARI) cases and healthy children. We aimed to assess the correlation of bacterial load of specific serotypes/serogroups with the prevalence and compare the prevalence of co-colonization of multiple serotypes between these two groups of children.

Methods

Study design

Acute respiratory infections (ARI) cases, as defined by World Health Organization (WHO), were recruited in the Department of Pediatrics, Khanh Hoa General Hospital, Nha Trang City, Vietnam from 07/04/2008 to 31/03/2009. The hospital has 750 beds, and is the only hospital that provides inpatient care for sick children in Nha Trang City. The participants were children under 5 years old from the study area, who were admitted to the pediatric ward during the study period with acute respiratory infections (ARI) defined by cough and/or difficulty in breathing (WHO). We also included healthy children to compare bacterial load and serotype distribution with ARI cases. Healthy children, who did not have fever, signs of respiratory infections or history of antibiotic intake in the month preceding the day of enrollment, were recruited from two communes in the study area. They were selected randomly during January 2008 from the under 5 years old children using the census data. Informed written consent was taken from the parents of the hospital admitted ARI cases and the healthy children. Details of the study site were described elsewhere [18].

Sample collection, storage and DNA extraction

A nasopharyngeal sample (NPS), (about 100 microliter in volume) was collected flexible dacron-tipped aluminum-shafted swabs (Copan, Brescia, Italy) from each participant according to the WHO protocol [19]. The samples were taken from ARI cases at the time of admission before they were treated with antibiotics. The samples were divided into two aliquots. One aliquot was sub-cultured onto 5% sheep blood agar and incubated overnight with 5% CO_2 at 37°C. Alpha hemolytic colonies with morphology suggestive of *S. pneumoniae* and positive Optochin test were considered potential *S. pneumoniae* isolates. The other aliquot was stored at −80°C. At a later stage DNA was extracted, following the protocol of QIAGEN kit for the Gram-positive bacteria, directly from the nasopharyngeal samples of the children from whom potential *S. pneumoniae* had been cultured. DNA was stored at -80°C, except for transportation to Nagasaki on dry ice, till used for the lytA PCR and the nanofluidic real time PCR system.

Identification of pneumococcus, its serotypes, quantification of bacterial load and definition of co-colonization of multiple serotypes

The DNA extract of the NPS from children with a potential *S. pneumoniae* culture positive isolate was analyzed by a lytA PCR that targeted the autolysin gene using the Light cycler II (Roche). Carriage of pneumococcus is defined as having positive lytA PCR NPS. The lytA positive samples were subjected to the nanofluidic real time PCR system for molecular serotyping. The nanofluidic real time PCR system can identify 50 serotypes in 29 groups, and it can detect minor population of multiple serotypes in co-colonization of pneumococci with the minimum level of detection of 30 to 300 copies. Total and specific serotype/serogroup bacterial loads were quantified using the standard curves. Details of the nanofluidic real time PCR system has been described elsewhere [20]. Samples positive for lytA and negative for all serotype/serogroup primer-pairs were grouped as non-typeable (NT). Co-colonization with multiple serotypes was defined as the presence of two or more serotypes/serogroups in a sample. In co-colonization the first serotype and second serotype were defined according to their bacterial loads; a serotype with the highest load was assigned as first serotype, with the second highest load as second serotype.

Statistical analysis

The data of pneumococcal loads, DNA copies, were changed into log10 scale. To compare the groups, Wilcoxon rank sum test was used for the continuous variables and Chi-square or Fisher exact test was used for categorical variables. Logistic regression was used to test the effects of pneumococcal load and co-colonization as risk factors for hospitalized children due to ARI. Odds ratios were adjusted for age, sex and daycare attendance. To test the correlation of bacterial load and prevalence of individual serotypes, Spearman's correlation was used. Analyses were performed using Stata v12.1 (StataCorp, College Station, Taxes, USA). The database for the analysis was submitted as (Table S1, S2).

Ethical approval

This study was approved by all the concerned research review boards: Nagasaki University Institutional Review Board Nagasaki, Japan; the National Institute of Hygiene and Epidemiology Scientific Review Committee, Hanoi and the Khanh Hoa Provincial Health Service Ethical Review Board, Nha Trang, Vietnam.

Results

Basic characteristics of ARI cases and healthy children

Among the hospital admitted ARI cases, 88.6% (527/595) were children less than 2 years old, proportion of male was 62% (369/595), and the median age was 10 months. Almost half, 45.5% of

ARI cases had history of antibiotic use before admission. The proportion of chest X-ray confirmed pneumonia among them was 22.8% (136/595). Among healthy children, 55.4% (194/350) were under 2 years of old, proportion of male was 52.6% (184/350), and the median age was 19 months.

Pneumococcal colonization and serotype distribution

Pneumococcal carriage rate was 32.6% (194/595) in ARI cases and 40% (140/350) in healthy children (figure 1). The proportion of typeable serotypes in ARI cases and healthy children were 95.9% (186/194) and 82.1% (115/140) respectively. Thirteen serotypes/serogroups of pneumococcus were detected in ARI cases and healthy children (figure 2). Serotypes/serogroups 19F, 6A/6B, 23F and 6C/6D were more prevalent in hospitalized ARI cases while serotypes/serogroups 14, 6A/6B, 19F, 15B/15C, 11 and non-typeables (NT) were common in healthy children. The proportion of serotypes/serogroups covered by pneumococcal conjugate vaccines: 7-valent (PCV7), 10-valent (PCV10) and 13-valent (PCV13) were approximately equal to one another, which was about 74% in ARI cases and 55% in healthy children (this was an approximate estimation as a serogroup was treated as a serotype as required).

Pneumococcal bacterial load

Higher bacterial load was associated with hospitalization due to ARI. The median bacterial load (total) was 6.61 log10/ml in ARI cases and 4.36 log10/ml in healthy children (OR = 9.96, 95%CI: 6.39–15.52; P<0.0001 and aOR = 9.07, 95%CI: 5.69–14.4; P< 0.0001). There was no difference in median bacterial load between males and females both in ARI cases (6.62 log10 in male Vs. 6.59 log10 in female; p-value: 0.76) and healthy children (4.36 log10 in male Vs. 4.32 log10 in female; p-value: 0.86). Bacterial loads of specific serotypes/serogroups were higher in ARI cases than healthy children in all detected serotypes (Figure 3). Serotypes 14,

19F, 23F, 6A/6B had higher median bacterial load than other serotypes in ARI cases while serotypes 14, 19F, 23A, 23F had higher load in healthy children. The bacterial load of serotype 6C/6D was found to be lower than other common serotypes in ARI cases.

Serotype/serogroup specific bacterial load was significantly higher in vaccine serotypes. When we compared the bacterial load of vaccine specific serotypes and non-vaccine serotypes, the load was higher in vaccine serotypes both in ARI cases: 6.61 log10 in vaccine serotypes and 5.51 log10 in non-vaccine serotypes (P< 0.0001), and in healthy children: 4.68 log10 in vaccine serotypes and 3.81 log10 in non-vaccine serotypes (P = 0.0001).

Correlation between bacterial load of serotypes and their prevalence

Serotype/serogroup specific bacterial load was positively correlated with serotype/serogroup prevalence. Serotype/serogroup specific bacterial load of individual NPS samples from ARI cases and healthy children were plotted against the prevalence of individual serotype/serogroup (i.e., proportion of the serotypes/serogroups in carriage positive samples). We found that the serotype/serogroup specific bacterial load had positive correlation with its prevalence, both in ARI cases (Spearman's rho = 0.44, n = 186, P<0.0001) and healthy children (Spearman's rho = 0.41, n = 115, P<0.0001) (Figure 4).

Co-colonization with multiple serotypes

Co-colonization of multiple serotypes of pneumococci was associated with ARI. Co-colonization of multiple-serotypes was detected in 18.5% (n = 36/194) in ARI cases and 7.1% (n = 10/140) in healthy children (OR 2.96, 95%CI 1.41–6.19; P = 0.004). When adjusted for age, sex and daycare, the adjusted odds ratio (aOR) was 2.92 (95%CI 1.27–6.71; P = 0.012). Co-colonization of serotypes 19F and 11, 19F and 15B/15C, 23F and 6A/6B

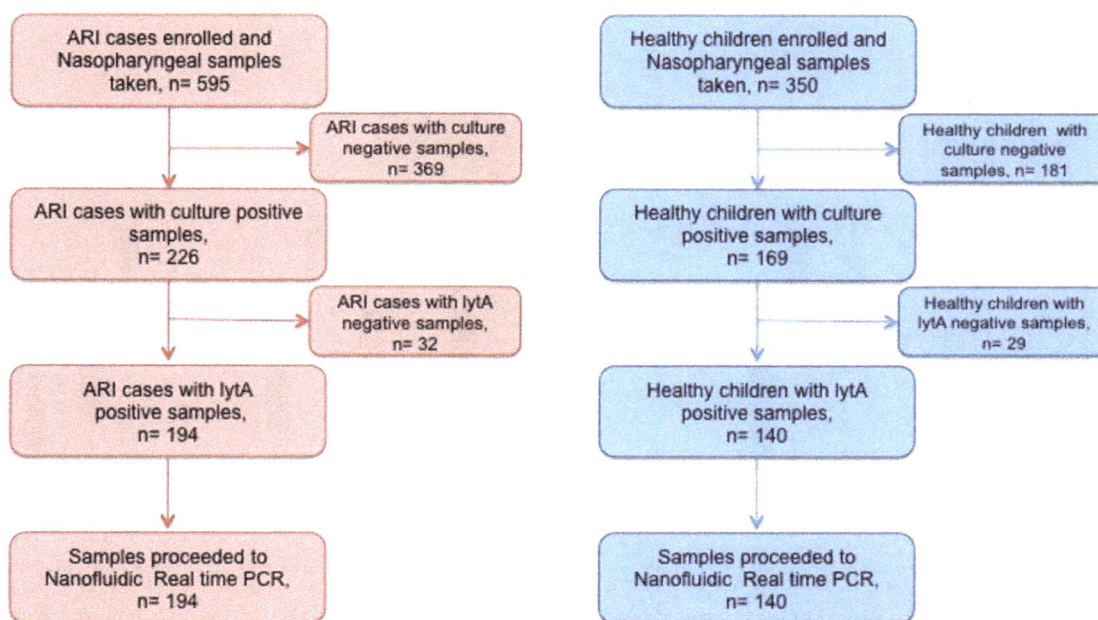

Figure 1. Participants recruited into the study, and their nasopharyngeal samples. Half of the aliquot of nasopharyngeal samples were cultured overnight in 5% sheep blood agar with 5% CO_2 at 37°C. DNA was extracted directly from the other half of the aliquot of the nasopharyngeal samples which yielded alpha hemolytic colonies and positive Optochin test. DNA was subjected to lytA PCR to confirm pneumococcus; and lytA positive samples were then processed for molecular serotyping in the nanofluidic real time PCR system.

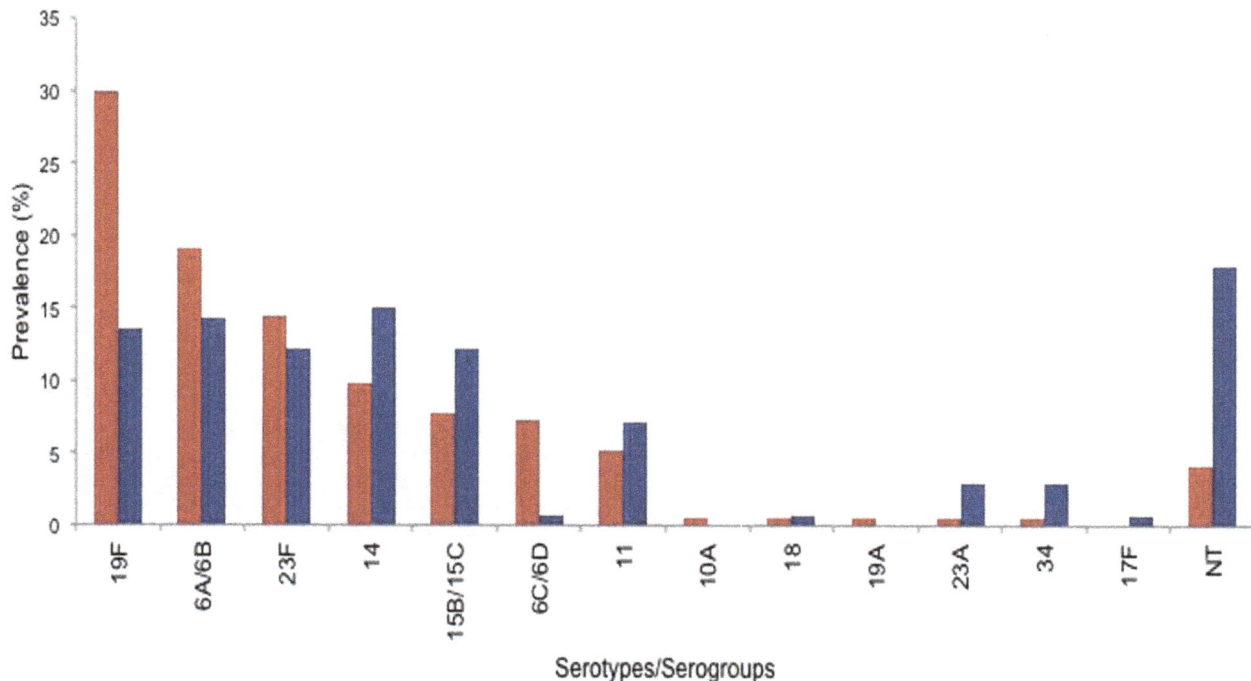

Figure 2. Distribution of serotypes/serogroups of pneumococcus in ARI cases and healthy children. Thirteen different serotypes/serogroups were detected; DNA samples which were positive for lytA (pneumococcus positive), but negative for tested 29 serotypes/serogroups were assigned as non-typeable (NT). Prevalence of each serotype/serogroup was calculated as proportion of total number of a serotype/serogroup to the total number of the lytA positive samples. Serotype/serogroup of ARI cases and healthy children were plotted in red and blue respectively. Proportion of serotype/serogroup covered by 13-valent conjugated vaccine (PCV13) was 74% in ARI cases and 55% in healthy children.

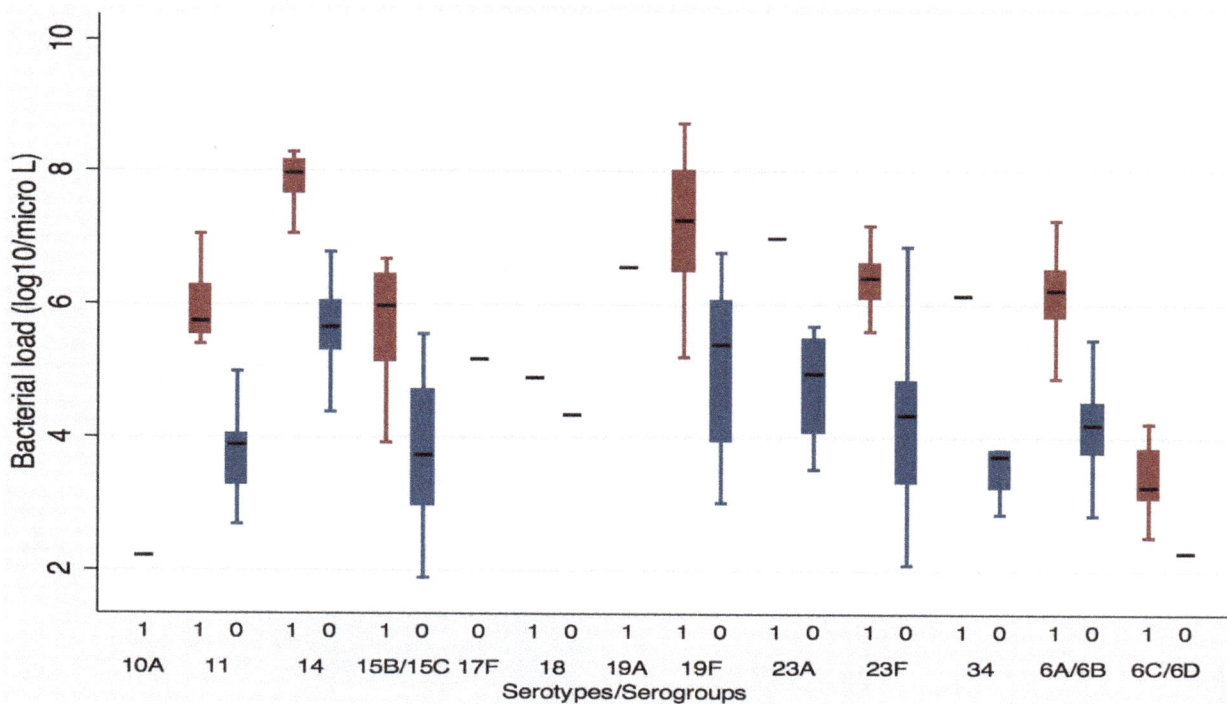

Figure 3. Bacterial load of specific serotypes/serogroups of pneumococcus in ARI cases and healthy children. Bacterial load of ARI cases (denoted by "1" in each serotype/serogroup) in red and healthy children (denoted by "0" in each serotype/serogroup) in blue, showed that the common serotypes 19F, 14, 23F, 6A/6B, 15B/15C had high bacterial load.

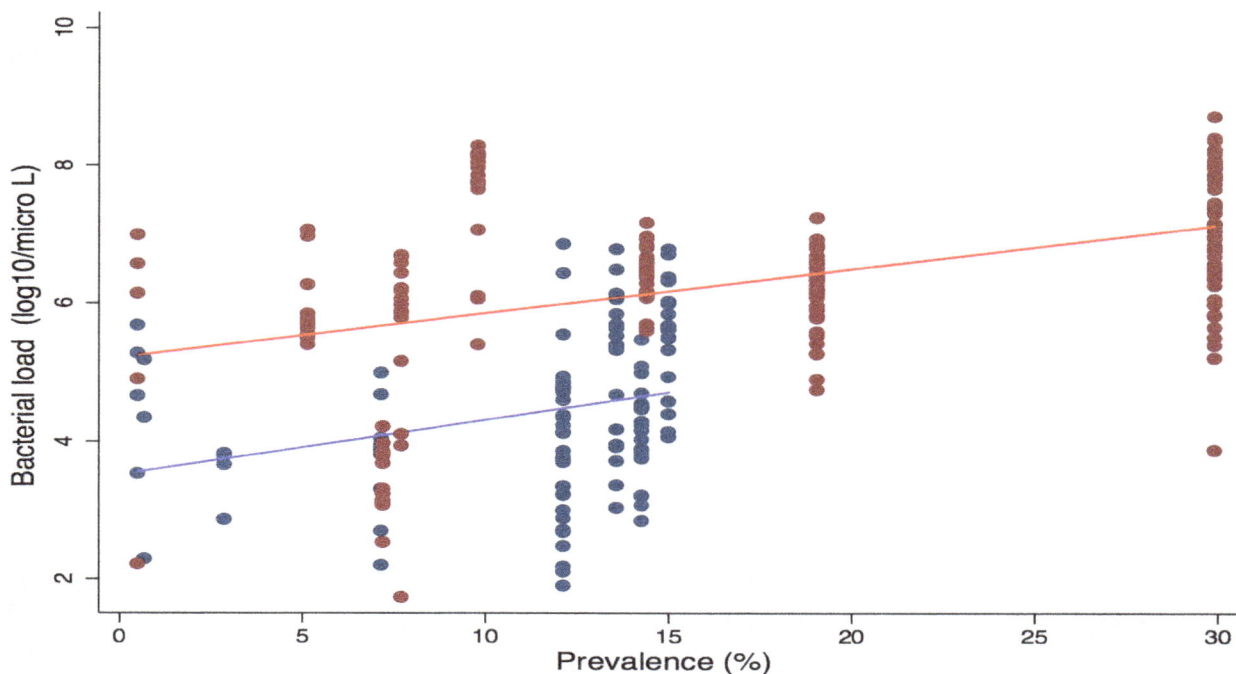

Figure 4. Relationship between bacterial load of specific serotypes/serogroups and their prevalence. Bacterial load of each of specific serotypes/serogroups was plotted against its prevalence. Both in ARI cases (red) and in healthy children (blue), a positive correlation was found. Each dot represents an ARI case or a healthy child in the plot, and the red and blue lines are the fitted values for ARI cases and healthy children respectively. Spearman's rho was 0.44 (n = 186; P<0.0001) and 0.41 (n = 115; P<0.0001) for ARI cases and healthy children respectively.

occurred more frequently in ARI cases. We observed none of the serotypes involved in co-colonization were 19A or 35B (Figure 5). Co-colonization of pneumococcus occurred in 18.56% (18/97) of ARI cases when pre-hospital antibiotics had been used and 38.71% (12/31) when no antibiotics were used (P = 0.002) [Unknown antibiotic status in 9.09% (6/66) of ARI cases]. The prevalence of co-colonization was found to be higher 32.5% (13/40) in age group of less than 6 months of age than 14.94% (23/154) in age group of 6 or more than 6 months of age in ARI cases (P = 0.01). But, we did not find any such difference in healthy children among these age groups, 0% (0/16) versus 7.04% (10/124) (P = 0.60).

One serotype/serogroup dominated the other serotype/serogroups in co-colonization. In co-colonization, the serotype/serogroup specific bacterial load was 2.45 log10 higher in the dominant serotypes than the subdominant serotypes in ARI cases, while it was 2.04 log10 higher in healthy children (Figure 6). The dominant serotype was a vaccine serotype in 100% (10/10) of co-colonization in healthy children (P = 0.003); while it was vaccine serotypes only in 72.22% (26/36) of co-colonization in ARI cases (P = 0.76). The median total bacterial load was higher, 4.81 log10 versus 4.31 log10 (P = 0.03), when co-colonization of multiple serotypes was present as compared to single serotype colonization in healthy children; however, no significant difference was found among them in ARI cases (6.65 log10 versus 6.58 log10, P = 0.59).

Discussion

Our data suggest two major findings. First, a positive correlation of serotype/serogroup specific bacterial load with prevalence of serotypes/serogroups, which may help to understand why some serotypes of pneumococcus are successful for colonization and

maintenance of the carriage for longer time. The second finding, an association of co-colonization of multiple serotypes with acute respiratory infections in children may infer a role of multiple serotypes of pneumococci in pathogenesis of ARI in children. Both of these findings are novel in pneumococcal pathogenesis and epidemiology in humans.

It is known that the prevalence of serotypes is inversely correlated with their serotype specific invasiveness [5]. It is found that some serotypes/serogroups: 1, 4, 5, 7F are more invasive but less prevalent in the nasopharynx than other serotypes/serogroups: 6A, 6B, 19F, 23F, which are more prevalent but less invasive [5]. Contributing factors for this inverse relationship of prevalence and invasiveness remains to be fully explained. It is found that colonizing serotypes: 19F, 6A, 6B, 23F have higher serotype specific rates of acquisition of colonization and longer duration of carriage than invasive serotypes: 1, 4, 5, 7F in children [6,7]. This shows that the colonizing serotypes are more capable to colonize and maintain the carriage than invasive serotypes. In this regard, our finding of positive correlation of serotype/serogroup specific bacterial load with prevalence of serotype/serogroup may explain that the higher numbers of bacteria in the nasopharynx may help them to transmit from one host to other, so that they have higher chance of colonization, and their ability to grow in number may help to maintain the carriage for longer time against the normal mucosal clearance of the host.

Some in vitro studies show that serotype specific growth of pneumococcus is positively correlated with prevalence of the serotype [8,9]. Hathaway et al found that high carriage prevalence serotypes (6B, 9V, 19F, 23F) can produce their capsules that are less metabolically demanding, and they can grow even in nutritionally poor environment [9]. These in vitro findings match with our in vivo findings of high bacterial load of common

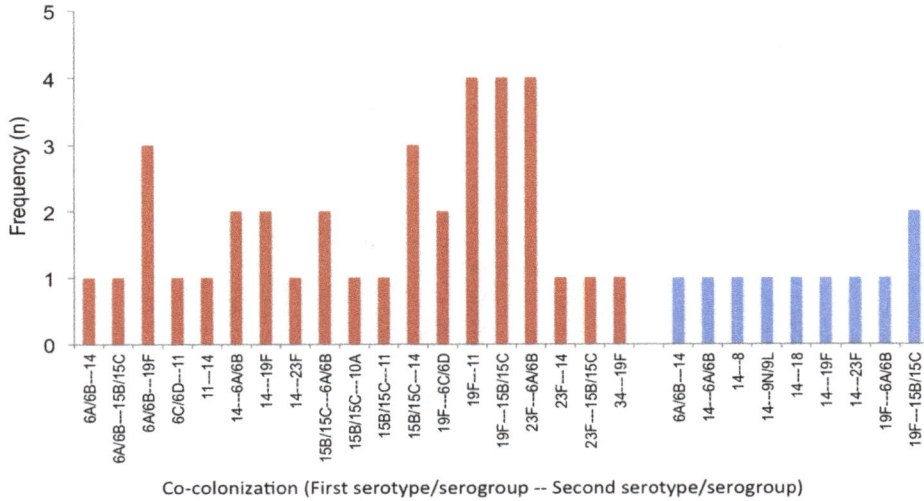

Figure 5. Distribution of co-colonization of multiple serotypes of pneumococcus. In ARI cases (red) co-colonization was detected in 36 samples out of 194 lytA positive samples (18.5%), while in healthy children (blue) it was detected in 10 samples out of 140 (7.1%) lytA positive samples. The odds ratio, adjusted for age, sex and daycare, was 2.92 (95%CI 1.27–6.71; P = 0.012). The serotypes/serogroups were positioned first and second according to their bacterial load.

serotypes/serogroups and their correlation with prevalence. Less prevalent but more invasive serotypes are characterized by poor growth, longer lag phase in bacterial growth [21], thinner capsule size and more prone to be killed by neutrophils than high prevalence serotypes [8].

We found the occurrence of co-colonization with multiple serotypes of pneumococcus was twice as common in hospitalized ARI cases as in healthy children. This is the first time to our knowledge that such an association of co-colonization of multiple

serotypes of pneumococci with ARI is reported. Although prevalence of co-colonization has been reported to occur from 1.3% to 39% in children by using different methods in various settings [11–15], none has reported an association with a clinical outcome. Non-vaccine serotypes such as 19A and 35B, which have emerged after the introduction of PCV7 vaccine [3,4], were not detected in co-colonization both in ARI cases and healthy children in our study. Although the number of children with co-colonization was relatively small, our data discourage the

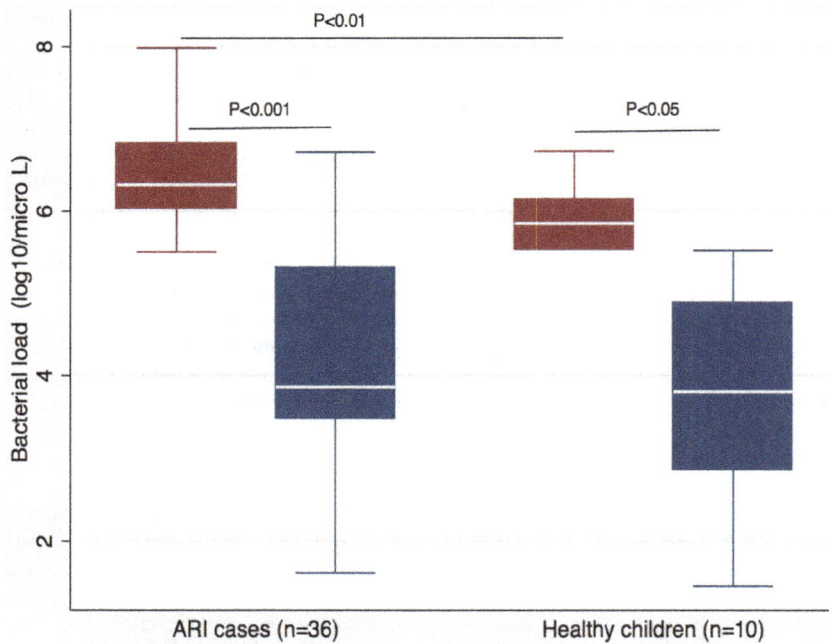

Figure 6. Dominance of one serotype/serogroup over the other in co-colonization of multiple serotypes/serogroups. Among two serotypes/serogroups present in a co-colonization, one serotype/serogroup (red) was found to be dominant by having 100 folds (2 log10) higher bacterial load than the other subdominant (blue) serotype/serogroup both in ARI cases and healthy children.

"unmasking phenomena" for emergence of non-vaccine serotypes [22]. The potential role of co-colonization in the emergence of 19A due to serotype replacement is partly explained by capsule switching phenomenon at the capsular locus by recombination [23,24]. As pneumococcus is highly recombinogenic and transformable bacteria, probability is high for genetic exchange when two or more pneumococcal serotypes inhabit at the same time in the nasopharynx [10]. This is true for evolution of not only vaccine-escape serotypes but also for the antibiotic resistant serotypes [24]. When multiple serotypes co-colonize, the genetic reservoir expands so called "Supragenome" will advance the microevolution of the pathogen and allow continued survival by evasion of serotype-specific immune response and adaptation by genetic change, which is demonstrated by the co-colonization of penicillin sensitive and penicillin resistance pneumococci at the same time [25]. Besides, it is found that in mouse model, pneumococci form a biofilm in the nasopharynx when multiple strains are present. The transformation efficiency becomes very high in the biofilm with multiple serotypes, so that the antibiotic resistance can easily be spread among the serotypes. Hence, co-colonization of multiple serotypes confers the development of supra-virulence and fitness in the pathogen for survival in the harsh environment of host [26].

We have further demonstrated the dominance of one serotype over the other in bacterial load when co-colonization is present. This difference in pneumococcal load among serotypes/serogroups in a co-colonization may suggest that there may be a competition among the serotypes for their growth due to limited nutrients and space. In mouse model, intra-species competition among pneumococci is demonstrated and found mediated by bacteriocin [27,28]. Epidemiological models also suggest the existence of competition among serotypes for initiation and persistence of colonization in children [16,17]. A study with mathematical modeling shows that direct (physical) competition and indirect (antibody mediated) competition do exit among the serotypes of pneumococcus in co-colonization [29]. We considered the 100 fold higher bacterial load, which we found in the dominant serotype, is due to direct competition as naturally acquired immune response due to colonization lasts for a short duration in unvaccinated young children. This is consistent with the finding of the mathematical modeling [29].

This study has limitations. Due to logistic problems, we were unable to bring all nasopharyngeal samples to Nagasaki from

Vietnam for DNA extraction and nanofluidic real time PCR. First, we screened all the samples by culture, and only samples that grew alpha hemolytic colonies and Optochin sensitive isolates were brought to Nagasaki for molecular assays. It may have decreased the overall sensitivity of detection of pneumococcus and carriage rate. Minimum level of detection of the nanofluidic real time PCR was 30-300 copies per reaction; other limitations of the nanofluidic real time PCR have been described elsewhere [20].

Conclusions

This study shows a positive correlation of serotype/serogroup specific bacterial load with serotype/serogroup prevalence of pneumococcus in children. Higher bacterial load of a serotype in the nasopharynx may be an attributing factor for higher transmission of the serotype. The association of multiple serotypes of pneumococcus with ARI shows its link with increased pathogenicity, and dominance of one serotype over the other may infer the competition among serotypes when multiple serotypes are present in the nasopharynx.

Acknowledgments

We are grateful to children and their parents who participated in this study. We would like to thank the staffs from Khanh Hoa Health Service and the medical staff in Khanh Hoa General Hospital who helped to carry out this research. BGD is grateful to the Government of Japan, Ministry of Education, Culture, Sports, Science, and Technology for Monbukagakusho (MEXT) scholarship.

Author Contributions

Conceived and designed the experiments: LMY KA MY MS DAD. Performed the experiments: BGD MY HAN THV ATTN LMY. Analyzed the data: BGD MS KA MY LMY. Contributed reagents/materials/analysis tools: BGD HAN ATTN THV MS KA MY LMY. Wrote the paper: BGD KA MS LMY MY HAN THV ATTN DAD.

References

1. O'Brien KL, Wolfson LJ, Watt JP, Henkle E, Deloria-Knoll M, et al. (2009) Burden of disease caused by Streptococcus pneumoniae in children younger than 5 years: global estimates. Lancet 374: 893–902.

2. Simell B, Auranen K, Kayhty H, Goldblatt D, Dagan R, et al. (2012) The fundamental link between pneumococcal carriage and disease. Expert Rev Vaccines 11: 841–855.

3. Weinberger DM, Malley R, Lipsitch M (2011) Serotype replacement in disease after pneumococcal vaccination. Lancet 378: 1962–1973.

4. Huang SS, Hinrichsen VL, Stevenson AE, Rifas-Shiman SL, Kleinman K, et al. (2009) Continued impact of pneumococcal conjugate vaccine on carriage in young children. Pediatrics 124: e1–11.

5. Brueggemann AB, Peto TE, Crook DW, Butler JC, Kristinsson KG, et al. (2004) Temporal and geographic stability of the serogroup-specific invasive disease potential of Streptococcus pneumoniae in children. J Infect Dis 190: 1203–1211.

6. Abdullahi O, Karani A, Tigoi CC, Mugo D, Kungu S, et al. (2012) Rates of acquisition and clearance of pneumococcal serotypes in the nasopharynges of children in Kilifi District, Kenya. J Infect Dis 206: 1020–1029.

7. Tigoi CC, Gatakaa H, Karani A, Mugo D, Kungu S, et al. (2012) Rates of acquisition of pneumococcal colonization and transmission probabilities, by serotype, among newborn infants in Kilifi District, Kenya. Clin Infect Dis 55: 180–188.

8. Weinberger DM, Trzcinski K, Lu YJ, Bogaert D, Brandes A, et al. (2009) Pneumococcal capsular polysaccharide structure predicts serotype prevalence. PLoS Pathog 5: e1000476.

9. Hathaway LJ, Brugger SD, Morand B, Bangert M, Rotzetter JU, et al. (2012) Capsule type of Streptococcus pneumoniae determines growth phenotype. PLoS Pathog 8: e1002574.

10. Shak JR, Vidal JE, Klugman KP (2013) Influence of bacterial interactions on pneumococcal colonization of the nasopharynx. Trends Microbiol 21: 129–135.

11. Hare KM, Morris P, Smith-Vaughan H, Leach AJ (2008) Random colony selection versus colony morphology for detection of multiple pneumococcal serotypes in nasopharyngeal swabs. Pediatr Infect Dis J 27: 178–180.

12. Huebner RE, Dagan R, Porath N, Wasas AD, Klugman KP (2000) Lack of utility of serotyping multiple colonies for detection of simultaneous nasopharyngeal carriage of different pneumococcal serotypes. Pediatr Infect Dis J 19: 1017–1020.

13. Hansman D, Morris S, Gregory M, McDonald B (1985) Pneumococcal carriage amongst Australian aborigines in Alice Springs, Northern Territory. J Hyg (Lond) 95: 677–684.

14. Brugger SD, Hathaway LJ, Muhlemann K (2009) Detection of Streptococcus pneumoniae strain cocolonization in the nasopharynx. J Clin Microbiol 47: 1750–1756.

15. Ercibengoa M, Arostegi N, Marimon JM, Alonso M, Perez-Trallero E (2012) Dynamics of pneumococcal nasopharyngeal carriage in healthy children attending a day care center in northern Spain. Influence of detection techniques on the results. BMC Infect Dis 12: 69.

16. Lipsitch M, Abdullahi O, D'Amour A, Xie W, Weinberger DM, et al. (2012) Estimating rates of carriage acquisition and clearance and competitive ability for

pneumococcal serotypes in Kenya with a Markov transition model. Epidemiology 23: 510–519.

17. Auranen K, Mehtala J, Tanskanen A, S Kaltoft M (2010) Between-strain competition in acquisition and clearance of pneumococcal carriage–epidemiologic evidence from a longitudinal study of day-care children. Am J Epidemiol 171: 169–176.

18. Vu HT, Yoshida LM, Suzuki M, Nguyen HA, Nguyen CD, et al. (2011) Association between nasopharyngeal load of Streptococcus pneumoniae, viral coinfection, and radiologically confirmed pneumonia in Vietnamese children. Pediatr Infect Dis J 30: 11–18.

19. O'Brien KL, Nohynek H (2003) Report from a WHO working group: standard method for detecting upper respiratory carriage of Streptococcus pneumoniae. Pediatr Infect Dis J 22: 133–140.

20. Dhoubhadel BG, Yasunami M, Yoshida LM, Thi HA, Thi TH, et al. (2014) A novel high-throughput method for molecular serotyping and serotype-specific quantification of Streptococcus pneumoniae using a nanofluidic real-time PCR system. J Med Microbiol 63: 528–539.

21. Battig P, Hathaway LJ, Hofer S, Muhlemann K (2006) Serotype-specific invasiveness and colonization prevalence in Streptococcus pneumoniae correlate with the lag phase during in vitro growth. Microbes Infect 8: 2612–2617.

22. Azzari C, Resti M (2008) Reduction of carriage and transmission of Streptococcus pneumoniae: the beneficial "side effect" of pneumococcal conjugate vaccine. Clin Infect Dis 47: 997–999.

23. Brueggemann AB, Pai R, Crook DW, Beall B (2007) Vaccine escape recombinants emerge after pneumococcal vaccination in the United States. PLoS Pathog 3: e168.

24. Croucher NJ, Harris SR, Fraser C, Quail MA, Burton J, et al. (2011) Rapid pneumococcal evolution in response to clinical interventions. Science 331: 430–434.

25. Leung MH, Oriyo NM, Gillespie SH, Charalambous BM (2011) The adaptive potential during nasopharyngeal colonisation of Streptococcus pneumoniae. Infect Genet Evol 11: 1989–1995.

26. Marks LR, Reddinger RM, Hakansson AP (2012) High levels of genetic recombination during nasopharyngeal carriage and biofilm formation in Streptococcus pneumoniae. MBio 3.

27. Lipsitch M, Dykes JK, Johnson SE, Ades EW, King J, et al. (2000) Competition among Streptococcus pneumoniae for intranasal colonization in a mouse model. Vaccine 18: 2895–2901.

28. Dawid S, Roche AM, Weiser JN (2007) The blp bacteriocins of Streptococcus pneumoniae mediate intraspecies competition both in vitro and in vivo. Infect Immun 75: 443–451.

29. Zhang Y, Auranen K, Eichner M (2004) The influence of competition and vaccination on the coexistence of two pneumococcal serotypes. Epidemiology and Infection 132: 1073–1081.

12

HIV in Children in a General Population Sample in East Zimbabwe: Prevalence, Causes and Effects

Erica L. Pufall[1]*, Constance Nyamukapa[1,2], Jeffrey W. Eaton[1], Reggie Mutsindiri[2], Godwin Chawira[2], Shungu Munyati[2], Laura Robertson[1], Simon Gregson[1]

1 Department of Infectious Disease Epidemiology, Imperial College London, St. Mary's Campus, Norfolk Place, London, United Kingdom, 2 Biomedical Research and Training Institute, Avondale, Harare, Zimbabwe

Abstract

Background: There are an estimated half-million children living with HIV in sub-Saharan Africa. The predominant source of infection is presumed to be perinatal mother-to-child transmission, but general population data about paediatric HIV are sparse. We characterise the epidemiology of HIV in children in sub-Saharan Africa by describing the prevalence, possible source of infection, and effects of paediatric HIV in a southern African population.

Methods: From 2009 to 2011, we conducted a household-based survey of 3389 children (aged 2–14 years) in Manicaland, eastern Zimbabwe (response rate: 73.5%). Data about socio-demographic correlates of HIV, risk factors for infection, and effects on child health were analysed using multi-variable logistic regression. To assess the plausibility of mother-to-child transmission, child HIV infection was linked to maternal survival and HIV status using data from a 12-year adult HIV cohort.

Results: HIV prevalence was (2.2%, 95% CI: 1.6–2.8%) and did not differ significantly by sex, socio-economic status, location, religion, or child age. Infected children were more likely to be underweight (19.6% versus 10.0%, p = 0.03) or stunted (39.1% versus 30.6%, p = 0.04) but did not report poorer physical or psychological ill-health. Where maternal data were available, reported mothers of 61/62 HIV-positive children were deceased or HIV-positive. Risk factors for other sources of infection were not associated with child HIV infection, including blood transfusion, vaccinations, caring for a sick relative, and sexual abuse. The observed flat age-pattern of HIV prevalence was consistent with UNAIDS estimates which assumes perinatal mother-to-child transmission, although modelled prevalence was higher than observed prevalence. Only 19/73 HIV-positive children (26.0%) were diagnosed, but, of these, 17 were on antiretroviral therapy.

Conclusions: Childhood HIV infection likely arises predominantly from mother-to-child transmission and is associated with poorer physical development. Overall antiretroviral therapy uptake was low, with the primary barrier to treatment appearing to be lack of diagnosis.

Editor: Delmiro Fernandez-Reyes, Brighton and Sussex Medical School, United Kingdom

Funding: ELP received a Doctoral Foreign Study Award from the Canadian Institutes for Health Research (http://www.cihr-irsc.gc.ca/e/193.html). JWE thanks the Bill and Melinda Gates foundation for funding support via a grant to the HIV Modelling Consortium (http://www.gatesfoundation.org/). The Manicaland HIV/STD Prevention Project is supported by a grant from the Wellcome Trust (grant 050517/z/97abc, http://www.wellcome.ac.uk/). The funders had no role in study design, data collection and analysis, decision to publish, or preparation of the manuscript.

Competing Interests: The authors have declared that no competing interests exist.

* Email: e.pufall11@imperial.ac.uk

Introduction

In 2012, it was estimated that over 85% of children who became infected with HIV were living in sub-Saharan Africa (SSA) [1]. However, general population data about epidemiology and health effects of paediatric HIV in SSA are sparse. The most common data about HIV prevalence in SSA, Demographic and Health Surveys (DHS) and community-based cohort studies, have typically only included persons over age 15 years. As a result, estimates for HIV in children are generally extrapolated from data about pregnant women using mathematical models [2]. In Zimbabwe, UNAIDS estimated that 2.8% (95% CI: 1.6–3.7%)

of children 0–14 were HIV-positive in 2012 [2,3]. Direct empirical data about the epidemiology, sources and impacts of HIV in children will improve confidence in estimates and ensure that health and social care systems are able to meet the needs of infected children.

Most infected children are believed to have acquired HIV perinatally from their HIV-positive mothers. Untreated HIV infection in infants is typically characterised by rapid disease progression and death at a median of two years of age or less, with survival depending at what stage (*e.g.* perinatally, breastfeeding) the infant becomes vertically infected [4,5], but it is estimated that perhaps up to a third of vertically infected children survive into adolescence [6–8] and clinical reports have provided evidence of non-sexually acquired infections in adolescents [9–12]. However, debate continues as to whether or not these children are actually long-term survivors of mother-to-child transmission (MTCT) or have acquired HIV horizontally. Other studies have reported instances of horizontal HIV transmission in children · [13–15]; however, these studies used non-representative samples or were conducted in highly localised areas.

In this study, we aim to: (i) describe patterns of HIV infection in a representative general population sample of children aged 2–14 years in a large-scale generalised HIV epidemic in rural areas of eastern Zimbabwe; (ii) investigate possible sources of horizontal HIV transmission in childhood; (iii) assess whether the observed age-pattern of HIV-positive children is consistent with that expected from survival of children infected from MTCT (given recent trends in adult prevalence and prevention of mother-to-child transmission (PMTCT) program scale-up); (iv) assess the impact of HIV on children's mental and physical health and nutritional status; and (v) investigate the levels and determinants of antiretroviral treatment (ART) coverage in children.

Methods

Study Population and Data Collection

The Manicaland HIV/STD Prevention Project is a population-based, open cohort study in eastern Zimbabwe [16–18]. Each round of the survey involves a census of all households in the 12 study sites (4 subsistence farming areas; 4 large-scale commercial estates; 2 small towns; and 2 roadside settlements), followed by interviews with individual household members and collection of dried blood spot samples for HIV testing.

In the most recent round (2009–2011) of the Manicaland survey, all children (aged 2–14 years) in a randomly selected 1/3 of households were invited to participate in an investigation of HIV prevalence amongst children. Children were interviewed about their welfare, health, and healthcare using a structured questionnaire. Children under seven answered with assistance from their primary caregiver. Questions on HIV testing and knowledge of HIV status were addressed to the child's primary caregiver in the presence of the child if he or she was over the age of seven. Additionally, the questionnaire was administered by a nurse who had HIV Testing and Counselling certificates, which include training in how to respond if a child becomes distressed. More sensitive questions were asked only of older children and were answered without their caregiver being present: children aged 7–14 years were asked questions on sexual abuse and on psychological health. If a child reported abuse then the interviewer notified the supervising nurse who would subsequently investigate in the company of a social worker. The information from the supervisor and social worker was then fed back to the Child Protection committee in the study area. All maternal data (religion and HIV status) were collected in the general (adult) survey and linked to child data based on children reporting who their biological mother was, and confirmed through fertility histories and the household roster. In cases where a link could not be made, or if the child was a maternal orphan, maternal data was coded as missing. Dried blood spot samples were collected and tested for HIV in an offsite laboratory using the COMBAIDS-RS HIV 1+2 Immunodot Assay (Span Diagnostics, India); for cases in which the child tested HIV-positive but had an uninfected mother, the HIV test results were confirmed using Vironostika HIV Uni-form II Plus O (Biomérieux, France) ELISA tests. Data used in the manuscript are provided in the supporting information file Dataset S1.

Ethics Statement

Ethical approval for the Manicaland HIV/STD Prevention Project was obtained from the Research Council of Zimbabwe (Number 02187), the Biomedical Research and Training Institute Zimbabwe's institutional review board (Number AP6/97), and the Imperial College London Research Ethics Committee (Number ICREC 9_3_13). Written informed consent was obtained prior to survey participation from each child's primary caregiver. In addition, children aged 7–14 years provided verbal or written assent, respectively. Participants and guardians were informed that, at any point, they could refuse to answer a question or decline to continue the interview.

Data Analysis

In this analysis of children aged 2–14 years old, we tested for associations of HIV infection with socio-demographic characteristics (sex, age-group, household socio-economic status (SES), community type, and mother's religion) using logistic regression. Socio-economic status was measured using a summed asset-based wealth index developed for the study population in Manicaland [19]. The mother's self-reported religious affiliation was classified into "Christian", "Traditional", "Spiritual", "Other", or "none", as in previous analyses of Manicaland data [20].

To test the hypothesis that HIV infection in children occurs primarily through MTCT, where available, we examined maternal survival/infection status (deceased, alive and HIV-negative, alive and HIV-positive, alive with unknown HIV status) by child HIV status to establish the plausibility of vertical HIV transmission. The odds ratios of being a maternal orphan and of being a maternal orphan or having an HIV-positive mother amongst infected and uninfected children were evaluated using a one-sided Fisher's exact test. We tested for associations between HIV infection and risk factors for horizontal HIV transmission, which included blood transfusion, vaccination, non-vaccination medical injections, breastfed by a non-biological mother, cared for a sick relative, and sexual abuse.

To assess whether the observed age-pattern of HIV prevalence in children is consistent with that which would be expected in Zimbabwe if infections were due to mother-to-child transmission, we compared the age-specific HIV prevalence data to national estimates of child HIV prevalence reported by UNAIDS [1]. These estimates are derived using the Spectrum model [21–23], which assumes MTCT is the source of paediatric HIV and reflects the declining trends in HIV prevalence recorded in pregnant women, rates of mother-to-child transmission, patterns of paediatric survival by time of infection, national data on PMTCT and anti-retroviral therapy (ART) scale-up, and effectiveness of PMTCT regimens [4]. The Spectrum file that we used in this analysis can be downloaded from http://apps.unaids.org/spectrum/.

The impact of HIV on measures of physical and mental health was evaluated using linear (continuous outcomes) or logistic (binary outcomes) regression, adjusting for age. Z-scores for height- and weight-for-age and weight-for-height were calculated using WHO child growth standards [24,25]. Z-scores below -2 were considered to indicate stunting (low height-for-age), being underweight (low weight-for-age) and wasting (low weight-for-height). Comparisons were made for stunting and being underweight for all children, while wasting was only compared in children aged 2–5 years, as these were the ages for which reference data were available [24]. Psychological wellbeing scores were calculated in children aged 7–14 years using principal components analysis of psychological distress measures as described by

Nyamukapa *et al.*, 2010 [26]. All analyses were conducted in Stata version 12.1 (StataCorp LP, USA).

Results

Demographic Profile of Infected Children

Four thousand six hundred and eleven children aged 2–14 years were enumerated and selected for inclusion in the study, of which 3389 (73.5%) completed the survey and gave a dried blood spot for HIV testing. Children who did not complete the survey did not have significantly different age or gender distributions and their household of residence did not have significantly different mean SESs than those who completed the questionnaire (all p>0.05). Reasons given for non-response included: away from home for work (7.4%), away from home for school (7.0%), another reason for being away from home (67.1%), whereabouts unknown (1.1%), refused (12.3%), and other (5.0%). Seventy-three (2.2%, 95% CI: 1.7–2.6%) were HIV-positive. Prevalence was 1.6% (11/688), 2.5% (33/1296), and 1.8% (25/1405) among children aged 2–4 years, 5–9 years, and 10–14 years, respectively. Demographic characteristics of children aged 2–14 years by HIV status are presented in Table 1. HIV prevalence did not differ significantly (p<0.05) by sex, age-group, or any other demographic characteristics (household SES, community type, and maternal religion).

Sources of HIV Infection

All but one HIV-positive child were either maternal orphans or had an HIV-positive surviving mother, consistent with the primary source of childhood infection being MTCT (Table 2). HIV-positive children were significantly more likely to be a maternal orphan (OR: 6.56, 95% CI: 4.03–10.66) and/or have an HIV-positive mother (OR: 76.03, 95% CI: 18.54–311.79)) than HIV-negative children. The one child who was HIV-positive but for whom the woman identified as his biological mother was HIV-negative (Table 2) was a three year-old male reported to be living with both biological parents. He did not report any of the risk factors for non-sexual horizontal transmission (blood transfusions, non-medical injections, breastfeeding by a non-biological mother, caring for a sick relative, or child abuse). Overall, 26.9% (902/3360) of participants who answered the survey questions reported any of the selected risk factors for horizontal HIV transmission (Table 3), excluding vaccination-related injections, of which 99.7% (3364/3374) of children reported having had. Item non-response ranged from 0.1% (ever cared for a sick relative) to 27.1% (ever had a blood transfusion) and did not differ between HIV-negative and HIV-positive children (all p>0.05). HIV-positive children were significantly more likely to report non-vaccination injections than HIV-negative children (41.1% vs. 26.2%, p = 0.01). Otherwise, no significant differences in reporting of risk factors (blood transfusions, breastfeeding by a non-biological mother, caring for a sick relative, child abuse or sexual activity) were found between HIV-positive and uninfected children.

Comparison of Observed Age-Specific HIV Prevalence with National Estimates from the Spectrum Model

HIV prevalence in children aged 2–14 observed in Manicaland was lower than the national estimates for Zimbabwe as a whole in 2010 from the Spectrum model (3.6%). However, the age-pattern of HIV prevalence amongst children observed in the data was consistent with the model estimates (Figure 1). This suggests that the age-patterns of HIV in Manicaland are in line with what would be expected if MTCT were the main source of child

Table 1. Association between demographic characteristics and HIV infection in children.

Category	Sub-category	HIV+	N in Sub-category	OR (95% CI)[†]	*p*-value[‡]
Gender	Male	2.34%	1712	Referent	0.21
	Female	1.73%	1677	0.75 (0.46–1.21)	
Age Group	2–4	1.60%	688	Referent	0.27
	5–9	2.54%	1296	1.61 (0.81–3.20)	
	10–14	1.78%	1405	1.11 (0.55–2.28)	
Household SES	Poorest quintile	1.75%	688	Referent	0.33
	Second quintile	2.38%	632	1.37 (0.64–2.95)	
	Middle quintile	0.70%	143	0.40 (0.05–3.07)	
	Fourth quintile	2.70%	1063	1.58 (0.80–3.13)	
	Least poor quintile	1.85%	863	1.06 (0.50–2.26)	
Community type	Subsistence farming	2.44%	1391	Referent	0.38
	Roadside trading	1.93%	671	0.79 (0.41–1.50)	
	Agricultural estate	1.36%	811	0.54 (0.27–1.08)	
	Commercial centre	2.13%	516	0.87 (0.44–1.73)	
Mother's religion[a]	Christian	1.44%	967	Referent	0.95
	Traditional	0%	13	N/A	
	Spiritual	1.53%	849	1.02 (0.48–2.19)	
	Other	1.69%	301	1.15 (0.41–3.21)	
	None	0%	67	N/A	

[†]Unadjusted odds ratio.
[‡]Fisher's exact test for difference of proportions.
[a]Total respondents (N = 2206) is lower than other categories due to maternal orphans (n = 348), unlinked records (n = 722) and question non-response (n = 113).

Table 2. Maternal mortality and HIV status in children.

	Child HIV status	
Maternal status	**HIV- (N = 3316)**	**HIV+ (N = 73)**
Mother deceased	318 (9.59%)	30 (41.09%)
Mother alive, HIV+	390 (11.76%)	31 (42.47%)
Mother alive, HIV-	1765 (53.23%)	1 (1.37%)
Mother alive, unknown HIV status	843 (25.42%)	11 (15.07%)

infections, accounting for the declining trend in adult HIV prevalence and the scale-up of PMTCT programmes in Zimbabwe.

HIV Status and Child Health

HIV-positive children were significantly more likely to be underweight (low weight-for-age) (AOR: 2.20; 95% CI: 1.08–4.47) and stunted (AOR: 1.69; 95% CI: 1.02–2.81) than HIV-negative children, but were not more likely to be wasted (low weight-for-height) (AOR: 0.43; 95% CI: 0.05–3.34) or to report a recent illness (AOR: 1.31; 95% CI: 0.64–2.66) (Table 4). HIV status was also not associated with psychological wellbeing (Coefficient: −0.06; 95% CI: −0.21 – +0.09) (Table 4).

Of the 73 HIV-positive children, 26.0% (19/73) reported that they knew their HIV status. Of the HIV-negative children, 114/3309 (3.5%) had had an HIV test, significantly less than reported testing prevalence in HIV-positive children (p<0.001). Children of mothers who reported that they knew they were HIV-positive were 5.17 times (95% CI: 2.27–11.76) more likely to have had an HIV test and know the result than children of mothers who self-reported as HIV-negative. Knowledge of HIV status was not associated with psychological wellbeing score for HIV-positive children (change in psychological wellbeing score: +0.01; 95% CI: −0.131– +0.33). All but two of the children (17/19) who were aware of their HIV-positive status reported taking drugs that stop HIV from causing AIDS (*i.e.* were on anti-retroviral therapy

(ART)). Despite high ART coverage when HIV status is known, overall, less than a quarter (23.3%, 17/73) of the HIV-positive children was receiving ART.

Discussion

This study describes the prevalence and consequences of HIV in children living in a rural area of southern Africa. In eastern Zimbabwe, from 2009–2011, 2.2% (95% CI: 1.7–2.6%) of children aged 2–14 years tested positive for HIV, at a time when HIV prevalence was 11% and 17%, respectively, amongst male and female adults (15–54 years) in the same population. This estimate, from a representative general-population sample, is lower than those from a sample of children in 2005 in Chimanimani district in southern Manicaland, where HIV prevalence was 3.2% (41/1290) in children aged 2–14 years [27]. Such a reduction between 2005 and 2010 is expected based on the decline in adult HIV prevalence and the increase in PMTCT coverage since 2005. A study conducted with 4,386 primary school children in Harare in 2010 found an HIV prevalence of 2.7% (95% CI: 2.2–3.1%) in children aged 6–13 years [28], which is close to the prevalence of 2.2% found in our study for a slightly different age-group in a different region. As was the case in the Chimanimani study [27] and in studies in similar age-groups elsewhere in SSA [29–31], including a large national population survey in South Africa conducted in 2008 [32], we

Table 3. Association between HIV status and potential horizontal risk factors for HIV.

Horizontal risk factors	Exposure	N	HIV+%	AOR (95% CI) [†]	*p*-value[‡]
Ever had a blood transfusion	No	3,355	2.15%	Referent	0.14
	Yes	7	14.3%	6.51 (0.80–53.34)	
Lifetime number of non-vaccination injections	0	2491	1.73%	Referent	0.004
	>0	873	3.44%	2.19 (1.23–3.89)	
Received tuberculosis, polio, measles, and/or diphtheria vaccination	No	10	0%	Referent	0.81
	Yes	3364	2.11%	N/A	
Breastfed by non-biological mother	No	3359	2.14%	Referent	0.71
	Yes	16	0%	N/A	
Cared for a sick relative (ages 6–14)	No	2403	2.29%	Referent	0.45
	Yes	35	0%	N/A	
Ever been sexually abused (ages 7–14)	No	2180	2.25%	Referent	N/A
	Yes	4	0%	N/A	

[†]Adjusted odds ratio; adjusted for age, gender, SES, and site type.
[‡]Fisher's exact test for difference of proportions.
NB: Different Ns are due to different question non-response rates.

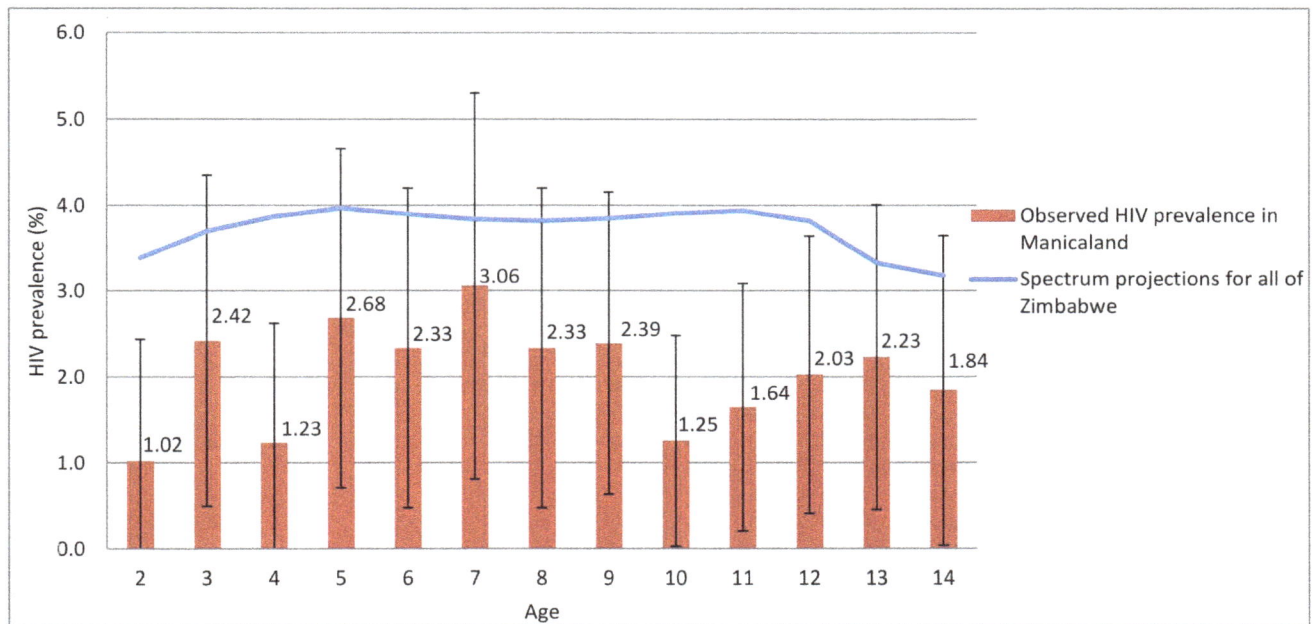

Figure 1. Comparison of observed HIV prevalence by age in Manicaland, with 95% confidence intervals, to the Zimbabwe national HIV estimates from UNAIDS and the Zimbabwe Ministry of Health and Child Welfare.

found no significant differences in HIV prevalence with respect to sex or age.

Our finding of a relatively even pattern of HIV prevalence by age is consistent with official national estimates derived from the Spectrum model. Survival data for children infected with HIV through MTCT suggest high mortality [7] and, in a stable epidemic with little horizontal transmission and no PMTCT intervention, HIV prevalence will decline as children age into adolescence. However, the decline in HIV prevalence in pregnant women since the late 1990s (from 25.7% in 2002 to 16.1% 2009 [33]) and the scale-up of PMTCT services from the mid-2000s explain reduced prevalence in younger children to the levels observed in the current study. The pattern of HIV prevalence we saw with age is also consistent with that reported by Eaton et al. in

15–17 year-olds in the same population at different time points (2009–2011 here and 2006–2008 in Eaton et al.) [12]. That is, it supports the hypothesis that MTCT is the main source of HIV infection in children and adolescents in this population.

Our data further confirm the belief that MTCT is the primary mode of HIV transmission in children in eastern Zimbabwe [12]. Mothers of HIV-infected children were significantly more likely than mothers of uninfected children to be deceased or HIV-positive. One child, for whom we could not identify a plausible source of infection, did not report any vertical, sexual, or other horizontal risk factors for transmission. Exposure to potential modes of transmission may have been under-reported and data were not collected on all possible sources of infection, such as scarification and hospital and dental visits, which have previously

Table 4. Effects of HIV status on physical and mental health outcomes in children and adolescents.

Health outcome	HIV status	N	%	AOR (95% CI)[†]	p-value
Ill in last two weeks	HIV−	3320	11.55%	Referent	0.11
	HIV+	69	19.61%	1.31 (0.64–2.66)	
Low height-for-age	HIV−	3222	30.60%	Referent	0.04
	HIV+	69	39.13%	1.69 (1.02–2.81)	
Low weight-for-age	HIV−	2225	9.97%	Referent	0.03
	HIV+	51	19.61%	2.20 (1.08–4.47)	
Low weight-for-height[‡]	HIV−	833	11.64%	Referent	0.42
	HIV+	16	6.25%	0.43 (0.05–3.34)	
Psychological wellbeing score[a]	HIV−	2385	0.01	Referent	0.45
	HIV+	55	−0.05	−0.06 (−0.21–+0.09)	

[†]Adjusted odds ratio; adjusted for age, gender, SES, and community type.
[‡]Children 2–5 only.
[a]Mean and change in score between HIV− and HIV+; ages 6–14 only.

been identified as sources of HIV in children [13–15]. Sexual abuse has also been identified as a potential mode of HIV acquisition in select cases in children [34–39], however, due to ethical reasons, little research has been conducted into the proportion of children infected with HIV through sexual abuse, even though sexual abuse has been reported to be common in South Africa [40,41]. While we cannot be certain about the accuracy of reporting about the child's biological mother, without biological tests, for which this study did not have consent, the identification of the biological mother was consistent with information reported on the household roster and the child was named on the mother's fertility history.

The need to understand HIV infection in children is particularly important given that HIV is increasingly becoming a cause of hospitalisation amongst adolescents in SSA [11] and this trend is likely to continue as more HIV-positive children age into adolescence. We found that HIV-positive children were significantly more likely to report non-vaccination medical injections than HIV-negative individuals, most likely because HIV-positive children are more likely to seek healthcare for managing their infection or to treat HIV-associated illnesses [11]. Thus, this association should therefore not be misconstrued as evidence for medical injections as a source of horizontal transmission, particularly as 27 of the 30 (90%) of the HIV-positive children who reported having had medical injections also reported being a maternal orphan or having a mother who was HIV-positive. Stunting and wasting in HIV-positive children, as well as being underweight, have been reported previously in SSA [11,42,43]. We found HIV-positive children to be significantly more likely to be underweight and stunted, indicative of the long-term harm of HIV infection on health and nutritional status. Perhaps unsurprisingly, we did not find a significant relationship with wasting, which measures recent severe weight loss, often associated with acute starvation and severe disease.

There are few data from SSA on the psychological manifestations of HIV infection in children, although studies from developed countries report significantly higher incidence of psychiatric admissions for HIV-positive children than HIV-negative children, with knowledge of HIV status increasing the risk of admission [44]. A previous study in Zimbabwe found that 56% of HIV-positive adolescents reported psychosocial problems, but that these problems were not common in younger children [45]. These data, however, were collected from children and adolescents visiting facilities offering HIV care services, and many respondents were already presenting with AIDS-related illnesses. Because the results were from a clinical study and were not compared to an HIV-negative population, it is not possible to conclude that there was a significant increase in psychosocial distress based on HIV status. Although we found no significant association between HIV status and psychological wellbeing, the lack of data from SSA in this area and the findings of Ferrand et al. (2010) [45] suggest that this is an important topic for future investigation.

Only a quarter of HIV-positive children in our study were aware of their HIV status. Across southern and eastern Africa, ART coverage among children is a major problem and high priority for many governments as it continues to lag behind adult coverage (33% versus 65% in the 22 priority countries, of which 21 are in Africa) [46]. So long as they remain undiagnosed, and therefore untreated, HIV-positive children are at higher risk for AIDS-related illnesses and early mortality. In the longer term, knowledge of HIV status is important to mitigate the risk of passing the infection on to sexual partners. Despite the low coverage of HIV testing, we found that if children or their guardians were aware of the child's HIV-positive status there was a 90% chance that the child would be on ART. This suggests that, despite the fear, potential stigma and associated costs, a positive diagnosis does result in the initiation of treatment. One way to help increase treatment amongst children might be to increase HIV-testing of women, as we found that when a mother knew herself to be HIV-positive, her child was significantly more likely to have had an HIV test themselves – suggesting that getting more mothers diagnosed through PMTCT programs will improve child testing. Other possible ways to increase infant diagnosis of HIV in this population are the new point-of-care tests currently being developed. New tests include a rapid p24 antigen test and a nucleic-acid amplification test, both of which can be performed in under half an hour [47]. Currently, many infants go undiagnosed due to the long turnaround times or poor infrastructure associated with dried blood spot sample testing [48]. Early infant HIV diagnosis is important, as the high ART coverage when children are aware of their status implies that lack of knowledge of HIV status is a contributing factor to the low coverage of ART in children that has been noted in Zimbabwe (39.5% according to the 2011 national estimates [49]) and more broadly in most of sub-Saharan Africa.

Conclusion

These findings provide evidence that MTCT is the principal source of HIV infection in children in southern Africa and that current initiatives to increase the availability and effectiveness of PMTCT should result in reductions in HIV prevalence in children over time. Effort should be made to encourage HIV testing in children because, despite low overall ART coverage, children who are aware of their HIV status were highly likely to be on treatment.

Acknowledgments

We thank Janet Dzangare and Elizabeth Gonese (Zimbabwe Ministry of Health and Child Welfare) and Mary Mahy (UNAIDS) for assistance with the Zimbabwe Spectrum file. We thank John Stover for advice regarding HIV prevalence estimates from the Spectrum software. We are grateful to all participants in the Manicaland HIV/STD Prevention Project.

Author Contributions

Conceived and designed the experiments: ELP CN JWE SM LR SG. Analyzed the data: ELP JWE. Wrote the paper: ELP CN JWE RM LR SG SM GC. Organised the data collection: CN RM GC SG.

References

1. UNAIDS (2013) Global report: UNAIDS report on the global AIDS epidemic 2013.
2. Zimbabwe National Statistics Agency (ZIMSTAT), ICF International. (2012) Zimbabwe demographic and health survey 2010–11.
3. UNAIDS (2012) Global AIDS response progress report 2012: Follow-up to the 2011 political declaration on HIV/AIDS: Intensifying our efforts to eliminate HIV/AIDS: Zimbabwe country report.
4. Rollins N, Mahy M, Becquet R, Kuhn L, Creek T, et al. (2012) Estimates of peripartum and postnatal mother-to-child transmission probabilities of HIV for

use in spectrum and other population-based models. Sex Transm Infect (Suppl 2): i44–i51.

5. Becquet R, Marston M, Dabis F, Moulton LH, Gray G, et al. (2012) Children who acquire HIV infection perinatally are at higher risk of early death than those acquiring infection through breastmilk: A meta-analysis. PLOS One 7(2): e28510.

6. Newell ML, Coovadia H, Cortina-Borja M, Rollins N, Gaillard P, et al. (2004) Mortality of infected and uninfected infants born to HIV-infected mothers in Africa: A pooled analysis. Lancet 364(9441): 1236–1243.

7. Ferrand RA, Corbett EL, Wood R, Hargrove J, Ndhlovu CE, et al. (2009) AIDS among older children and adolescents in southern Africa: Projecting the time course and magnitude of the epidemic. AIDS 23(15): 2039–2046.

8. Marston M, Zaba B, Salomon JA, Brahmbhatt H, Bagenda D (2005) Estimating the net effect of HIV on child mortality in African populations affected by generalized HIV epidemics. J Acquir Immune Defic Syndr 38(2): 219–227.

9. Ferrand RA, Luethy R, Bwakura F, Mujuru H, Miller RF, et al. (2007) HIV infection presenting in older children and adolescents: A case series from Harare, Zimbabwe. Clin Infect Dis 44(6): 874–878.

10. Ferrand RA, Munaiwa L, Matsekete J, Bandason T, Nathoo K, et al. (2010) Undiagnosed HIV infection among adolescents seeking primary health care in Zimbabwe. Clin Infect Dis 51(7): 844–851.

11. Ferrand RA, Bandason T, Musvaire P, Larke N, Nathoo K, et al. (2010) Causes of acute hospitalization in adolescence: Burden and spectrum of HIV-related morbidity in a country with an early-onset and severe HIV epidemic: A prospective survey. PLoS Med 7(2): e1000178.

12. Eaton J, Garnett GP, Takavarasha F, Mason P, Robertson L, et al. (2013) Increasing adolescent HIV prevalence in eastern zimbabwe - evidence of long-term survivors of mother-to-child transmission? PLoS One 8(8): e70447.

13. Okinyi M, Brewer DD, Potterat JJ (2009) Horizontally-acquired HIV infection in kenyan and swazi children. Int J STD AIDS 20(12): 852–857.

14. Gomo E, Chibatamoto PP, Chandiwana SK, Sabeta CT (1997) Risk factors for HIV infection in a rural cohort in Zimbabwe: A pilot study. Cent Afr J Med 43(12): 350–354.

15. Shisana O, Connolly C, Rehle TM, Mehtar S, Dana P (2008) HIV risk exposure among South African children in public health facilities. AIDS Care 20(7): 755–763.

16. Gregson S, Garnett GP, Nyamukapa CA, Hallett TB, Lewis JJ, et al. (2006) HIV decline associated with behaviour change in eastern Zimbabwe. Science 311(5761): 664–666.

17. Lopman B, Nyamukapa CA, Mushati P, Wambe M, Mupambireyi Z, et al. (2008) HIV incidence after 3 years follow-up in a cohort recruited between 1998 and 2000 in Manicaland, Zimbabwe: Contributions of proximate and underlying determinants to transmission. Int J Epidemiol 37(1): 88–105.

18. Gregson S, Nyamukapa C, Garnett GP, Mason PR, Zhuwau T, et al. (2002) Sexual mixing patterns and sex-differentials in teenage exposure to HIV infection in rural Zimbabwe. Lancet 359: 1896–1903.

19. Lopman B, Lewis JJ, Nyamukapa CA, Mushati P, Chandiwana SK, et al. (2007) HIV incidence and poverty in Manicaland, Zimbabwe. AIDS 21(Supplement 7): S57–S66.

20. Manzou R, Schumacher C, Gregson S (2014) Temporal dynamics of religion as a determinant of HIV infection in East Zimbabwe: A serial cross-sectional analysis. PLoS One 9(1): e86060.

21. Stover J (2009) AIM: A computer program for making HIV/AIDS projections and examining the demographic and social impacts of AIDS.

22. Stover J, Kirmeyer S (2009) DemProj: A computer program for making population projections.

23. Stover J, Brown T, Marston M (2012) Updates to the spectrum/estimation and projection package (EPP) model to estimate HIV trends for adults and children. Sex Transm Infect (Suppl 2): i11–i16.

24. WHO Multicentre Growth Reference Study Group (2006) WHO child growth standards: Length/height-for-age, weight-for-age, weight-for-length, weight-for-height and body mass index-for-age: Methods and development: 312.

25. de Onis M, Onyango AW, Borghi E, Siyam A, Nishida C, et al. (2007) Development of a WHO growth reference for school-aged children and adolescents. Bull World Health Organ 85(9): 660–667.

26. Nyamukapa CA, Gregson S, Wambe M, Mushore P, Lopman B, et al. (2010) Causes and consequences of psychological distress among orphans in eastern Zimbabwe. AIDS Care 22(8): 988–996.

27. Gomo E, Rusakaniko S, Mashange W, Mutsvangwa J, Chandiwana B, et al. (2006) Household survey of HIV-prevalence and behaviour in Chimanimani district, Zimbabwe, 2005.

28. Bandason T, Langhaug LF, Makamba M, Laver S, Hatzold K, et al. (2013) Burden of HIV among primary school children and feasibility of primary school-linked HIV testing in Harare, Zimbabwe: A mixed methods study. AIDS Care 25(12): 1520–1526.

29. [Anonymous] (2005) South African national HIV prevalence, HIV incidence, behaviour and communication survey, 2005.

30. Tsheko GN, Odirile LW, Segwabe M, Bainame K (2005) A census of orphans and vulnerable children in two villages in Botswana.

31. Munyati S, Rusakaniko S, Mupambireyi PF, Mahati ST, Chibatamoto PP, et al. (2006) A census of orphans and vulnerable children in two zimbabwean districts.

32. Shisana O, Rehle T, Simbayi LC, Zuma K, Jooste S, et al. (2009) South african national HIV prevalence, incidence, behaviour and communication survey 2008: A turning tide among teenagers?

33. Zimbabwe Ministry of Health and Child Welfare (2010) Antenatal clinic HIV surveillance report 2009.

34. Bechtel K (2010) Sexual abuse and sexually transmitted infections in children and adolescents. Curr Opin Pediatr 22(1): 94–99.

35. Girardet RG, Lahoti S, Howard LA, Fajman NN, Sawyer MK, et al. (2009) Epidemiology of sexually transmitted infections in suspected child victims of sexual assault. Pediatrics 124(1): 79–86.

36. Gellert GA, Durfee MJ, Berkowitz CD, Higgins KV, Tubiolo VC (1993) Situational and sociodemographic characteristics of children infected with human immunodeficiency virus from pediatric sexual abuse. Pediatrics 91(1): 39–44.

37. Hammerschlag MR (1998) Sexually transmitted diseases in sexually abused children: Medical and legal implications. Sex Transm Infect 74(3): 167.

38. Lindegren ML, Hanson IC, Hammett TA, Beil J, Fleming PL, et al. (1998) Sexual abuse of children: Intersection with the HIV epidemic. Pediatrics 102(4): E461–E4610.

39. Schaaf HS (2004) Human immunodeficiency virus infection and child sexual abuse. S Afr Med J 94(9): 782–785.

40. Jewkes R, Levin J, Mbananga N, Bradshaw D (2002) Rape of girls in South Africa. Lancet 359(9303): 319–320.

41. Meel BL (2003) A study on the prevalence of HIV-seropositivity among rape survivals in Transkei, South Africa. J Clin Forensic Med 10(2): 65–70.

42. Nalwoga A, Maher D, Todd J, Karabarinde A, Biraro S, et al. (2012) Nutritional status of children living in a community with high HIV prevalence in rural Uganda: A cross-sectional population-based survey. Trop Med Int Health 15(4): 414–422.

43. Chiabi A, Lebela J, Kobela M, Mbuagbaw L, Obama MT, et al. (2012) The frequency and magnitude of growth failure in a group of HIV-infected children in Cameroon. Pan Afr Med J 11: 15.

44. Gaughan DM, Hughes MD, Oleske JM, Malee K, Gore CA, et al. (2004) Psychiatric hospitalizations among children and youths with human immuno-deficiency virus infection. Pediatrics 113(6): e544–e551.

45. Ferrand RA, Lowe S, Whande B, Munaiwa L, Langhaug L, et al. (2010) Survey of children accessing HIV services in a high prevalence setting: Time for adolescents to count? Bull World Health Organ 88(6): 428–434.

46. WHO UNICEF, UNAIDS (2013) Global update on HIV treatment 2013: Results, impact and opportunities.

47. Haleyur Giri Setty MK, Hewlett IK (2014) Point of care technologies for HIV. AIDS Res Treat 2014(497046).

48. Mori Y, Kitao M, Tomita N, Notomi T (2004) Real-time turbidimetry of LAMP reaction for quantifying template DNA. J Biochem Biophys Methods 59(2): 145–157.

49. Zimbabwe Ministry of Health and Child Welfare (2012) Zimbabwe national HIV and AIDS estimates 2011 (draft).

13

Corticosteroids and Pediatric Septic Shock Outcomes: A Risk Stratified Analysis

Sarah J. Atkinson[1,2], Natalie Z. Cvijanovich[3], Neal J. Thomas[4], Geoffrey L. Allen[5], Nick Anas[6], Michael T. Bigham[7], Mark Hall[8], Robert J. Freishtat[9], Anita Sen[10], Keith Meyer[11], Paul A. Checchia[12], Thomas P. Shanley[13], Jeffrey Nowak[14], Michael Quasney[13], Scott L. Weiss[15], Sharon Banschbach[1], Eileen Beckman[1], Kelli Howard[1], Erin Frank[1], Kelli Harmon[1], Patrick Lahni[1], Christopher J. Lindsell[16], Hector R. Wong[1,17]*

1 Division of Critical Care Medicine, Cincinnati Children's Hospital Medical Center and Cincinnati Children's Research Foundation, Cincinnati, OH, United States of America, 2 Department of Surgery, University of Cincinnati, Cincinnati, OH, United States of America, 3 UCSF Benioff Children's Hospital Oakland, Oakland, CA, United States of America, 4 Penn State Hershey Children's Hospital, Hershey, PA, United States of America, 5 Children's Mercy Hospital, Kansas City, MO, United States of America, 6 Children's Hospital of Orange County, Orange, CA, United States of America, 7 Akron Children's Hospital, Akron, OH, United States of America, 8 Nationwide Children's Hospital, Columbus, OH, United States of America, 9 Children's National Medical Center, Washington, DC, United States of America, 10 Morgan Stanley Children's Hospital, Columbia University Medical Center, New York, NY, United States of America, 11 Miami Children's Hospital, Miami, FL, United States of America, 12 Texas Children's Hospital, Houston, TX, United States of America, 13 C. S. Mott Children's Hospital at the University of Michigan, Ann Arbor, MI, United States of America, 14 Children's Hospital and Clinics of Minnesota, Minneapolis, MN, United States of America, 15 The Children's Hospital of Philadelphia, Philadelphia, PA, United States of America, 16 Department of Emergency Medicine, University of Cincinnati College of Medicine, Cincinnati, OH, United States of America, 17 Department of Pediatrics, University of Cincinnati College of Medicine, Cincinnati, OH, United States of America

Abstract

Background: The potential benefits of corticosteroids for septic shock may depend on initial mortality risk.

Objective: We determined associations between corticosteroids and outcomes in children with septic shock who were stratified by initial mortality risk.

Methods: We conducted a retrospective analysis of an ongoing, multi-center pediatric septic shock clinical and biological database. Using a validated biomarker-based stratification tool (PERSEVERE), 496 subjects were stratified into three initial mortality risk strata (low, intermediate, and high). Subjects receiving corticosteroids during the initial 7 days of admission (n = 252) were compared to subjects who did not receive corticosteroids (n = 244). Logistic regression was used to model the effects of corticosteroids on 28-day mortality and complicated course, defined as death within 28 days or persistence of two or more organ failures at 7 days.

Results: Subjects who received corticosteroids had greater organ failure burden, higher illness severity, higher mortality, and a greater requirement for vasoactive medications, compared to subjects who did not receive corticosteroids. PERSEVERE-based mortality risk did not differ between the two groups. For the entire cohort, corticosteroids were associated with increased risk of mortality (OR 2.3, 95% CI 1.3–4.0, p = 0.004) and a complicated course (OR 1.7, 95% CI 1.1–2.5, p = 0.012). Within each PERSEVERE-based stratum, corticosteroid administration was not associated with improved outcomes. Similarly, corticosteroid administration was not associated with improved outcomes among patients with no comorbidities, nor in groups of patients stratified by PRISM.

Conclusions: Risk stratified analysis failed to demonstrate any benefit from corticosteroids in this pediatric septic shock cohort.

Editor: Lyle L. Moldawer, University of Florida College of Medicine, United States of America

Funding: This study was supported by National Institutes of Health grants RO1GM064619, RO1GM099773, and R01GM108025, and supported in part by an Institutional Clinical and Translational Science Award, NIH/NCRR 8UL1 TR000077. Dr. Atkinson is supported by a training grant from the National Institutes of Health, T32GM008478. The funders had no role in study design, data collection and analysis, decision to publish, or preparation of the manuscript.

Competing Interests: Dr. Wong and the Cincinnati Children's Hospital Research Foundation have submitted a provisional patent application for PERSEVERE. PCT/US2013/025233 (published 8/15/13 as WO 2013/119871), entitled "Biomarkers of Septic Shock", filed 2/7/13 and claiming priority to U.S. Provisional application 61/595,996, filed 2/7/12. Dr. Lindsell is named as a co-inventor in the above patent application. The remaining authors have no competing interests to report.

* Email: hector.wong@cchmc.org

Introduction

The controversy surrounding corticosteroid use in septic shock has yielded multiple adult randomized controlled trials, yet their results are conflicting and a consensus has yet to be reached [1–6]. The Surviving Sepsis Campaign guidelines recommend considering corticosteroid usage in patients with refractory shock, defined as those who continue to require vasopressors despite adequate fluid resuscitation [7]. However, physician practices surrounding adjunctive corticosteroid administration vary significantly [8,9]. Practitioners must weigh the potential hemodynamic improvements seen with corticosteroids against the risks of diminished wound healing, gastrointestinal bleeding, hyperglycemia, and immune suppression [4,6,10].

Studies examining corticosteroid use in pediatric septic shock are less abundant than adult studies, but currently the use of corticosteroids is recommended for children with fluid-resuscitated septic shock and evidence of catecholamine resistance or adrenal insufficiency, although these conditions are not evidence- or consensus-defined for children [11]. No large randomized controlled trials examining corticosteroids use in pediatric septic shock have been completed. However, a meta-analysis of small trials showed no benefit attributable to corticosteroids [12]. In addition, two large retrospective observational studies did not show any survival benefit with corticosteroid use in children with septic shock [13,14]. One of these studies normalized for illness severity and organ failure burden, but did not specifically conduct a risk-stratified analysis [14]. Consequently, the lack of any survival benefit from corticosteroids may be a reflection of the fact that those children who received corticosteroids had a higher initial mortality risk than those who did not receive corticosteroids.

The Surviving Sepsis Campaign guidelines report on an analysis of "low risk" (placebo mortality rate <50%) and "high risk" (placebo mortality >60%) patients, demonstrating no benefit in low risk patients receiving corticosteroids, but a trend toward lower mortality in high risk patients receiving corticosteroids [15]. A recent retrospective, multicenter, propensity-matched study stratified patients with septic shock using the Acute Physiology and Chronic Health Evaluation II (APACHE II) score and reported that corticosteroids were associated with a survival benefit in patients occupying the upper quartile of APACHE II scores for that cohort [16]. Accordingly, the potential benefit of adjunctive corticosteroids for septic shock would be better understood in the context of mortality risk stratification.

Recently, a biomarker-based stratification tool was derived and validated for children with septic shock (Pediatric Sepsis Biomarker Risk Model, PERSEVERE), allowing for stratification into mortality risk categories upon pediatric intensive care unit (PICU) admission [17–21]. A potential application of PERSEVERE is to enable stratified analysis of clinical data [22]. We explored the association between corticosteroids and outcomes in children with septic shock stratified by risk of mortality. We hypothesized that, similar to previous reports in adults with septic shock, any potential benefit of corticosteroids in pediatric septic shock is dependent on the initial mortality risk as determined by PERSEVERE. We secondarily hypothesized that the potential benefit of corticosteroids would also be dependent on illness severity as determined by the Pediatric Risk of Mortality (PRISM) score.

Materials and Methods

Ethics statement

All study subjects were enrolled after written informed consent from parents or legal guardians. The Institutional Review Boards (IRB) of each participating institution approved secondary use of biological specimens and clinical data: Cincinnati Children's Hospital Medical Center, UCSF Benioff Children's Hospital Oakland, Penn State Hershey Children's Hospital, Children's Mercy Hospital, Children's Hospital of Orange County, Akron

Table 1. Clinical and demographic data for the study subjects.

	No Corticosteroids (n = 244)	Corticosteroids (n = 252)	P value
Age in years, median (IQR)	2.8 (0.7–7.1)	3.4 (1.3–7.0)	0.097
Males, N (%)	137 (56)	140 (56)	0.966
Deaths, N (%)	21 (9)	43 (17)	0.005
Complicated course, N (%)	53 (22)	80 (32)	0.016
PRISM score, median (IQR)	11 (7–18)	15 (10–22)	<0.001
Mean days to death ± SD	5.4±6.8	5.4±5.7	0.955
Median days to death (IQR)	3 (1–17)	4 (1–12)	0.553
PERSEVERE-based mortality probability, mean (95% C.I.)	9.8 (7.9–11.7)	12.7 (10.6–14.8)	0.090
Maximum number of organ failures, median (IQR)	2 (1–3)	2 (2–3)	0.025
Gram-positive bacteria, N (%)	60 (25)	58 (23)	0.759
Number of vasoactive agents at the time of corticosteroid initiation, median (IQR)	–	2 (1–2)	–
Maximum number of simultaneous vasoactive agents during the first 7 days, median (IQR)	1 (1–2)	2 (1–3)	<0.001
Gram-negative bacteria, N (%)	45 (18)	58 (23)	0.252
Other organism, N (%)	19 (8)	25 (10)	0.525
Negative cultures, N (%)	120 (49)	111 (44)	0.291
Comorbidity, N (%)	70 (29)	105 (42)	0.003

Table 2. Association between corticosteroids and mortality.

Group	# of deaths	Subjects receiving ≥2 vasoactive medications # (%)	OR	95% C.I.	P value
All subjects (n = 496)	64	242 (49)	2.304	1.312–4.046	0.004
Low risk subjects (n = 323)	7	132 (41)	6.898	0.821–57.595	0.075
Intermediate risk subjects (n = 117)	27	66 (56)	1.371	0.563–3.343	0.487
High risk subjects (n = 56)	30	44 (79)	2.333	0.780–6.980	0.130

Children's Hospital, Nationwide Children's Hospital, Children's National Medical Center, Morgan Stanley Children's Hospital, Columbia University Medical Center, Miami Children's Hospital, Texas Children's Hospital, CS Mott Children's Hospital at the University of Michigan, Children's Hospital and Clinics of Minnesota, and The Children's Hospital of Philadelphia.

Study and Data Collection

The patient cohort (n = 496) was derived from an ongoing multicenter pediatric septic shock database, which has been previously described in detail [23–25]. Briefly, children admitted to the PICU meeting pediatric-specific criteria for septic shock were eligible for enrollment [26]. After informed consent from parents or legal guardians, blood samples were obtained as close to the time of meeting criteria for septic shock as possible (<24 hours). Clinical and laboratory data were collected through the first seven days of PICU admission. Mortality was tracked for 28 days after enrollment and organ failure was defined using pediatric-specific criteria [26]. Any neonates (subjects less than 28 days of age) included in the study were full term and admitted to the PICU with septic shock following discharge to home after birth. Subjects were enrolled between May 2002 and May 2013.

Patient Classification and Stratification

We surveyed the medication fields of the clinical database to determine if the study subjects received systemic corticosteroids. Subjects receiving any formulation of systemic corticosteroids during the first 7 days of meeting criteria for septic shock were classified in the corticosteroid group. The one exception was subjects who received dexamethasone for less than 48 hours for airway edema. These patients were classified in the no corticosteroid group (13 subjects). All other subjects were classified in the no corticosteroid group. We were unable to consistently determine dosages or the clinical indications for corticosteroids in all subjects.

The blood sample was used to stratify subjects into mortality risk strata using PERSEVERE [18,19]. Based on a histogram showing three main bins, we stratified subjects into low, intermediate, or high risk categories. The "low risk" population was defined as those subjects with a mortality probability ≤2.5%. The "inter-

mediate risk" group was defined as those subjects with a mortality probability >2.5% up to and including 26.7%. The "high risk" group was defined as subjects with a mortality probability > 26.7%. All subjects in this study were previously included in the derivation (n = 353) and validation (n = 114) of PERSEVERE.

In a sensitivity analysis, we included only the subjects without comorbidities as an indirect means of selecting only those subjects who received corticosteroids for the indication of refractory shock. In a secondary analysis, subjects were stratified based on the PRISM score tertiles for this cohort. The first tertile contained subjects with PRISM scores ≤10, the second tertile contained subjects with PRISM scores from 11 through 17, and the third tertile contain subjects with PRISM scores >17. We selected this approach to mirror the three PERSEVERE-based risk strata.

Data Analysis

Statistical analyses were conducted using SigmaStat Software (Systat Software, Inc., San Jose, CA). Initially, data are described using medians, interquartile ranges, frequencies, and percentages. Comparisons between study groups used the Mann-Whitney U-test, Chi-square, or Fisher's Exact tests, as appropriate.

The association between corticosteroids and outcome was modeled using logistic regression. First, we modeled the probability of all cause 28-day mortality. Second, we modeled the probability of a composite endpoint termed "complicated course", which is defined as either death within the 28-day study period, or persistence of two or more new organ failures at 7 days after meeting criteria for septic shock, as previously described [20,22,27]. Complicated course is not a validated endpoint, but is intended to serve as a pragmatic clinical endpoint that captures both septic shock-related morbidity and mortality.

Results

Demographics and clinical characteristics

Among the subjects who received corticosteroids, 78% were prescribed hydrocortisone, 16% were prescribed methylprednisolone, and 6% were prescribed dexamethasone. The median duration of corticosteroid prescription was 5 days (maximum days

Table 3. Association between corticosteroids and complicated course (CC).

Group	# with CC	OR	95% C.I.	P value
All subjects (n = 496)	133	1.676	1.119–2.510	0.012
Low risk subjects (n = 323)	37	1.735	0.865–3.482	0.121
Intermediate risk subjects (n = 117)	54	1.000	0.481–2.078	1.000
High risk subjects (n = 56)	42	2.667	0.773–9.194	0.120

Table 4. Clinical and demographic data for the study subjects without comorbidities.

	No Corticosteroids (n = 174)	Corticosteroids (n = 147)	P value
Age in years, median (IQR)	2.4 (0.6–6)	2.2 (1.0–5.5)	0.952
Males, N (%)	92 (52.9)	83 (56.5)	0.595
Deaths, N (%)	14 (8)	27 (18.4)	0.010
Complicated course, N (%)	37 (21.2)	51 (34.7)	0.010
PRISM score, median (IQR)	11 (7–17.3)	16 (11–22)	<0.001
Mean days to death ± SD	5.9±7.7	4.7±4.9	0.540
Median days to death (IQR)	3 (1–6)	3 (2–6)	0.759
PERSEVERE-based mortality probability, mean (95% C.I.)	11.2% (8.7–13.7)	14.8% (11.7–17.9)	0.191
Maximum number of organ failures, median (IQR)	2 (1–3)	2 (2–3)	0.020
Number of vasoactive agents at the time of corticosteroid initiation, median (IQR)	–	2 (1–3)	–
Maximum number of simultaneous vasoactive agents during the first 7 days, median (IQR)	1 (1–2)	2 (1–3)	<0.001
Gram-positive bacteria, N (%)	44 (25.3)	36 (24.7)	1.000
Gram-negative bacteria, N (%)	24 (13.8)	29 (19.9)	0.192
Other organism, N (%)	10 (5.7)	16 (11)	0.135
Negative cultures, N (%)	95 (54.6)	66 (45.2)	0.118

recorded = 7, interquartile range [IQR], 3–7). The median day of septic shock at which corticosteroids were initially prescribed was day 1 (IQR, 1–1).

Table 1 describes the demographic and clinical characteristics of subjects who received corticosteroids (n = 252) and subjects who did not receive corticosteroids (n = 244). Subjects who received corticosteroids had higher rates of complicated course and mortality, a higher median PRISM score, a higher median number of organ failures, and a greater requirement for vasoactive medications, when compared to subjects who did not receive corticosteroids. A greater proportion of subjects who received corticosteroids had a comorbidity (Table S1). PERSEVERE-based mortality risk did not differ between the two groups. No other differences were noted.

Association between corticosteroids and mortality

Table 2 shows the association between corticosteroids and mortality. In the overall cohort, there were 64 deaths (13%) and the use of corticosteroids was associated with an increased risk of death (OR 2.3, 95% CI 1.3–4.0, p = 0.004). Within each risk stratum, there was no association between the use of corticosteroids and mortality.

Association between corticosteroids and complicated course

Table 3 shows the association between corticosteroids and a complicated course. Overall, there were 133 (27%) subjects with a complicated course and the use of corticosteroids was associated with an increased risk of a complicated course (OR 1.7, 95% CI 1.1–2.5, p = 0.012). When stratified into the three PERSEVERE-based mortality risk strata, there was no association between the use of corticosteroids and the risk for a complicated course.

Analysis of subjects without comorbidities

Since we were unable to consistently determine the clinical indications for corticosteroids in all subjects, we conducted a sensitivity analysis limiting the dataset to patients without comorbidities (n = 321). We reasoned that the majority of these subjects were administered corticosteroids for the indication of refractory shock.

Table 5. Association between corticosteroids and mortality in subjects without comorbidities.

Group	# of deaths	Subjects Receiving ≥2 vasoactive medications # (%)	OR	95% C.I.	P value
All subjects (n = 321)	41	162 (50)	2.571	1.293–5.114	0.007
Low risk subjects (n = 202)[1]	1	85 (42)	–	–	–
Intermediate risk subjects (n = 71)	14	40 (56)	1.707	0.524–5.558	0.375
High risk subjects (n = 48)	26	37 (77)	2.700	0.828–8.807	0.100

[1]The number of deaths is too small to estimate the odds ratio.

Table 6. Association between corticosteroids and complicated course (CC) in subjects without comorbidities.

Group	# with CC	OR	95% C.I.	P value
All subjects (n = 321)	88	1.967	1.196–3.234	0.008
Low risk subjects (n = 202)	21	2.404	0.949–6.090	0.064
Intermediate risk subjects (n = 71)	30	1.013	0.394–2.604	0.978
High risk subjects (n = 48)	37	3.231	0.795–13.123	0.101

Among the subjects without comorbidities who received steroids, 79% were prescribed hydrocortisone, whereas 15% were prescribed methylprednisolone, and 6% were prescribed dexamethasone. The median duration of steroid prescription was 4 days (maximum days recorded = 7, IQR, 3–7). The median day of septic shock at which corticosteroids were initially prescribed was day 1 (IQR, 1–1).

Table 4 describes subjects without comorbidities grouped by whether or not they received corticosteroids. Subjects who received corticosteroids had higher rates of complicated course and mortality, higher PRISM scores, higher median number of organ failures, and a greater requirement for vasoactive medications, compared to subjects who did not receive corticosteroids. PERSEVERE-based mortality risk did not differ between the two groups. No other differences were noted.

Table 5 shows the association between corticosteroids and mortality in the subjects without comorbidities. There were 41 deaths (13%) and the use of corticosteroids was associated with an overall increased risk of death (OR 2.6, 95% CI 1.3–5.1, p = 0.007). Within mortality risk strata, no benefit of corticosteroids was observed.

Table 6 shows the associations between corticosteroid use and complicated course among subjects without comorbidities. Within this population, there were 88 subjects (27%) with a complicated course and the use of corticosteroids was associated with an increased risk of a complicated course (OR 2.0, 95% CI 1.2–3.2, p = 0.008). When stratified into the three PERSEVERE-based mortality risk strata, there was no association between corticosteroid use and complicated course.

Association between corticosteroids and outcomes using PRISM-based stratification

Because PRISM scores are more familiar to the critical care medicine field than PERSEVERE, we conducted a secondary regression analysis using subjects grouped into low, medium, and high risk based on PRISM score tertiles. For all subjects, higher PRISM scores were associated with increased risk of mortality (OR 1.09, 95% CI 1.07–1.12, p<0.001) and complicated course (OR 1.08, 95% CI 1.06–1.11, p<0.001). Table 7 shows the association between corticosteroids and mortality within each

PRISM-based stratum. There was no association between the use of corticosteroids and mortality within each risk stratum. Similarly, Table 8 shows the association between corticosteroids and a complicated course within each risk stratum. There was no association between the use of corticosteroids and a complicated course within each risk stratum.

Discussion

We examined the association between corticosteroid administration and outcomes in a large, heterogeneous cohort of children with septic shock from multiple institutions across the United States. When including all subjects regardless of initial mortality risk, corticosteroids were associated with poorer outcomes. We note that subjects who received corticosteroids had greater illness severity as measured by PRISM score, mortality, organ failure burden, and requirement for vasoactive medications. Thus, the finding that corticosteroids were associated with poorer outcomes in the overall cohort is likely confounded by illness severity.

To account for this important confounder, we stratified the subjects into three mortality risk strata using PERSEVERE. Within each mortality risk strata, we observed no benefits associated with corticosteroid use. These findings are consistent with previous studies showing no outcome benefit associated with corticosteroid administration in children with septic shock [12–14].

Menon et al. conducted a meta-analysis of 447 selected cases and found no survival benefit associated with corticosteroids in children with septic shock [12]. Markovitz et al. studied over 6,000 subjects using the Pediatric Health Information System administrative database and reported that corticosteroids were associated with increased mortality, although they were not able to account for illness severity [13]. Zimmerman et al. analyzed the results of the largest interventional clinical trial in pediatric sepsis and found that corticosteroids were not associated with improved outcomes [14]. The subjects in the study by Zimmerman et al. had similar PRISM scores and organ failure burden in the two treatment groups, but the study did not explicitly stratify for initial mortality risk as done here.

Table 7. Association between corticosteroids and mortality based on PRISM tertiles.

PRISM Tertile	# of deaths	Subjects receiving ≥2 vasoactive medications # (%)	OR	95% C.I.	P value
1st (n = 172)	7	61 (35)	4.048	0.762–21.494	0.101
2nd (n = 169)	13	89 (53)	1.651	0.477–5.710	0.428
3rd (n = 155)	44	92 (59)	1.633	0.781–3.412	0.192

Table 8. Association between corticosteroids and complicated course (CC) based on PRISM tertiles.

PRISM Tertile	# with CC	OR	95% C.I.	P value
1st (n = 172)	20	2.571	0.991–6.671	0.052
2nd (n = 169)	41	0.901	0.444–1.825	0.771
3rd (n = 155)	72	1.355	0.709–2.590	0.358

An important limitation of this retrospective study is that the indication for corticosteroids was not standardized across the study subjects, nor was the general clinical care for sepsis. Corticosteroid administration was at the discretion of the attending physician, therefore some corticosteroid administration might have been for indications other than septic shock. We note, however, that 78% of the overall cohort was prescribed hydrocortisone and the median day of hydrocortisone administration was "day 1" of meeting criteria for septic shock. In addition, subjects who received corticosteroids had a greater requirement for vasoactive medications. These observations are consistent with the Surviving Sepsis Campaign recommendations for adjunctive corticosteroid administration in patients with septic shock. To further account for this confounder, we conducted a sensitivity analysis that excluded subjects with comorbidities. By limiting subjects to those without comorbidities, we hoped to exclude subjects who received corticosteroids for chronic diseases and indications other than septic shock. Similar to the overall cohort, the subjects who received corticosteroids in this cohort with no comorbidity had greater illness severity and the use of corticosteroids was associated with worse outcomes overall. When this cohort with no comorbidity was stratified by initial mortality risk using PERSEVERE, there was no benefit associated with corticosteroid use in any risk stratum. The same pattern was observed using the more familiar PRISM score to stratify patients: we found no survival benefit associated with the use of corticosteroids in any PRISM-based risk stratum.

The timing of corticosteroids was not standardized for patients included in this analysis. This may be important because a recent, small study suggests that administration of corticosteroids within nine hours of vasopressor initiation leads to improved outcomes [28]. Conversely, a much larger study by Casserly et al. showed that adjunctive corticosteroids are associated with increased adjusted hospital mortality even when prescribed within eight hours of vasopressor initiation [3]. It is unclear, then, how variable timing of corticosteroids might have influenced our findings.

Another limitation of our study is that we could not determine whether patients were diagnosed with relative adrenal insufficiency. It has been suggested that patients with relative adrenal insufficiency may benefit the most from corticosteroid administration [1]. While relative adrenal insufficiency has been shown to exist in critically ill children depending on the definition used, there is little data on the association between corticosteroids and pediatric outcomes in the context of relative adrenal insufficiency [29]. Therefore, relative adrenal insufficiency may remain a confounder in our study and should be incorporated in future studies. Finally, the retrospective design of our study makes it impossible to determine whether associations between corticosteroid use and poorer outcomes in the overall cohort are causal or simply associated with initial mortality risk. To explore this relationship further, a randomized controlled trial using mortality risk-stratification at study entry is warranted.

In conclusion, risk stratified analysis failed to demonstrate any benefit from corticosteroids in this pediatric septic shock cohort. Thus, apart from children receiving chronic steroids and children with "classic" adrenal insufficiency, the accumulating evidence does not support the routine use of corticosteroids in children with septic shock in the absence of a randomized trial.

Author Contributions

Conceived and designed the experiments: SJA CJL HRW. Performed the experiments: SJA SB EB K. Howard EF K. Harmon PL CJL HRW. Analyzed the data: SJA CJL HRW. Contributed reagents/materials/analysis tools: NZC NJT GLA NA MTB MH RJF AS KM PAC TPS JN MQ SLW. Contributed to the writing of the manuscript: SJA CJL HRW.

References

1. Annane D (2011) Corticosteroids for severe sepsis: an evidence-based guide for physicians. Ann Intensive Care 1: 7.
2. Annane D, Sebille V, Charpentier C, Bollaert PE, Francois B, et al. (2002) Effect of treatment with low doses of hydrocortisone and fludrocortisone on mortality in patients with septic shock. JAMA 288: 862–871.
3. Casserly B, Gerlach H, Phillips GS, Lemeshow S, Marshall JC, et al. (2012) Low-dose steroids in adult septic shock: results of the Surviving Sepsis Campaign. Intensive Care Med 38: 1946–1954.
4. Patel GP, Balk RA (2012) Systemic steroids in severe sepsis and septic shock. Am J Respir Crit Care Med 185: 133–139.
5. Sprung CL, Annane D, Keh D, Moreno R, Singer M, et al. (2008) Hydrocortisone therapy for patients with septic shock. N Engl J Med 358: 111–124.
6. Hanna W, Wong HR (2013) Pediatric sepsis: challenges and adjunctive therapies. Crit Care Clin 29: 203–222.
7. Dellinger RP, Levy MM, Rhodes A, Annane D, Gerlach H, et al. (2013) Surviving sepsis campaign: international guidelines for management of severe sepsis and septic shock: 2012. Crit Care Med 41: 580–637.
8. Menon K, McNally JD, Choong K, Ward RE, Lawson ML, et al. (2013) A survey of stated physician practices and beliefs on the use of steroids in pediatric fluid and/or vasoactive infusion-dependent shock. Pediatr Crit Care Med 14: 462–466.
9. McIntyre LA, Hebert PC, Fergusson D, Cook DJ, Aziz A, et al. (2007) A survey of Canadian intensivists' resuscitation practices in early septic shock. Crit Care 11: R74.
10. Wong HR, Cvijanovich NZ, Allen GL, Thomas NJ, Freishtat RJ, et al. (2014) Corticosteroids are associated with repression of adaptive immunity gene programs in pediatric septic shock. Am J Respir Crit Care Med: 140320091249000.
11. Brierley J, Carcillo JA, Choong K, Cornell T, Decaen A, et al. (2009) Clinical practice parameters for hemodynamic support of pediatric and neonatal septic shock: 2007 update from the American College of Critical Care Medicine. Crit Care Med 37: 666–688.
12. Menon K, McNally D, Choong K, Sampson M (2013) A systematic review and meta-analysis on the effect of steroids in pediatric shock. Pediatr Crit Care Med 14: 474–480.

13. Markovitz BP, Goodman DM, Watson RS, Bertoch D, Zimmerman J (2005) A retrospective cohort study of prognostic factors associated with outcome in pediatric severe sepsis: what is the role of steroids? Pediatr Crit Care Med 6: 270–274.

14. Zimmerman JJ, Williams MD (2011) Adjunctive corticosteroid therapy in pediatric severe sepsis: observations from the RESOLVE study. Pediatr Crit Care Med 12: 2–8.

15. Dellinger RP, Levy MM, Rhodes A, Annane D, Gerlach H, et al. (2013) Surviving sepsis campaign: international guidelines for management of severe sepsis and septic shock: 2012. Crit Care Med 41: 580–637.

16. Funk D, Doucette S, Pisipati A, Dodek P, Marshall JC, et al. (2014) Low-Dose Corticosteroid Treatment in Septic Shock: A Propensity-Matching Study. Crit Care Med.

17. Kaplan JM, Wong HR (2011) Biomarker discovery and development in pediatric critical care medicine. Pediatr Crit Care Med 12: 165–173.

18. Wong HR, Salisbury S, Xiao Q, Cvijanovich NZ, Hall M, et al. (2012) The pediatric sepsis biomarker risk model. Crit Care 16: R174.

19. Wong HR, Weiss SL, Giuliano JS Jr, Wainwright MS, Cvijanovich NZ, et al. (2014) Testing the prognostic accuracy of the updated pediatric sepsis biomarker risk model. PLoS One 9: e86242.

20. Wong HR, Weiss SL, Giuliano JS Jr, Wainwright MS, Cvijanovich NZ, et al. (2014) The temporal version of the pediatric sepsis biomarker risk model. PLoS One 9: e92121.

21. Alder MN, Lindsell CJ, Wong HR (2014) The pediatric sepsis biomarker risk model: potential implications for sepsis therapy and biology. Expert Rev Anti Infect Ther.

22. Abulebda K, Cvijanovich NZ, Thomas NJ, Allen GL, Anas N, et al. (2014) Post-ICU admission fluid balance and pediatric septic shock outcomes: a risk-stratified analysis. Crit Care Med 42: 397–403.

23. Wong HR (2013) Genome-wide expression profiling in pediatric septic shock. Pediatr Res 73: 564–569.

24. Wong HR, Cvijanovich N, Wheeler DS, Bigham MT, Monaco M, et al. (2008) Interleukin-8 as a stratification tool for interventional trials involving pediatric septic shock. Am J Respir Crit Care Med 178: 276–282.

25. Wong HR, Shanley TP, Sakthivel B, Cvijanovich N, Lin R, et al. (2007) Genome-level expression profiles in pediatric septic shock indicate a role for altered zinc homeostasis in poor outcome. Physiol Genomics 30: 146–155.

26. Goldstein B, Giroir B, Randolph A, International Consensus Conference on Pediatric S (2005) International pediatric sepsis consensus conference: definitions for sepsis and organ dysfunction in pediatrics. Pediatr Crit Care Med 6: 2–8.

27. Mickiewicz B, Vogel HJ, Wong HR, Winston BW (2013) Metabolomics as a novel approach for early diagnosis of pediatric septic shock and its mortality. Am J Respir Crit Care Med 187: 967–976.

28. Katsenos CS, Antonopoulou AN, Apostolidou EN, Ioakeimidou A, Kalpakou GT, et al. (2014) Early administration of hydrocortisone replacement after the advent of septic shock: impact on survival and immune response. Crit Care Med 42: 1651–1657.

29. Menon K, Ward RE, Lawson ML, Gaboury I, Hutchison JS, et al. (2010) A prospective multicenter study of adrenal function in critically ill children. Am J Respir Crit Care Med 182: 246–251.

14

Impact of NGO Training and Support Intervention on Diarrhoea Management Practices in a Rural Community of Bangladesh: An Uncontrolled, Single-Arm Trial

Ahmed S. Rahman[1]*, Mohammad Rafiqul Islam[2], Tracey P. Koehlmoos[3], Mohammad Jyoti Raihan[1], Mohammad Mehedi Hasan[1], Tahmeed Ahmed[1], Charles P. Larson[4]

1 Centre for Nutrition and Food Security, International Centre for Diarrhoeal Diseases Research, Bangladesh (icddr,b), Dhaka, Bangladesh, 2 CCEB, School of Medicine and Public Health, University of Newcastle, Newcastle, Australia, 3 Department of Health Administration and Policy, College of Health and Human Services, George Mason University, Fairfax, Virginia, United States of America, 4 Department of Pediatrics, University of British Columbia and Centre for International Child Health, BC Children's Hospital, Vancouver, British Columbia, Canada

Abstract

Purpose/Objective: The evolving Non-Governmental Organization (NGO) sector in Bangladesh provides health services directly, however some NGOs indirectly provide services by working with unlicensed providers. The primary objective of this study was to examine the impact of NGO training of unlicensed providers on diarrhoea management and the scale up of zinc treatment in rural populations.

Methods: An uncontrolled, single-arm trial for a training and support intervention on diarrhoea outcomes was employed in a rural sub-district of Bangladesh during 2008. Two local NGOs and their catchment populations were chosen for the study. The intervention included training of unlicensed health care providers in the management of acute childhood diarrhoea, particularly emphasizing zinc treatment. In addition, community-based promotion of zinc treatment was carried out. Baseline and endline ecologic surveys were carried out in intervention and control villages to document changes in treatments received for diarrhoea in under-five children.

Results: Among surveyed household with an active or recent acute childhood diarrhoea episode, 69% sought help from a health provider. Among these, 62.8% visited an unlicensed private provider. At baseline, 23.9% vs. 22% of control and intervention group children with diarrhoea had received zinc of any type. At endline (6 months later) this had changed to 15.3% vs. 30.2%, respectively. The change in zinc coverage was significantly higher in the intervention villages (p<0.01). Adherence with giving zinc for 10 days or more was significantly higher in the intervention households (9.2% vs. 2.5%; p<0.01). Child's age, duration of diarrhoea, type of diarrhoea, parental year of schooling as well as oral rehydration solution (ORS) and antibiotic usage were significant predictors of zinc usage.

Conclusion: Training of unlicensed healthcare providers through NGOs increased zinc coverage in the diarrhoea management of under-five children in rural Bangladesh households.

Trial Registration: ClinicalTrials.gov NCT02143921

Editor: Susanna Esposito, Fondazione IRCCS Ca' Granda Ospedale Maggiore Policlinico, Università degli Studi di Milano, Italy

Funding: This study was funded by a grant from the Bill & Melinda Gates Foundation (contract # HRN-AA-00-98-00047-00.) The funders had no role in study design, data collection and analysis, decision to publish, or preparation of the manuscript.

Competing Interests: The authors have declared that no competing interests exist.

* Email: ashafiq@icddrb.org

Introduction

Even a decade after into the 21st century and the proven efficacy of oral rehydration salts and zinc therapy, diarrhoea still remains the second leading cause of mortality among under-five children globally [1–4]. It has been estimated that diarrhoea has accounted for about 800,000 out of the total 7.6 million under-five child death globally with the highest contribution from the developing countries [5]. The comparison of 69,000 child death attributed to diarrhoea in Bangladesh in a year [6] to the US child mortality of 300 [7], portrays the ravaging effect of diarrhoea in developing countries. A recent estimate has shown that diarrhoea is responsible for 22% of all under-five child deaths in Africa and 23% in South Asia [6]. Therefore, 'one out of every nine under-5 child death is due to diarrhoea', is a statement bold enough to illustrate the impact of diarrhoea on child mortality. Despite the huge burden of diarrhoea among under-five children, most do not receive appropriate treatment [8]. WHO diarrhoeal management guidelines include treating patients with hypo-osmolar oral rehydrating salt (ORS) and zinc along with recommendation to avoid unnecessary use of pharmacological agents. Continued feeding has also been suggested [9]. Meta-analyses of several randomized controlled trials have confirmed the preventive and prophylactic effects of zinc on diarrhoeal episodes among under-five children [10–12], which complements the WHO guidelines on zinc usage for diarrhoea. It has been estimated that globally, the successful scaling up of zinc treatment for childhood diarrhoea could potentially save 400,000 under-five deaths per year [13]. Antibiotics, on other hand, is indicated in certain types of diarrhoea such as confirmed or suspected cholera, invasive diarrhoea caused by Shigella and E coli. and dysentery induced by other organisms such as Campylobacter spp. [14]. The European Society for Paediatric Gastroenterology, Hepatology and Nutrition (ESPGHAN) has suggested nine components for good diarrhoeal management, which includes, use of oral rehydration solution, use of hypotonic solution (Na 60 mmol/L, glucose 74–111 mmol/L), fast oral rehydration over of the period of 3 to 4 hours followed by normal feeding, avoid using special formula unless justified, avoid using diluted formula unless justified, continued breastfeeding all the time, supplementation with oral rehydration solution and avoid using unnecessary medication [15]. The guideline also stated that more than 8 episodes/day with substantial stool volumes, persistent vomiting, severe underlying disease and age less than 2 months as indications for medical visits for diarrhoeal patients, whereas, telephone consultation is recommended for uncomplicated diarrhoea. As for hospitalization criteria, ESPGHAN recommended the presence of at least one of the following abnormality/condition: shock, severe dehydration (>9% body weight), any neurological abnormalities, intractable or bilious vomiting, ORS treatment failure, failure of caregivers to provide adequate care at home and/or concerns on social/logistic scenario and suspected surgical condition [16]. It is needed to be pointed out that ESPGHAN recommendation for diarrhoeal management does not include zinc therapy, indicating the European population, specifically children may not be zinc deficient like that of many developing nations such as Bangladesh [17]. Bangladesh also do not have a national guideline for child diarrhoeal management, similar to most developing countries. Most hospitals have developed their own protocol which are adopted from WHO guidelines on diarrhoeal management and therefore includes ORS for rehydration, zinc therapy and careful using antibiotics. Additionally, like most of its poor neighbors, Bangladesh do not have a robust health system and telephone consultation as exists in more developed nation, is an usual practice for general practitioners or even visit to qualified doctors is not always possible due to many access barriers especially in lowest rural tier [18]. Under such drawbacks, it is crucial to train and integrate paramedical workforce such as NGO workers in current health system to increase ORS and zinc therapy coverage in the country and provide effective management of diarrhoea to the rural population.

In Bangladesh, following the launch of the national zinc scale-up campaign in late 2006, repeat impact surveys were carried out in order to monitor diarrhoea management practices especially ORS and zinc usage in under-five children [19]. Before the initiation of the mass media campaign, caretakers' awareness of zinc as a treatment for childhood diarrhoea was under 5% in rural areas, however, increased to 55% by 12 months and 75% by 24 months [20]. On the other hand, zinc usage (any amount) as a treatment of childhood diarrhoea increased from under 5% to 13% during the same time period in rural areas.

Being a low income country, Bangladesh, since its independence in 1971, has been observed to have a pluralistic health system with a large segment of rural population still inclined to seek care from informal health sector providers such as traditional healers, pharmacists and 'village doctors' [21–23]. The fragmented health system also relies heavily on the several hundred or so local and national NGOs who have been playing a significant role in the health sector since the independence of the nation [24]. Under the latest national health, population and nutrition development program strategy of Bangladesh, which follows a sector-wide approach, the role of NGOs are recognized as more pivotal than ever, with increased Government-NGO collaboration [25]. Within the NGO sector, health services is directly provided in the community; however some NGOs also work closely with private sector unlicensed providers who are the preferred source of care seeking in rural communities in Bangladesh for childhood diarrhoea [26]. Involvements of NGOs working through networking with unlicensed providers are therefore a potentially important strategy to be included in the effort to bring zinc treatment of childhood diarrhoea to scale in Bangladesh.

The primary objective of the study was to determine whether a training intervention given to unlicensed health service providers by NGO providers' increases zinc coverage as an adjunct to ORS for the management of childhood diarrhoea in rural communities of Bangladesh.

Materials and Methods

Design and site

The protocol for this trial and supporting CONSORT checklist are available as supporting information; see Checklist S1 and Protocol S1. This uncontrolled, single-arm trial for a training and support intervention on diarrhoea outcomes was employed in a rural sub-district of Bangladesh during 2008. The study was conducted in Sreepur sub-district under Gazipur district of Bangladesh.

Two local NGOs with long working experience on providing health services in the chosen community were selected along with their catchment areas for the purpose of this study. The intervention area included 53 villages having a population of ~95,000 against 49 villages in the control area with a population of ~76,000. The curative health services in these sites were provided by unlicensed (local drug vendors, village practitioners, traditional healers), and licensed government, private or NGO health service providers. A cluster sampling design was employed and the required number of clusters (villages) was randomly selected from the total listed villages in both the intervention and control areas using a random number generating software/calculator. Baseline data was collected during February 2008 and endline data in August 2008.

The study evaluated the effect of intervention primarily on zinc coverage and secondarily on ORS and antibiotic use in childhood diarrhoea through community surveys. The study design was such that the participants (mothers/caretakers) were not aware of the intervention and hence was blinded. A baseline survey was conducted in the intervention and control villages concomitantly with the training of the health service providers in the intervention area and an endline survey around six months following the training. We have hypothesized that greater increased change in zinc coverage for diarrhoea management would be observed in the intervention when compared to control villages six months following the training.

Intervention. The intervention included orientation and training of the unlicensed health care providers (village doctors, drug vendors and traditional healers) regarding zinc treatment in childhood diarrhoea through NGO health care providers. In addition, the NGO conducted community-based promotion of zinc treatment in the intervention villages.

A package of training materials custom designed for the scale up of zinc for young children plus ORS was delivered using a training of the trainers' strategy. The package is described in Table 1.

After the initial training to NGO service providers in the intervention areas, subsequent training was delivered by the NGOs done through quarterly meetings and follow-up sessions with village practitioners throughout the intervention areas. This work was conducted by Sub-Assistant Medical Officers (SAC-MOs). In intervention villages there are at least four SACMOs who have training experience with village practitioners.

Ethical approval

The study was reviewed and approved by the Research Review and Ethical Review Committees of the International Centre for Diarrhoeal Diseases Research, Bangladesh (icddr,b). Informed written consent was obtained in a prescribed form from the caretakers of the enrolled children. The Trial Registration number for this protocol is NCT02143921. It is to be mentioned that due to procedural and institutional reasons, we were only able to register the trial after completing the study.

Sample size estimation

To detect a minimum 50% increase in zinc coverage for childhood diarrhoea in the intervention area with a level of confidence of 0.95, a power of 0.9 and assuming a 1.5 design effect adjustment for clustering, it was estimated 580 cases of childhood diarrhoea per group would be required.

We have randomly selected 28 out of 49 villages from the control NGO's catchment area and 28 out of 53 villages in the intervention NGO's catchment area to meet the sample size requirement during the baseline survey, whereas; 26 and 29 villages respectively were again randomly selected during the endline survey.

Sampling. Baseline and endline data has been collected from all households from the selected villages in both control and intervention areas. Within each village, a central starting point was chosen and door-to-door survey technique of households was implemented for screening and recruiting children with a current or recent episode of diarrhoea (lasting for ≥ 2 days) within two weeks prior to the survey. Thus, information from all children with diarrhoea in the selected clusters was recorded. However, if more than one child in the household was eligible, one was randomly chosen. The respondents of the survey were the mothers or other caretakers of the identified children of the selected households.

Statistics

Data were entered and verified using SPSS version 10.5 and converted to Stata version 11.5 for all analyses. Data were checked for missing values and recoded to generate new categorical variables using cut-off values. The analyses carried out were both stratified by time of the survey (baseline and endline) and location of residence (intervention and control) and without any stratification. To assess differences in categorical outcomes, chi-square statistical comparisons of proportions with 95% confidence intervals, were calculated. Of particular interest was the identification of disparities in the use of zinc, ORS and antibiotic by area. Age of child, gender, type of diarrhoea, duration of diarrhoea, age of mother, parental year of schooling, parental occupation, type of toilet facility and weekly expenditure on food (own production/ purchase) as proxy indicator of financial status were included in the bivariate analysis in order to identify significant predictors of zinc and antibiotic usage. Variables that were significant ($p < 0.05$) in bivariate analyses were included in the multiple logistic regression analyses after controlling for area and time in order to assess independent association of the variables with zinc and antibiotic usage. All the analyses were done by taking cluster effect into account using '*svy*' command in Stata.

Results

The survey result shows that at baseline, data of 630 and 612 children were collected from the control and intervention areas with current or recent episode of diarrhoea, whereas; at endline the figure was 650 and 612 children respectively. The trial flow chart is shown in Figure 1. Among the total cases (n = 2504), the most prevalent type of diarrhoea was 'predominantly mucoid' (63.7%) whereas 20.6% cases were 'watery/loose' and 15.7% cases had predominantly bloody diarrhoea. Among all cases, 71% children received ORS during diarrhoeal illness.

Table 1. Training Package for health care providers in the intervention area.

For licensed providers
• Refresher course and up-date on WHO/UNICEF guidelines for treatment of childhood diarrhea
• Training videos (docu-drama)
• Orientation/training materials (zinc babohar nirdeshika)
• Frequently asked questions booklet
• Follow-up support
For unlicensed community health care providers
• Orientation/training materials (flip chart)
• Training videos (docu-drama)
• Zinc commercial (mass media campaign)
• Refresher training and up-date on WHO/UNICEF guidelines for treatment of childhood diarrhea
• Frequently asked questions booklet
• Follow-up support

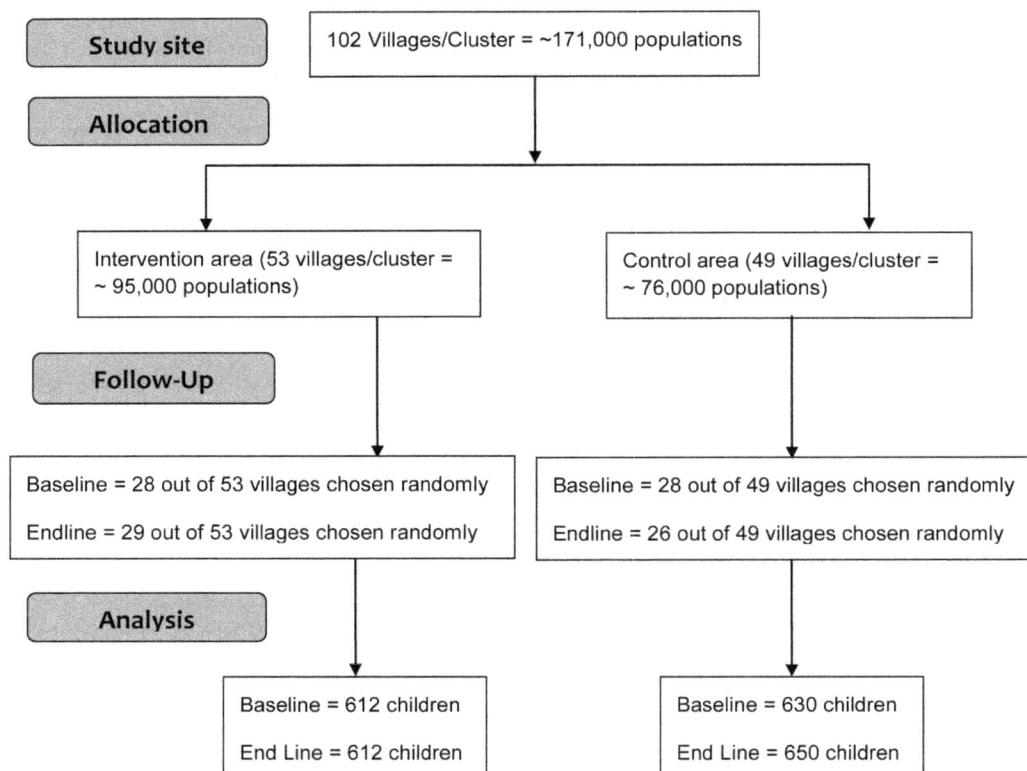

Figure 1. Trial Flowchart.

Descriptive statistics of selected socio-demographic characteristics of households are presented in Table 2. No significant differences were found between control and intervention areas at baseline and endline in terms of age and sex of the study children, age of the mothers and type of toilet facility used by the household. Overall, irrespective of study area and time of the survey, 31% of the children did not seek treatment for diarrhoeal illness from any health service providers (Figure 2). Among the children who did seek treatment from service providers, most of them received treatment from unlicensed (e.g. village doctor, drug vendor, and traditional healers) private providers (68.7%). Almost 16% received treatment from licensed (MBBS) private providers whereas, only 1.6% and 2.1% went to NGO and government facilities respectively to receive treatment for their illness.

Table 3 presents the usage of ORS, zinc and antibiotic usage among children in the control and intervention areas. Compared to control area, ORS usage was significantly higher in the intervention area after 6 months of intervention (65.1 vs. 72.2%, p<0.01). Similarly, there was a significant difference in zinc usage between control and intervention areas (15.3% vs. 30.2%; p< 0.01). After 6 months of intervention, the recommended usage of zinc for 10 days or more in under-5 diarrhoea was significantly higher among children in the intervention area compared to the control area (9.2% vs. 2.5%, p<0.01). Compared to the baseline prevalence, antibiotic usage increased more in the intervention area compared to control area at the endline.

Table 4 depicts the results of multiple logistic regression analyses exploring the relationship of potential factors with zinc usage. The older children aged 25–59 months were less likely to use zinc during diarrhoeal illness compared to younger children aged 6–12 months. On the other hand, children with a higher duration (4 to 10+ days) of diarrhoeal illness were more likely to use zinc compared to children with lower duration of illness (1–3 days). The other significant predictors of zinc usage were type of diarrhoea, parental year of schooling as well as ORS and antibiotic usage whereas, age of mother, mother occupation, sex of child, father occupation, type of toilet facility and weekly expenditure on food were insignificant to predict zinc usage.

The results of multiple logistic regression analyses showing significant predictors of antibiotic usage are presented in Table 5. The children aged over 12 months were less likely to use antibiotic during diarrhoeal illness compared to younger children aged 6–12 months. However, children were more likely to use antibiotic who suffered predominately from bloody diarrhoea compared to watery/loose diarrhoea as well as with duration of diarrhoea for 4–9 days compared to 1–3 days. The other significant predictors of antibiotic usage were father's year of schooling, ORS usage and zinc usage.

Discussion

A simple training intervention to unlicensed private providers on diarrhoeal management by local NGOs had significantly increased zinc usage in a rural community compared to nonintervened control area. The study was conducted in 2008 after launching in late 2006 of the national campaign to scale up zinc treatment of childhood diarrhoea in Bangladesh. Two years after the inauguration of zinc program, the national prevalence of zinc usage in under-5 children was 9–13% in rural areas [19]. While in this study, we found that after 6 months of training intervention and community sensitization, zinc usage was

Table 2. Socio-demographic characteristics of the Control and Intervention areas.*

Variable	Baseline		Endline	
	Control Total n = 630	Intervention Total n = 612	Control Total n = 650	Intervention Total n = 612
	%	%	%	%
Age of child in months				
6–12	27.0	23.4	21.2	19.8
13–24	29.1	31.3	25.7	27.3
25–36	18.7	23.2	20.8	18.8
37–59	25.2	22.1	32.3	34.1
Sex of child				
Male	54	52.1	52.9	55.6
Female	46	47.9	47.1	44.4
Age of mother in years				
≤20	15.6	18.6	17.5	20.1
21–25	36.4	40.7	37.1	40.0
26–30	28.1	24.2	28.8	24.8
31–49	19.8	16.2	16.5	14.9
Missing	0.1	0.3	0.1	0.2
Mother's year of schooling				
No education	20.5	13.4	26.8	21.1
1–4 years	18.3	15.7	16.6	12.4
5–9 years	53.3	60.5	47.7	58.8
10–11 years	4.9	5.7	6.2	6.1
> = 12 years	2.9	4.4	2.6	1.3
Missing	0.1	0.3	0.1	0.3
Father's year of schooling				
No education	32.1	24.2	35.7	33.0
1–4 years	14.4	11.2	13.5	11.6
5–9 years	36.0	46.8	33.5	38.9
10–11 years	8.4	8.7	8.9	9.3
> = 12 years	7.3	8.9	8.0	6.5
Don't Know	1.8	0.2	0.3	0.7
Type of toilet facility				
No facility	3.8	5.7	2.8	2.3
Unimproved	65.9	59.2	62.0	59.0
Improved	30.3	35.1	35.2	38.7
Weekly expenditure on food in BDT (Bangladesh Taka)				
< = 500	6.8	4.4	2.0	2.6
501–1000	56.7	46.9	44.2	43.5
1001–1500	25.7	31.5	39.2	34.3
> = 1501	10.8	17.2	14.6	19.6

*Cluster adjusted analyses of all variables.

increased to 30% in the intervention area from the baseline usage of 22% and in the non-intervention area it was reduced to 15% from the baseline usage of 24%. More importantly, the recommended 10 days zinc usage for diarrhoeal management was increased by 7% in the intervention area at the endline. As expected, we demonstrated a significant improvement in ORS usage following the NGO's training intervention to the unlicensed Health Care Providers.

Our finding clearly states the importance of training to the informal health care providers for overall zinc treatment and compliance to 10 days zinc treatment in addition to ORS for childhood diarrhoea management in the rural areas. Rural Bangladesh is facing a shortage of qualified physician (MBBS or above) over a long period of time and the shortage is less likely to be filled in near future [27]. Therefore, most people in the rural communities had to rely on privately owned local drug outlets where unlicensed health care providers such as drug sellers/

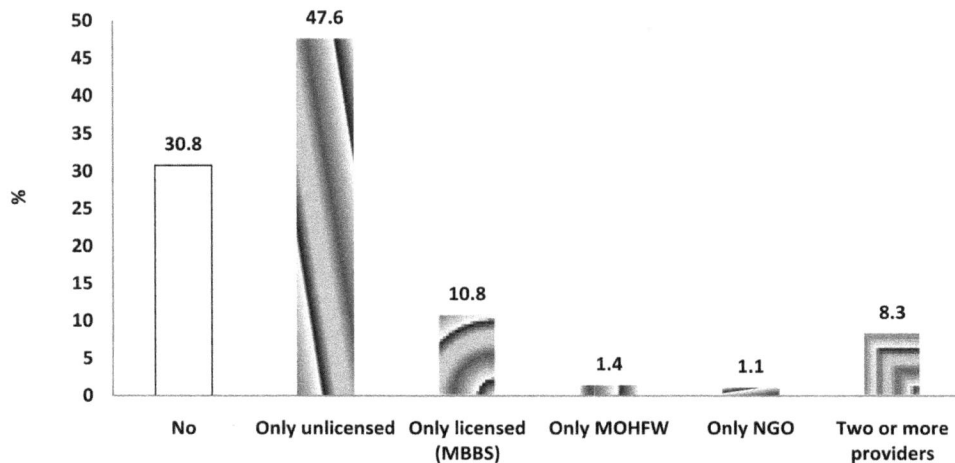

Figure 2. Health seeking behaviour during diarrhoeal illness among children 6–59 months by type of service providers.

vendors and village doctors are providing services. In 2006, Larson CP et al.; reported a dominance of private sector in providing health care delivery for diarrhoeal diseases both in urban and rural communities [26] while unlicensed health care providers remains the first point of privately delivering any health care services in most cases in the rural areas [27]. Training intervention to the unlicensed health care providers and community health workers for improving health is well acknowledged in many developing

countries including Bangladesh [28]. Successful training and involvement of these health cadres are now a national policy for tuberculosis control in Bangladesh [29,30].

It can be assumed that there is a difference in knowledge and awareness between unlicensed urban and rural health care providers as well as the urban and rural population. A previous study demonstrates a difference in awareness about zinc treatment for diarrhoeal diseases in children between urban and rural

Table 3. ORS, zinc and antibiotic usage in Control and Intervention areas.*

Variables	Baseline			Endline		
	Control % (95% CI)	Intervention % (95% CI)	p-value	Control % (95% CI)	Intervention % (95% CI)	p-value
ORS usage						
	n=630	n=612		n=650	n=612	
Yes	73.2 (69.1, 77.2)	74.4 (70.3, 78.3)	0.67	65.1 (61.2, 68.9)	72.2 (69, 75.4)	<0.01
Zinc usage of any duration (Tablet or Syrup)						
	n=594	n=608		n=636	n=609	
Yes	23.9 (19.2, 28.7)	22 (17.2, 26.9)	0.57	15.3 (13.1, 17.4)	30.2 (25.2, 35.3)	<0.01
Duration of zinc usage (Tablet or Syrup)						
	n=594	n=608		n=636	n=609	
No use	76.9 (72.2, 81.6)	78.5 (73.7, 83.3)	0.83	84.8 (82.6, 86.9)	69.8 (64.7, 74.8)	<0.01
1–3 day	8.8 (6.7, 10.9)	8.4 (5.7, 11.1)		6.6 (4.8, 8.5)	9.2 (7.1, 11.3)	
4–9 day	11.3 (8.4, 14.2)	9.7 (6.5, 12.9)		6.1 (4.3, 8)	11.8 (8.7, 15)	
≥10 day	3 (1.4, 4.7)	3.5 (1.7, 5.2)		2.5 (0.9, 4.2)	9.2 (6.9, 11.5)	
Duration of zinc usage (Tablet)						
	n=594	n=608		n=636	n=609	
No use	84.5 (80.2, 88.8)	83.9 (79.4, 88.3)	0.78	87.7 (85.6, 89.9)	76.4 (71.8, 80.9)	<0.01
1–3 day	5.7 (3.5, 7.9)	7.1 (4.2, 9.9)		6 (4.7, 7.3)	8.9 (6.7, 11)	
4–9 day	7.6 (4.7, 10.4)	6.6 (3.9, 9.2)		3.9 (2.5, 5.4)	6.9 (4.5, 9.3)	
≥10 day	2.2 (0.9, 3.5)	2.5 (1.2, 3.7)		2.4 (0.8, 3.9)	7.9 (5.4, 10.3)	
Antibiotic usage						
	n=623	n=611		n=639	n=606	
Yes	24.7 (20.5, 28.9)	23.6 (19.2, 27.9)	0.70	28.8 (26.2, 31.4)	36.3 (31.6, 41)	<0.01

*Cluster adjusted analyses of all variable.

Table 4. Predictors of zinc usage in childhood diarrhoea after controlling area and time variation.[*]

Variable[#]	OR (95% CI)	p-value
Age of child in months		
6–12	Reference	
13–24	1.13 (0.86, 1.48)	0.37
25–36	0.74 (0.55, 0.98)	0.04
37–60	0.39 (0.26, 0.59)	<0.01
Type of diarrhoea		
Watery/Loose	Reference	
Predominantly mucoid	0.0.6 (0.47, 0.78)	<0.01
Predominantly bloody	0.65 (0.48, 0.89)	<0.01
Duration of diarrhoea		
1–3 days	Reference	
4–9 days	1.89 (1.49, 2.4)	<0.01
>=10 days	3.76 (2.41, 5.88)	<0.01
Father's year of schooling		
No education	Reference	
1–4 years	0.93 (0.66, 1.3)	0.67
5–9 years	1.07 (0.82, 1.4)	0.62
10–11 years	1.71 (1.16, 2.53)	<0.01
>=12 years	1.03 (0.67, 1.58)	0.9
Mother's year of schooling		
No education	Reference	
1–4 years	1.11 (0.75, 1.66)	0.59
5–9 years	1.55 (1.1, 2.19)	0.01
10–11 years	2.1 (1.34, 3.29)	<0.01
>=12 years	3.36 (1.8, 6.26)	<0.01
ORS usage		
No	Reference	
Yes	5.83 (3.96, 8.61)	<0.01
Antibiotic usage		
No	Reference	
Yes	1.75 (1.35, 2.26)	<0.01

*All analyses were adjusted for cluster effect.
#Variables (age of child, type of diarrhoea, duration of diarrhoea, age of mother, Father's year of schooling, Mother's year of schooling, mother occupation, ORS usage and antibiotic usage) significant (p<0.05) in bivariate analysis (simple logistic regression) were used in multiple logistic regression analyses.

caregivers [20]. Since, the study area is very close to the capital city of the country therefore, it is more likely that the unlicensed health care providers in these areas are privileged for exchanging updated health related information including zinc treatment for diarrhoea in children. Also, the community dwellers are similarly privileged for receiving mass media and other sources of information compared to other rural, remote hard to reach areas. Despite, the above mentioned minor limitations, the findings can be generalized in context of Bangladesh. As the population in Bangladesh is rather homogenous in terms of culture and social characteristics, we do not expect too much variation in statistical findings if any other intervention areas are chosen. It is also to be notified that our study staff has confirmed no report of adverse effect occurred to any participants during the trial period due to the intervention.

We found 12.7% increment in antibiotic usage at endline in the intervention area vs. 4.1% increment in the control area compared

to the baseline usage (23.6% in intervention vs. 24.7% in control area). The rate of antibiotic use was not much different in comparison to national usage of antibiotic for diarrhoeal diseases which was 31 and 36% in female and male children respectively in the rural areas [26]. In this study, the use of antibiotic was higher among younger children and those who were suffering from bloody diarrhoea. However, rational use of antibiotic is indicated in bloody diarrhoea while the reason for higher use of antibiotic in younger children is unclear.

The training intervention repeatedly emphasized that zinc treatment is an adjunct therapy to ORS for the management of childhood diarrhoea. Given this, we observed an increased utilization of ORS in the intervention area (72%) than control area (65%). As illustrated before that the intervention and control areas are rural settings though very close to the capital city and ORS usage in both these areas were comparable to the overall

Table 5. Predictors of antibiotic usage in childhood diarrhoea after controlling area and time variation.[*]

Variable[#]	OR (95% CI)	p-value
Age of child in months		
6–12	Reference	
13–24	0.66 (0.48, 0.91)	0.01
25–36	0.69 (0.51, 0.93)	0.02
37–60	0.55 (0.37, 0.84)	<0.01
Type of diarrhoea		
Watery/Loose	Reference	
Predominantly mucoid	1.02 (0.79, 1.3)	0.9
Predominantly bloody	1.79 (1.33, 2.43)	<0.01
Duration of diarrhoea		
1–3 days	Reference	
4–9 days	1.92 (1.58, 2.33)	<0.01
>=10 days	2.78 (1.99, 3.87)	<0.01
Father's year of schooling		
No education	Reference	
1–4 years	1.04 (0.71, 1.51)	0.84
5–9 years	1.43 (1.07, 1.92)	0.02
10–11 years	1.83 (1.24, 2.72)	<0.01
>=12 years	1.62 (1.07, 2.47)	0.02
ORS usage		
No	Reference	
Yes	2.07 (1.64, 2.63)	<0.01
Zinc usage		
No	Reference	
Yes	1.75 (1.36, 2.27)	<0.01

*All analyses were adjusted for cluster effect.
#Variables (age of child, type of diarrhoea, duration of diarrhoea, age of mother, father education, mother education, mother occupation, ORS usage and antibiotic usage) significant (p<0.05) in bivariate analysis (simple logistic regression) were included in multiple logistic regression analyses.

national ORS usage during concurrent time period (52–68%) in rural areas of Bangladesh [19].

Overall, the training intervention to the unlicensed health care providers is very effective in terms of zinc treatment coverage and compliance to 10 days zinc treatment, increasing ORS usage. This training intervention, can be seen as capacity building for non-professionals, who would be able to provide diarrhoeal management for established cases, and for more complicated cases referral would be done to nearest Government Health Care facility, and hence would provide sufficient pace, if scaled-up, to the nation's target to reduce childhood diarrhoeal mortality and morbidity and to achieve Millennium Development Goal (MDG) 4. Nevertheless, training intervention should be critically emphasized on the rational use of antibiotic in diarrhoea in young children.

Conclusions

The study results shows that, a simple inexpensive training intervention for the unlicensed health care providers through NGO network increases the use of zinc for diarrhoea management. These efforts therefore need to continue with non-sector (Partnership of NGOs and Private Health Care Providers) provider for successful nationwide zinc scaling up.

Learning

This study will contribute to effort of scaling up zinc by employing an existing network of NGO providers in the training of unlicensed providers.

Acknowledgments

This research was funded by Bill and Melinda Gates Foundation (contract # HRN-AA-00-98-00047-00). icddr,b acknowledges with gratitude the commitment of Bill and Melinda Gates Foundation to its research efforts.

Author Contributions

Conceived and designed the experiments: CPL ASR TPK MRI. Performed the experiments: ASR MRI TPK. Analyzed the data: ASR MRI MJR MMH. Contributed reagents/materials/analysis tools: ASR MRI TPK. Wrote the paper: ASR MRI MJR TA TPK CPL MMH.

References

1. Walker CLF, Perin J, Aryee MJ, Boschi-Pinto C, Black RE (2012) Diarrhoea incidence in low-and middle-income countries in 1990 and 2010: a systematic review. BMC Public Health 12: 220.

2. Bajait C, Thawani V (2011) Role of zinc in pediatric diarrhoea. Indian journal of pharmacology 43: 232.

3. Walker CLF, Black RE (2010) Zinc for the treatment of diarrhoea: effect on diarrhoea morbidity, mortality and incidence of future episodes. International Journal of Epidemiology 39: i63–i69.

4. Wardlaw T, Salama P, Brocklehurst C, Chopra M, Mason E (2010) Diarrhoea: why children are still dying and what can be done. Lancet 375: 870–872.

5. Liu L, Johnson HL, Cousens S, Perin J, Scott S, et al. (2012) Global, regional, and national causes of child mortality: an updated systematic analysis for 2010 with time trends since 2000. The Lancet 379: 2151–2161.

6. Boschi-Pinto C, Velebit L, Shibuya K (2008) Estimating child mortality due to diarrhoea in developing countries. Bulletin of the World Health Organization 86: 710–717.

7. Farthing M, Lindberg G, Dite P (2010) World gastroenterology organisation practice guideline: acute diarrhoea. 2008. Available: http://www.worldgastro enterology. org/assets/downloads/en/pdf/guidelines/01_acute_diarrhoea. pdf. Accessed 29.

8. Ahs JW, Tao W, Löfgren J, Forsberg BC (2010) Diarrhoeal Diseases in Low- and Middle-Income Countries: Incidence, Prevention and Management. The Open Infectious Diseases Journal 4: 113–124.

9. WHO U (2004) WHO-UNICEF Joint statement on the clinical management of acute diarrhoea. World Health Assembly Geneva.

10. Bhutta Z, Black R, Brown K, Gardner JM, Gore S, et al. (1999) Prevention of diarrhoea and pneumonia by zinc supplementation in children in developing countries: pooled analysis of randomized controlled trials. The Journal of pediatrics 135: 689–697.

11. Bhutta ZA, Bird SM, Black RE, Brown KH, Gardner JM, et al. (2000) Therapeutic effects of oral zinc in acute and persistent diarrhoea in children in developing countries: pooled analysis of randomized controlled trials. The American journal of clinical nutrition 72: 1516–1522.

12. Lazzerini M, Ronfani L (2008) Oral zinc for treating diarrhoea in children. Cochrane Database Syst Rev 3.

13. Jones G, Steketee RW, Black RE, Bhutta ZA, Morris SS (2003) How many child deaths can we prevent this year? Lancet 362: 65–71.

14. Thapar N, Sanderson IR (2004) Diarrhoea in children: an interface between developing and developed countries. The Lancet 363: 641–653.

15. Szajewska H, Hoekstra JH, Sandhu B (2000) Management of acute gastroenteritis in Europe and the impact of the new recommendations: a multicenter study. Journal of Pediatric Gastroenterology and Nutrition 30: 522–527.

16. Guarino A, Albano F, Ashkenazi S, Gendrel D, Hoekstra JH, et al. (2008) European Society for Paediatric Gastroenterology, Hepatology, and Nutrition/

European Society for Paediatric Infectious Diseases evidence-based guidelines for the management of acute gastroenteritis in children in Europe: executive summary. Journal of pediatric gastroenterology and nutrition 46: 619–621.

17. Ahmed T, Mahfuz M, Ireen S, Ahmed AS, Rahman S, et al. (2012) Nutrition of children and women in Bangladesh: trends and directions for the future. Journal of health, population, and nutrition 30: 1.

18. Parkhurst JO, Rahman SA, Ssengooba F (2006) Overcoming access barriers for facility-based delivery in low-income settings: insights from Bangladesh and Uganda. Journal of health, population, and nutrition 24: 438.

19. Larson CP, Saha UR, Nazrul H (2009) Impact monitoring of the national scale up of zinc treatment for childhood diarrhoea in Bangladesh: repeat ecologic surveys. PLoS medicine 6: e1000175.

20. Larson CP, Koehlmoos TP, Sack DA (2012) Scaling up zinc treatment of childhood diarrhoea in Bangladesh: theoretical and practical considerations guiding the SUZY Project. Health policy and planning 27: 102–114.

21. Ahmed SM (2005) Exploring health-seeking behaviour of disadvantaged populations in rural Bangladesh: Institutionen för folkhälsovetenskap/Department of Public Health Sciences.

22. Ahmed SM, Evans TG, Standing H, Mahmud S (2013) Harnessing pluralism for better health in Bangladesh. The Lancet 382: 1746–1755.

23. Ahmed SM, Hossain MA, Chowdhury MR (2009) Informal sector providers in Bangladesh: how equipped are they to provide rational health care? Health Policy and Planning 24: 467–478.

24. Mercer A, Khan MH, Daulatuzzaman M, Reid J (2004) Effectiveness of an NGO primary health care programme in rural Bangladesh: evidence from the management information system. Health Policy and Planning 19: 187–198.

25. Ministry of Health and Family Welfare B (2011) Health, Population and Nutrition Sector Development Program (2011–2016) Program Implementation Plan. In: Welfare PWMoHaF, editor: Government of the People's Republic of Bangladesh.

26. Larson CP, Saha UR, Islam R, Roy N (2006) Childhood diarrhoea management practices in Bangladesh: private sector dominance and continued inequities in care. International Journal of Epidemiology 35: 1430–1439.

27. Mahmood SS, Iqbal M, Hanifi S, Wahed T, Bhuiya A (2010) Are 'Village Doctors' in Bangladesh a curse or a blessing? BMC international health and human rights 10: 18.

28. Oshiname FO, Brieger WR (1992) Primary care training for patent medicine vendors in rural Nigeria. Social science & medicine 35: 1477–1484.

29. Chowdhury AMR, Chowdhury S, Islam MN, Islam A, Vaughan JP (1997) Control of tuberculosis by community health workers in Bangladesh. The Lancet 350: 169–172.

30. Salim H, Uplekar M, Daru P, Aung M, Declercq E, et al. (2006) Turning liabilities into resources: informal village doctors and tuberculosis control in Bangladesh. Bulletin of the World Health Organization 84: 479–484.

15

Maternal Obesity Is Associated with Alterations in the Gut Microbiome in Toddlers

Jeffrey D. Galley[1], Michael Bailey[1,2]*, Claire Kamp Dush[3], Sarah Schoppe-Sullivan[3], Lisa M. Christian[2,4,5,6]

1 Division of Biosciences, College of Dentistry, Ohio State University, Columbus, Ohio, United States of America, 2 The Institute for Behavioral Medicine Research, The Ohio State University Wexner Medical Center, Columbus, Ohio, United States of America, 3 Department of Human Science, The Ohio State University, Columbus, Ohio, United States of America, 4 Department of Psychiatry, The Ohio State University Wexner Medical Center, Columbus, Ohio, United States of America, 5 Department of Obstetrics and Gynecology, The Ohio State University Wexner Medical Center, Columbus, Ohio, United States of America, 6 Psychology, The Ohio State University, Columbus, Ohio, United States of America

Abstract

Children born to obese mothers are at increased risk for obesity, but the mechanisms behind this association are not fully delineated. A novel possible pathway linking maternal and child weight is the transmission of obesogenic microbes from mother to child. The current study examined whether maternal obesity was associated with differences in the composition of the gut microbiome in children in early life. Fecal samples from children 18–27 months of age (n = 77) were analyzed by pyro-tag 16S sequencing. Significant effects of maternal obesity on the composition of the gut microbiome of offspring were observed among dyads of higher socioeconomic status (SES). In the higher SES group (n = 47), children of obese (BMI≥30) versus non-obese mothers clustered on a principle coordinate analysis (PCoA) and exhibited greater homogeneity in the composition of their gut microbiomes as well as greater alpha diversity as indicated by the Shannon Diversity Index, and measures of richness and evenness. Also in the higher SES group, children born to obese versus non-obese mothers had differences in abundances of *Faecalibacterium* spp., *Eubacterium* spp., *Oscillibacter* spp., and *Blautia* spp. Prior studies have linked some of these bacterial groups to differences in weight and diet. This study provides novel evidence that maternal obesity is associated with differences in the gut microbiome in children in early life, particularly among those of higher SES. Among obese adults, the relative contribution of genetic versus behavioral factors may differ based on SES. Consequently, the extent to which maternal obesity confers measureable changes to the gut microbiome of offspring may differ based on the etiology of maternal obesity. Continued research is needed to examine this question as well as the relevance of the observed differences in gut microbiome composition for weight trajectory over the life course.

Editor: Kartik Shankar, University of Arkansas for Medical Sciences, United States of America

Funding: This study was supported by an Innovative Initiative Award to MTB and LMC from the Food Innovation Center at The Ohio State University. This study was also supported by awards from NINR (R01NR01366) and NICHD (R21HD067670) to LMC, NCCAM (R01AT006552) to MTB and NIDCR (T32 DE014320). The content is solely the responsibility of the authors and does not necessarily represent the official views of the National Center for Research Resources or the National Institutes of Health. The sponsors did not participate in study design, data collection and analysis, decision to publish, or preparation of the manuscript.

Competing Interests: The authors have declared that no competing interests exist.

* Email: Michael.Bailey@osumc.edu

Introduction

Obesity is a substantial public health problem globally. In the US, it is estimated that 16.9% of children ages 2–19 years and 33.8% of adults ≥20 years are obese [1,2]. However, early life antecedents of obesity are not well delineated. In children under 3 years of age, the strongest predictor of obesity in adolescence and adulthood is parental obesity [3]. Compared to paternal obesity, maternal obesity has greater predictive value for body mass index (BMI) of offspring through adolescence [4,5]. However, the relative influence of genetics versus environmental pathways in the transgenerational transmission of obesity from parent to child is unknown.

A novel possible mechanistic pathway linking parental and child weight is the transmission of commensal microbiota via parental exposures, particularly maternal. The microbiota are a consortium of trillions of bacteria that are resident to a variety of human body niches [6]. The vast majority of these microbes reside within the gastrointestinal (GI) tract where they form microbial communities whose structures are stable during periods of homeostasis and heavily involved in host metabolic and nutritional functions, including food digestion and vitamin synthesis [7,8].

Disruptions in the relative abundances of microbes that comprise these communities have been associated with obesity and high-fat diets [9–14]. For example, obese mice have abnormal levels of GI *Firmicutes* and *Bacteroidetes*, two primary phyla of the GI tract microbiota [12]. Such skewed bacterial abundances may lead to alterations in energy procurement from food and related propensity toward obesity. When microbiota from obese mice are transferred into germ-free mice, recipient mice have increased body fat, providing strong evidence of a causal link between the microbiota and obesity [14].

Factors affecting the establishment of bacterial abundances in early life are not well understood. During birth, the neonate is rapidly colonized by maternal bacteria via vertical transmission from the gastrointestinal and reproductive tracts as well as environmental microbes [15–17]. In very early life, mothers are likely to be primary donors of bacteria through physical contact and breast milk. Demonstrating such maternal influence, at one and six months of age, infants of obese mothers have significantly different bacterial population abundances compared to infants of non-obese mothers [18]. Importantly, during the first year of life, the microbiota show great transience and volatility [19]. As solid foods are introduced to the diet, the structure of the microbiota stabilizes and begins to reflect the adult profile [20]. Thus, it is important to determine if maternal influences on gut microbial groups persist in children past early infancy despite competing factors.

In addition, the recent advent of next generation pyrosequencing allows for wider study of microbial communities than permitted by earlier methods, including denaturing gradient gel electrophoresis (DGGE) and polymerase chain reaction (PCR). Utilization of this technology permits the analyses of entire bacterial communities rather than examination of smaller classification subsets selected by a priori hypotheses. To our knowledge, pyrosequencing has not been used in studies associating parental obesity to child microbiota communities.

Addressing these gaps in the literature, the current study examined the association between maternal obesity and the gut microbiota profiles of toddlers at approximately two years of age using pyrosequencing technology. We hypothesized that the microbiota of children born to obese mothers would have a significantly different gastrointestinal microbiota, as assessed using alpha and beta diversity measurements, when compared to children born to normal weight mothers. We also hypothesized that differences in abundances of bacterial populations previously associated with obesity would be observed in children of obese versus non-obese mothers.

Methods

Study Design

We recruited 79 women with children approximately two years of age from the general community of Columbus, Ohio. Children were excluded if their mother reported the child had a major health condition or developmental delay. Children were also excluded if they were already toilet trained. Each woman completed an online questionnaire which included assessment of her health behaviors and exposures (e.g., medications) during pregnancy as well as health and feeding behaviors in her child.

Within 7 days of completing the online questionnaire, each woman collected a stool sample from her child per the protocol detailed below. Two samples were removed from statistical analyses due to low sequence count (<5108), resulting in final sample of 77 mother-child pairs. This study was approved by the Ohio State University Biomedical Institutional Review Board. All women completed written informed consent for themselves and provided written consent on behalf of their children. Women received modest compensation for their participation. Data collection occurred from May 2011 to December 2012.

Parental Characteristics

Women reported information about their age, race (self and child's father), marital status, education level (self and child's father), and total family income per year. Body mass index (BMI; kg/m^2) was calculated based on the provided maternal and paternal heights and weights. BMI values ≥ 30 were classified as obese.

Perinatal Health Information

Self-report data was collected regarding exposure to antibiotics during pregnancy and while breastfeeding (if applicable). With regard to birth outcomes, women reported the route of delivery (vaginal versus C-section), gestational age at the time of delivery and the child's sex.

Child Diet and Growth

Women reported the occurrence and duration of breastfeeding and the age at which formula (if applicable), cereals/grains, fruits/vegetables, and meats were introduced as part of the child's diet. The current frequency of each food type was also reported, from less than once per month to two or more times per day. Women reported the number of times their child had been exposed to antibiotic medications, with completion of a full prescription course (e.g., 10 days) considered as one exposure. Women also reported child exposure to probiotics in capsule/supplement form or in formula or food which specified it contained probiotics.

Finally, to determine the child's growth trajectory, women reported their child's height and weight percentile at the most recent well-visit to the pediatrician. A weight/height ratio was calculated and children were categorized into three groups: those whose weight percentile was greater than their height percentile (n = 11), those in the same percentile bracket (n = 31), and those whose weight percentile was lower than their height percentile (n = 33).

Stool Sample Collection and Storage

Women were provided with sterile wooden applicators and sterile 50 ml plastic conical collection tubes for collection. They were instructed to sterilely collect the stool sample from child's soiled diaper with the wooden applicator and place in the collection tube. Samples were then stored at 4°C (i.e., refrigerated) for up to 24 hours until collection by study personnel from the participant's home or delivery by the participant to OSUWMC. In the latter case, women were instructed to transport samples in a cooler with ice. Upon arrival at the Wexner Medical Center, samples were placed in long-term storage at −80°C until pyrosequencing was conducted.

bTEFAP

Bacterial tag-encoded FLX-Amplicon Pyrosequencing (bTE-FAP) was performed as previously described [21,22]. The 16 s rrn universal primers 27f (AGA GTT TGA TCM TGG CTC AG) and 519r (GWATTACCGCGGCKGCTG) were used for specific 16S rrn targeting.

These primers were used for single-step 30 cycle PCR. The following thermoprofile was used: a single cycle of 94°C for 3 minutes, then 28 cycles of: 30 seconds at 94°C; 40 seconds at 53°C, 1 minute at 72°C, with a single 5 minute cycle at 72°C for 5 minutes for elongation. Amplicons were pooled at equivalent concentrations and purified (Agencourt Bioscience Corporation, MA, USA). Sequencing was performed with the Roche 454 FLX Titanium system using manufacturer's guidelines.

Sequencing Analysis

Analysis was performed using the open-source software package, Quantitative Insights Into Microbial Ecology (QIIME), v.1.7.0. [23]. Sequences were provided via.fasta file and sequence quality was denoted with a.qual file. Barcodes were trimmed and low-quality reads were removed. An average quality score of 25 was used. Minimum sequence length of 200 and maximum length of 1000 were used. No mismatches were allowed in the primer sequence. An average of 14862 sequences were attained per sample, and a total of 77.06% of sequences passed quality filtering.

Sequences were clustered based upon 0.97 similarity using UClust into operational taxonomic units (OTUs) [24]. A representative sequence was selected from each OTU and the RDP classifier was used to assign taxonomy to the representative sequence [25]. Sequences were aligned using PyNAST [26] against a Greengenes core reference alignment database [27] and an OTU phylogenetic tree was assembled based upon this alignment [28].

Phylogenetic Investigation of Communities by Reconstruction of Unobserved States, or PiCRUST, was used to identify differences in predictive metagenome function [29]. In summary, OTUs were picked from a demultiplexed fasta file containing the sequences for all 77 subjects using the closed-reference procedure, against the GreenGenes 13_5 reference database [30]. These OTUs were normalized by the predicted 16 s copy number, and functions were predicted from these normalized OTUs with the use of GreenGenes 13_5 database for KEGG Orthologs. From this, a BIOM table containing the predicted metagenome for each sample was attained. Each sample was rarefied at 2,000,000 before further analysis. Downstream statistical analysis was performed using STAMP [31].

Statistical Analysis

The Shannon Diversity Index (SDI), a measurement of within-sample (alpha-diversity) community diversity, as well as Chao1 (estimates richness), equitability (measures evenness), and observed_species (calculates unique OTUs) were used to ascertain differences in alpha diversity based on maternal obesity status [32]. All alpha-diversity measurements were calculated with QIIME and significance was measured using a parametric t-test at a depth of 5930 sequences for comparison of all obese vs non-obese groups. Depths of 4534 sequences for comparison of maternal obesity among the high income group alone, and 5126 sequences for comparison among the low income group alone were also used. UniFrac unweighted distance matrices were calculated from the OTU phylogenetic tree for beta diversity analyses [33]. A sampling depth of 5108 sequences/sample was used for beta diversity for all groups.

The adonis statistic, available through the vegan package on the open-source statistical program R, and further employed in QIIME, was used to measure differences in variance between two groups based upon their microbiota UniFrac distance matrices [34,35]. Groups were split based upon maternal and paternal BMI, as well as by income level and differences in community structure were determined using adonis. The permdisp statistic, also available through vegan, was then performed to verify equal variances between groups dichotomized by obesity.

Chi-square analyses and two-sample t-tests were used to determine the demographic and behavioral similarity between the maternal obesity groups to identify possible confounding factors. Additionally, Pearson's correlations, univariate analysis of variance (ANOVA) and regression analyses were used to examine associations between variables including maternal BMI, child's weight/height ratio and the SDI. The relative abundance of bacterial groups in samples from children of obese and non-obese mothers were compared using Mann-Whitney U-tests. All analyses were performed using SPSS v.21 (IBM, Chicago, IL). For predictive functional group analysis in STAMP, Welch's t-tests were used for two group comparisons, while Kruskal-Wallis H-tests were used for multiple group comparisons. P-values were corrected for multiple-tests using the Benjamini-Hochberg method [36], with a q-value of 0.10.

Results

Participant Characteristics

This study included 77 mother-child pairs. Children were 18–27 months at the time of assessment (Mean = 23.14, SD = 2.00), with 91% falling between 21–26 months. In this sample, 87.0% (n = 67) of mothers were White, 9.1% (n = 7) were Black and 3.9% (n = 3) were Asian. The mean maternal age at the time of delivery was 31.10±5.43 and 87.0% of women (n = 67) were married. In this sample, 66.2% of mothers (n = 51) were non-obese (BMI <30) and 33.8% (n = 26) were obese (BMI ≥30) based self-reported height and weight prior to pregnancy. The mean BMI among the obese women was 35.13±4.48 compared to 22.65±2.85 among the non-obese (t(75) = 15.3, $p < 0.001$).

To identify potential factors which may confound the relationship between maternal obesity and the composition of the child microbiome, we examined the demographic and behavioral similarity between obese and non-obese women (Tables 1 & 2). Obese and non-obese women did not differ significantly in race, marital status, maternal age at the time of delivery, antibiotic exposure during pregnancy or breastfeeding, or delivery route (vaginal versus C-section). Obese women had heavier male partners than did non-obese women, with BMIs of 31.20±5.98 vs. 26.91±4.60, respectively (t(75) = 3.49, $p = 0.001$). Obese women and their partners had completed less education than non-obese women and their partners ($ps \leq 0.014$). However, women did not differ in annual household income based on obesity status ($X^2(3) = 1.92$, $p = .59$), although household income was significantly correlated with both maternal (r = .65, $p < 0.001$) and paternal education (r = .52, $p < 0.001$).

Maternal obesity and beta diversity in the child gut microbiome

Unweighted UniFrac distance matrices were used to assess differences between the microbial communities, known as beta diversity, in children of obese compared to non-obese mothers. Permutational multivariate ANOVA using adonis showed that children of obese versus non-obese mothers had a different microbiota community structure ($r^2 = 0.01539$, $p = 0.044$). However, this did not result in clustering of two distinct populations using a principle coordinate analysis (PCoA) (Fig. 1). To further explain the significant adonis statistic in the absence of obvious clustering, permdisp, a statistic that measures the extent to which variances in different populations are equivalent, was used to compare the two groups. Dispersion of the community structures of children born to obese versus non-obese mothers differed signficantly, with greater variance among children of non-obese mothers ($p = 0.035$, $F = 4.843$). In contrast, there was no difference in between-sample community structure as measured via adonis in children of obese versus non-obese fathers ($r^2 = 0.01214$, $p = 0.801$).

Next, we examined whether the strength of the association between beta diversity and maternal obesity differed among children of mothers from higher versus lower socioeconomic backgrounds. Analyses showed no main effects of socioeconomic indicators; neither maternal education ($r^2 = 0.01267$, $p = 0.615$) nor income level ($r^2 = 0.01331$, $p = 0.409$) were associated with shifts in the offspring microbial profile. Similarly, neither maternal education nor income were associated with clustering on a PCoA (Fig. S1). Next, the interaction between obesity status with both

Table 1. Demographic Characteristics.

	Total (n = 77)	Obese (n = 26)	Non-Obese (n = 51)	Obese vs. Non-Obese
Maternal BMI [Mean (SD)]	26.86 (6.83)	35.13 (4.48)	22.65 (2.85)	$t(75) = 15.3$, $p = .000*$
Paternal BMI [Mean (SD)]	28.34 (5.47)	31.2 (5.98)	26.89 (4.92)	$t(75) = 3.49$, $p = .001*$
Maternal Age [Mean (SD)]	31.10 (5.43)	31.96 (6.02)	30.67 (5.11)	$t(75) = 0.99$, $p = .33$
Child Sex [n (%)]				$X^2(1) = 0.79$, $p = .37$
Male	41 (53.2%)	12 (46.2%)	29 (56.9%)	
Female	36 (46.8%)	14 (53.8%)	22 (43.1%)	
Maternal Race				$X^2(1) = 0.47$, $p = .47@$
White	67 (87.0%)	21 (80.8%)	46 (90.2%)	
Black/African-American	7 (9.1%)	5 (19.2%)	2 (3.9%)	
Asian	3 (3.9%)	0 (0%)	3 (5.9%)	
Marital Status [n (%)]				$X^2(1) = 3.54$, $p = .06$
Married	67 (87.0%)	20 (76.9%)	47 (92.2%)	
Unmarried	10 (13%)	6 (23.1%)	4 (7.8%)	
Maternal Education [n (%)]				$X^2(2) = 10.67^\ddagger$, $p = .005*$
High school graduate or less	19 (24.7%)	12 (46.2%)	7 (13.7%)	
College graduate (2 or 4 yr)	26 (33.8%)	8 (30.8%)	18 (35.3%)	
Some graduate school or higher	32 (41.6%)	6 (23.1%)	26 (51.0%)	
Paternal Education [n (%)]				$X^2(2) = 8.51$, $p = .014*$
High school graduate or less	29 (37.6%)	12 (46.2%)	17 (33.3%)	
College graduate (2 or 4 yr)	30 (39.0%)	12 (46.2%)	18 (35.3%)	
Some graduate school or higher	18 (23.3%)	2 (7.7%)	16 (31.4%)	
Income [n (%)]				$X^2(3) = 1.92$, $p = .59$
< $ 30,000	15 (19.5%)	7 (26.9%)	8 (15.7%)	
$30,000–49,999	15 (19.5%)	5 (19.2%)	10 (19.6%)	
$50,000–99,999	30 (39.0%)	10 (38.4%)	20 (39.2%)	
≥ $100,000	17 (22.0%)	4 (15.4%)	13 (25.5%)	

*$p < .05$.
@White versus non-white.

education (high school graduate or less versus college graduate or more) and income (<$50 k versus ≥$50 k) was examined. An interaction effect between income and obesity status was observed; in the high-income group, a different microbiota community structure was seen in the children of obese versus non-obese mothers ($r^2 = 0.02547$, $p = 0.041$). However, in the lower-income group, no significant effects of maternal obesity on beta diversity were observed ($r^2 = 0.03798$, $p = 0.139$). Also, in dyads from high-income households, the microbiota of children of obese mothers had greater homogeneity among the samples compared to those from non-obese mothers ($F = 11.942$, $p = 0.003$). Furthermore, clustering based on obesity status was observed using a PCoA in the high income group only (Fig. 2A–B).

Similar effects were seen when using education as an indicator of socioeconomic status. Among mothers with a high education, children born to obese mothers had a different community structure than those born to non-obese mothers ($r^2 = 0.02049$, $p = 0.045$) and this was partly explained by significantly greater homogeneity in variance ($F = 6.215$, $p = 0.02$). In contrast, among children born to women with less education, there were no significant differences in beta diversity based on maternal obesity status ($r^2 = 0.05327$, $p = 0.61$). Thus, similar results were observed in relation to income and education as indicators of socioeconomic

status. Compared to education level, income was more evenly distributed in the obese and non-obese groups, providing greater statistical power. Thus, all downstream analyses focused on income.

Maternal obesity and alpha diversity in the child gut microbiome

We next examined the relationship between maternal BMI and alpha diversity of the child microbiota. First, we examined the Shannon Diversity Index (SDI), a measure of the overall diversity within a microbial community. Two samples were below the threshold for SDI, resulting in a sample of 75 for these analyses. Results showed that children of obese mothers had a significantly higher SDI than children of non-obese mothers ($t(73) = 2.1$, $p = 0.04$; Fig. 3A). Greater alpha diversity in children born to obese mothers was associated with greater equitability ($t(73) = 1.96$, $p = 0.05$; Fig. 3B) and a trend towards greater richness as estimated by Chao1 ($t(73) = 1.83$, $p = 0.07$; Fig. 3C). Furthermore, children of obese mothers had higher number of unique OTUs as defined by QIIME variable observed_species ($t(73) = 2.25$, $p = 0.03$; Fig. 3D).

Next, we examined interactions between maternal socioeconomic status and obesity on alpha diversity of the child gut

Table 2. Health/Behavioral Characteristics.

	Total (n = 77)	Obese (n = 26)	Non-Obese (n = 51)	Obese vs. Non-Obese
Route of delivery [n (%)]				X2(1) = 0.17, p = .68
C-Section	33 (42.9%)	12 (46.2%)	21 (41.2%)	
Vaginal	44 (57.1%)	14 (53.8%)	30 (58.8%)	
Breastfeeding duration [n (%)]				$X^2(2) = 3.84$, $p = .147^\#$
Never	5 (6.5%)	4 (15.4%)	1 (2%)	
<3 months	7 (9.1%)	3 (11.5%)	4 (7.8%)	
3 to 11 months	38 (49.4%)	11 (42.3%)	27 (52.9%)	
≥12 months	27 (35.1%)	8 (30.8%)	19 (37.2%)	
Grains/Cereals introduced [n (%)]				$X^2(1) = 0.06$, $p = .812^\wedge$
≤4 months	30 (39.0%)	12 (46.2%)	18 (35.3%)	
5–6 months	41 (53.2%)	11 (42.3%)	30 (58.8%)	
≥7 months	6 (7.8%)	3 (11.5%)	3 (5.9%)	
Vegetables, fruits, and/or meats introduced [n (%)]				$X^2(2) = 0.17$, $p = .92$
≤4 months	17 (22.1%)	6 (23.1%)	11 (21.6%)	
5–6 months	38 (49.4%)	12 (46.2%)	26 (51.0%)	
≥7 months	22 (28.6%)	8 (30.8%)	14 (27.5%)	
Meat frequency [n (%)]				$X^2(2) = 2.24$, $p = .33$
Less than once per day	25 (32.5%)	6 (23.1%)	19 (37.3%)	
Once per day	27 (35.1%)	9 (34.6%)	18 (35.3%)	
More than once per day	25 (32.5%)	11 (42.3%)	32 (27.5%)	
Vegetable frequency [n (%)]				$X^2(2) = 0.30$, $p = .86$
Less than once per day	17 (22.1%)	5 (19.2%)	12 (23.5%)	
Once per day	24 (31.2%)	9 (34.6%)	15 (29.4%)	
More than once per day	36 (46.8%)	12 (46.2%)	24 (47.1%)	
Antibiotic use in pregnancy [n (%)]				X2(1) = 1.07, $p = .30$
No	64 (83.1%)	20 (76.9%)	44 (86.3%)	
Yes	13 (16.9%)	6 (23.1%)	7 (13.7%)	
Antibiotic use while breastfeeding [n (%)]				X2(1) = .056, $p = .81$
No	69 (89.6%)	23 (88.5%)	46 (90.2%)	
Yes	8 (10.4%)	3 (11.5%)	5 (9.8%)	
Antibiotic exposure in child [n (%)]				X2(2) = 2.30, $p = .317$
None	23 (29.9%)	5 (19.2%)	18 (35.3%)	
One or two courses	29 (37.7%)	12 (46.2%)	17 (33.3%)	
More than two courses	25 (32.4%)	9 (34.6%)	16 (31.4%)	

#Never and <3 months combined in analyses due to low occurrence.
^5–6 months and ≥7 months combined in analyses due to low occurrence.

microbiome. As with beta diversity, results indicated that effects of maternal obesity on alpha diversity were driven by the high-income group. Specifically, in high income households, SDI (t(73) = 2.30, p = 0.026), Chao1 (t(73) = 2.08, p = 0.043), equitability (t(73) = 2.20, p = 0.033), and observed OTUs (t(73) = 2.30, p = 0.029) were all higher in children of obese versus non-obese mothers. However, among children in lower income households, no differences in alpha diversity were detected in relation to maternal obesity status [SDI (t(73) = 0.537, p = 0.595), Chao1 (t(73) = −0.018, p = 0.992), equitability (t(73) = 0.498, p = 0.619), observed OTUs (t(73) = 0.674, p = 0.515)] (Fig. 4A–H).

Further analyses demonstrated that the SDI was higher in children of obese versus non-obese fathers (t(73) = 1.99, $p = 0.05$) which corresponded to greater equitability (t(73) = 2.10, p = 0.04).

However, there were no significant differences in either the Chao1 estimation or OTUs (i.e., observed_species in QIIME) between children born to obese or non-obese fathers (data not shown). When entered into a regression model together, maternal BMI remained a significant predictor of the SDI ($\beta = 0.324$, $p = 0.008$) while paternal BMI was no longer significantly associated ($\beta = 0.085$, $p = 0.48$) suggesting that maternal BMI was the critical predictor. In addition, univariate ANOVA demonstrated that the child weight/height ratio showed no association with the toddler SDI (F(2,72) = 0.58, $p = .565$). Moreover, maternal BMI remained a significant predictor after including the child's WHR in the model ($\beta = 3.178$, $p = 0.002$), indicating an effect of maternal BMI that was independent of the child's current body composition.

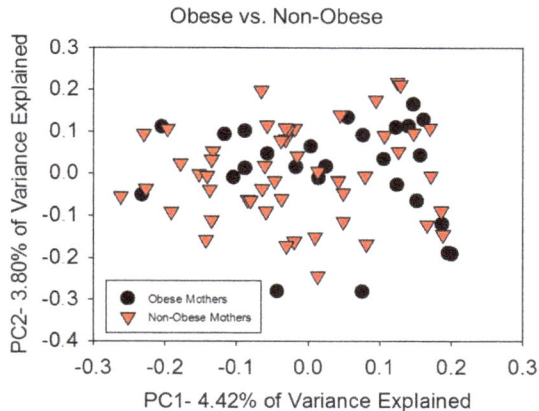

Figure 1. In the overall sample, datapoints did not cluster on a principle coordinate analysis (PCoA) scatter-plot as a function of maternal obesity. The beta-diversity non-parametric statistic adonis showed that children born to obese (n = 26) versus non-obese mothers (n = 51) had unique microbial profiles (p = 0.044). However, this was due to greater homogeneity among the obese group as measured with permdisp (p = 0.035).

Maternal obesity and phylogenetic shifts in child gut microbiome

We next examined phylogenetic shifts in the fecal microbiome of the children, to determine if differences in abundances of given genera were evident. An area graph of the phyla present in all subjects indicated that considerable variability existed across children in the abundances of the highly abundant phyla, wherein a wide range of ratios between *Firmicutes:Bacteroidetes* was observed (Fig. 5). Mann-Whitney U-tests revealed no significant differences in the two largest bacterial phyla in the gut, *Firmicutes* (p = 0.667) and *Bacteroidetes* (p = 0.914) when the relative abundances found in children from obese versus non-obese mothers were compared. When analyses were conducted separately among higher versus lower income groups, no significant effects of

maternal obesity on the child gut microbiome at the phyla level were observed that withstood multiple test correction.

Next, genera-level abundances were examined. The Mann-Whitney U test was used due to the skewed distributions of the population abundances. Benjamini-Hochberg tests for multiple comparisons were used, with a q-value set at 0.10. In the overall sample, there were limited significant differences between children born to obese versus non-obese mothers after multiple test correction (Table 3). However, examination of interactions between SES and obesity status revealed multiple associations. Among children of high-income mothers, abundances of the genera *Parabacteroides* (p = 0.008, q<0.10), *Eubacterium* (p = 0.021, q<0.10), *Blautia* (p = 0.025, q<0.10), and *Oscillibacter* (p = 0.011, q<0.010), as well as an undefined genus in *Bacteroidales* (p = 0.005, q<0.10) differed significantly based on maternal obesity status (Table 4). In contrast, after correction for multiple tests, there were no significant differences between children born to obese versus non-obese mothers in the low-income group (Table 5).

Other behavioral and environmental influences upon the microbiota

In addition to influence by exposure to maternal bacteria, mothers could affect the toddler microbiome via control of the toddler diet, as diet is a primary factor in determining population abundances of the GI microbiota. In chi-square analyses, we found no significant differences in dietary patterns in children of obese versus non-obese women (Table 2). Specifically, children did not differ significantly in duration of breastfeeding, age at which grains/cereals or other foods were introduced, or the frequency of consuming meat or vegetables (p's≥0.15). Children of obese versus non-obese mothers also did not differ in the extent to which they had been exposed to antibiotic medications (during pregnancy, breastfeeding, or directly during childhood) or probiotics in food or supplement form (p's≥ .34).

Because significant results in this study were found predominately in high-income dyads, we further examined potential dietary differences in children born to obese versus non-obese mothers in the high income group. Results also showed no

A. Obese vs. Non-Obese among High-Income Participants

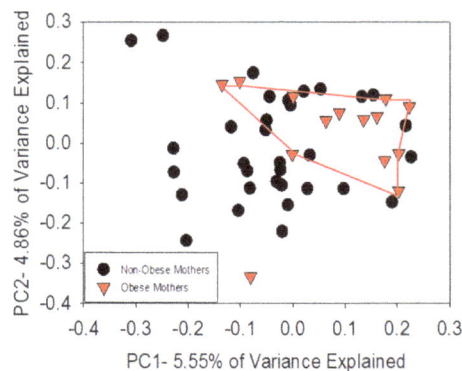

B. Obese vs. Non-Obese among Low-Income Participants

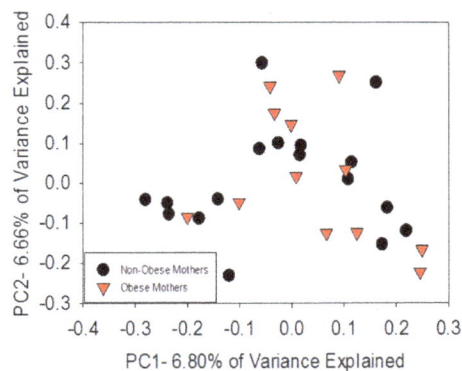

Figure 2. Interactive effects of maternal obesity and socioeconomic status were observed; effects of maternal obesity on the child microbiome were primarily seen among the higher SES group. A) In the higher income group, children born to obese versus non-obese mothers clustered (adonis, p = 0.041) and had higher homogeneity (permdisp, p = 0.003). B) These effects of maternal obesity were not seen in children in the lower income group.

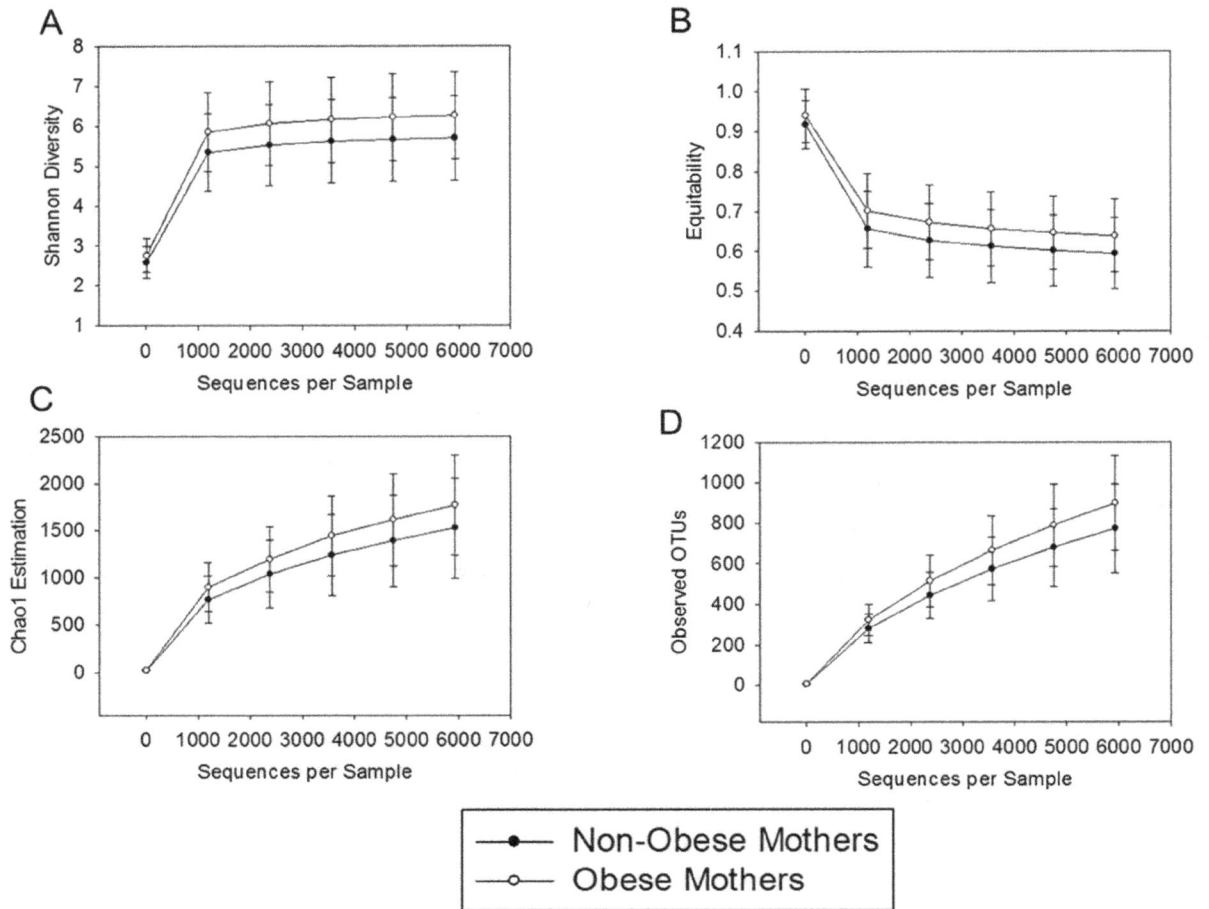

Figure 3. In the overall sample, children born to obese versus non-obese mothers had significantly greater alpha diversity as indicated by A) Shannon Diversity Index (SDI), a measure of overall alpha diversity; B) equitability, a measurement of evenness; C) Chao1, an estimation of richness; and D) the total observed operational taxonomic units (OTUs) (ps <.05; Means ±1 SE).

differences in breastfeeding duration, age at which grains/cereals or other foods were introduced, or the frequency of consuming meat or vegetables among children of obese versus non-obese mothers in this group ($p's \geq 0.13$).

We also examined the potential role of three key environmental factors that may covary with maternal obesity status and SES: route of delivery (vaginal versus C-section), duration of breastfeeding, and antibiotic exposure in mothers and children. Analyses showed no significant associations between these factors and the community structure of the child gut microbiome (Table S1), and no clustering observed using PCoA (Fig. S2). Also, as described earlier, these exposures did not differ based on maternal obesity status (Table 2). Further analyses among the high-income group also showed that route of delivery, maternal antibiotic use in pregnancy/breastfeeding (combined due to low occurrence), and antibiotic exposure in the child did not differ significantly based on maternal obesity status ($ps \geq .12$).

Predictive metagenome

The predictive metagenome program, PiCrust, was used to examine if maternal obesity and other factors (duration of breastfeeding, maternal use of antibiotics during breastfeeding or pregnancy, child use of antibiotics, and birth route) were associated with altered functioning of the microbial groups.

Abundances of Kyoto Encyclopedia of Genes and Genomes (KEGG) Orthologies, or KOs, were highly similar across children (Fig. S3). Deeper analysis of the KOs revealed that carbohydrate metabolism was significantly lower in children born to obese mothers. However, these differences in KO abundances did not pass correction for multiple tests, due to low effect sizes (Table S2). Likewise, when high and low-income participants were examined separately, maternal obesity was not associated with any significant differences in functional group abundance after multiple test correction (Table S3), nor were differences detected in functional groups based upon breastfeeding duration, antibiotic use by mother or child, and birth route (Tables S4–S6).

Discussion

Children born to obese mothers are at greater risk for obesity in adulthood compared to children of non-obese mothers, with odds ratios ranging from 1.23 to 6.12 depending on sex and age [3,37,38]. Factors including diet and genetics contribute to, but do not fully explain this increased risk [39]. The gut microbiome may play a clinically meaningful role; bacteria that affect metabolic processes are transmitted from the mother to the infant during birth and subsequently through physical contact and, in many cases, breastfeeding [15–17]. Obese adults have different

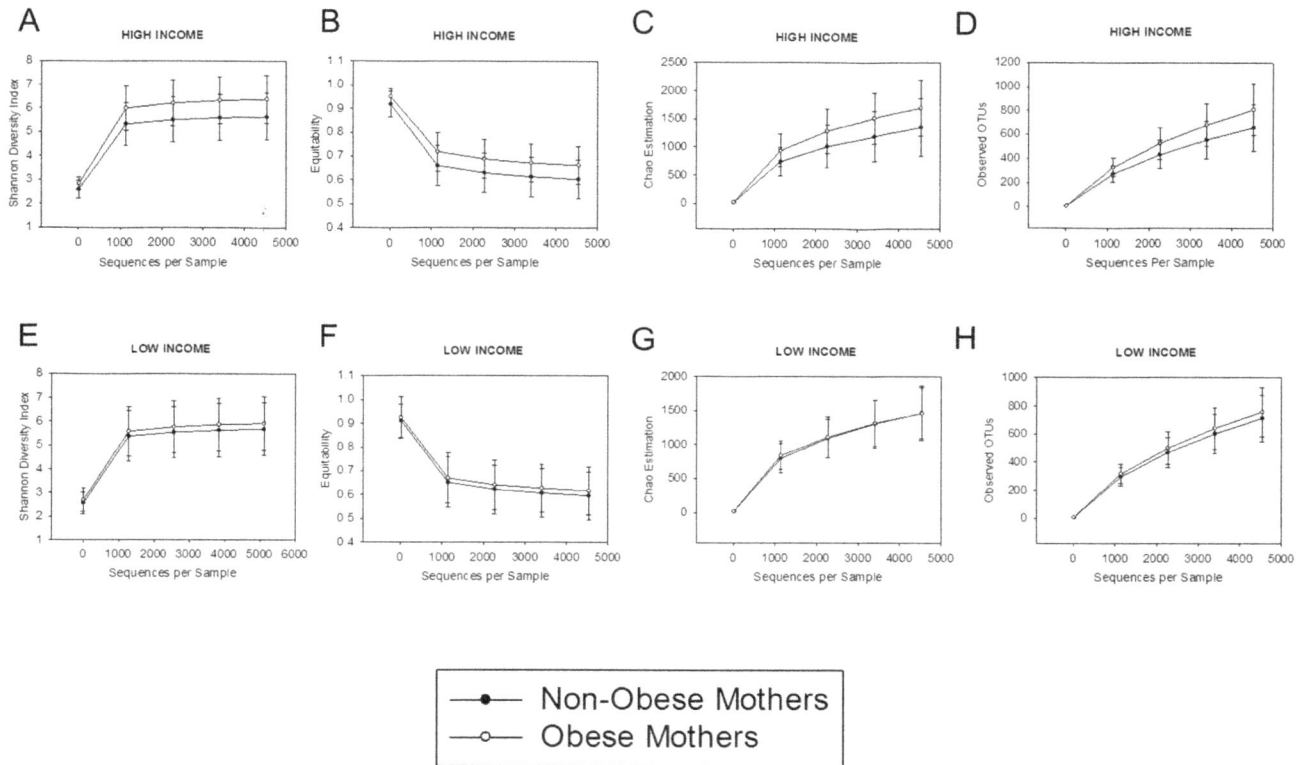

Figure 4. As with measures of beta diversity, differences in alpha diversity in relation to maternal obesity were seen predominately in the higher SES group. In the higher-income group, children born to obese versus non-obese mothers had significantly higher A) Shannon Diversity Index, B) equitability, C) Chao1 estimation, and D) observed operational taxonomic units (OTUs) ($ps \leq 0.05$). In contrast, in the lower-income group, no significant effects of maternal obesity on alpha diversity indicators were observed (E–H).

microbial community profiles in the gut [9–11], and studies show that transplanting microbiota from obese mice into germ-free mice can lead to increased body fat [14], illustrating that altered profiles of microbiota can be both obesogenic and transmittable. However, the extent to which the microbiome may contribute to the intergenerational transmission of obesity in humans is not known.

This study provides novel evidence that maternal obesity is related to measurable differences in the composition of the gut microbiome in offspring, as reflected by measures of both alpha (Shannon Diversity Index, equitability, unique OTUs) and beta diversity (per adonis). Despite the lack of group clustering on a PCoA, differences in beta diversity were explained using permdisp, which indicated increased homogeneity among the microbiomes of the obese-group and increased dispersion among the non-obese group. Our results suggest that the relationship between maternal obesity and the composition of the child gut microbiome remain after accounting for paternal BMI and indicators of child body composition, supporting an exposure rather than purely genetic pathway. This is consistent with epidemiological studies showing that maternal BMI is more strongly associated with obesity in offspring than is paternal BMI [4,5]. In addition, in metagenome function analyses using PiCRUST, lower abundances of communities related to carbohydrate metabolism were observed in children born to obese versus non-obese mothers, although this result did not remain significant after statistical correction for multiple comparisons.

Importantly, effects of maternal obesity on the composition of the gut microbiome in offspring were stronger and more consistent among those born to mothers of higher socioeconomic status (SES)

as defined by income and/or education. Specifically, when higher and lower income groups were examined separately, differences in beta diversity in relation to maternal obesity (per adonis/permdisp and PCoA) were evident only in the higher income group, as were multiple measures of alpha diversity. Less dispersion of profiles among children born to obese compared to non-obese mothers, particularly among those of high SES, indicates that these children are developing microbial profiles typified by greater homogeneity of community structures. Additional studies are needed to determine if similar effects are present in older children, adolescents, and adults.

Also demonstrating effects of socioeconomic status, among the high-income group only, children born to obese versus non-obese mothers had greater abundances of *Parabacteroides* spp., *Oscillibacter* spp., and an unclassified genus of the order *Bacteroidales* as well as lower *Blautia* spp., and *Eubacterium* spp. Of note, differences in *Eubacteriaceae, Oscillibacter* and *Blautia* have been found in prior studies of diet and obesity [40–42], but the clinical relevance of these bacterial types in affecting obesity risk is not fully understood. Also, when PiCRUST was used to examine metagemone function based on obesity status in the higher income group only, no significant differences were found.

The mechanisms underlying the interaction between maternal obesity and SES in predicting the composition of the child gut microbiome are not known. Obesity is a health condition with multifactorial origins, both genetic and behavioral (i.e., diet, physical activity). Research on the true interaction between social-environmental and genetic factors (i.e., moderating effects) is sparse. However, among obese adults, the relative contribution of

Children born to Obese Mothers

Children born to Non-Obese Mothers

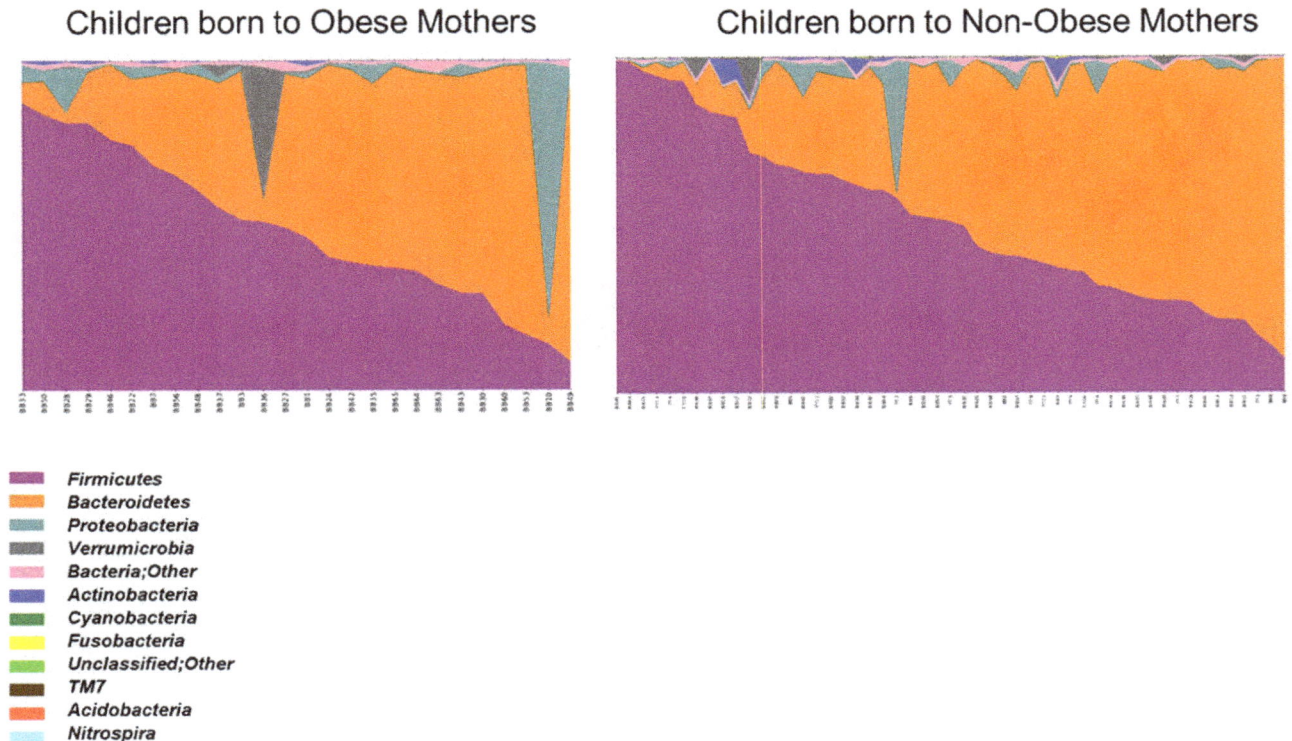

- ■ *Firmicutes*
- ■ *Bacteroidetes*
- ■ *Proteobacteria*
- ■ *Verrumicrobia*
- ■ *Bacteria;Other*
- ■ *Actinobacteria*
- ■ *Cyanobacteria*
- ■ *Fusobacteria*
- ■ *Unclassified;Other*
- ■ *TM7*
- ■ *Acidobacteria*
- ■ *Nitrospira*

Figure 5. Across individuals, there was considerable variance in the *Firmicutes:Bacteroidetes* **ratio, as shown.** However, there were no differences between the children born to obese versus non-obese mothers in abundances of the major phyla, *Firmicutes* ($p = 0.667$) and *Bacteroidetes* ($p = 0.914$).

genetic versus behavioral factors may differ in those from higher versus lower socioeconomic backgrounds [43]. Relatedly, the extent to which maternal obesity confers measureable changes to the gut microbiome of offspring may differ based on the etiology of maternal obesity.

Our finding of higher SDI among children of obese versus non-obese mothers contrasts prior research linking obesity with lower alpha diversity [9,44]. However, previous studies have focused on adults or used mouse models with experimentally-induced obesity. This is one of the first studies to ascertain SDI among toddlers as a function of maternal obesity. Higher SDI in children born to obese mothers may reflect interactions between their unique beta-diversity community profile and age-related effects, possibly down-regulated immune surveillance or reduced GI motility, which could result in greater growth and diversification of microbial groups. Due to the novelty of the study, further investigation is required.

In early life, parents largely control the diet of the child, and tend to offer solid foods that reflect their own adult diets [45]. Diet can substantially affect the composition of the gut microbiome [40,46,47]. In our sample, we found no differences in the children from obese and non-obese mothers in terms of breastfeeding behavior, age at which solid foods were introduced, or the current frequency of consumption of meat, vegetables, and cereals/grains regardless of maternal SES. This suggests that diet did not explain the observed differences in the children's gut microbiome related to maternal obesity and SES. However, this study did not include detailed food diaries that would capture the volume and quality of foods (e.g., high versus low fat meats) consumed. Thus, the possibility remains that differences in feeding behaviors contribute

to the observed association with maternal obesity and/or the interaction between maternal obesity and SES.

In addition, other key factors that can affect the gut microbiome including antibiotic exposure, breastfeeding, and route of delivery were examined, but did not account for the observed effects of maternal obesity, or the interaction between maternal obesity and SES. After correction for multiple comparisons, there were not significant differences in individual KOs based upon these factors. Moreover, as described, these factors did not differ significantly based on obesity status, regardless of maternal SES. However, the role of such factors requires further attention.

If continued research supports the notion that obese mothers may pass obesogenic microbiota to their infants, interventions could target manipulation of maternal vaginal and gut micro-biome. Prior research has shown that administration of antibiotics during the delivery process reduces vaginal *Lactobacillus* spp. levels in the mother and corresponds to lower levels of lactobacilli in oral samples from newborns [48]. In this case, these effects are potentially detrimental, as early colonization with *Lactobacillus* spp. may have a preventative role in the development of allergic diseases. However, such studies demonstrate that interventions that affect population abundances in the mother can have downstream effects in the neonate's own microbial structure.

A strength of this study is a focus on children between 18 and 27 months of age. Prior studies have shown that infants of obese mothers have differences in the gut microbiota, specifically the numbers of *Bacteroides* spp. and *Staphylococcus* spp. in the stool [18]. However, the microbiota are characterized by a lack of consistency and high volatility during the first year of life [19]. These profiles generally stabilize and increase in diversity, more

Table 3. Top 20 Most Abundant Genera.

	Normal Weight	Obese
Bacteroides spp.	36.24±3.76	27.35±4.33
Lachnospiraceae; Other	19.31±2.89	13.37±2.44
Dialister spp.	5.51±1.67	7.71±2.05
Faecalibacterium spp.	5.60±1.46	6.96±2.24*
Prevotella spp.	2.85±1.44	9.46±3.94
Unclassified Clostridiales	5.22±0.60	4.44±0.73
Roseburia spp.	2.97±0.41	4.52±1.21
Veillonella spp.	3.31±0.93	2.25±1.62
Ruminococcaceae; Other	2.00±0.61	2.42±0.91
Parabacteroides spp.	1.78±0.61	2.04±0.57
Escherichia/Shigella spp.	1.54±0.79	1.09±0.46
Alistepes spp.	1.11±0.34	1.88±0.92
Ruminococcus spp.	1.70±0.86	0.61±0.30
Unclassified Bacteria	1.09±0.09	1.44±0.17
Akkermansia spp.	0.60±0.27	1.88±1.54
Klebsiella spp.	0.03±0.02	2.81±2.65
Unclassified Bacteroidales	0.67±0.09	0.82±0.11
Eubacterium spp.	0.80±0.26	0.34±0.13**
Oscillibacter spp.	0.43±0.09	1.00±0.35
Coprobacillus spp.	0.28±0.13	1.00±0.81

Data are the mean relative abundance ± standard error.
**p<.05 vs. Non-Obese, passed correction for multiple comparisions.
*p<.05 vs. Non-Obese.

Table 4. Top 20 Most Abundant Genera Among High-Income Subjects.

	Normal Weight	Obese
Bacteroides spp.	30.65±4.59	31.24±5.86
Lachnospiraceae; Other	20.94±3.99	11.13±2.71
Dialister spp.	6.85±2.50	5.61±2.66
Faecalibacterium spp.	5.83±1.86	5.92±1.64
Prevotella spp.	3.06±1.90	11.79±6.71
Unclassified Clostridiales	5.85±0.86	3.87±0.66
Roseburia spp.	3.68±0.57	6.09±2.12
Veillonella spp.	4.55±1.36	3.41±3.00
Parabacteroides spp.	1.66±0.91	3.03±0.94**
Ruminococcaceae spp.	1.28±0.25	3.10±1.67
Escherichia/Shigella spp.	2.24±1.21	0.66±0.34
Alistepes spp.	0.93±0.45	2.14±1.52
Ruminococcus spp.	1.40±1.02	0.96±0.55
Unclassified Bacteria	1.07±0.12	1.36±0.19
Eubacterium spp.	0.92±0.38	0.41±0.23**
Unclassified Bacteroidales	0.53±0.08	1.01±0.14**
Akkermansia spp.	0.70±0.41	0.45±0.26
Oscillibacter spp.	0.28±0.08	1.18±0.60**
Blautia spp.	0.53±0.23	0.32±0.25**
Unclassified Peptostreptococcaceae	0.53±0.30	0.32±0.22

Data are the mean relative abundance ± standard error.
**p<.05 vs. Non-Obese, passed correction for multiple comparisions.

Table 5. Top 20 Most Abundant Genera Among Low-Income Subjects.

	Normal Weight	Obese
Bacteroides spp.	46.49±5.97	22.81±6.47*
Lachnospiraceae; Other	16.33±3.74	15.99±4.25
Faecalibacterium spp.	5.19±2.42	8.19±4.58
Dialister spp.	3.05±1.06	10.16±3.14
Unclassified *Clostridiales*	4.06±0.57	5.12±1.39
Prevotella spp.	2.46±2.19	6.76±4.79
Ruminococcaceae; Other	3.34±1.64	1.64±0.45
Klebsiella spp.	0.01±0.00	5.76±5.75
Roseburia spp.	1.65±0.35	2.69±0.63
Akkermansia spp.	0.42±0.18	3.55±3.33
Parabacteroides spp.	1.99±0.49	0.87±0.34
Alistepes spp.	1.42±0.52	1.58±1.00
Ruminococcus spp.	2.23±1.61	0.20±0.08
Unclassified *Bacteria*	1.13±0.13	1.55±0.30
Veillonella spp.	1.03±0.50	0.89±0.41
Coprobacillus spp.	0.11±0.05	1.88±1.75
Escherichia/Shigella spp.	0.27±0.14	1.60±0.92
Unclassified *Bacteroidales*	0.92±0.19	0.59±0.15
Oscillibacter spp.	0.72±0.18	0.78±0.34
Megasphaera spp.	1.06±0.85	0.02±0.02

Data are the mean relative abundance ± standard error.
*p<.05 vs. Non-Obese; did not pass correction for multiple comparisons.

closely resembling adult profiles, when the range of dietary exposures for the child expands [20,49]. Thus, the current data extend prior findings and support the hypothesis that early life exposures may have lasting effects on the gut microbiota. However, considerable variability of the major phyla is still a hallmark of the 18–27 month old child microbiota. In future studies, long-term and longitudinal examination through early childhood and adolescence would be highly valuable in explicating the extent to which observed effects persist and ultimately influence weight.

This study utilized deep pyrosequencing technology which adds upon prior studies by allowing for whole bacterial community profiling of the toddler microbiome. Utilization of this technology allowed increased sensitivity in detecting differences in the gastrointestinal microbiota community structure between children born to obese and non-obese mothers. PiCRUST was used for prediction of metagenome function based upon 16 s rRNA abundances. As reviewed, some effects in relation to maternal obesity were suggested, but these did not remain significant after correction for multiple tests. Unique microbial profiles would be expected to result in differences in microbiome function. True metagenomic shotgun sequencing will likely provide greater power to examine effects of factors such as maternal obesity on the function of the microbiota in children.

In this study, parental BMI as well as children's body composition indicators (height and weight percentile) were collected via maternal report rather than direct measurement. Current maternal BMI was not the focus because 1) maternal BMI may have changed considerably since the target pregnancy (e.g., due to weight retention after the target pregnancy or subsequent weight gain) and 2) women were of childbearing age, thus a meaningful proportion were pregnant with another child at the time of data collection. Prior studies suggest that among women of reproductive age, BMI classified by self-reported height and weight is generally accurate, resulting in correct categorization of 84%–87% and an underestimate in BMI of 0.8 kg/m² [50,51]. Because BMI by self-report tends to be slightly lower than true BMI, effects of maternal obesity on outcomes of interest may be underestimated in the current study. In addition, this study did not include collection of maternal specimens, such as vaginal or fecal samples, which would permit profiling of maternal microbial communities. This is clearly a critical next step in establishing a direct link from maternal to child microbial profiles.

In conclusion, obesity is a worldwide public health issue. Identification of modifiable early life antecedents is key to addressing this disease process. A rapidly growing body of literature indicates that the gut microbiome plays a critical role in the development of obesity. Adding to this literature, the current study provides novel evidence that maternal obesity is associated with different microbial profiles in offspring 18–27 months of age. The potential role of the gut microbiome in this intergenerational transmission of obesity risk warrants further attention. In particular, the stability of such effects into later childhood and adolescence, the clinical relevance of abundances of specific bacteria in conferring risk for obesity, and the ultimate impact of early life microbial profiles on long-term weight trajectory remains to be explicated.

Supporting Information

Figure S1 Indicators of socioeconomic status (SES), maternal education (A) and income (B) did not predict

differences in the offspring microbiota community structure.

Figure S2   Other key factors which may impact the gut microbiome were not associated with differences in community structure, including (A) birth route (B) antibiotic use by the mother while breastfeeding (C) antibiotic use during pregnancy (D), child antibiotic use or (E) duration of breastfeeding.

Figure S3   KEGG Orthologues (KOs) were highly similar across individuals. PiCRUST was used to predict metagenomic function of the child microbiome. An area graph produced by QIIME indicated that overall abundances of KOs were similar across samples.

Table S1   Potential Impacts Upon the Offspring Microbiota.

Table S2   KEGG Orthologues.

Table S3   KEGG Orthologues among High-Income Subjects.

Table S4   KEGG Orthologues.

Table S5   KEGG Orthologues.

Table S6   KEGG Orthologues.

Acknowledgments

The content is solely the responsibility of the authors and does not necessarily represent the official views of the National Center for Research Resources or the National Institutes of Health.

Author Contributions

Conceived and designed the experiments: JG MB LC. Performed the experiments: JG MB LC. Analyzed the data: JG MB LC. Contributed reagents/materials/analysis tools: MB CKD SSS LC. Contributed to the writing of the manuscript: JG MB CKD SSS LC.

References

1. Ogden CL, Carroll MD, Kit BK, Flegal KM (2012) Prevalence of obesity and trends in body mass index among US children and adolescents, 1999–2010. JAMA 307: 483–490.
2. Flegal KM, Carroll MD, Ogden CL, Curtin LR (2010) Prevalence and trends in obesity among US adults, 1999–2008. JAMA 303: 235–241.
3. Whitaker RC, Wright JA, Pepe MS, Seidel KD, Dietz WH (1997) Predicting obesity in young adulthood from childhood and parental obesity. N Engl J Med 337: 869–873.
4. Linabery AM, Nahhas RW, Johnson W, Choh AC, Towne B, et al. (2013) Stronger influence of maternal than paternal obesity on infant and early childhood body mass index: the Fels Longitudinal Study. Pediatr Obes 8: 159–169.
5. Whitaker KL, Jarvis MJ, Beeken RJ, Boniface D, Wardle J (2010) Comparing maternal and paternal intergenerational transmission of obesity risk in a large population-based sample. Am J Clin Nutr 91: 1560–1567.
6. Backhed F, Ley RE, Sonnenburg JL, Peterson DA, Gordon JI (2005) Host-bacterial mutualism in the human intestine. Science 307: 1915–1920.
7. Backhed F, Ding H, Wang T, Hooper LV, Koh GY, et al. (2004) The gut microbiota as an environmental factor that regulates fat storage. Proc Natl Acad Sci U S A 101: 15718–15723.
8. Coates ME, Ford JE, Harrison GF (1968) Intestinal synthesis of vitamins of the B complex in chicks. Br J Nutr 22: 493–500.
9. Verdam FJ, Fuentes S, de Jonge C, Zoetendal EG, Erbil R, et al. (2013) Human intestinal microbiota composition is associated with local and systemic inflammation in obesity. Obesity (Silver Spring) 21: E607–615.
10. Ley RE, Turnbaugh PJ, Klein S, Gordon JI (2006) Microbial ecology: human gut microbes associated with obesity. Nature 444: 1022–1023.
11. Bervoets L, Van Hoorenbeeck K, Kortleven I, Van Noten C, Hens N, et al. (2013) Differences in gut microbiota composition between obese and lean children: a cross-sectional study. Gut Pathog 5: 10.
12. Ley RE, Backhed F, Turnbaugh P, Lozupone CA, Knight RD, et al. (2005) Obesity alters gut microbial ecology. Proc Natl Acad Sci U S A 102: 11070–11075.
13. Park DY, Ahn YT, Park SH, Huh CS, Yoo SR, et al. (2013) Supplementation of Lactobacillus curvatus HY7601 and Lactobacillus plantarum KY1032 in diet-induced obese mice is associated with gut microbial changes and reduction in obesity. PLoS One 8: e59470.
14. Turnbaugh PJ, Ley RE, Mahowald MA, Magrini V, Mardis ER, et al. (2006) An obesity-associated gut microbiome with increased capacity for energy harvest. Nature 444: 1027–1031.
15. Favier CF, de Vos WM, Akkermans ADL (2003) Development of bacterial and bifidobacterial communities in feces of newborn babies. Anaerobe 9: 219–229.
16. Dominguez-Bello MG, Costello EK, Contreras M, Magris M, Hidalgo G, et al. (2010) Delivery mode shapes the acquisition and structure of the initial microbiota across multiple body habitats in newborns. Proc Natl Acad Sci U S A 107: 11971–11975.
17. Makino H, Kushiro A, Ishikawa E, Kubota H, Gawad A, et al. (2013) Mother-to-infant transmission of intestinal bifidobacterial strains has an impact on the early development of vaginally delivered infant's microbiota. PLoS One 8: e78331.
18. Collado MC, Isolauri E, Laitinen K, Salminen S (2010) Effect of mother's weight on infant's microbiota acquisition, composition, and activity during early infancy: a prospective follow-up study initiated in early pregnancy. Am J Clin Nutr 92: 1023–1030.
19. Palmer C, Bik EM, DiGiulio DB, Relman DA, Brown PO (2007) Development of the human infant intestinal microbiota. PLoS Biol 5: e177.
20. Koenig JE, Spor A, Scalfone N, Fricker AD, Stombaugh J, et al. (2011) Succession of microbial consortia in the developing infant gut microbiome. Proc Natl Acad Sci U S A 108 Suppl 1: 4578–4585.
21. Dowd SE, Callaway TR, Wolcott RD, Sun Y, McKeehan T, et al. (2008) Evaluation of the bacterial diversity in the feces of cattle using 16S rDNA bacterial tag-encoded FLX amplicon pyrosequencing (bTEFAP). BMC Microbiol 8: 125.
22. Dowd SE, Wolcott RD, Sun Y, McKeehan T, Smith E, et al. (2008) Polymicrobial nature of chronic diabetic foot ulcer biofilm infections determined using bacterial tag encoded FLX amplicon pyrosequencing (bTEFAP). PLoS One 3: e3326.
23. Caporaso JG, Kuczynski J, Stombaugh J, Bittinger K, Bushman FD, et al. (2010) QIIME allows analysis of high-throughput community sequencing data. Nat Methods 7: 335–336.
24. Edgar RC (2010) Search and clustering orders of magnitude faster than BLAST. Bioinformatics 26: 2460–2461.
25. Wang Q, Garrity GM, Tiedje JM, Cole JR (2007) Naive Bayesian classifier for rapid assignment of rRNA sequences into the new bacterial taxonomy. Appl Environ Microbiol 73: 5261–5267.
26. Caporaso JG, Bittinger K, Bushman FD, DeSantis TZ, Andersen GL, et al. (2010) PyNAST: a flexible tool for aligning sequences to a template alignment. Bioinformatics 26: 266–267.
27. DeSantis TZ, Hugenholtz P, Larsen N, Rojas M, Brodie EL, et al. (2006) Greengenes, a chimera-checked 16S rRNA gene database and workbench compatible with ARB. Appl Environ Microbiol 72: 5069–5072.
28. Price MN, Dehal PS, Arkin AP (2010) FastTree 2–approximately maximum-likelihood trees for large alignments. PLoS One 5: e9490.
29. Langille MG, Zaneveld J, Caporaso JG, McDonald D, Knights D, et al. (2013) Predictive functional profiling of microbial communities using 16S rRNA marker gene sequences. Nat Biotechnol 31: 814–821.
30. McDonald D, Price MN, Goodrich J, Nawrocki EP, DeSantis TZ, et al. (2012) An improved Greengenes taxonomy with explicit ranks for ecological and evolutionary analyses of bacteria and archaea. ISME J 6: 610–618.
31. Parks DH, Tyson GW, Hugenholtz P, Beiko RG (2014) STAMP: Statistical analysis of taxonomic and functional profiles. Bioinformatics.
32. Shannon CE, Weaver W (1949) The mathematical theory of communication. Urbana,: University of Illinois Press. v (i.e. vii), 117 p. p.
33. Lozupone C, Knight R (2005) UniFrac: a new phylogenetic method for comparing microbial communities. Appl Environ Microbiol 71: 8228–8235.
34. Oksanen J BF, Kindt R, Legendre R, Minchin PR, O'Hara RB, Simpson GL, Solymos P, Stevens MHH, Wagner H. Vegan: community ecology package. pp. R package version 2.0–3.
35. Development RCT R: a language and environment for statistical computing. Coventry, United Kingdom R Foundation for Statistical Computing.

36. Benjamini YH, Y. (1995) Controlling the False Discovery Rate: A Practical and Powerful Approach to Multiple Testing. Journal of the Royal Statistical Society Series B (Methodological) 57: 289–300.

37. Koupil I, Toivanen P (2008) Social and early-life determinants of overweight and obesity in 18-year-old Swedish men. Int J Obes (Lond) 32: 73–81.

38. Stuebe AM, Forman MR, Michels KB (2009) Maternal-recalled gestational weight gain, pre-pregnancy body mass index, and obesity in the daughter. Int J Obes (Lond) 33: 743–752.

39. Thompson AL (2013) Intergenerational impact of maternal obesity and postnatal feeding practices on pediatric obesity. Nutr Rev 71 Suppl 1: S55–61.

40. Lam YY, Ha CW, Campbell CR, Mitchell AJ, Dinudom A, et al. (2012) Increased gut permeability and microbiota change associate with mesenteric fat inflammation and metabolic dysfunction in diet-induced obese mice. PLoS One 7: e34233.

41. Clarke SF, Murphy EF, O'Sullivan O, Ross RP, O'Toole PW, et al. (2013) Targeting the microbiota to address diet-induced obesity: a time dependent challenge. PLoS One 8: e65790.

42. Martinez I, Lattimer JM, Hubach KL, Case JA, Yang J, et al. (2013) Gut microbiome composition is linked to whole grain-induced immunological improvements. ISME J 7: 269–280.

43. Faith MSaKTVE (2006) Social, Environmental, and Genetic Influences on Obesity and Obesity-Promoting Behaviors: Fostering Research Integration. In: Hernandez LMaBDG, editor. Genes, Behavior, and the Social Environment: Moving Beyond the Nature/Nurture Debate: National Academies Press. pp. 232–235.

44. Turnbaugh PJ, Hamady M, Yatsunenko T, Cantarel BL, Duncan A, et al. (2009) A core gut microbiome in obese and lean twins. Nature 457: 480–484.

45. Anzman SL, Rollins BY, Birch LL (2010) Parental influence on children's early eating environments and obesity risk: implications for prevention. Int J Obes (Lond) 34: 1116–1124.

46. Walker AW, Ince J, Duncan SH, Webster LM, Holtrop G, et al. (2011) Dominant and diet-responsive groups of bacteria within the human colonic microbiota. ISME J 5: 220–230.

47. Kim KA, Gu W, Lee IA, Joh EH, Kim DH (2012) High fat diet-induced gut microbiota exacerbates inflammation and obesity in mice via the TLR4 signaling pathway. PLoS One 7: e47713.

48. Keski-Nisula L, Kyynarainen HR, Karkkainen U, Karhukorpi J, Heinonen S, et al. (2013) Maternal intrapartum antibiotics and decreased vertical transmission of Lactobacillus to neonates during birth. Acta Paediatr 102: 480–485.

49. Yatsunenko T, Rey FE, Manary MJ, Trehan I, Dominguez-Bello MG, et al. (2012) Human gut microbiome viewed across age and geography. Nature 486: 222–227.

50. Brunner Huber LR (2007) Validity of self-reported height and weight in women of reproductive age. Matern Child Health J 11: 137–144.

51. Holland E, Moore Simas TA, Doyle Curiale DK, Liao X, Waring ME (2013) Self-reported pre-pregnancy weight versus weight measured at first prenatal visit: effects on categorization of pre-pregnancy body mass index. Matern Child Health J 17: 1872–1878.

36. Benjamini YH, Y. (1995) Controlling the False Discovery Rate: A Practical and

44. Turnbaugh PJ, Hamady M, Yatsunenko T, Cantarel BL, Duncan A, et al.

16

Parental Socioeconomic Status, Childhood Asthma and Medication Use – A Population-Based Study

Tong Gong[1]*, **Cecilia Lundholm**[1], **Gustaf Rejnö**[1], **Carina Mood**[2], **Niklas Långström**[1], **Catarina Almqvist**[1,3]

1 Department of Medical Epidemiology and Biostatistics, Karolinska Institutet, Stockholm, Sweden, **2** Swedish Institute for Social Research, Stockholm University, Stockholm, Sweden, **3** Astrid Lindgren Children's Hospital, Lung and Allergy Unit, Karolinska University Hospital, Stockholm, Sweden

Abstract

Background: Little is known about how parental socioeconomic status affects offspring asthma risk in the general population, or its relation to healthcare and medication use among diagnosed children.

Methods: This register-based cohort study included 211,520 children born between April 2006 and December 2008 followed until December 2010. Asthma diagnoses were retrieved from the National Patient Register, and dispensed asthma medications from the Prescribed Drug Register. Parental socioeconomic status (income and education) were retrieved from Statistics Sweden. The associations between parental socioeconomic status and outcomes were estimated by Cox proportional hazard regression.

Results: Compared to the highest parental income level, children exposed to all other levels had increased risk of asthma during their first year of life (e.g. hazard ratio, HR 1.19, 95% confidence interval, CI 1.09–1.31 for diagnosis and HR 1.17, 95% CI 1.08–1.26 for medications for the lowest quintile) and the risk was decreased after the first year, especially among children from the lowest parental income quintile (HR 0.84, 95% CI 0.77–0.92 for diagnosis, and HR 0.80, 95% CI 0.74–0.86 for medications). Further, compared to children with college-educated parents, those whose parents had lower education had increased risk of childhood asthma regardless of age. Children with the lowest parental education had increased risk of an inpatient (HR 2.07, 95% CI 1.61–2.65) and outpatient (HR 1.32, 95% CI 1.18–1.47) asthma diagnosis. Among diagnosed children, those from families with lower education used fewer controller medications than those whose parents were college graduates.

Conclusions: Our findings indicate an age-varying association between parental income and childhood asthma and consistent inverse association regardless of age between parental education and asthma incidence, dispensed controller medications and inpatient care which should be further investigated and remedied.

Editor: Yang-Ching Chen, Taipei City Hospital, Taiwan

Funding: Financial support was provided from the Swedish Research Council (grant no 2011-3060) and through the Swedish Initiative for Research on Microdata in the Social And Medical Sciences (SIMSAM) framework grant no 340-2013-5867, the Swedish Heart Lung foundation, the Strategic Research Program in Epidemiology at Karolinska Institutet, and through the regional agreement on medical training and clinical research (ALF) between Stockholm County Council and Karolinska Institutet. The funders had no role in study design, data collection and analysis, decision to publish, or preparation of the manuscript.

Competing Interests: The authors have declared that no competing interests exist.

* Email: tong.gong@ki.se

Introduction

Asthma is the most prevalent chronic disease among children and is associated with morbidity, substantial healthcare resource use and parental absence from work [1,2]. Following an increase in prevalence over the last decades, recent data suggest that the prevalence has plateaued at 6–9% [3]. Despite the considerable genetic contribution [4], there are likely several additional social and environmental factors involved in the cause and exacerbation of childhood asthma [5,6]. Several studies have tried to explain how socioeconomic status (SES) influences the development of asthma but with discrepant results. Most studies have reported that children in families with low SES (measured by parental occupation, education or family income), have an increased asthma risk even after adjustment for known confounders such as prenatal maternal smoking, indoor allergens, and maternal stress [7–9]. Other studies, however, found no relationship with parental

SES [10–12]. These diverse results could be due to different study designs, small sample sizes, or varying measures of SES [13].

Current global and national treatment guidelines emphasize use of controller medications such as inhaled corticosteroids (ICS) or leukotriene receptor antagonists (LTRA) for asthma control [14,15]. However, clinical research has shown that parental SES strongly impacts their offspring's quality of care and asthma control [16–18]. Among studies investigating SES and asthma pharmacotherapy, none have been done in children younger than age 5.

In this study we investigated whether parental income and education were associated with the risk of childhood asthma in a nationwide register-based cohort of preschool children. We also investigated whether parental income and education were associated with an inpatient or outpatient diagnosis and use of controller medications among all diagnosed children identified from the cohort.

Methods

The Swedish National Board of Health and Welfare holds a number of registers covering health information. The universal use of the Personal Identity Number (PIN), a unique identifier for each resident, enables unambiguous linkage between these registers and those covering socioeconomic information held by Statistics Sweden. We conducted a prospective population-based cohort study among children aged 0–4 years in Sweden, using data from the Medical Birth Register (MBR), the Multi-Generation Register (MGR), the National Patient Register (NPR), the Prescribed Drug Register (PDR), and the longitudinal integration database for health insurance and labour market studies (LISA by Swedish acronym), linked through each individual's unique PIN. The regional ethical review board in Stockholm, Sweden granted permission for the study and all individual's information was anonymized and de-identified prior to analysis.

Study design and participants

From the MBR (reporting more than 99% of all births in Sweden since 1973 [19]), we included all children born between 1 April 2006 and 31 December 2008 (n = 288,872) in the cohort; this ensured full coverage of dispensed medications for children since birth and their mothers' pregnancy period from the PDR (established on 1 July 2005). Fathers were linked to their children through the MGR. Children of parents who were born abroad and migrated to Sweden after 15 years of age were excluded from the study (n = 77,352, 26.8%) to ensure full information on highest attained level of education in Statistics Sweden. The children included in the study were followed from birth to 31 December 2010.

Measurements of socioeconomic status

Parental SES (annual disposable income and education) data were obtained from the LISA database at yearly intervals from the child's birth year. LISA includes all individuals 16 years and older living in Sweden and integrates labour market, educational and social sector data from several nationwide, annually updated registers. Firstly, parental SES was measured by annual disposable income, which includes individual net benefits after deduction of debits such as taxes, repaid study allowance, and paid maintenance support. The household level disposable incomes were summed up and adjusted for consumption weights [20] to calculate the disposable income per consumption unit, make it comparable for different family sizes and compositions, and converted to euros [21]. Annual disposable incomes per consumption unit were finally divided into quintiles. Secondly, parental SES was also measured by highest education attained within each couple and categorized as compulsory school (≤9 years of education), high school (10–12 years), some college (13–14 years), and college graduate or higher education (≥15 years).

Outcome measures

There are two common care-seeking pathways for asthma conditions, one of which is a primary care physician occasionally followed by referral to a hospital specialist and the other contact with a specialist directly depending on symptoms and availability. Incident asthma was defined either by diagnosis from the NPR, which covers more than 99% of all hospital discharges and about 80% of all outpatient specialist visits, or by filling two prescriptions for asthma medication from the PDR, which contains data on all

prescribed medication dispensed in Swedish pharmacies since 1 July 2005. Both asthma measures have been previously validated in population-based analyses [22]. From the NPR, asthma was ascertained if there was at least one hospital admission or outpatient department visit containing a primary diagnosis of asthma (code J45–46 according to the 10th version of the International Classification of Diseases (ICD-10)). The level of healthcare resource used at diagnosis was categorized as inpatient or outpatient care. Time to the next visit at inpatient care after the first diagnosis was measured as time from the first visit at inpatient (discharge date) or outpatient (visit date) care to the date of the next admission to in-patient care with an asthma diagnosis. From the PDR, incidence date of asthma medication was defined as the date of the first dispensed medication followed by at least one more record of any of the four anti-asthma medications within 24 months: ICS, β2 agonists, combination products or LTRA (identified by Anatomical Therapeutic Chemical (ATC) codes R03AC, R03AK, R03BA, and R03DC, respectively). The average daily dose was defined and categorized in each of three groups: ICS, β2-agonists, and LTRA. The combination products (R03AK) were split into both ICS and β2-agonists according to corresponding proportion of active ingredients. The daily dose of each type of medication was calculated as the total amount of active ingredients across all dispensed packages of this medication divided by number of days from the date of first asthma diagnosis to end of follow-up.

Covariates

Other independent variables included were the child's age, gender, number of children born in the family during the study period, metropolitan areas (Stockholm, Gothenburg, Malmö vs the rest of Sweden) and healthcare regions based on residential addresses at birth year (Stockholm-Gotland, Uppsala-Örebro, Northern, Western, Southeastern, and Southern Sweden), to account for shared healthcare resources between counties and regional differences of asthma prevalence. Maternal characteristics included were age at first antenatal care visit, marital status (single, married/cohabiting), maternal smoking during pregnancy (0, 1–9 or ≥10 cigarettes per day). Delivery characteristics included were preterm birth (≤37 weeks of gestational age), low birth weight (< 2,500 grams) and parity (first child or not first child). Maternal and delivery characteristics were retrieved from the MBR.

Statistical analyses

Cox proportional hazards regression was used for the following (yes/no) endpoints: asthma diagnosis, at least two dispensed asthma medications (since the first active prescription), an inpatient asthma diagnosis, and an outpatient asthma diagnosis. Observations were censored at the date of death, migration, or end of follow-up (31 Dec 2010). Parental income and education were modelled as time-dependent variables, with yearly updates. Cumulative hazards for childhood-onset asthma and SES indicators were estimated with the Nelson–Aalen method. In order to examine the independent and joint effects of each SES indicator on asthma outcomes, we performed all analyses with adjustment for one single indicator, mutual adjustment (education in models of income and income in models of education) and interaction terms for education and income. Wald test was used to test for interaction between education and income and between SES measures and preterm birth. Attained age was the underlying analysis time scale. The proportional hazards assumption was checked with a test based on the Schoenfeld residuals as well as graphical examination. When the proportional hazards assumption was violated for the exposure variables, time (age) dependent

Table 1. Study population and background characteristics related to childhood asthma (diagnosis and $> = 2$ medications) in a Swedish cohort of 211,520 children aged 0–4.5 years.

		All children born during 2006.04.01 –2008.12.31	Children with ≥1 asthma diagnosis	Children with ≥2 asthma medications within 2 years
N		211,520	13,990	22,520
Person-years at risk till end of follow-up			683,448	670,107
Child's characteristics		n (%)*		
Gender	Male	109,012 (51.5)	8,978 (64.2)	13,934 (61.9)
	Female	102,508 (48.5)	5,012 (35.8)	8,587 (38.1)
Age (end of follow-up or time at first event)*	Mean± SD	2.9±0.8	3.1±0.8	3.0±0.8
Preterm birth	Yes (≤37 weeks)	12,876 (6.1)	1,485 (10.6)	2,295 (10.2)
	No (>37 weeks)	198,534 (93.9)	12,500 (89.4)	20,211 (89.8)
	Missing	110 (0.1)	5 (0.0)	14 (0.1)
Low birth weight	Yes (<2,500 g)	8,801 (4.2)	977 (7.0)	1,598 (7.1)
	No (≥2,500 g)	202,438 (95.7)	12,989 (92.8)	20,884 (92.7)
	Missing	281 (0.1)	24 (0.2)	38 (0.2)
Parity	First	95,394 (45.1)	5,410 (38.7)	9,465 (42.0)
	Not first	116,126 (54.9)	8,580 (61.3)	13,055 (57.9)
Living in metropolitan areas at age 1	Yes	80,806 (38.2)	5,690 (40.7)	9,001 (40.0)
	No	129,153 (61.1)	8,282 (59.2)	13,494 (59.9)
	Missing	1,561 (0.7)	18 (0.1)	25 (0.1)
Healthcare regions	Stockholm-Gotland	46,571 (22.0)	3,584 (25.6)	5,563 (24.7)
	Uppsala-Örebro	49,586 (23.4)	2,836 (20.3)	4,465 (19.8)
	Southeast	22,456 (10.6)	1,294 (9.3)	2,408 (10.7)
	South	40,668 (19.2)	3,064 (21.9)	5,100 (22.7)
	West	35,873 (17.0)	2,220 (15.9)	3,424 (15.2)
	North	14,805 (7.0)	974 (7.0)	1,535 (6.8)
	Missing	1,561 (0.7)	18 (0.1)	25 (0.1)
Asthma medications (≥2 medications)	No	189,000 (89.4)	3,102 (22.2)	-
	Yes	22,520 (10.6)	10,888 (77.8)	-
Any asthma diagnosis (≥1 diagnosis)	No	197,530 (93.4)	-	11,632 (51.6)
	Yes	13,990 (6.6)	-	10,888 (48.4)
Family characteristics				
Annual disposable income per consumption unit at child birth	Lowest (≤13,942 EUR)	42,329 (20.0)	3,116 (22.3)	4,517 (20.1)
	Lower middle (13,942–16,725 EUR)	42,244 (20.0)	3,085 (22.1)	4,787 (21.3)
	Middle (16,725–19,490 EUR)	42,289 (20.0)	2,873 (20.5)	4,568 (20.3)
	Upper middle (19,490–23,750 EUR)	42,268 (20.0)	2,582 (18.5)	4,427 (19.6)
	Highest (>20,093 EUR)	42,269 (20.0)	2,332 (16.7)	4,216 (18.7)
	Missing	121 (0.0)	2 (0.0)	5 (0.0)
Income quintile changes during follow-up	Yes	135,755 (64.2)	9,281 (66.3)	14,770 (65.6)
	No	75,218 (35,6)	4,682 (33.5)	7,723 (34.3)
	Missing	547 (0.3)	27 (0.2)	27 (0.1)
Highest education between parents at child birth	Compulsory school	5,591 (2.6)	532 (3.8)	713 (3.2)
	High school	81,206 (38.4)	6,037 (43.2)	9,377 (41.7)
	Some college (<3 years)	28,903 (13.7)	1,817 (13.0)	2,956 (13.1)

Table 1. Cont.

		All children born during 2006.04.01 –2008.12.31	Children with ≥1 asthma diagnosis	Children with ≥2 asthma medications within 2 years
	College graduates or higher	95,630 (45,2)	5,597 (40.0)	9,462 (42.0)
	Missing	190 (0.1)	7 (0.1)	12 (0.1)
Education changes during follow-up	Yes	3,969 (1.9)	296 (2.1)	430 (1.9)
	No	206,935 (97.8)	13,660 (97.6)	22,056 (97.9)
	Missing	616 (0.3)	34 (0.2)	34 (0.2)
Maternal age at delivery*	Mean± SD	30.4±5.1	30.0±5.0	30.3±5.0
Mother's smoking during pregnancy	Not smoking	186,093 (88.0)	11,690 (83.6)	19,195 (85.2)
	1–9 cigarettes/day	10,651 (5.0)	1,049 (7.5)	1,456 (6.5)
	≥10 cigarettes/day	3,185 (1.5)	368 (2.6)	487 (2.2)
	Missing	11,591 (5.5)	883 (6.3)	1,382 (6.1)
Mother's marital status	Single	16,064 (7.6)	1,168 (8.4)	1,794 (8.0)
	Married or cohabiting	194,107 (91.8)	12,766 (91.3)	20.639 (91.7)
	Missing	1,349 (0.6)	56 (0.4)	87 (0.4)
Family history of asthma	Yes (either parent)	32,822 (15.5)	3,619 (25.9)	5,811 (25.8)
	No	178,698 (84.5)	10,371 (74.1)	16,709 (74.2)
Number of children born in the family during the study period	1	179,665 (84.9)	11,705 (83.7)	19,050 (84.6)
	2	30,983 (14.7)	2.198 (15,7)	3,347 (14.9)
	≥3	872 (0.4)	87 (0.6)	123 (0.5)

*n (%) indicated the frequency and percentage for relevant subgroups, unless otherwise specified.

hazard ratios (HR) were estimated. In the sub-cohort of children with at least one asthma diagnosis from NPR or at least 2 dispensed asthma medications regardless of diagnosis, the associations between parental income and education at the time of first diagnosis/medication and medication dosage, were analysed using linear regression with logarithmic transformed daily average dose of medication as outcome variables (among those with the corresponding medication). Children with at least one asthma diagnosis from NPR were further analysed using Cox regression model with parental income and education as time-dependent variables for the risk of a visit at inpatient care after a first diagnosis, with time from first inpatient/outpatient diagnosis as analysis time scale. Directed acyclic graph was used to determine potential confounders for different models [23]. For all regression analyses we presented the estimates adjusted for child's gender, parity, maternal age and marital status during pregnancy, healthcare regions, and metropolitan areas. We also fitted models with further adjustment for maternal smoking during pregnancy, low birth weight, and preterm birth. Analyses of parental SES and next visit at inpatient care after first diagnosis as well as of parental SES and average doses of controller medications were further adjusted for levels of healthcare use at previous hospital visit. Sensitivity analysis was performed for severe asthma defined as ≥3 medications within 12 months. As some families contribute more than one child, robust standard errors were used to account for family clustering. The measures of associations presented were hazard ratios (HR) for Cox regression models and exp(β) for linear regression models on log transformed data together with 95%

confidence intervals (CI). Stata 12.0 was used for all analyses and a 5% significance level.

Results

Table 1 shows characteristics at birth and follow-up in the full cohort of 211,520 children and among those diagnosed with asthma. The average person-years at risk were 3.2 in the study population. The cumulative incidence of an asthma diagnosis was 6.6% during the study period and that of having at least two dispensed asthma medications was 10.6%. Mean annual disposable income at child birth was 192,436 SEK (20,169 EUR, 2010 annual exchange rate). There were 2.6% of households that had compulsory schooling as their highest education, 38.4% had high school, 13.7% had some college and 45.2% had completed college or a higher level of education. Children diagnosed with asthma were more often male, born preterm or with low birth weight and had more often been exposed to maternal smoking during pregnancy.

Figure 1 displays the association between current parental SES and childhood-onset asthma. The proportional hazard assumption did not hold for either asthma definitions (p<0.001). Therefore, we estimated separate effects for the first year of life and the time after the first year for both asthma definitions. During a child's first year of life, those from the lowest compared to the highest income families were more likely to be diagnosed with asthma (fully adjusted HR 1.19, 95% CI 1.09–1.31) or to dispense ≥2 asthma medications (HR 1.17, 95% CI 1.08–1.26). This association turned negative after the first year of life for lowest income families

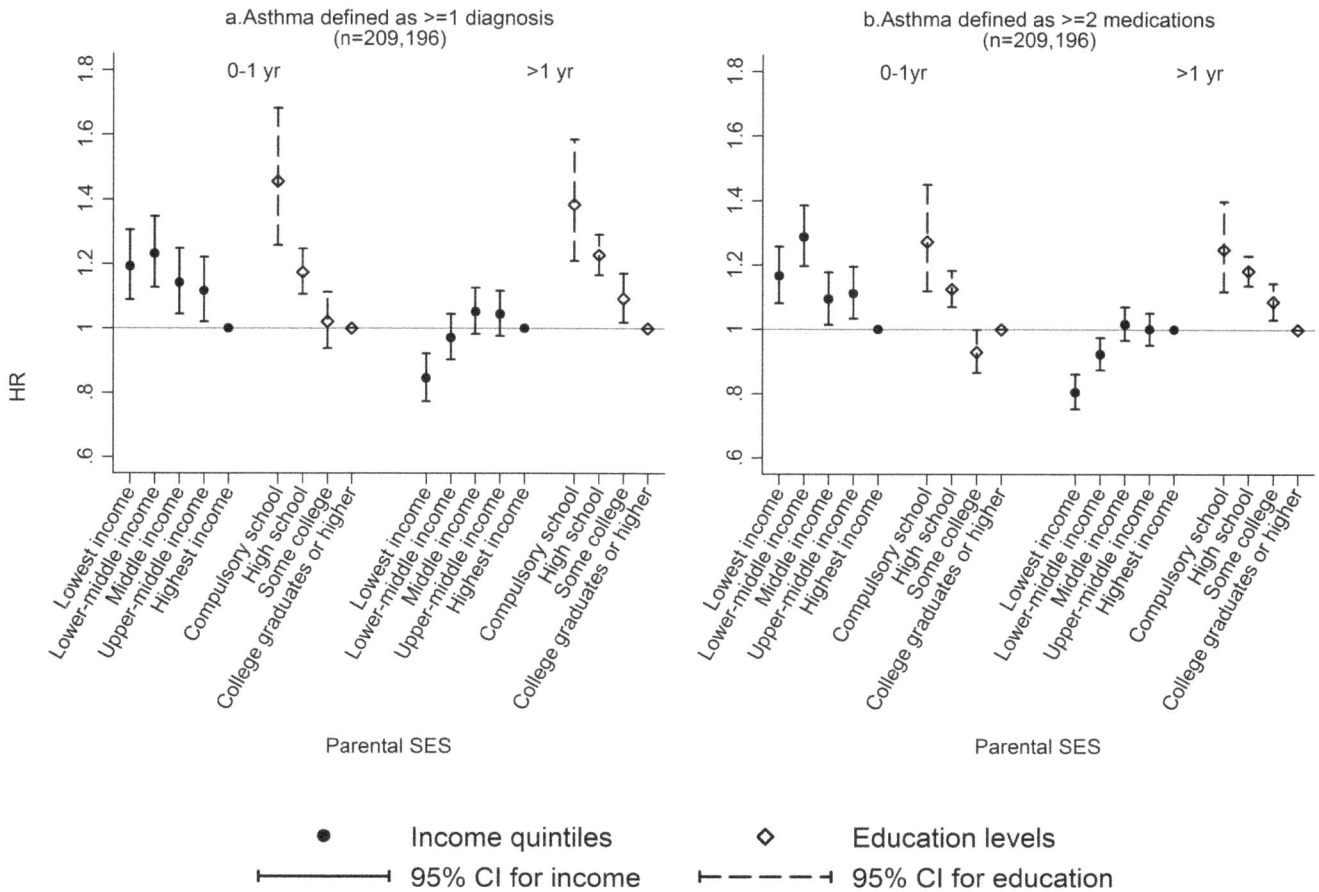

Figure 1. Hazard ratios of childhood-onset asthma by parental SES. Association between parental SES (income and education) and childhood-onset asthma (diagnosis or ≥2 medications) in first year of life and up to 4.5 years.

compared to the highest (fully adjusted HR 0.84, 95% CI 0.77–0.92 for diagnosis, and HR 0.80, 95% CI 0.74–0.86 for medications, both p-values for trend <0.001). Furthermore, children from the lowest compared to the highest educated families were consistently at increased risk of asthma, independent of definition and regardless of age (fully adjusted HR 1.46, 95% CI 1.26–1.68 for children up to 1 year of age and HR 1.39, 95% CI 1.21–1.59 for children aged one or older for asthma diagnosis, all p-values for trend <0.001).

The cumulative hazards curves for asthma defined as ≥1 diagnosis and as ≥2 prescriptions by income groups (Figure 2 a–b) show that the children in the lowest income group get diagnosis and medications earlier than the others, with a catch up by other income groups around the age of 4 years. Regarding parental education levels (Figure 2 c–d) the initial differences on asthma incidence between SES groups are preserved throughout the follow up. Estimates were similar with adjustment for maternal smoking during pregnancy, low birth weight and preterm birth and there was no effect modification through preterm birth. Risk estimates were also similar for severe asthma defined as ≥3 filled prescriptions within 12 months (data not tabulated). There was no interaction between income and education (lowest p = 0.50).

Figure 3 shows the association between parental SES and risk of receiving an inpatient or outpatient asthma diagnosis. There was no difference in the risk of receiving an inpatient or outpatient diagnosis for children from the lowest income group compared to

the highest income group. For parental education, the finding was consistent for both inpatient and outpatient diagnoses, with increased risk of an asthma diagnosis in inpatient care (adjusted HR 2.07, 95% CI 1.61–2.65) as well as outpatient care (adjusted HR 1.32, 95% CI 1.18–1.47) for the lowest education group, compared to the highest education group (both p-values for trend <0.001). There was no effect of parental income or education on risk of a next visit at inpatient care after first diagnosis (results not shown).

Table 2 displays dispensed asthma medications by parental SES among children diagnosed with asthma. Overall, 1,349 out of the 13,990 (9.6%) diagnosed children had not had any dispensed asthma medication since their first asthma diagnosis from NPR, with the highest percentages in the highest income (11.3%) and lowest education groups (9.8%). The percentages of diagnosed patients that had filled prescriptions of ICS and β2-agonists were slightly over 60% and 80%. Around one fifth of diagnosed patients had dispensed medications of LTRA and 2% had combination products. Figure 4 graphically depicts the association between parental SES and average daily doses of different asthma medications among children diagnosed with asthma and children with at least 2 dispensed prescriptions of asthma medications. There was no statistically significant effect of income on average dose of dispensed asthma medication. However, children from less educated families had lower daily doses of dispensed ICS and LTRA, compared to those from the most educated families

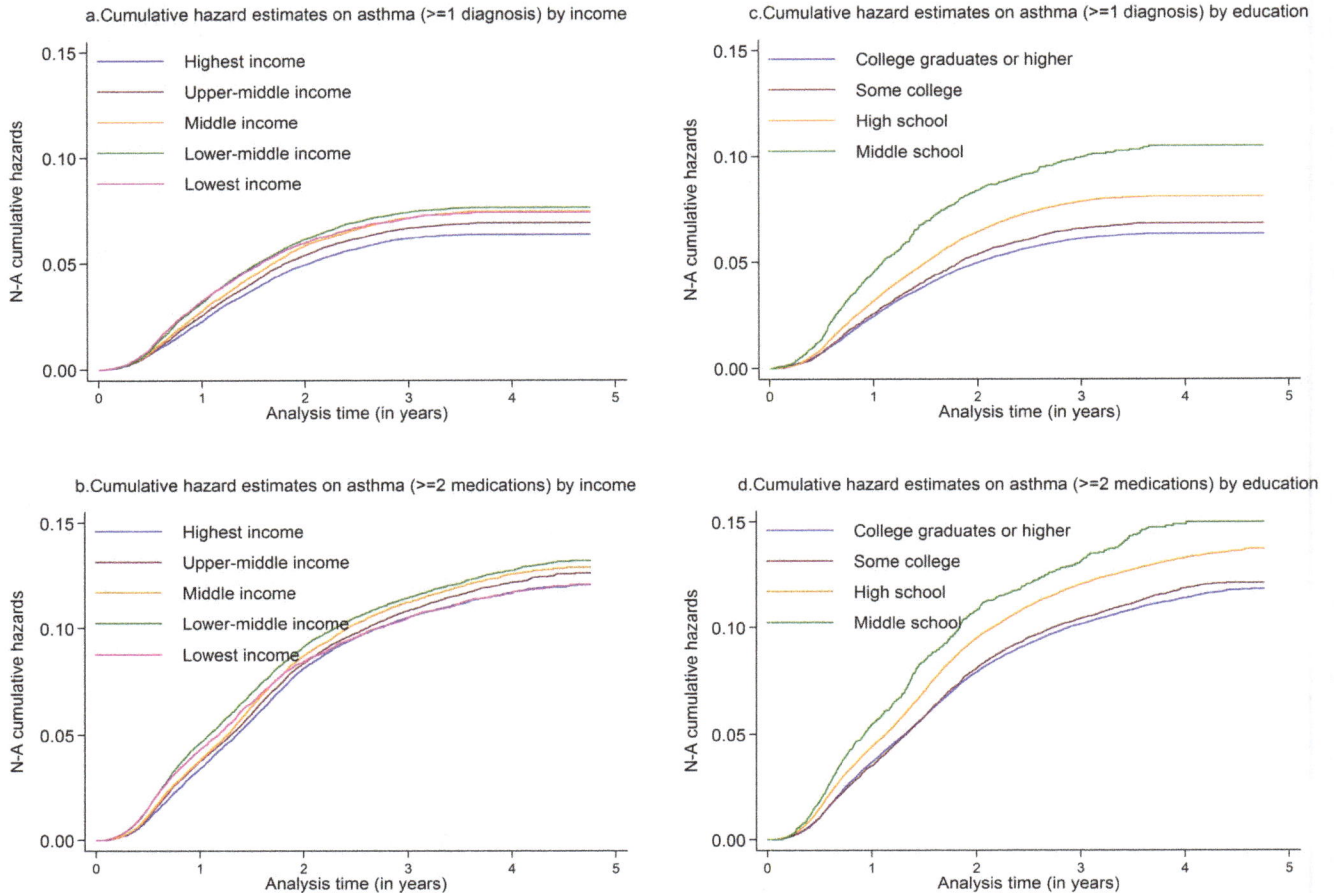

Figure 2. Cumulative hazards of childhood-onset asthma by parental SES. Cumulative hazards of childhood asthma (diagnosis and ≥2 medications) in different SES groups (parental income and education). Estimates adjusted for gender, parity, maternal age, marital status at delivery, healthcare regions, and metropolitan areas.

(college degree or higher). For example, the average (geometric mean) daily dose of ICS was 15% lower (exp(β) = 1.15, p-value for trend = 0.002) in the compulsory school groups compared to children of college graduates, while there was no difference in average daily dose of β2- agonists. Furthermore, among children with at least 2 dispensed medications, the average doses of ICS tended to be lower in families with lower parental education background after adjusting for individual β2- agonist use and diagnostic status (p-value for trend <0.001).

Discussion

In this population-based cohort of 211,520 pre-school children, the study results support our hypotheses that there is an association between parental SES and childhood asthma occurrence, level of healthcare use at diagnosis and pattern of medication usage. Interestingly, parental income and education seem to affect asthma outcomes in different ways. Firstly, children from families with lower income or education had higher incidence rates of asthma measured by specialist diagnosis or medication. However, there was a lower incidence in the lowest income group after one year of age, to such an extent that there was a catch-up by the other groups. Secondly, those in families from the lowest education group had an increased risk of in- and outpatient asthma diagnosis and asthma medication. Finally, lower amounts of controller

medications were dispensed for children from families with lower parental education.

Although the effect of SES on the development of childhood asthma has been observed in hospital-based and other epidemiological studies [7,24,25], asthma diagnosis and medications in relation to age, income and/or education in the general population have not been previously characterized. Reviews conducted by Mielck et al [26] and Rona et al [27] have demonstrated inconsistent findings on the association between SES and childhood asthma overall. However, more recent findings focusing on children at preschool age [8,9,28–33] showed that those from low SES familial background are more likely to develop asthma, which is partially in line with our result.

Based on our finding on the association between different SES indicators and incident asthma, one possibility is that parental healthcare seeking behaviour, i.e. the income gradient of parents' request for diagnosis and treatment, differs between the first year of life and later in childhood. Halldórsson et al. found no difference in using primary healthcare for children above 2 years of age, but less specialist care and more inpatient care for those from the lowest income group [34]. Another recent study from Eastern Sweden showed that low-income families received equal child health services from birth until 4 years of age [35]. Thus, the age-varying effect on income in our study remains a challenge

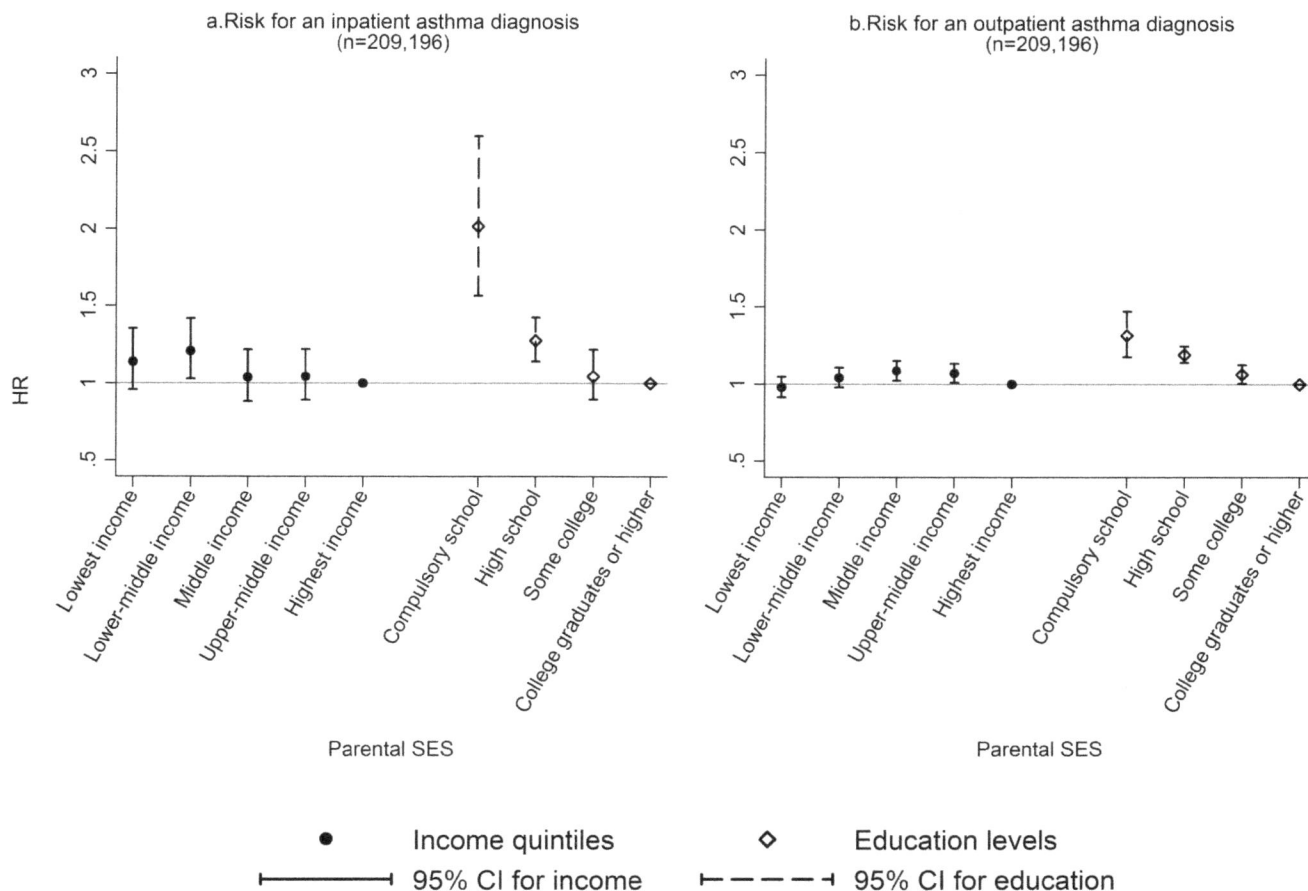

Figure 3. Hazard ratios of inpatient and outpatient asthma diagnosis by parental SES. Hazard ratios and 95% confidence intervals for the association between parental SES (income and education) and inpatient or outpatient asthma diagnoses. The estimates have been adjusted for gender, parity, maternal age, marital status at delivery, healthcare regions, and metropolitan areas.

Table 2. Frequency of medications consumptions among diagnosed children from different SES groups (parental income and education at diagnosis) from date of first diagnosis of asthma in a Swedish cohort of 211,520 children age 0–4.5.

SES	Number of patients	No. (%) of ICS	No. (%) of β2-agonists	No. (%) of LTRA	No. (%) of Combination products	No. (%) of no medications at all
Income						
Lowest	2,235	2,004 (64.3)	2,583 (82.9)	661 (21.2)	83 (2.7)	265 (8.5)
Lower-middle	2,980	2,744 (67.7)	2,583 (83.7)	690 (22.4)	86 (2.8)	229 (7.4)
Middle	3,095	1,972 (68.6)	2,430 (84.6)	640 (22.3)	74 (2.6)	247 (8.6)
Upper-middle	2,952	1,781 (69.0)	2,162 (83.7)	591 (22.9)	52 (2.0)	251 (9.7)
Highest	2,720	1,515 (65.0)	1,918 (82.3)	521 (22.3)	46 (2.0)	264 (11.3)
Total	13,990	9,360	11,678	3,103	341	1,349
Education						
Compulsory school	508	309 (58.1)	436 (82.0)	111 (20.9)	11 (2.1)	52 (9.8)
High school	6,021	3,970 (65.8)	5,050 (83.7)	1,331 (22.0)	156 (2.6)	495 (8.2)
Some college	1,808	1,224 (67.4)	1,504 (83.6)	379 (20.9)	54 (3.0)	175 (9.6)
College graduate or higher	5,640	3,853 (68.8)	4,681 (83.6)	1,280 (22.9)	119 (2.1)	534 (9.5)
Total	13,990	9,360	11,678	3,103	341	1,256

Definition of abbreviations: SES = socioeconomic status; ICS = inhaled corticosteroids; LTRA = leukotriene receptor antagonist.

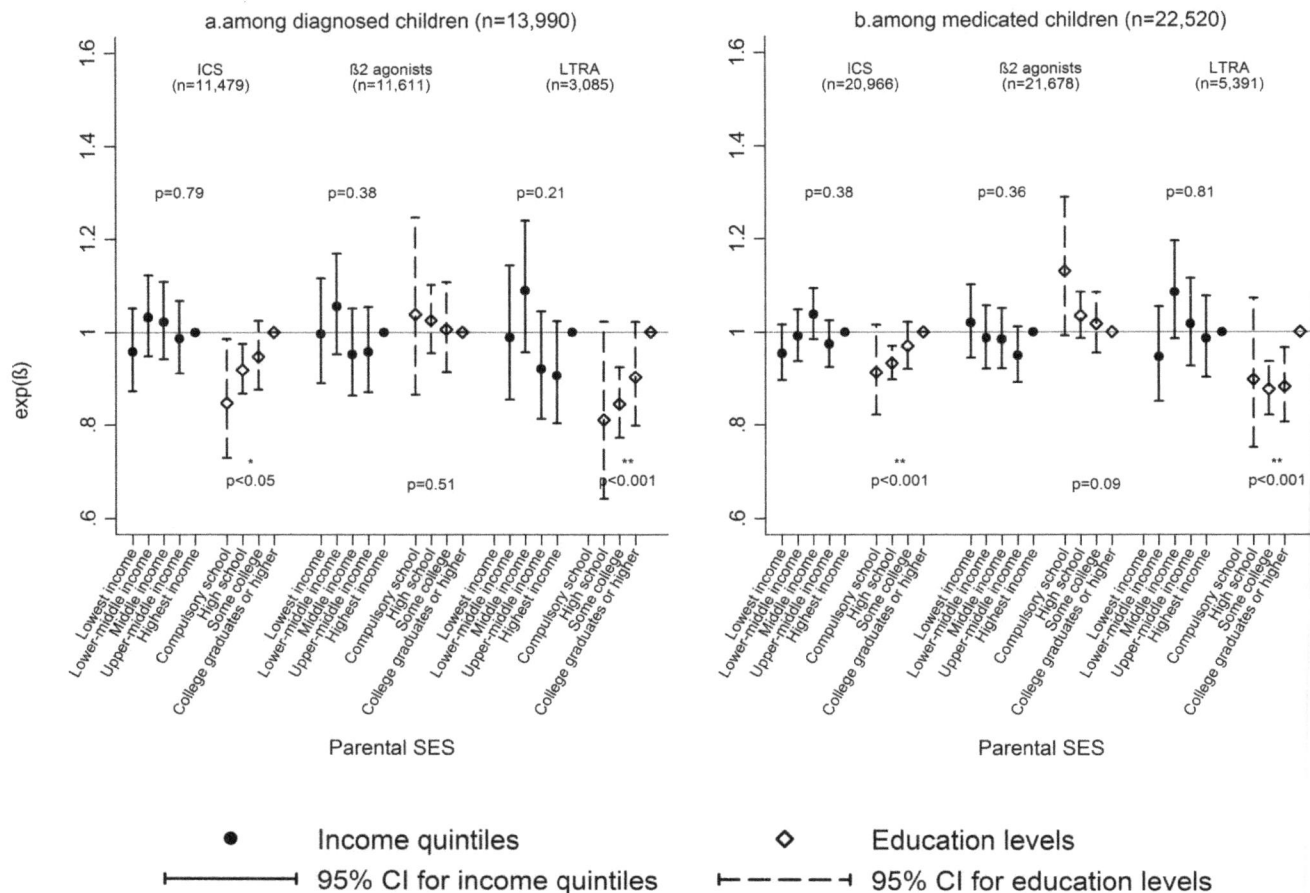

Figure 4. Average doses of asthma medications by parental SES. Average doses (log transformed) of asthma medications (ICS, b-agonists and LTRA) predicted by parental SES (income and education) in the group of children with asthma (diagnosis or ≥2 medications). Estimates in 4a have been adjusted for child age, gender, parity, maternal age, marital status at delivery, healthcare regions, metropolitan areas and those in 4b have been additionally adjusted for asthma diagnosis (yes/no).

because of lacking information on parental choice of healthcare-related cost over time.

Furthermore, as consistent with previous literature [36,37], our data support the hypothesis that there was an effect of parental education level on asthma diagnosis and medication use among preschool children. However, the question remains why children of more educated parents have less asthma. Admittedly, the mechanism of association has been hypothesized to involve multidimensional factors and only a small part of the education gradient could be attributed to years of parental schooling alone. Despite factors that we controlled for, there are still other potential covariates that are difficult to measure including life style (e.g. breastfeeding) [38] and health literacy [39] in this total population.

Our results also indicated an effect of lower parental income and education on level of healthcare use at asthma diagnosis. This may reflect a tendency for less advantaged groups to seek care at emergency units due to parental stress and need of healthcare services [34,40], while more advantaged groups may be more prone to have an established relation with a general practitioner or a private outpatient specialist, which is not recorded in the NPR. On the other hand, it is also possible that groups with lower parental education and income are more often admitted to hospital due to their offspring's symptoms and severity at the first occasion they seek healthcare [41]. Additional analyses, however,

did not support any evidence of disparities for a next visit at inpatient care after first diagnosis.

Among children with diagnosed asthma, we found that parental income did not have any influence on average daily doses of all types of medications, which was in contrast to previous findings [16,42]. This could be due to the equity-promoting medication benefits in Sweden: pharmaceutical expenses for all children under 18 years old are fully reimbursed over a total annual cost of 189 EURO per family [43]. However, there was a worrisome association between parental education and dispenses of controller medications. Less ICS and LTRA were consumed by children in families with lower parental education background, and dispenses of ICS were even lower when adjusting for use of quick-relief medication (for those with confirmed diagnosis and/or at least 2 dispensed medications in whom they should be strongly indicated). Established asthma guidelines [15] and patient education on the importance of adherence to controller medications in young children should be provided and followed up by both clinicians and parents, in order to reduce asthma exacerbation and avoidable healthcare costs. A recent review on adherence to paediatric asthma treatment indicates inconsistent result on non-adherence with familial socioeconomic indicators [44]. However, we did not have access to issued prescription records but only dispensed medications so we were not able to compare the degree of non-adherence through the rate of proper information, prescriptions' initiating, filling or usage.

The present study is the first to show an association between parental SES and asthma medication purchases for children in a general population. By using register based information on filled prescriptions in pharmacy and diagnosis records from inpatient and outpatient care, we obtained objective measurements on childhood asthma occurrence, healthcare resource usage, and quantities of medication consumption [45]. We also collected register based information on SES and potential confounders, which preclude recall bias.

The current study also has limitations. Firstly, using the NPR for ascertainment of asthma diagnoses has its drawback on differentiating asthma from transient wheezing in preschool children and missing information on children diagnosed in the primary care setting. Instead, we added the alternative definition on dispensed asthma medication as an additional proxy of asthma [22]. However, we cannot rule out the potential misclassification on asthma and bronchitis/bronchiolitis by measuring asthma medications. Secondly, children of parents who were born abroad and migrated to Sweden after 15 years of age were excluded, since their parental education levels may be underestimated systematically from the register. Thus, the results of this study may not apply to these groups of immigrant families in Sweden. Thirdly, parents with illicit working conditions or tax evasion (estimated to 6%) would result in underestimation of income [46], and

consequently some of those would be wrongly classified into lower quintiles and we might not capture their actual income.

In conclusion, our population-based study shows that there is an increased risk of early childhood asthma diagnosis among families with lower income and education. Even though it appears that liberal prescription drug benefits in Sweden promote equal use of total medications between lower and higher SES families, the fact that lower SES families dispense fewer of the controller medications and are more often hospitalized at first diagnosis suggests obstacles more subtle than simply cost. The findings call for improved clinical measures to reach all young children in early stage of asthma development. Such approaches might include information and well maintained surveillance of asthma control therapy, asthma severity assessment and improved adherence to international guidelines targeted especially towards groups with lower SES over a long period.

Acknowledgments

Christina Norrby and Marcus Boman have contributed with excellent database managing. Valuable dialogue with Sandra Ganrud Tedner, Anne Örtqvist and Vilhelmina Ullemar has enriched this work.

Author Contributions

Conceived and designed the experiments: TG CL GR CM CA. Analyzed the data: TG CL GR CA. Contributed reagents/materials/analysis tools: CL GR CM NL CA. Wrote the paper: TG CL GR CM NL CA.

References

1. Fleming L, Wilson N, Bush A (2007) Difficult to control asthma in children. Current opinion in allergy and clinical immunology 7: 190–195.
2. Braman SS (2006) The global burden of asthma. Chest 130: 4S–12S.
3. Asher MI, Montefort S, Bjorksten B, Lai CK, Strachan DP, et al. (2006) Worldwide time trends in the prevalence of symptoms of asthma, allergic rhinoconjunctivitis, and eczema in childhood: ISAAC Phases One and Three repeat multicountry cross-sectional surveys. Lancet 368: 733–743.
4. Martel MJ, Rey E, Malo JL, Perreault S, Beauchesne MF, et al. (2009) Determinants of the incidence of childhood asthma: a two-stage case-control study. American journal of epidemiology 169: 195–205.
5. Melen E, Wickman M, Nordvall SL, van Hage-Hamsten M, Lindfors A (2001) Influence of early and current environmental exposure factors on sensitization and outcome of asthma in pre-school children. Allergy 56: 646–652.
6. Braun-Fahrlander C, Riedler J, Herz U, Eder W, Waser M, et al. (2002) Environmental exposure to endotoxin and its relation to asthma in school-age children. The New England journal of medicine 347: 869–877.
7. Kozyrskyj AL, Kendall GE, Jacoby P, Sly PD, Zubrick SR (2010) Association between socioeconomic status and the development of asthma: analyses of income trajectories. American journal of public health 100: 540–546.
8. Lindbaek M, Wefring KW, Grangard EH, Ovsthus K (2003) Socioeconomical conditions as risk factors for bronchial asthma in children aged 4–5 yrs. The European respiratory journal 21: 105–108.
9. Almqvist C, Pershagen G, Wickman M (2005) Low socioeconomic status as a risk factor for asthma, rhinitis and sensitization at 4 years in a birth cohort. Clinical and experimental allergy: journal of the British Society for Allergy and Clinical Immunology 35: 612–618.
10. Poyser MA, Nelson H, Ehrlich RI, Bateman ED, Parnell S, et al. (2002) Socioeconomic deprivation and asthma prevalence and severity in young adolescents. The European respiratory journal: official journal of the European Society for Clinical Respiratory Physiology 19: 892–898.
11. Hancox RJ, Milne BJ, Taylor DR, Greene JM, Cowan JO, et al. (2004) Relationship between socioeconomic status and asthma: a longitudinal cohort study. Thorax 59: 376–380.
12. Mitchell EA, Stewart AW, Pattemore PK, Asher MI, Harrison AC, et al. (1989) Socioeconomic status in childhood asthma. International journal of epidemiology 18: 888–890.
13. Braveman PA, Cubbin C, Egerter S, Chideya S, Marchi KS, et al. (2005) Socioeconomic status in health research: one size does not fit all. JAMA: the journal of the American Medical Association 294: 2879–2888.
14. Bateman ED, Hurd SS, Barnes PJ, Bousquet J, Drazen JM, et al. (2008) Global strategy for asthma management and prevention: GINA executive summary. The European respiratory journal: official journal of the European Society for Clinical Respiratory Physiology 31: 143–178.
15. Socialstyrelsen (2004) The guidelines for the care of asthma and chronic obstructive pulmonary disease by the Swedish National Board of Health and Social Welfare. Available: http://www.socialstyrelsen.se/Lists/Artikelkatalog/Attachments/10272/2004-102-6_20041027.pdf. Accessed 08 June 2014.
16. Bloomberg GR, Banister C, Sterkel R, Epstein J, Bruns J, et al. (2009) Socioeconomic, family, and pediatric practice factors that affect level of asthma control. Pediatrics 123: 829–835.
17. Fiks AG, Localio AR, Alessandrini EA, Asch DA, Guevara JP (2010) Shared decision-making in pediatrics: a national perspective. Pediatrics 126: 306–314.
18. Morse RB, Hall M, Fieldston ES, McGwire G, Anspacher M, et al. (2011) Hospital-level compliance with asthma care quality measures at children's hospitals and subsequent asthma-related outcomes. JAMA: the journal of the American Medical Association 306: 1454–1460.
19. Socialstyrelsen (2005). The Medical Birth Register 2003. Available: http://www.socialstyrelsen.se/Lists/Artikelkatalog/Attachments/10204/2005-42-4_2005424.pdf. Accessed 20 July 2012.
20. Disposable income per consumption weight for household aged 20–64 years by type in 2010. Statistics Sweden. Available: http://www.scb.se/Pages/ThematicAreaTableAndChart____334774.aspx. Accessed 30 November 2012.
21. Riksbanken. Annual avarage exchange rates (aggregate). Available: http://www.riksbank.se/en/Interest-and-exchange-rates/Annual-aggregate-Exchange-rates/. Accessed 22 July 2012.
22. Ortqvist AK, Lundholm C, Wettermark B, Ludvigsson JF, Ye W, et al. (2013) Validation of asthma and eczema in population-based Swedish drug and patient registers. Pharmacoepidemiology and drug safety 22: 850–860.
23. Greenland S, Pearl J, Robins JM (1999) Causal diagrams for epidemiologic research. Epidemiology 10: 37–48.
24. To T, Wang C, Guan J, McLimont S, Gershon AS (2010) What is the lifetime risk of physician-diagnosed asthma in Ontario, Canada? American journal of respiratory and critical care medicine 181: 337–343.
25. Braback L, Hjern A, Rasmussen F (2005) Social class in asthma and allergic rhinitis: a national cohort study over three decades. The European respiratory journal 26: 1064–1068.
26. Mielck A, Reitmeir P, Wjst M (1996) Severity of childhood asthma by socioeconomic status. International journal of epidemiology 25: 388–393.
27. Rona RJ (2000) Asthma and poverty. Thorax 55: 239–244.
28. Seguin L, Xu Q, Gauvin L, Zunzunegui MV, Potvin L, et al. (2005) Understanding the dimensions of socioeconomic status that influence toddlers' health: unique impact of lack of money for basic needs in Quebec's birth cohort. Journal of epidemiology and community health 59: 42–48.
29. Seguin L, Nikiema B, Gauvin L, Zunzunegui MV, Xu Q (2007) Duration of poverty and child health in the Quebec Longitudinal Study of Child Development: longitudinal analysis of a birth cohort. Pediatrics 119: e1063–1070.
30. Crighton EJ, Wilson K, Senecal S (2010) The relationship between socio-economic and geographic factors and asthma among Canada's Aboriginal populations. International journal of circumpolar health 69: 138–150.

31. Midodzi WK, Rowe BH, Majaesic CM, Saunders LD, Senthilselvan A (2010) Early life factors associated with incidence of physician-diagnosed asthma in preschool children: results from the Canadian Early Childhood Development cohort study. The Journal of asthma: official journal of the Association for the Care of Asthma 47: 7–13.

32. Hafkamp-de Groen E, van Rossem L, de Jongste JC, Mohangoo AD, Moll HA, et al. (2012) The role of prenatal, perinatal and postnatal factors in the explanation of socioeconomic inequalities in preschool asthma symptoms: the Generation R Study. Journal of epidemiology and community health 66: 1017–1024.

33. Violato M, Petrou S, Gray R (2009) The relationship between household income and childhood respiratory health in the United Kingdom. Social science & medicine 69: 955–963.

34. Halldorsson M, Kunst AE, Kohler L, Mackenbach JP (2002) Socioeconomic differences in children's use of physician services in the Nordic countries. Journal of epidemiology and community health 56: 200–204.

35. Wallby T, Hjern A (2011) Child health care uptake among low-income and immigrant families in a Swedish county. Acta paediatrica 100: 1495–1503.

36. Spencer N (2005) Maternal education, lone parenthood, material hardship, maternal smoking, and longstanding respiratory problems in childhood: testing a hierarchical conceptual framework. Journal of epidemiology and community health 59: 842–846.

37. Cesaroni G, Farchi S, Davoli M, Forastiere F, Perucci CA (2003) Individual and area-based indicators of socioeconomic status and childhood asthma. The European respiratory journal: official journal of the European Society for Clinical Respiratory Physiology 22: 619–624.

38. Kull I, Wickman M, Lilja G, Nordvall SL, Pershagen G (2002) Breast feeding and allergic diseases in infants-a prospective birth cohort study. Archives of disease in childhood 87: 478–481.

39. Curtis LM, Wolf MS, Weiss KB, Grammer LC (2012) The impact of health literacy and socioeconomic status on asthma disparities. The Journal of asthma: official journal of the Association for the Care of Asthma 49: 178–183.

40. Mangrio E, Hansen K, Lindstrom M, Kohler M, Rosvall M (2011) Maternal educational level, parental preventive behavior, risk behavior, social support and medical care consumption in 8-month-old children in Malmo, Sweden. BMC public health 11: 891.

41. Fergusson DM, Horwood LJ, Shannon FT (1986) Social and family factors in childhood hospital admission. Journal of epidemiology and community health 40: 50–58.

42. Ungar WJ, Paterson JM, Gomes T, Bikangaga P, Gold M, et al. (2011) Relationship of asthma management, socioeconomic status, and medication insurance characteristics to exacerbation frequency in children with asthma. Annals of allergy, asthma & immunology: official publication of the American College of Allergy, Asthma, & Immunology 106: 17–23.

43. The Dental and Pharmaceutical Benefits Agency (2007) The Swedish Pharmaceutical Reimbursement System. Available: http://www.tlv.se/Upload/English/ENG-swe-pharma-reimbursement-system.pdf. Accessed 01 June 2014.

44. Drotar D, Bonner MS (2009) Influences on adherence to pediatric asthma treatment: a review of correlates and predictors. Journal of developmental and behavioral pediatrics: JDBP 30: 574–582.

45. Osterberg L, Blaschke T (2005) Adherence to medication. The New England journal of medicine 353: 487–497.

46. (2012) Taxes in Sweden: An English Summary of Tax Statistical Yearbook of Sweden.. Swedish Tax Agency.

17

Caregivers' Health Literacy and Gaps in Children's Medicaid Enrollment: Findings from the Carolina Oral Health Literacy Study

Jessica Y. Lee[1,2]*, Kimon Divaris[1,3], Darren A. DeWalt[4], A. Diane Baker[1], Ziya Gizlice[5], R. Gary Rozier[2], William F. Vann, Jr.[1]

1 Department of Pediatric Dentistry, School of Dentistry, University of North Carolina at Chapel Hill, Chapel Hill, NC, United States of America, 2 Department of Health Policy and Management, UNC Gillings School of Global Public Health, University of North Carolina at Chapel Hill, Chapel Hill, NC, United States of America, 3 Department of Epidemiology, UNC Gillings School of Global Public Health, University of North Carolina at Chapel Hill, Chapel Hill, NC, United States of America, 4 School of Medicine and Cecil G. Sheps Center for Health Services Research, University of North Carolina at Chapel Hill, Chapel Hill, NC, United States of America, 5 Center for Health Promotion and Disease Prevention, University of North Carolina at Chapel Hill, Chapel Hill, NC, United States of America

Abstract

Background and Objectives: Recent evidence supports a link between caregivers' health literacy and their children's health and use of health services. Disruptions in children's health insurance coverage have been linked to poor health care and outcomes. We examined young children's Medicaid enrollment patterns in a well-characterized cohort of child/caregivers dyads and investigated the association of caregivers' low health literacy with the incidence of enrollment gaps.

Methods: We relied upon Medicaid enrollment data for 1208 children (mean age = 19 months) enrolled in the Carolina Oral Health Literacy project during 2008–09. The median follow-up was 25 months. Health literacy was measured using the Newest Vital Sign (NVS). Analyses relied on descriptive, bivariate, and multivariate methods based on Poisson modeling.

Findings: One-third of children experienced one or more enrollment gaps; most were short in duration (median = 5 months). The risk of gaps was inversely associated with caregivers' age, with a 2% relative risk decrease for each added year. Low health literacy was associated with a modestly elevated risk increase [Incidence Rate Ratio (IRR) = 1.17 (95% confidence interval (CI) 0.88–1.57)] for enrollment disruptions; however, this estimate was substantially elevated among caregivers with less than a high school education [IRR = 1.52 (95% CI 0.99–2.35); homogeneity p<0.2].

Conclusions: Our findings provide initial support for a possible role of caregivers' health literacy as a determinant of children's Medicaid enrollment gaps. Although the association between health literacy and enrollment gaps was not confirmed statistically, we found that it was markedly stronger among caregivers with low educational attainment. This population, as well as young caregivers, may be the most vulnerable to the negative effects of low health literacy.

Editor: Gozde Ozakinci, University of St Andrews, United Kingdom

Funding: The Carolina Oral Health Literacy Study is supported by a grant from the National Institute of Dental and Craniofacial Research of the National Institutes of Health (RO1DE018045). The funders had no role in study design, data collection and analysis, decision to publish, or preparation of the manuscript.

Competing Interests: The authors have declared that no competing interests exist.

* Email: Jessica_Lee@unc.edu

Introduction

Health Insurance Coverage Affects Appropriate Health Care during the First Years of Life

Children's health insurance coverage is a major determinant of preventive and continuous health care [1–3]. Low-income children enrolled in Medicaid are more likely to receive timely preventive care, including well-child visits, compared with their counterparts without insurance coverage [4–8]. Nationally representative US data confirm that being uninsured is associated with low levels of adherence to professional recommendations for well-child visits, with the lowest rates found among children eligible but not enrolled in public insurance [9]. This is an important observation because well-child visits and preventive care during the first years of life have demonstrable benefits [10–12]. Similarly, continuity of care has been linked to favorable health outcomes, including lower emergency department utilization [13]. These observations are aligned with the concept of a 'medical home' which, according to the American Academy of Pediatrics, encompasses the characteristics of pediatric care considered essential for all children" and is defined as a "model of primary care that is accessible, continuous, comprehensive, family-centered, coordinated, compassionate, and culturally effective" [14–15].

Current legislation supports the expansion in Medicaid coverage in 2014 [16] and has the potential to benefit a large and vulnerable component of the US population. Insurance coverage is an important enabling factor for health care use overall and its absence leads to under-utilization and unmet medical needs [8]; however, its availability is not sufficient for enrollment or the establishment of a medical home [10]. To affect health outcomes, the expansion of coverage must be met with adequate enrollment.

To What Extent are Disruptions in Health Insurance Detrimental for Children?

Current evidence demonstrates that disruptions ("gaps") in coverage are likely to decrease both access to a medical home and the likelihood of seeking routine care for young children [17–19]. A 2006 report [20] found that between 18–36% of children in four states had insurance gaps over a period of up to 2 years. Other recent studies confirmed that insurance gaps may be frequent, with 25% of children experiencing a gap in Medicaid enrollment over a 12-month period in Oregon [17], and 14–61% of children in five other states experiencing similar gaps over a 4-year period [21]. Because of its frequency and negative effects, unstable health insurance coverage is a phenomenon that needs further investigation as a risk factor for children's health [2,22–23].

What is known about the Correlates of Health Insurance Enrollment Gaps?

State Medicaid programs have a compelling interest in enrolling and maintaining coverage for eligible children but there is a paucity of evidence to inform policy makers on relevant strategies and best practices to accomplish these goals [24]. Although state programs strive to keep enrollment and renewal procedures simple, most reports on enrollment gaps implicate caregiver-related factors. For example, studies by DeVoe et al. [17] and Satchell and Pati [22] relied upon nationally representative data and found that poverty and maternal education were the strongest correlates of enrollment gaps. Gaps may be attributed to changes in family circumstances that render parents and children ineligible; nevertheless, caregivers' difficulty in navigating the complex administrative processes can also explain why those eligible for public or private insurance are challenged to enroll and maintain enrollment. The challenges of the required forms and paperwork are well-documented [20,25–26]. As one example, recent findings indicate that Medicaid enrollment forms may be excessively demanding to read and comprehend [27]; in fact, most states fail to meet their self-established readability criteria [28].

The Role of Health Literacy

A recent report [29] identified low health literacy as a risk factor for lack of adult health insurance and outlined the direct implications for the anticipated Medicaid expansion and implementation under the Affordable Care Act (ACA). Several studies have documented an association between caregiver health literacy and child health and services' use [30–33]. Health literacy's relationship to Medicaid enrollment gaps may offer one potential explanation of the relationship between parental health literacy and child health outcomes. To the best of our knowledge, no data exist to date regarding the possible association between caregivers' health literacy and gaps in their children's public health insurance enrollment. Our aims were to 1) describe and characterize gaps in Medicaid enrollment of young, low-income children of English-speaking families in North Carolina, and 2) identify caregiver factors associated with this phenomenon, including health literacy.

Methods

Ethics statement

Written consent and HIPPA approval were obtained by all participants and the study was approved by the Biomedical Institutional Review Board at the University of North Carolina-Chapel Hill (approval #07-0837).

Parent study sampling frame

This investigation utilizes data obtained in the context of the Carolina Oral Health Literacy (COHL) Study, which initially enrolled 1,405 clients of the Special Supplemental Nutrition Program for Women, Infants and Children (WIC) in seven counties in NC: Brunswick, Buncombe, Burke, New Hanover, Orange, Robeson, and Wake [34]. The study's aim was to investigate the impact of caregivers' health literacy on their children's oral health and use of services. The study population consisted of low-income predominantly female caregivers who were 18 years of age or older, English-speaking, and the primary caregiver of a Medicaid-eligible healthy child. Purposeful quota sampling [35] was used to ensure adequate representation of African American (AA; 40%) and American Indian (AI; 20%) participants. Detailed descriptions of the study procedures, interview instruments and baseline outcomes have been reported previously [36–38]. In brief, non-random WIC sites were selected based on geographic region, rural or urban makeup, population demographics, existence of very active WIC clinics, and established working relationship with the investigators [34]. Consecutive WIC-attending clients were approached by study personnel while in the waiting areas and asked if they would to 8 questions included in the study's eligibility screener. Caregivers who were determined to be eligible and agreed to participate were accompanied to a private area to complete the in-person study interview. Of note, to qualify for WIC, caregivers must have an income <185 percent of the federal poverty level.

Data Sources

Data were collected in 30-minute in-person interviews with one of the two trained study interviewers between July 2008-July 2009 in the domains of socio-demography, caregivers' self-reported personal and children's general and dental health status, dental knowledge and behaviors, quality of life, dental neglect, general self-efficacy, and health literacy. Study personnel screened eligible participants to ensure that unique children were enrolled in the cohort. In June 2011, we obtained Medicaid enrollment and claims files for children from the NC Division of Medical Assistance, ranging from January 2004 to December 2010, a period that covered the lifetime Medicaid enrollment history for all children up to the end of CY-2010. We merged these files with interview data that were obtained at baseline using the children's unique Medicaid identification number that was provided by the caregivers at study enrollment. All COHL children were Medicaid-eligible or enrolled at baseline, as per our inclusion requirements. Of the 1405 caregivers recruited, 1242 had children with a Medicaid identification number at the baseline interview. Children's unique Medicaid identification number was used to link interview and Medicaid claims data. Subsequently, we excluded dyads wherein children had no Medicaid data (n = 31; 2% of total), caregivers under 18 years old (n = 2; 0.2%), and one caregiver (0.1%) who had missing information on health literacy. Thus, the final analytical sample included 1208 child/caregiver dyads.

Outcome Definition and Covariates

The study's primary analytical endpoint was the incidence of Medicaid enrollment disruptions or "gaps". During the study period (2004–2010) Medicaid eligibility criteria in NC, as well as procedures of enrollment and re-enrollment varied for different categories of child/caregiver dyads; however, these criteria included, among others, income, resources, residence, and proof of citizenship. Re-enrollment processes included periodic verifications of eligibility criteria at intervals ranging between 3–12 months, unless changes were self-reported by the beneficiaries. The current list of eligibility criteria and required documentation can be found at: http://www.ncdhhs.gov/dma/forms/famchld.pdf. For the purposes of this study we defined gap as a period during which a child was Medicaid-eligible but not enrolled, which was preceded *and* followed by periods of enrollment, as described by Copper et al. [39]. This definition of enrollment disruption was conservative, in a manner that prevented children with a permanent change in Medicaid-eligibility from being classified as having a gap. In such instances, there would be no subsequent re-enrollment in the NC files and the child would be labeled "lost to follow-up" rather than having an enrollment gap.

Apart from caregivers' difficulty with necessary forms and processes and administrative reasons, there are several other reasons why enrollment interruptions occur for children covered by Medicaid. Among others, these include: a child/family moving out of state, a child's acquisition of comprehensive private health insurance, a caregiver's request for termination of coverage, and family income changes. Any of these result in permanent eligibility changes without subsequent re-enrollment. We cannot ascertain with certainty the reason for permanent eligibility changes and some may be due to difficulty in processes/procedures; however, our goal for using a conservative definition of gaps was to ensure we were capturing administrative-related lapses due to parental actions that resulted in an interruption in enrollment.

Enumeration of enrolled/non-enrolled months began at the month of the baseline COHL interview and ended in December 2010. For each child, we identified and counted enrolled/non-enrolled periods and calculated their duration in months. We calculated 'enrollment proportion' as the ratio of months enrolled divided by months eligible with a range of 0–100. History of Medicaid enrollment was available from January 2004-December 2010, a period that included all available Medicaid data up to 2010 for all children. To further characterize patterns of Medicaid enrollment, we calculated periods of non-enrollment, enrollment gaps, and percent time enrolled both during the study duration and the entire period available.

We measured health literacy using a comprehension and numeracy-based instrument, the Newest Vital Sign (NVS). The NVS is a nutritional label accompanied by six questions, requiring approximately three minutes for completion. The NVS is a validated test with good psychometric properties and it has been used extensively since its introduction [40–41]. According to Weiss et al. [40] who developed and tested the NVS, the instrument is reliable (Cronbach alpha >0.76 in English), correlates with the test of functional health literacy in adults (TOFHLA), requires 3 minutes for administration and, thus, is suitable for use as a quick screening test for limited health literacy. According to Osborn et al. [42], the NVS is able to reliably identify individuals with limited literacy skills, which was the group of interest in this study (vs. the upper end of the literacy spectrum). In the context of our study, the NVS's Cronbach's *alpha* was 0.75. The NVS score ranges from 0–6, wherein values of 0–1 are indicative of "low", 2–3 "moderate" and 4–6 "higher health literacy" [42]. We used this 3-level categorical classification as well as a dichotomous one

where NVS score 0–1: "low health literacy" and 2–6: "higher health literacy". The examination of the latter dichotomy was driven by our working hypothesis which considered low caregiver health literacy as a predictor of children's Medicaid enrollment gap; in this scenario, a contrast between the lowest category of the NVS index (containing individuals most likely to face difficulties with forms and administrative processes) and higher ones was the most meaningful one.

Socio-demographic covariates included caregivers' race, sex, age, education, marital status, number of children, and child's age. Race was self-reported and categorized as white, African American (AA), and American Indian (AI). Caregivers' age was measured in years and classified as a tertile-categorical variable for descriptive purposes and a continuous variable for analytical purposes. Education was grouped in four categories: less than high school (HS) education, HS/General Education Diploma (GED), some technical or college training, and college or higher education. Marital status was classified as single, married, and divorced/separated/other. Children's age was measured in months and was categorized in five groups: 0–11, 12–23, 24–25, 36–47, and 48–59 months.

As a measure of caregivers' self-perceived health status, we used the National Health and Nutrition Examination Study (NHANES) self-reported item containing five possible answers: excellent, very good, good, fair, and poor. For analytical purposes, the responses were converted to a dichotomous variable, excellent/very good/good *versus* fair/poor.

Data availability

We have created and made available a de-identified dataset to accompany this manuscript, as supplemental material available online. This tab-delimited dataset (Dataset S1) contains all original and derived variables described and used for this study's analyses, including a data dictionary as a separate spreadsheet.

Statistical Analyses

We used descriptive statistics for our initial data presentation and χ^2 tests to compare the distribution of low/adequate health literacy and Medicaid enrollment gaps across strata of covariates. Because the occurrence of enrollment gaps is a time-dependent event, ignoring the time at-risk could introduce bias of substantial magnitude and unknown direction. For this reason, we used multivariate Poisson regression models that accounted for time at risk using months enrolled as the exposure and a log-link function. Although our modeling approach did not consider the length of each gap, we support that it is superior to the enumeration of months not enrolled due to reasons outlined above. To identify a final model, we employed a backward hierarchical variable selection strategy [43], starting with a full model that included all covariates and a p<0.2 criterion. We included caregivers' race, age, and general health status *a priori* in all models and obtained exponentiated model coefficients corresponding to Incidence Rate Ratios (IRR) and 95% confidence intervals (CI). For the interpretation of results, we followed an effect-estimation (estimation of the magnitude and precision of the association) *versus* hypothesis-testing (determination of the presence of an association or not) approach [44].

For sensitivity analysis, we developed a second identical model considering all Medicaid enrollment history available, prior to and after enrollment in the COHL study. All Medicaid enrollment history covered the lifetime period for all enrolled children, up to December 2010. In addition, to explore for potential vulnerable sub-groups, we conducted a *post hoc* homogeneity analysis to determine whether educational attainment and race modified the association between caregivers' health literacy and insurance gaps. To do so, we compared education level and race-specific estimates against the main effect estimate using a homogeneity χ^2 test. Because these *post hoc* stratified analyses are *de facto* underpowered, we used an a priori p value criterion of <0.2 for the detection of heterogeneity [45]. We used Stata version 12.1 (StataCorp LP, College Station, TX) and SAS version 9.3 (SAS Institute, Cary, NC) software for data analyses.

Results

The primary caregivers' socio-demographic characteristics and responses to the self-reported health status items, both overall and stratified by health literacy group, are presented in Table 1. There was a 2:2:1 distribution of white, AA, and AI participants with the vast majority of all participants being female. Caregivers' and children's mean age at the baseline interview was 27 years and 17 months, respectively. A small proportion (11%) of caregivers reported their general health as fair or poor. Fifteen percent of participants were classified as low health literacy based on their NVS score. This proportion was higher among AA and AI participants and among those who were younger, had lower educational attainment, and worse self-reported health status.

The median follow-up time was 25 months (mean = 24; range = 18–29), with 11% of children experiencing an interruption of Medicaid enrollment with no subsequent re-enrollment. This latter phenomenon was almost twice as high among children of caregivers with some technical/college or higher education *versus* those with less than high school education (15% *versus* 8%). Thirty percent of children experienced at least one enrollment gap (Table 2). Relative to gaps, the majority of the children (90%) experienced only one, 9% had two, and 1% had three. Twenty percent of these interruptions had duration of one month, 50% four months or less, while 21% were 12 months or longer. As anticipated, children with no gaps were enrolled longer, on average for six more months compared to those with gaps. Relative to bivariate associations, continuous enrollment was more frequent among children of older caregivers, older children, and those with more siblings (Table 2). Continuous enrollment was more frequent among children whose caregivers reported having better health but the difference was small (3%).

We present the final Poisson regression model (A) for enrollment gap incidence in Table 3. After adjusting for race, education, gender, and all other covariates, inclusion in the low health literacy group was associated with a modestly elevated risk for an enrollment gap (adjusted IRR = 1.17; 95% CI 0.89–1.54). The risk of gaps was inversely associated with caregivers' age, with a 2% relative risk decrease for each added year. An association between female gender and decreased risk of enrollment gaps was also noted; however, this finding was based on an analysis including only 46 male caregivers and thus should be viewed with caution. Stratified analyses (Table 4) revealed that educational attainment significantly modified the association between literacy and gaps (homogeneity p<0.2), with the highest risk estimates found among caregivers with less than high school education (IRR = 1.52; 95% CI 0.99–2.35). Race-stratified estimates did not depart substantially from homogeneity. Inspection of the exploratory models (B) that considered all available Medicaid enrollment history did not reveal any important differences compared to our main analyses.

Discussion

In this study of approximately 1200 young children of low-income predominantly female caregivers enrolled in WIC, 30%

had a gap in Medicaid enrollment over 25 months. Most experienced only one gap of short duration. Our findings revealed a weak association between caregivers' health literacy and their children's Medicaid enrollment gaps; in the entire cohort, independent of race, education, and age, low health literacy was associated with a non-significant gap risk increase of about 20%. Nevertheless, this effect was substantially elevated among caregivers with less than high school education compared to those with high school or higher education; caregivers with low education may be the most vulnerable to the effects of low health literacy. Moreover, above and beyond other caregiver factors, caregivers' age was inversely associated with the risk of gaps.

The concept of Medicaid's serving as a revolving-door for some children has been recognized and more steps must be taken by state Medicaid programs to alleviate this problem. While we cannot confirm it using our data, this phenomenon may be more closely related to administrative issues (i.e. difficulty with the enrollment and maintenance process) rather than eligibility disruptions. States are required to record and report on children's coverage stability but this has generally not been undertaken [46]. It is not uncommon for children who are uninsured for less than a full year to be reported as insured and this cohort of children has received less attention in public health research and policy discussions [23]. Olson [2] found that children insured for part of the previous year had higher proportions of delayed care and unmet medical care *versus* those uninsured for the full year. A similar finding was reported by DeVoe and colleagues [17], who compared children with gaps longer than six months *versus* those never insured.

Children from poor and near-poor families have been reported to be 4–5 times more likely to have lapsed coverage than those from high-income families [22]. At the same time, decreased preventive care utilization among children who had Medicaid insurance gaps was irrespective of their insurance status after discontinued enrollment [47]. Taken together, these findings underscore the dramatic effects that interruptions may have for children, their families, and the health care system. The association between Medicaid interruptions and subsequent children's health outcomes and related costs is fertile ground for future research.

As more health literacy findings are reported, the multi-level effects of health literacy are becoming increasingly evident. Health literacy is recognized already as having a pivotal role in numerous health outcomes [48–49], insurance status [29], and health disparities [50–51], and recently was termed the "sixth vital sign" [52]. Strategies that attempt to circumvent or mitigate the effects of low health literacy, such as the Federal Plain Language Act and simplification of enrollment procedures are promising [53], but more steps towards implementation are necessary. Although it is impossible to quantify the precise contributors to the relationship between health literacy and Medicaid enrollment gaps from our data, it appears that the readability of Medicaid forms [27] and user-friendliness of the enrollment renewal process [26,54–55] are potential targets for addressing literacy-sensitive concerns. This notion was recently mirrored by findings reported by Pati et al. [56] who found that mothers with inadequate health literacy were less likely to receive child care subsidy than those with adequate health literacy, implicating the application processes as health literacy-sensitive step.

Our findings on the incidence of enrollment gaps are consistent with previous reports of Medicaid insurance gaps among young children. Previously published estimates [20,46,57] of any gap of enrollment were 25% over a 12-month period in Oregon, 26–35% over 18 months in Ohio, 18% over a 2-year period in Louisiana,

Table 1. Distribution of Health Literacy Estimates (NVS) across Levels of Caregivers' Characteristics, in the COHL Study Follow-up Cohort, North Carolina, 2008–2010.

	No.ª (%) or mean (median)	Health Literacy (NVS)				χ²; p
		NVS score (95% CI)	Low n (row %)	Moderate n (row %)	Higher n (row %)	
All	1208	3.1 (3.0, 3.2)	199 (16)	508 (42)	501 (41)	
Race						<0.001
White	484 (40)	3.8 (3.6, 3.9)	45 (9)	162 (33)	277 (57)	
African American	478 (40)	2.7 (2.6, 2.9)	96 (20)	239 (50)	143 (30)	
American Indian	236 (20)	2.8 (2.6, 3.0)	51 (22)	106 (45)	79 (33)	
Caregiver's sex						0.6
Male	46 (4)	3.3 (2.7, 3.8)	9 (20)	16 (35)	21 (46)	
Female	1162 (96)	3.1 (3.0, 3.2)	190 (16)	492 (42)	480 (41)	
Caregiver's age (years, tertiles; range)						<0.001
Q1 (18.0, 23.0)	20.8 (20.9)	2.8 (2.7, 3.0)	71 (18)	202 (50)	130 (32)	
Q2 (23.1, 28.4)	25.5 (25.3)	3.4 (3.3, 3.6)	51 (13)	155 (38)	197 (49)	
Q3 (28.5, 65.6)	35.0 (33.2)	3.2 (3.0, 3.4)	77 (19)	151 (38)	174 (43)	
Education						<0.001
Did not finish high school	288 (24)	2.2 (2.1, 2.4)	87 (30)	143 (50)	58 (20)	
High school diploma or GED	467 (39)	3.0 (2.8, 3.1)	80 (17)	212 (45)	175 (37)	
Some technical/college or higher	453 (37)	3.9 (3.8, 4.1)	32 (7)	153 (34)	268 (59)	
Marital status						<0.001
Single	772 (64)	2.9 (2.7, 3.0)	149 (19)	363 (47)	260 (34)	
Married	316 (26)	3.7 (3.5, 3.9)	33 (10)	103 (33)	180 (57)	
Divorced/separated/other	120 (10)	3.5 (3.2, 3.8)	17 (14)	42 (35)	61 (51)	
Number of children						0.6
1	479 (40)	3.2 (3.1, 3.4)	73 (15)	204 (43)	202 (42)	
2	395 (33)	3.1 (3.0, 3.3)	62 (16)	173 (44)	160 (41)	
3	196 (16)	3.2 (2.9, 3.4)	34 (17)	76 (39)	86 (44)	
≥4	136 (11)	2.9 (2.6, 3.2)	29 (21)	55 (40)	52 (38)	
Caregiver general health						0.4
Excellent/Very good/Good	1076 (89)	3.2 (3.1, 3.3)	173 (16)	451 (42)	452 (42)	
Fair/Poor	132 (11)	2.9 (2.6, 3.2)	26 (20)	57 (43)	49 (37)	

Note. NVS = Newest Vital Sign; COHL = Carolina Oral Health Literacy; CI = Confidence Interval; HS = High School; GED = General Educational Development. The sample size was n = 1208.
ªColumn figures may not add up to total because of missing values.

25% over 12 months in Rhode Island, and 33% over an 18-month period in in Virginia. State, community, and local population-specific parameters may account for these relatively small variations. Our finding of increased risk for children's enrollment gaps among younger caregivers is a likely reflection of additional stressors and strains experienced by young parents/caregivers compared to older ones that could include education, employment, transportation, or others.

The finding of a weak association between enrollment gaps and literacy in the full cohort analysis requires further investigation. First, it must be acknowledged that in absence of statistical confirmation, an association may in fact be non-existent. Further, it is possible that the negative effects of low health literacy are manifested only among vulnerable subsets of the population, including those with low educational attainment, a scenario supported by our data. It is also possible that truly a weak

association exists; this result might be a reflection of the NC Medicaid Program's success in addressing issues with the enrollment and maintenance processes and caregiver community support (i.e. an effect of WIC and practice health coordinators). In fact, while NC had the highest readability level goal (6–8 grade) for enrollment forms among all states with such guidelines, it was 40th in terms of actual readability level [28]. This parallels our finding of a 52% risk increase for enrollment gaps among caregivers in the lowest educational attainment group. Nevertheless, other differences in caregivers' age, family conditions, or children's health care needs may influence the likelihood to enroll in Medicaid and remain continuously enrolled. As an example, Cooper et al. [39] found that among children with asthma, those without insurance gaps had more hospitalizations compared with those with insurance gaps. This finding was a possible consequence of health

Table 2. Medicaid Enrollment Estimates (Children with and without Gaps in Enrollment) by Caregiver Characteristics among the COHL Study Follow-up Cohort during the Follow-up Period (Median 25 Months), North Carolina, 2008–2010.

	No enrollment gap[a]			χ²; p[c]	One or more enrollment gaps[a]			
		Enrollment (months)				Enrollment (months)		
	No.[b] (row %)	Mean	Median (range)		No.[b] (row %)	Mean	Median (range)	Enrollment Proportion[d] (95% CI)
Total	846 (70)	24	25 (8–30)		362 (30)	18	19 (1–29)	0.71 (0.68–0.74)
Race				0.2				
White	329 (68)	25	25 (8–30)		155 (32)	18	19 (2–29)	0.71 (0.66–0.75)
African American	334 (70)	25	27 (18–30)		144 (30)	18	19 (1–29)	0.71 (0.66–0.75)
American Indian	177 (75)	22	21 (11–29)		59 (25)	17	18 (4–29)	0.76 (0.70–0.81)
Caregiver's sex				.02				
Male	25 (54)	26	27 (18–30)		21 (46)	17	17 (3–29)	0.64 (0.51–0.78)
Female	821 (71)	24	25 (8–30)		341 (29)	18	19 (1–29)	0.71 (0.69–0.74)
Caregiver's age (tertiles)				0.03				
Q1	264 (66)	24	24 (18–30)		139 (34)	19	20 (3–29)	0.76 (0.72–0.80)
Q2	284 (70)	24	25 (8–30)		119 (30)	17	18 (3–29)	0.70 (0.65–0.75)
Q3	298 (74)	25	25 (18–30)		104 (26)	17	18 (1–29)	0.66 (0.60–0.71)
Child's age (months; at baseline interview)				0.05				
0–11	347 (66)	25	25 (18–30)		182 (34)	17	18 (2–28)	0.69 (0.65–0.73)
12–23	177 (72)	25	25 (11–30)		70 (28)	19	20 (1–29)	0.75 (0.69–0.81)
24–35	154 (74)	24	23 (8–30)		55 (26)	18	20 (3–29)	0.74 (0.68–0.81)
36–47	146 (75)	24	25 (18–30)		48 (25)	17	17 (3–28)	0.69 (0.62–0.76)
48–59	22 (76)	21	19 (18–30)		7 (24)	16	17 (7–25)	0.73 (0.50–0.95)
Education				0.8				
<HS	204 (71)	24	25 (8–30)		84 (29)	19	21 (3–29)	0.79 (0.74–0.84)
HS/GED	330 (71)	24	25 (18–30)		137 (29)	18	19 (3–29)	0.72 (0.68–0.77)
Some college/technical or more	312 (69)	25	25 (18–30)		141 (31)	16	18 (1–29)	0.65 (0.61–0.70)
Marital status				0.5				
Single	537 (70)	24	25 (8–30)		235 (30)	19	20 (2–29)	0.75 (0.72–0.78)
Married	221 (70)	24	25 (18–30)		95 (30)	16	16 (2–29)	0.63 (0.57–0.68)
Divorced/separated/other	88 (73)	24	25 (18–30)		32 (27)	16	17.5 (1–26)	0.67 (0.56–0.78)
Number of children				0.03				
1	313 (65)	24	24 (18–30)		166 (35)	18	19 (2–29)	0.71 (0.67–0.75)
2	294 (74)	25	25 (18–30)		101 (26)	18	18 (1–29)	0.72 (0.67–0.77)
3	139 (71)	24	25 (11–30)		57 (29)	17	19 (3–29)	0.69 (0.62–0.76)
≥4	98 (72)	25	26 (8–30)		38 (28)	19	19.5 (6–29)	0.74 (0.65–0.82)

Table 2. Cont.

| | No enrollment gap[a] | | | | One or more enrollment gaps[a] | | | |
| | | Enrollment (months) | | | | Enrollment (months) | | |
	No.[b] (row %)	Mean	Median (range)	χ²; p[c]	No.[b] (row %)	Mean	Median (range)	Enrollment Proportion[d] (95% CI)
Caregiver general health				0.4				
Excellent/Very good/Good	758 (70)	24	25 (8–30)		318 (30)	18	19 (1–29)	0.71 (0.69–0.74)
Fair/Poor	88 (67)	25	25 (18–30)		44 (33)	17	17.5 (2–29)	0.69 (0.61–0.77)
Health Literacy (NVS)				0.8				
Low[e]	137 (69)	24	24 (8–30)		62 (31)	19	19 (4–29)	0.77 (0.72–0.83)
Moderate[f]	360 (71)	24	25 (18–30)		148 (29)	18	19 (1–29)	0.71 (0.67–0.75)
Higher[g]	349 (70)	25	25 (11–30)		152 (30)	17	18 (2–29)	0.69 (0.65–0.73)

Note. COHL = Carolina Oral Health Literacy; CI = Confidence Interval; HS = High School; GED = General Educational Development; NVS = Newest Vital Sign. The sample size was n = 1208.
[a] Enrollment gap was defined as any disruption in Medicaid enrollment within a period of eligibility, preceded and superseded by periods of enrollment.
[b] Column figures may not add up to total because of missing values.
[c] Corresponds to X² tests of the equality of distribution of participants with and without enrollment gap across categories of caregiver characteristics.
[d] Enrollment proportion was calculated for children with enrollment gaps as the ratio of months enrolled over months eligible.
[e] Defined as NVS score: 0–1.
[f] Defined as NVS score: 2–3.
[g] Defined as NVS score: 4–6.

Table 3. Results of Multivariate Poisson Regression Modeling of Medicaid Enrollment Gap Incidence on Caregiver and Child Characteristics, among the COHL Study Follow-up Cohort in North Carolina, during the Study Period (A) and Using all Available Medicaid History (B) between January 2004 and December 2010.

	Model A[a]: COHL study follow-up period			Model B[a]: All available Medicaid history		
	IRR	95% CI	p	IRR	95% CI	p
Health literacy (NVS)						
Low[b]	1.17	0.89–1.54	0.3	1.10	0.87–1.38	0.4
Moderate-Higher[c]	1.00	*referent*		1.00	*referent*	
Race						
White	1.00	*referent*		1.00	*referent*	
African American	0.91	0.73–1.13	0.4	0.93	0.77–1.12	0.4
American Indian	0.86	0.64–1.15	0.3	0.94	0.75–1.18	0.6
Education (ordinal categorical)	1.10	0.96–1.26	0.2	1.08	0.96–1.21	0.2
Caregiver's sex						
Male	1.00	*referent*		1.00	*referent*	
Female	0.53	0.35–0.80	0.003	0.62	0.43–0.90	0.01
Caregiver's age (years; continuous)	0.98	0.96–1.00	0.01	0.98	0.96–0.99	<0.001
Child's age (years; ordinal categorical)	0.93	0.86–1.02	0.1	0.99	0.93–1.06	0.9
Caregiver general health						
Excellent/Very good/Good	0.83	0.61–1.12	0.2	0.88	0.69–1.14	0.3
Fair/Poor	1.00	*referent*		1.00	*referent*	

Note. NVS = Newest Vital Sign; COHL = Carolina Oral Health Literacy; IRR = Incidence Rate Ratio; CI = Confidence Interval. The sample size was n = 1208.
[a]Variable selection was based on a backward hierarchical procedure starting from a full model and a P<.2 criterion; caregivers' race, age and general health were included a priori in the models; time at risk for a gap was considered time (months) of Medicaid enrollment.
[b]Defined as NVS score: 0–1.
[c]Defined as NVS score: 2–6.

Table 4. Estimates of the Association between Caregivers' Low Health Literacy (Defined as NVS Score of less than 2) and the Incidence of Children's Medicaid Enrollment Gaps, Overall and Stratified by Educational Attainment, among the COHL Study Follow-up Cohort in North Carolina, during the Study Period (A) and Using all Available Medicaid History (B) between January 2004 and December 2010.

	Model A[a]: COHL study follow-up period		Model B[a]: All available Medicaid history	
	IRR	95% CI	IRR	95% CI
All	1.17	0.89–1.54	1.10	0.86–1.40
Race				
Whites	1.23	0.73–2.06	1.29	0.85–1.96
African American	1.14	0.76–1.69	1.05	0.75–1.48
American Indian	1.18	0.64–2.16	0.96	0.58–1.57
Homogeneity (χ^2)[b] P	0.97		0.63	
Education				
Did not finish high school	1.52	0.99–2.35	1.36	0.97–1.92
High school diploma or GED	1.07	0.68–1.69	1.07	0.73–1.58
Some technical/college training or higher	0.67	0.31–1.45	0.65	0.34–1.24
Homogeneity (χ^2)[b] P	0.17		0.13	

Note. NVS = Newest Vital Sign; COHL = Carolina Oral Health Literacy; IRR = Incidence Rate Ratio; CI = Confidence Interval; GED = General Educational Development. The sample size was n = 1208.
[a]Variable selection was based on a backward hierarchical procedure starting from a full model and a P<.2 criterion; caregivers' race, age and general health were included a priori in the models; time at risk for a gap was considered time (months) of Medicaid enrollment.
[b]Wald χ^2 test of a common IRR (across-strata homogeneity).

problem-initiated and enrollment pattern driven care-seeking behavior.

Evidence supporting an association between parental health literacy and child health insurance status has been reported by large, rigorous studies, including those by Pati et al. [56] and Yin et al. [58]. Although these studies did not investigate enrollment gaps, they add to the growing evidence base linking health literacy with children's insurance status. The findings of the DeVoe et al. [17] and Satchell and Pati [22] studies underscored the importance of socio-economic stressors, including poverty and maternal education as strong predictors of enrollment gaps. This effect was reflected in our study's stratified analyses, wherein the effect of low health literacy varied significantly according to education level, with the largest estimates found among the lowest-educated caregivers.

Our findings have limitations. This WIC study cohort was not a probability sample, an important factor because WIC enrollment alone has been shown to confer benefits for child health behaviors and outcomes [59–60]. The WIC program is the largest public health nutrition program in the US and, as such, serves a large percentage of low-income children and their mothers. To put this in perspective, in fiscal year 2013, more than 2 million women and infants nationwide participated in WIC, whereas there were 264,000 WIC participants in North Carolina. Our sample size was modestly sized, including approximately 1,200 dyads and 199 caregivers with low health literacy; however, it must be noted to the best of our knowledge no other cohorts to-date exist with person-level data on parents' health literacy and children's Medicaid enrollment information. For many practical reasons, our population was limited to English-speaking caregivers over the age of 18, limiting the generalizability of our findings beyond that demographic group. Although there is a Spanish version of the NVS tool, most of our survey instruments at the time of the study had not been developed for or validated in Spanish. Because Hispanic children are often the most likely to have insurance gaps [22], the absence of this demographic group is an obvious study limitation. Future studies among these high-risk, vulnerable groups are warranted. Another limitation that must be pointed out is that NVS is only one of many available instruments available to assess health literacy; as a comprehension and numeracy-based test, it is not a comprehensive health literacy assessment.

Understanding Medicaid enrollment gaps is a complex issue. State differences in the enrollment and re-enrollment processes warrant the investigation of the association between health literacy and enrollment gaps in diverse population-based samples in different states. It is possible that enrollment and re-enrollment in Medicaid require cognitive and/or executive functioning skills not well-captured by the instrument used in this study. Prolonged interruptions could be due to changes in eligibility, but gaps can be due to administrative issues on both the program and the client's sides. Our data included rich information from the perspective of the client, but lacked information from the perspective of the program.

Summary and implications

Health insurance gaps have been linked to increased health disparities [61], leading to a poorer quality of health care [62]. Accordingly, correcting problems with children's health insurance enrollment and coverage should be a priority for stakeholders. We found that 30% of young children experienced one or more enrollment gaps over a 2-year period. Our data did not reveal any important association between caregivers' health literacy and the incidence of these gaps; however, they indicated that low health literacy may be a risk factor for enrollment gaps among the lowest-educated caregivers, who may be the most vulnerable to its detrimental effects. Moreover, caregivers' young age showed an association with increased risk for enrollment gaps. Considering the economy of scale of the anticipated health insurance coverage expansion in 2014, insurance coverage and continuity issues are certain to become ever more important challenges. Because health literacy issues are, unlike many other social determinants, amenable to interventions, it is critical that they are kept on the agendas of policy makers. Although age is a non-intervenable factor, it may be pertinent to consider caregivers' (young) age as a possible additional risk factor for their children's public insurance enrollment disruptions.

The Congressional Budget Office projects that the currently 34 million people that are covered by Medicaid will increase to 47 million in 2014 with the implementation of the ACA [63]. Considering this huge expansion, health insurance coverage should be examined from a social and behavioral perspective to inform and guide states' actions in the implementation of the Medicaid coverage expansion [16,64–66]. Gaps in insurance coverage should be considered with a rigor similar to non-enrollment. More research is needed to comprehensively characterize health system and individual-level risk factors for public health insurance gaps; however, it must be acknowledged that population-wide, policy solutions such as continuous eligibility and automatic re-enrollment in public insurance may be more effective approaches compared to "individual risk factor" strategies. Beyond the obvious utility of identifying susceptible groups or individuals (i.e., young caregivers of children), it is critical that planned interventions are evidence-based with attention to the critical issues of health literacy and cultural appropriateness.

Author Contributions

Conceived and designed the experiments: JYL DAD RGR WFV. Performed the experiments: ADB. Analyzed the data: KD ZG. Contributed reagents/materials/analysis tools: JYL KD ZG. Wrote the paper: KD WFV. Conceived the study: JYL. Overviewed the data analysis: JYL. Contributed to the interpretation of results: JYL. Assisted in preparation of the first draft of the manuscript: JYL. Conducted the data analysis: KD. Prepared the first draft of the manuscript: KD. Participated in the study design: DAD RGR. Participated in results interpretation: DAD RGR ADB. Participated in data collection: ADB. Critically revised the manuscript: ADB ZG. Participated in the data management and data analysis: ZG. Contributed to the critical interpretation of results: JYL KD DAD ADB ZG RGR WFV. Substantially revised the initial manuscript draft for content and accuracy, confirm that they are responsible for the reported research, and meet all criteria for authorship: JYL KD DAD ADB ZG RGR WFV.

References

1. Chung PJ, Lee TC, Morrison JL, Schuster MA (2006) Preventive care for children in the United States: quality and barriers. Annu Rev Public Health 27: 491–515.

2. Olson LM, Tang SF, Newacheck PW (2005) Children in the United States with discontinuous health insurance coverage. N Engl J Med 353: 382–291.

3. Newacheck PW, Stoddard JJ, Hughes DC, Pearl M (1998) Health insurance and access to primary care for children. N Engl J Med 338: 513–519.

4. Fisher MA, Mascarenhas AK (2009) A comparison of medical and dental outcomes for Medicaid-insured and uninsured Medicaid-eligible children: a U.S. population-based study. J Am Dent Assoc 140: 1403–1412.

5. Fisher MA, Mascarenhas AK (2007) Does Medicaid improve utilization of medical and dental services and health outcomes for Medicaid-eligible children in the United States? Community Dent Oral Epidemiol 35: 263–271.

6. Freed GL, Clark SJ, Pathman DE, Schectman R (1999) Influences on the receipt of well-child visits in the first two years of life. Pediatrics 103: 864–869.

7. St Peter RF, Newacheck PW, Halfon N (1992) Access to care for poor children. Separate and unequal? JAMA 267: 2760–2764.

8. Newacheck PW, Halfon N (1988) Preventive care use by school-aged children: differences by socioeconomic status. Pediatrics 82: 462–468.

9. Selden TM (2006) Compliance with well-child visit recommendations: evidence from the Medical Expenditure Panel Survey, 2000–2002. Pediatrics 118: e1766–1778.

10. Starfield B, Shi L (2004) The medical home, access to care, and insurance: a review of evidence. Pediatrics 113: 1493–1498.

11. Savage MF, Lee JY, Kotch JB, Vann WF Jr (2004) Early preventive dental visits: effects on subsequent utilization and costs. Pediatrics 114: e418–423.

12. Hakim RB, Bye BV (2001) Effectiveness of compliance with pediatric preventive care guidelines among Medicaid beneficiaries. Pediatrics 108: 90–97.

13. Christakis DA, Wright JA, Koepsell TD, Emerson S, Connell FA (1999) Is greater continuity of care associated with less emergency department utilization? Pediatrics 103: 738–742.

14. Strickland BB, Jones JR, Ghandour RM, Kogan MD, Newacheck PW (2011) The medical home: health care access and impact for children and youth in the United States. Pediatrics 127: 604–611.

15. National Association of Pediatric Nurse Practitioners (2003) NAPNAP position statement on credentialing and privileging for pediatric nurse practitioners. J Pediatr Health Care 17: A22–23.

16. Landers RM (2012) The Dénouement of the Supreme Court's ACA Drama. N Engl J Med 367: 198–199.

17. DeVoe JE, Graham A, Krois L, Smith J, Fairbrother GL (2008) "Mind the Gap" in children's health insurance coverage: does the length of a child's coverage gap matter? Ambul Pediatr 8: 129–134.

18. Federico SG, Steiner JF, Beaty B, Crane L, Kempe A (2007) Disruptions in insurance coverage: patterns and relationship to health care access, unmet need, and utilization before enrollment in the State Children's Health Insurance Program. Pediatrics 120: e1009–1016.

19. Wise PH, Wampler NS, Chavkin W, Romero D (2002) Chronic illness among poor children enrolled in the temporary assistance for needy families program. Am J Public Health 92: 1458–1461.

20. Summer L, Mann C (2006) Instability of public health insurance coverage for children and their families: causes, consequences, and remedies. New York: The common wealth fund. Available: http://www.commonwealthfund.org/~/media/Files/Publications/Fund%20Report/2006/Jun/Instability%20of%20Public%20Health%20Insurance%20Coverage%20for%20Children%20and%20Their%20Families%20%20Causes%20%20Consequence/Summer_instabilitypubhltinschildren_935%20pdf.pdf. Accessed 2014 Sept 19.

21. Fairbrother GL, Emerson HP, Partridge L (2007) How stable is medicaid coverage for children? Health Aff (Millwood) 26: 520–528.

22. Satchell M, Pati S (2005) Insurance gaps among vulnerable children in the United States, 1999–2001. Pediatrics 116: 1155–1161.

23. Tang SF, Olson LM, Yudkowsky BK (2003) Uninsured children: how we count matters. Pediatrics 112: e168–173.

24. Wachino V, Weiss A (2009) Maximizing kids' enrollment in Medicaid and SCHIP: What works in reaching, enrolling, and retaining eligible children. National Academy for State Health Policy, Washington, DC. Available: http://nashp.org/sites/default/files/Max_Enroll_Report_FINAL.pdf?q=files/Max_Enroll_Report_FINAL.pdf. Accessed 2014 Sept 19.

25. Price J, Boswell J, Lessard M, Wood K (2006) Why Parents Disenroll Children from Public Health Insurance: The Case of Southeastern North Carolina. Journal of Applied Social Science 21: 92–106.

26. DeVoe JE, Westfall N, Crocker S, Eigner D, Selph S, et al. (2012) Why do some eligible families forego public insurance for their children? A qualitative analysis. Fam Med 44: 39–46.

27. Wilson JM, Wallace LS, DeVoe JE (2009) Are state Medicaid application enrollment forms readable? J Health Care Poor Underserved 20: 423–431.

28. Pati S, Kavanagh JE, Bhatt SK, Wong AT, Noonan K, et al. (2012) Reading level of medicaid renewal applications. Acad Pediatr 12: 297–301.

29. Sentell T (2012) Implications for reform: survey of California adults suggests low health literacy predicts likelihood of being uninsured. Health Aff (Millwood) 31: 1039–1048.

30. DeWalt DA, Hink A (2009) Health literacy and child health outcomes: a systematic review of the literature. Pediatrics 124 Suppl 3: S265–274.

31. Sanders LM, Federico S, Klass P, Abrams MA, Dreyer B (2009) Literacy and child health: a systematic review. Arch Pediatr Adolesc Med 163: 131–140.

32. Ferguson B (2008) Health literacy and health disparities: the role they play in maternal and child health. Nurs Womens Health 12: 286–298.

33. Sanders LM, Thompson VT, Wilkinson JD (2007) Caregiver health literacy and the use of child health services. Pediatrics 119: e86–92.

34. Lee JY, Divaris K, Baker AD, Rozier RG, Lee SY, et al. (2011) Oral health literacy levels among a low income population. J Public Health Dent 71: 152–160.

35. Kalton G (1983) Models in the practice of survey sampling. International Statistical Review 51: 175–188.

36. Lee JY, Divaris K, Baker AD, Rozier RG, Vann WF Jr (2012) The relationship of oral health literacy and self-efficacy with oral health status and dental neglect. Am J Public Health 102: 923–929.

37. Divaris K, Lee JY, Baker AD, Vann WF Jr (2011) The relationship of oral health literacy and oral health-related quality of life in a multi-racial sample of low-income female caregivers. Health Qual Life Outcomes 9: 108.

38. Vann WF Jr, Lee JY, Baker D, Divaris K (2010) Oral health literacy among female caregivers: impact on oral health outcomes in early childhood. J Dent Res 89: 1395–400.

39. Cooper WO, Arbogast PG, Hickson GB, Daugherty JR, Ray WA (2005) Gaps in enrollment from a Medicaid managed care program: effects on emergency department visits and hospitalizations for children with asthma. Med Care 43: 718–725.

40. Weiss BD, Mays MZ, Martz W, Castro M, DeWalt DA, et al. (2005) Quick assessment of literacy in primary care: the newest vital sign. Ann Fam Med 3: 514–522.

41. Welch VL, VanGeest JB, Caskey R (2011) Time, costs, and clinical utilization of screening for health literacy: a case study using the Newest Vital Sign (NVS) instrument. J Am Board Fam Med 24: 281–289.

42. Osborn CY, Weiss BD, Davis TC, Skripkauskas S, Rodrigue C, et al. (2007) Measuring adult literacy in health care: performance of the newest vital sign. Am J Health Behav 31 Suppl 1: S36–46.

43. Peixoto JL (1987) Hierarchical variable selection in polynomial regression models. The American Statistician 41: 311–313.

44. Gardner MJ, Altman DG (1986) Confidence intervals rather than P values: estimation rather than hypothesis testing. Br Med J (Clin Res Ed) 292: 746–750.

45. Greenland S, Rothman KJ (2008) Introduction to stratified analysis. In: Rothman KJ, Greenland S, Lash TL. Modern epidemiology. New York: Lippincott, Williams and Wilkins. pp. 258–282.

46. Fairbrother G, Madhavan G, Goudie A, Watring J, Sebastian RA, et al. (2011) Reporting on continuity of coverage for children in Medicaid and CHIP: what states can learn from monitoring continuity and duration of coverage. Acad Pediatr 11: 318–325.

47. Yu J, Harman JS, Hall AG, Duncan RP (2011) Impact of Medicaid/SCHIP disenrollment on health care utilization and expenditures among children: a longitudinal analysis. Med Care Res Rev 68: 56–74.

48. Sørensen K, Van den Broucke S, Fullam J, Doyle G, Pelikan J, et al. (2012) Health literacy and public health: a systematic review and integration of definitions and models. BMC Public Health 12: 80.

49. Berkman ND, Sheridan SL, Donahue KE, Halpern DJ, Crotty K (2011) Low health literacy and health outcomes: an updated systematic review. Ann Intern Med 155: 97–107.

50. Sentell TL, Halpin HA (2006) Importance of adult literacy in understanding health disparities. J Gen Intern Med 21: 862–866.

51. Parker RM, Ratzan SC, Lurie N (2003) Health literacy: a policy challenge for advancing high-quality health care. Health Aff (Millwood) 22: 147–153.

52. Heinrich C (2012) Health literacy: the sixth vital sign. J Am Acad Nurse Pract 24: 218–223.

53. Sheridan SL, Halpern DJ, Viera AJ, Berkman ND, Donahue KE, et al. (2011) Interventions for individuals with low health literacy: a systematic review. J Health Commun 16 Suppl 3: 30–54.

54. Flores G, Abreu M, Brown V, Tomany-Korman SC (2005) How Medicaid and the State Children's Health Insurance Program can do a better job of insuring uninsured children: the perspectives of parents of uninsured Latino children. Ambul Pediatr 5: 332–340.

55. Ross DC, Hill IT (2003) Enrolling eligible children and keeping them enrolled. Future Child 13: 81–97.

56. Pati S, Siewert E, Wong AT, Bhatt SK, Calixte RE, et al. (2014) The Influence of Maternal Health Literacy and Child's Age on Participation in Social Welfare Programs. Matern Child Health J 18: 1176–1189.

57. DeVoe JE, Krois L, Edlund T, Smith J, Carlson NE (2008) Uninsurance among children whose parents are losing Medicaid coverage: Results from a statewide survey of Oregon families. Health Serv Res 43: 401–418.

58. Yin HS, Johnson M, Mendelsohn AL, Abrams MA, Sanders LM, et al. (2009) The health literacy of parents in the United States: a nationally representative study. Pediatrics 124: S289–298.

59. Chatterji P, Brooks-Gunn J (2004) WIC participation, breastfeeding practices, and well-child care among unmarried, low-income mothers. Am J Public Health 94: 1324–1327.

60. Lee JY, Rozier RG, Norton EC, Kotch JB, Vann WF Jr (2004) Effects of WIC participation on children's use of oral health services. Am J Public Health 94: 772–777.

61. Lillie-Blanton M, Hoffman C (2005) The role of health insurance coverage in reducing racial/ethnic disparities in health care. Health Aff (Millwood) 24: 398–408.

62. Chassin MR, Galvin RW (1998) The urgent need to improve health care quality. Institute of Medicine National Roundtable on Health Care Quality. JAMA 280: 1000–1005.

63. Congressional Budget Office Bulletin (2012) "Updated Estimates for the Insurance Coverage Provisions of the Affordable Care Act". Available: http://cbo.gov/sites/default/files/cbofiles/attachments/03-13-Coverage%20Estimates.pdf. Accessed 2014 Sept 19.

64. Baicker K, Congdon WJ, Mullainathan S (2012) Health insurance coverage and take-up: lessons from behavioral economics. Milbank Q 90: 107–134.

65. Sommers BD, Tomasi MR, Swartz K, Epstein AM (2012) Reasons for the wide variation in Medicaid participation rates among states hold lessons for coverage expansion in 2014. Health Aff (Millwood) 31: 909–919.

66. Kronebusch K, Elbel B (2004) Simplifying children's Medicaid and SCHIP. Health Aff (Millwood) 23: 233–246.

18

Serotype Distribution and Antibiotic Susceptibility of *Streptococcus pneumoniae* Strains Carried by Children Infected with Human Immunodeficiency Virus

Dodi Safari[1]*, **Nia Kurniati**[2], **Lia Waslia**[3], **Miftahuddin Majid Khoeri**[1], **Tiara Putri**[4], **Debby Bogaert**[5], **Krzysztof Trzciński**[5]

1 Eijkman Institute for Molecular Biology, Jakarta, Indonesia, 2 Department of Child Health, Dr. Cipto Mangunkusumo Hospital/Faculty of Medicine Universitas Indonesia, Jakarta, Indonesia, 3 Eijkman Oxford Clinical Research Unit, Jakarta, Indonesia, 4 Faculty of Biology, Gajah Mada University, Yogyakarta, Indonesia, 5 Department of Pediatric Immunology and Infectious Diseases, Wilhelmina's Children Hospital, University Medical Center Utrecht, Utrecht, the Netherlands

Abstract

Background: We studied the serotype distribution and antibiotic susceptibility of *Streptococcus pneumoniae* isolates carried by children infected with HIV in Jakarta, Indonesia.

Methods: Nasopharyngeal swabs were collected from 90 HIV infected children aged 4 to 144 months. *S. pneumoniae* was identified by conventional and molecular methods. Serotyping was performed with sequential multiplex PCR and antibiotic susceptibility with the disk diffusion method.

Results: We identified *S. pneumoniae* carriage in 41 children (46%). Serotype 19F was most common among 42 cultured strains (19%) followed by 19A and 6A/B (10% each), and 23F (7%). Most isolates were susceptible to chloramphenicol (86%), followed by clindamycin (79%), erythromycin (76%), tetracycline (43%), and sulphamethoxazole/trimethoprim (41%). Resistance to penicillin was most common with only 33% of strains being susceptible. Strains of serotypes targeted by the 13-valent pneumococcal conjugate polysaccharide vaccine (PCV13) were more likely to be multidrug resistant (13 of 25 or 52%) compared to non-PCV13 serotype isolates (3 of 17 or 18%; Fisher exact test $p = 0.05$).

Conclusion: Our study provides insight into the epidemiology of pneumococcal carriage in young HIV patients in Indonesia. These findings may facilitate potential preventive strategies that target invasive pneumococcal disease in Indonesia.

Editor: Adam J. Ratner, Columbia University, United States of America

Funding: This study was supported by a small grant from International Society of Infectious Disease (ISID). The funders had no role in study design, data collection and analysis, decision to publish, or preparation of the manuscript.

Competing Interests: DB has received consulting fees from Pfizer. KT has received consulting fees from Pfizer and grant support for studies on pneumococcal carriage from Pfizer. All other authors report no potential conflicts.

* Email: safari@eijkman.go.id

Introduction

Streptococcus pneumoniae is a leading cause of bacterial pneumonia, meningitis, and sepsis worldwide. An estimated 1.6 million people die from invasive pneumococcal disease (IPD) each year, one million of whom are children [1]. Incidence of IPD varies substantially by age, genetic background, socioeconomic status, immune status, and geographical location [2]. Capsular polysaccharide is considered to be the ultimate virulence factor of *S. pneumoniae* as un-encapsulated strains are virtually absent among *S. pneumoniae* causing IPD [3,4]. Over 90 *S. pneumoniae* serotypes have been identified based on the capsule chemical structure and immunogenicity [5] and capsular oligosaccharides are used as vaccine antigens in pneumococcal vaccines.

Current pneumococcal conjugate vaccines cover only a selected set of serotypes, e.g. PCV7 (7 serotypes), PCV10 (10 serotypes) and PCV13 (13 serotypes). The introduction of the PCV7 vaccine targeting the serotypes 4, 6B, 9V, 14, 18C, 19F, and 23F significantly reduced the burden of pneumococcal disease in many

populations [6]. Despite high efficacy against disease caused by the vaccine serotypes (VTs), the net effect of vaccination is often reduced due to serotype replacement [6,7]. In a number of geographical locations including the USA, Germany, The Netherlands, England and Wales [8–11], serotype 19A was reported to be the most commonly emerging non-vaccine serotype (NVT) following PCV7 introduction. Colonization of the upper respiratory tract is the obligatory first step in the pathogenesis of pneumococcal disease, and therefore considered the most important risk factor for IPD [12]. It also provides the basis for horizontal spread of pneumococci in the community, making it an important target for preventive measures [13,14].

Currently, epidemiological data on *S. pneumoniae* carriage and invasive disease is limited for the Indonesian population. In 2001, Soewignjo *et al.* reported that the prevalence of *S. pneumoniae* carriage was 48% in healthy children in Lombok Island, Indonesia [15]. Recently, Farida *et al.* reported that in Semarang, Indonesia, prevalence of *S. pneumoniae* in 2010 was 43% and 11% in children aged 6–60 months and adults aged 45–75 years, respectively [17]. One of the risk factors for IPD is infection with human immunodeficiency virus (HIV) [16]. So far, no data are available on *S. pneumoniae* carriage in high-risk populations in Indonesia. Currently, pneumococcal vaccination is not part of the expanded program on immunization (EPI) for infants in Indonesia. Both the PCV13 (targeting all PCV7 serotypes plus serotypes 1, 3, 5, 6A, 7F and 19A) and the 23-valent pneumococcal polysaccharide vaccine (PPV23) are available at a commercial price. The use of pneumococcal vaccines is not monitored in any systemic way in Indonesia.

In this present study, we investigate the carriage of *S. pneumoniae* in children infected with HIV in Jakarta, Indonesia. We expect our results to guide the modification of existing, and the implementation of potentially new preventive strategies targeting pneumococcal disease in the country.

Methods

Study population

A cross-sectional study on *S. pneumoniae* nasopharyngeal colonization was performed from January to July 2012 among children infected with human immunodeficiency virus (HIV) during their routine clinic visits at the Cipto Mangunkusumo Hospital, Jakarta – Indonesia. The study has been reviewed and approved by the ethical committee of Faculty of Medicine, Universitas Indonesia, Jakarta, Indonesia. The children's parents signed informed consent forms and provided clinical and demographic information, such as age, sex, family size and in which region they were living. Detailed medical information on the CD4 lymphocyte count within the past 3 months and the use of antibiotics was recorded during the study. Parents were also asked whether any person living with a child is smoking. No other environmental exposure factors were recorded. According to the study's protocol children with symptoms of a respiratory tract infection and children who were immunized with one or more doses of any pneumococcal vaccine were excluded from the study.

Sample collection

Nasopharyngeal (NP) swabs were collected using a flexible nasopharyngeal flocked swab (Copan, Italy no 503SC01) as recommended by WHO [14,18]. Swabs were placed into 1.0 ml of skim milk tryptone glucose glycerol (STGG) transport medium, shipped on wet ice directly to the Eijkman Institute, Jakarta. Upon arrival at the lab, 20 µl of each STGG sample was plated onto a 5% sheep blood agar supplemented with 5 mg/L gentamicin (SB-Gent), and incubated at 35°C for 24 h with 5% CO_2. In the case of alpha-hemolytic colonies growth on the SB-Gent plate, a single colony was re-cultured and tested by Gram-staining, and also tested for susceptibility to optochin [13]. Gram-positive, optochin-sensitive isolates were stored in STGG at −80°C for further analysis.

DNA extraction

Bacterial DNA was extracted as described previously [19]. Briefly, pneumococcal isolates were retrieved from storage by subculture on the SB-Gent. The bacterial cells suspension was heated at 100°C for 10 minutes and instantly frozen at −20°C for 10 minutes. Lysates were centrifuged at 1000×g for 10 minutes, after which the supernatant was collected and stored at −20°C until further use.

Molecular detection of pneumococcal surface antigen A gene

The polymerase chain reaction (PCR) targeting the pneumococcal surface antigen A gene (*psa*A) was performed as described by Morrison et al. [20]. In short, the reaction mixture contained GoTaq Green Master Mix (Promega), forward (5′-CTTTCTGC-AATCATTCTTG-3′) and reverse (3′-GCCTTCTTTACCTT-GTTCTGC-5′) primers at 10 µM concentration, and 1.0 µl of DNA template. The presence of 838 bp amplicon was detected by electrophoresis of 5 µl of PCR product on 1% agarose gels stained with ethidium bromide, and visualized in UV light.

Serotyping

Serotype determination was performed by a sequential multiplex PCR (smPCR), as published by Pai et al. [19]. Briefly, seven smPCRs were performed, each in a 25 µl reaction mixture of GoTaq Green Master Mix (Promega) and up to five pairs of primers specific for a particular serotype or serotypes cluster and an internal positive control targeting 160 bp fragment of capsule transcriptional regulator gene *wzg* (*cps*A) universally present in *cps* operons of almost all serotypes and using 1.0 µl of cell lysate extract as DNA template. The primers set used in the study allowed for identification of 40 serotypes, including all serotypes targeted by PCV13 and were published by the CDC (USA) [21].

Antibiotic susceptibility testing

Antibiotic susceptibility tests were carried out for all of the pneumococcus isolates using the disk diffusion method according to CLSI standard [22], and antimicrobial disks (Oxoid) with chloramphenicol, clindamycin, erythromycin, sulfamethoxazole/trimethoprim, and tetracycline. Susceptibility to penicillin was tested with the oxacillin disk [22]. Strains expressing lack of susceptibility to three or more antimicrobial agents of different classes were considered multidrug resistant (MDR) in the study.

Statistical methods

Statistical analyses were conducted using GraphPad Prism V5.0 (GraphPad Software, San Diego, CA, USA).

Results

Streptococcus pneumoniae isolates were cultured from 41 of 90 (46%) nasopharyngeal samples collected in the study from children infected with HIV in Jakarta, Indonesia. All strains were susceptible to optochin and positive for the *psa*A gene by PCR. The patient characteristics are described in Table 1. There were no differences in carriage rates within gender, family size, use of antibiotics, or tobacco smoking in the household. Although, *S. pneumoniae* carriage rates were higher in children with a CD4 lymphocyte count less than 25% (59%), compared to children with a CD4 count >25% (37%) the difference did not reach statistical significance (Fisher exact test $p = 0.086$) (Table 1). There was no correlation between child age and CD4 count (Pearson; $r = 0.09$, $p = 0.46$) neither of the differences in carriage rates between age groups in the study were significant. There were no exclusions from the study based on a child's previous immunization with any pneumococcal vaccine.

Altogether, we cultured 42 *S. pneumoniae* strains from 41 samples, with a single sample from one child positive simultaneously for strains of serotype 3 and 9V. The most commonly observed was serotype 19F (8 of 42 cultured pneumococcal strains; 19%) followed by 9A and 6A/B (4 carriers each; 10%), 23F (3

Table 1. Patient characteristics related to pneumococcal carriage.

Characteristics		N	N (%) of children carrying *S. pneumoniae*
HIV-infected children		90	41 (46)
Age (month)			
	0–24	9	3 (33)
	25–60	33	15 (46)
	61–144	48	23 (48)
Sex			
	Male	44	18 (49)
	Female	46	23 (51)
Exposure to cigarette			
	Yes	41	18 (44)
	No	49	23 (47)
No of family member			
	[1–3]	34	17 (50)
	[4–6]	28	11 (39)
	[>7]	12	6 (50)
	no data	16	7 (44)
Current antibiotics use			
	Yes	20	9 (45)
	No	70	32 (46)
CD4 lymphocyte count[a]			
	<25%	34	20 (59)
	≥ 25%	30	11 (37)
	no data	26	10 (39)

[a]CD4 lymphocyte count measured within 3 months prior to nasopharyngeal sampling.

carriers; 7%), 9V, 35B, 11A (two carriers each; 5%) and serotypes 18C, 3, 12F, 15B/C and 35F (single carrier each; 2%) (Table 2). We found that eleven isolates (26%) were untypeable using the SM-PCR method, with six of those 11 (14% of all) also being PCR-negative for the *cpsA* gene. In this study, strains that could be covered by the pneumococcal conjugate vaccine varied between 45% to 60% for PCV7 and PCV13 vaccines, respectively.

The majority of strains were susceptible to chloramphenicol (86%), clindamycin (79%), erythromycin (76%), sulphamethoxazole/trimethoprim (41%) and tetracycline (43%) (Table 3). Meanwhile, only 33% of strains were susceptible to penicillin (Table 3). Use of the oxacillin disc to screen isolates for lack of susceptibility to penicillin could be considered as a limitation in our study as it does not allow to distinguish low level from high level resistance with low level resistant strains often retaining sensitivity to a range of beta-lactams, including aminopenicllins [22]. Compared to strains of other serotypes, isolates of PCV13 serotypes detected in the study (3, 6A/B, 7F, 9V, 14, 18C, 19A, 19F, and 23F) were less susceptible to any of the six antimicrobial agents tested, although the difference was significant only for penicillin (Table 3). In this study, we found 16 of isolates expressed a lack of susceptibility to three or more antimicrobial agents of different classes thus considered multi-drug resistant (MDR) (Table 4). With 13 (52%) of 25 strains of PCV13 serotypes versus three (18%) of 17 non-PCV13 serotype strains classified as MDR in our study, the multidrug resistance was more common, however the difference did not reach statistical significance (Fisher exact test $p = 0.0504$) among isolates of serotypes targeted by the vaccine.

Discussion

Since limited data was available on the epidemiology of *S. pneumoniae* carriage in the Indonesian population, especially in high-risk children, we studied *S. pneumoniae* carriage in children infected with HIV. Our findings of 46% of *S. pneumoniae* carriage in HIV-positive children (aged 4 to 144 months) in Jakarta are in line with a previously published report on carriage in healthy children in Lombok Island and Semarang, Indonesia, where 48% of children (aged 0–25 months) and 43% of children (aged 6–60 months) carried pneumococci [15,17]. *S. pneumoniae* carriage in children with this acquired immunodeficiency varies in different geographical locations. In comparison to other studies in which nasopharyngeal carriage of *S. pneumoniae* was detected in HIV-infected children using the WHO-recommended culture method, the prevalence of pneumococcal carriage in Jakarta was lower compared to 66% recorded in Tanzania (children aged 12–168 months) and 77% reported in Kenya (3–59 months) [23,24], but higher than in Romania (children aged 39–106 months), Brazil (0–228 months), and USA with the reported carriage rates of 30%, 29%, and 20%, respectively [25–27]. There is relatively little known about possible impact of the HIV infection on pneumococcal carriage. Abdullahi *et al.* [24] reported higher carriage prevalence in Kenya among HIV-positive versus HIV-negative children whereas infection with HIV has no effect on pneumococcal carriage reported in adults in South Africa by Shiri *et al.* [28]. Although we observed a trend towards higher *S. pneumoniae* carriage rates in children with lower CD4 lymphocyte count, both Mwenya, *et al.* [29] and Anthony *et al.* [23] reported lack of any

Table 2. Serotype distribution and vaccine coverage among 42 *S. pneumoniae* carriage isolates of HIV-infected children in Jakarta.

Serotype		N (%) of isolates
19F		8 (19)
19A		4 (10)
6A/B		4 (10)
23F		3 (7)
11A		2 (5)
9V		2 (5)
sg18		2 (5)
12F		1 (2)
15B/C		1 (2)
3		1 (2)
35B		1 (2)
35F		1 (2)
7F		1 (2)
untypeable		
	cps-positive	5 (12)
	cps-negative	6 (14)
PCV-7 coverage		19 (45)
PCV-13-coverage		25 (60)

association between CD4 levels and pneumococcal carriage in HIV-infected children.

Pneumococcal conjugate vaccines are reported to provide substantial protection against IPD and clinical pneumonia when given to HIV-infected infants [30]. Despite PCV7 vaccine being available in Indonesia since 2008 and PCV13 since 2011, their use is limited as it is evident from lack of any exclusion from the study based on child previous immunization against pneumococcal disease but also from a relatively high prevalence of vaccine serotypes in carriage. We observed that serotype 19F isolates were the most common in carriage in this study. Meanwhile in 2001, Soewignjo *et al.* reported that in healthy children from Lombok, Indonesia, the most common were strains of serogroup 6 (25%) followed by serogroup 23 (21%) and serogroup 19 (6%) [15]. Farida *et al.* reported that in healthy children from Semarang, Indonesia, the most common were strains of serotype 6A/B (19%) followed by serotype 15B/C and 11A (10%), 23F(9%), and

19F(8%) [17]. In our study, serogroup 19 isolates (serotypes 19F and 19A together) accounted for over a quarter (12 out of 42 or 29%) of all the pneumococcal strains cultured from HIV-infected children. Interestingly, eleven isolates were classified as untypeable in the study, with six strains of PCR-negative for the *cpsA* gene. It either indicates over-representation of untypeable strains when carriage is detected by conventional culture [31], reflects significant circulation of strains expressing capsular types not targeted by SM-PCR, or indicates low sensitivity of the protocol used to determine the serotype of pneumococcal strains.

We identified susceptibility to sulfamethoxazole/trimethoprim in 41%, and to penicillin in 33% carriage isolates in this study, whereas susceptibility to sulfamethoxazole/trimethoprim and penicillin was still common (91% and 100% respectively) in the study conducted in 1997 in Lombok [15]. Meanwhile in Semarang, Indonesia in 2010, 24% of *S. pneumoniae* strains were penicillin non-susceptible, and 45% were resistant to sulfamethoxazole/trimethoprim [17].

Table 3. Antimicrobial susceptibility of *Streptococcus pneumoniae* strains carried by children infected with HIV.

Antimicrobial Agent	Number (%) of susceptible isolates			p-Value (Fisher exact test)
	All (n = 42)	PCV13 serotype strains[a] (n = 25)	non-PCV13 serotype strains (n = 17)	
Chloramphenicol	36 (86)	20 (80)	16 (94)	0.3739
Clindamycin	33 (79)	18 (72)	15 (88)	0.2708
Erythromycin	32 (76)	16 (64)	16 (94)	0.0312
Sulphamethoxazole/ trimethoprim	17 (41)	7 (28)	10 (59)	0.0605
Penicillin[b]	14 (33)	5 (20)	9 (53)	0.0448
Tetracycline	18 (43)	8 (32)	10 (59)	0.1169

[a]Strains of serotypes targeted by thirteen-valent conjugated polysaccharide pneumococcal vaccine: 1, 3, 4, 5, 6A, 6B, 7F, 9V, 14, 18C, 19A, 19F, 23F.
[b]Susceptibility to penicillin was determined with oxacillin disk [22].

Table 4. Serotype of multi-drug resistant S. pneumoniae strains.

Isolate	Serotype	Antimicrobial susceptibility profile [22]					
		Chloramphenicol	Clindamycin	Erythromycin	Sulphamethoxazole/trimethoprim	Penicillin[a]	Tetracycline
ISID-77	19F	S	R	R	R	R	R
ISID-107	19F	S	S	R	R	R	R
ISID-1	19F	S	R	R	R	R	R
ISID-16	19F	S	R	R	R	R	R
ISID-31	19F	S	S	R	R	R	R
ISID-12	19F	S	R	R	R	R	R
ISID-8	19A	S	S	S	S	R	R
ISID-6	19A	S	S	S	R	R	R
ISID-24	19A	S	S	S	R	R	R
ISID-110	6A/B	S	R	R	R	R	R
ISID-11	6A/B	S	R	R	R	R	R
ISID-36	12 F	R	S	S	R	S	R
ISID-47	11A	S	R	R	R	S	R
ISID-104	23F	R	R	R	R	R	R
ISID-75-R	9V	R	S	S	R	R	R
ISID-111	untypeable	S	R	S	R	S	R

S – susceptible; R – non-suceptible.
[a]Susceptibility to penicillin was determined with oxacillin disk [22].

We also found that serotype 19F isolates along isolates of serogroup 6A/B were more frequently resistant to antimicrobial drugs tested in the study compared to strains of other serotypes. This is in agreement with ANSORP (Asian Network for Surveillance of Resistant Pathogens) data reporting a 59% multidrug resistance among *S. pneumoniae* invasive isolates collected in the region, with 19F being the major multidrug resistant serotype (24% of all MDR strains from IPD) [32]. Furthermore, recent Malaysian data showed that serotype 19F was correlated with increased resistance against penicillin [33].

We observed strains of serotypes targeted by PCV13 to be more frequently resistant to antipneumococcal drugs tested in the study compared to non-PCV13 strains. Immunization with PCVs would target not only serotypes common in carriage in the studied population, but also strains of serotypes less susceptible to antipneumococcal drugs. In geographical locations with high rates of antibiotics resistance among *S. pneumoniae* strains, introduction of PCVs lowered not only incidence of IPD, but also lowered (at least temporarily) rates of resistance to particular antimicrobial agents in strains circulating in carriage and causing pneumococcal diseases [34–36]. Similar effects could be expected in our study population. In conclusion, our study gives insight into the population of *S. pneumoniae* strains circulating in carriage in patients who are at high risk for IPD due to age and comorbidity. We expect our results to be helpful in shaping preventive strategies targeting IPD in Indonesia both on a national and local level.

Acknowledgments

We are grateful to the children and parents for participating in the study, and the staff of the Department of Child Health, Dr. Cipto Mangunkusumo Hospital, Jakarta. We also thank Dr. Decy Subekti, Siti Mudaliana, and Stephany Tumewu for technical assistance and discussion.

Author Contributions

Conceived and designed the experiments: DS NK DB KT. Performed the experiments: DS NK LW MMK TP. Analyzed the data: DS NK DB KT. Contributed reagents/materials/analysis tools: NK LW MMK TP. Wrote the paper: DS KT.

References

1. O'Brien KL, Wolfson LJ, Watt JP, Henkle E, Deloria-Knoll M, et al. (2009) Burden of disease caused by *Streptococcus pneumoniae* in children younger than 5 years: global estimates. Lancet 374: 893–902. doi:10.1016/S0140-6736(09)61204-6.

2. Van der Poll T, Opal SM (2009) Pathogenesis, treatment, and prevention of pneumococcal pneumonia. Lancet 374: 1543–1556. doi:10.1016/S0140-6736(09)61114-4.

3. Browall S, Norman M, Tångrot J, Galanis I, Sjöström K, et al. (2014) Intraclonal variations among *Streptococcus pneumoniae* isolates influence the likelihood of invasive disease in children. J Infect Dis 209: 377–388. doi:10.1093/infdis/jit481.

4. Jansen AGSC, Rodenburg GD, van der Ende A, van Alphen L, Veenhoven RH, et al. (2009) Invasive pneumococcal disease among adults: associations among serotypes, disease characteristics, and outcome. Clin Infect Dis 49: e23–e29. doi:10.1086/600045.

5. Oliver MB, van der Linden MPG, Küntzel SA, Saad JS, Nahm MH (2013) Discovery of *Streptococcus pneumoniae* serotype 6 variants with glycosyltransferases synthesizing two differing repeating units. J Biol Chem 288: 25976–25985. doi:10.1074/jbc.M113.480152.

6. Weinberger DM, Malley R, Lipsitch M (2011) Serotype replacement in disease after pneumococcal vaccination. Lancet 378: 1962–1973. doi:10.1016/S0140-6736(10)62225-8.

7. Feikin DR, Kagucia EW, Loo JD, Link-Gelles R, Puhan MA, et al. (2013) Serotype-specific changes in invasive pneumococcal disease after pneumococcal conjugate vaccine introduction: a pooled analysis of multiple surveillance sites. PLoS Med 10: e1001517. doi:10.1371/journal.pmed.1001517.

8. Van der Linden M, Reinert RR, Kern WV, Imöhl M (2013) Epidemiology of serotype 19A isolates from invasive pneumococcal disease in German children. BMC Infect Dis 13: 70. doi:10.1186/1471-2334-13-70.

9. Spijkerman J, van Gils EJM, Veenhoven RH, Hak E, Yzerman EPF, et al. (2011) Carriage of *Streptococcus pneumoniae* 3 years after start of vaccination program, the Netherlands. Emerg Infect Dis 17: 584–591. doi:10.3201/eid1704.101115.

10. Miller E, Andrews NJ, Waight PA, Slack MP, George RC (2011) Herd immunity and serotype replacement 4 years after seven-valent pneumococcal conjugate vaccination in England and Wales: an observational cohort study. Lancet Infect Dis 11: 760–768. doi:10.1016/S1473-3099(11)70090-1.

11. Kaplan SL, Barson WJ, Lin PL, Stovall SH, Bradley JS, et al. (2010) Serotype 19A Is the most common serotype causing invasive pneumococcal infections in children. Pediatrics 125: 429–436. doi:10.1542/peds.2008-1702.

12. Bogaert D, De Groot R, Hermans PWM (2004) *Streptococcus pneumoniae* colonisation: the key to pneumococcal disease. Lancet Infect Dis 4: 144–154. doi:10.1016/S1473-3099(04)00938-7.

13. Auranen K, Rinta-Kokko H, Goldblatt D, Nohynek H, O'Brien KL, et al. (2013) Colonisation endpoints in *Streptococcus pneumoniae* vaccine trials. Vaccine 32: 153–158. doi:10.1016/j.vaccine.2013.08.061.

14. Satzke C, Turner P, Virolainen-Julkunen A, Adrian PV, Antonio M, et al. (2013) Standard method for detecting upper respiratory carriage of *Streptococcus pneumoniae*: Updated recommendations from the World Health Organization Pneumococcal Carriage Working Group. Vaccine 32: 165–179. doi:10.1016/j.vaccine.2013.08.062.

15. Soewignjo S, Gessner BD, Sutanto A, Steinhoff M, Prijanto M, et al. (2001) *Streptococcus pneumoniae* nasopharyngeal carriage prevalence, serotype distribution, and resistance patterns among children on Lombok Island, Indonesia. Clin Infect Dis 32: 1039–1043. doi:10.1086/319605.

16. Gilks CF, Ojoo SA, Ojoo JC, Brindle RJ, Paul J, et al. (1996) Invasive pneumococcal disease in a cohort of predominantly HIV-1 infected female sex-workers in Nairobi, Kenya. Lancet 347: 718–723.

17. Farida H, Severin JA, Gasem MH, Keuter M, Wahyono H, et al. (2014) Nasopharyngeal carriage of *Streptococcus pneumoni*a in pneumonia-prone age groups in Semarang, Java Island, Indonesia. PLoS ONE 9: e87431. doi:10.1371/journal.pone.0087431.

18. O'Brien KL, Nohynek H, World Health Organization Pneumococcal Vaccine Trials Carriage Working Group (2003) Report from a WHO Working Group: standard method for detecting upper respiratory carriage of *Streptococcus pneumoniae*. Pediatr Infect Dis J 22: e1–e11. doi:10.1097/01.inf.0000049347.42983.77.

19. Pai R, Gertz RE, Beall B (2006) Sequential multiplex PCR approach for determining capsular serotypes of *Streptococcus pneumoniae* isolates. J Clin Microbiol 44: 124–131. doi:10.1128/JCM.44.1.124-131.2006.

20. Morrison KE, Lake D, Crook J, Carlone GM, Ades E, et al. (2000) Confirmation of psaA in all 90 serotypes of *Streptococcus pneumoniae* by PCR and potential of this assay for identification and diagnosis. J Clin Microbiol 38: 434–437.

21. CDC website. Available: http://www.cdc.gov/ncidod/biotech/files/pcr-oligonucleotide-primers.pdf. Accessed 2014 September 11.

22. Clinical and Laboratory Standards Institute (2007) Performance Standards for Antimicrobial Susceptibility Testing: Seventeenth Informational Supplement. Wayne, PA: CLSI.

23. Anthony L, Meehan A, Amos B, Mtove G, Mjema J, et al. (2012) Nasopharyngeal carriage of *Streptococcus pneumoniae*: prevalence and risk factors in HIV-positive children in Tanzania. Int J Infect Dis 16: e753–e757. doi:10.1016/j.ijid.2012.05.1037.

24. Abdullahi O, Karani A, Tigoi CC, Mugo D, Kungu S, et al. (2012) The prevalence and risk factors for pneumococcal colonization of the nasopharynx among children in Kilifi District, Kenya. PloS One 7: e30787. doi:10.1371/journal.pone.0030787.

25. Polack FP, Flayhart DC, Zahurak ML, Dick JD, Willoughby RE (2000) Colonization by *Streptococcus penumoniae* in human immunodeficiency virus-infected children. Pediatr Infect Dis J 19: 608–612.

26. Cardoso VC, Cervi MC, Cintra OAL, Salathiel ASM, Gomes ACLF (2006) Nasopharyngeal colonization with *Streptococcus pneumoniae* in children infected with human immunodeficiency virus. J Pediatr (Rio J) 82: 51–57. doi:10.2223/JPED.1437.

27. Leibovitz E, Dragomir C, Sfartz S, Porat N, Yagupsky P, et al. (1999) Nasopharyngeal carriage of multidrug-resistant *Streptococcus pneumoniae* in institutionalized HIV-infected and HIV-negative children in northeastern Romania. Int J Infect Dis 3: 211–215.

28. Shiri T, Auranen K, Nunes MC, Adrian PV, van Niekerk N, et al. (2013) Dynamics of pneumococcal transmission in vaccine-naive children and their HIV-infected or HIV-uninfected mothers during the first 2 years of life. Am J Epidemiol 178: 1629–1637. doi:10.1093/aje/kwt200.

29. Mwenya DM, Charalambous BM, Phillips PPJ, Mwansa JCL, Batt SL, et al. (2010) Impact of cotrimoxazole on carriage and antibiotic resistance of *Streptococcus pneumoniae* and *Haemophilus influenzae* in HIV-infected children in Zambia. Antimicrob Agents Chemother 54: 3756–3762. doi:10.1128/AAC.01409-09.

30. Bliss SJ, O'Brien KL, Janoff EN, Cotton MF, Musoke P, et al. (2008) The evidence for using conjugate vaccines to protect HIV-infected children against pneumococcal disease. Lancet Infect Dis 8: 67–80. doi:10.1016/S1473-3099(07)70242-6.

31. Valente C, de Lencastre H, Sá-Leão R (2013) Selection of distinctive colony morphologies for detection of multiple carriage of *Streptococcus pneumoniae*. Pediatr Infect Dis J 32: 703–704. doi:10.1097/INF.0b013e31828692be.

32. Kim SH, Song J-H, Chung DR, Thamlikitkul V, Yang Y, et al. (2012) Changing trends in antimicrobial resistance and serotypes of *Streptococcus pneumoniae* isolates in Asian countries: an Asian Network for Surveillance of Resistant Pathogens (ANSORP) study. Antimicrob Agents Chemother 56: 1418–1426. doi:10.1128/AAC.05658-11.

33. Le C-F, Palanisamy NK, Mohd Yusof MY, Sekaran SD (2011) Capsular serotype and antibiotic resistance of *Streptococcus pneumoniae* isolates in Malaysia. PloS One 6: e19547. doi:10.1371/journal.pone.0019547.

34. Kyaw MH, Lynfield R, Schaffner W, Craig AS, Hadler J, et al. (2006) Effect of introduction of the pneumococcal conjugate vaccine on drug-resistant *Streptococcus pneumoniae*. N Engl J Med 354: 1455–1463. doi:10.1056/NEJMoa051642.

35. Dagan R (2009) Impact of pneumococcal conjugate vaccine on infections caused by antibiotic-resistant *Streptococcus pneumoniae*. Clin Microbiol Infect 15 Suppl 3: 16–20. doi:10.1111/j.1469-0691.2009.02726.x.

36. Link-Gelles R, Thomas A, Lynfield R, Petit S, Schaffner W, et al. (2013) Geographic and temporal trends in antimicrobial nonsusceptibility in *Streptococcus pneumoniae* in the post-vaccine era in the United States. J Infect Dis 208: 1266–1273. doi:10.1093/infdis/jit315.

19

Persistence of Health Inequalities in Childhood Injury in the UK; A Population-Based Cohort Study of Children under 5

Elizabeth Orton[1]*, Denise Kendrick[2], Joe West[3], Laila J. Tata[4]

1 Lecturer and Specialty Registrar in Public Health, Division of Primary Care, University Park, University of Nottingham, Nottingham United Kingdom, **2** Professor of Primary Care Research, Division of Primary Care, University Park, University of Nottingham, Nottingham United Kingdom, **3** Clinical Associate Professor and Reader in Epidemiology; Consultant Gastroenterologist, Division of Epidemiology and Public Health, Nottingham City Hospital, University of Nottingham, Nottingham, United Kingdom, **4** Associate Professor in Epidemiology, Division of Epidemiology and Public Health, Nottingham City Hospital, University of Nottingham, Nottingham, United Kingdom

Abstract

Background: Injury is a significant cause of childhood death and can result in substantial long-term disability. Injuries are more common in children from socio-economically deprived families, contributing to health inequalities between the most and least affluent. However, little is known about how the relationship between injuries and deprivation has changed over time in the UK.

Methods: We conducted a cohort study of all children under 5 registered in one of 495 UK general practices that contributed medical data to The Health Improvement Network database between 1990–2009. We estimated the incidence of fractures, burns and poisonings by age, sex, socio-economic group and calendar period and adjusted incidence rate ratios (IRR) comparing the least and most socio-economically deprived areas over time. Estimates of the UK annual burden of injuries and the excess burden attributable to deprivation were derived from incidence rates.

Results: The cohort of 979,383 children experienced 20,804 fractures, 15,880 burns and 10,155 poisonings, equating to an incidence of 75.8/10,000 person-years (95% confidence interval 74.8–76.9) for fractures, 57.9 (57.0–58.9) for burns and 37.3 (35.6–38.0) for poisonings. Incidence rates decreased over time for burns and poisonings and increased for fractures (p< 0.001 test for trend for each injury). They were significantly higher in more deprived households (IRR test for trend p<0.001 for each injury type) and these gradients persisted over time. We estimate that 865 fractures, 3,763 burns and 3,043 poisonings could be prevented each year in the UK if incidence rates could be reduced to those of the most affluent areas.

Conclusions: The incidence of burns and poisonings declined between 1990 and 2009 but increased for fractures. Despite these changes, strong socio-economic inequalities persisted resulting in an estimated 9,000 additional medically-attended injuries per year in under-5s.

Editor: Claire Thorne, UCL Institute of Child Health, University College London, United Kingdom

Funding: The author(s) received no specific funding for this work.

Competing Interests: The authors have declared that no competing interests exist.

* Email: elizabeth.orton@nottingham.ac.uk

Introduction

Childhood injury is a major cause of preventable ill-health, disability and death, [1]. In England and Wales it is the second most common cause of childhood death (age 1–4) after cancer, [2] and results in substantial long term disability, [1]. Injuries disproportionately affect more socio-economically deprived families, [3–14]. Globally this health inequality is striking, with more than 95% of all injury-related child deaths around the world occurring in low and middle-income countries, [1]. However, health inequalities in injury persist within high income countries also. For example, a study in England and Wales showed that the average annual death rate from injury in 2001 for children under age 15 was more than 13 times higher for children whose parents were classed as never having worked compared to children whose parents were in managerial or professional occupations, [3].

Since the UK government has made clear its intention to reduce health inequalities (as indicated in the Health and Social Care Act 2012, [15]) and the inclusion of injury-related admissions in young people has been included as a key performance indicator in the Public Health Outcomes Framework for England, [16], monitoring changes in injury rates over time and across socio-economic groups has never been more important. However, whilst the European Union recommend that 'accidents and injuries' are included in the European Statistical System of Eurostat, [17], in the UK there are no national surveillance systems monitoring all medically-attended injuries and we do not currently have any audit data that allow exploration by socio-economic group at a population level. Available data on hospital admissions for injury are routinely available for England and Wales, but by definition comprise only the most severe injuries and do not contain information on socio-economic status. Many more injuries are likely to be attended to in primary care, walk-in centres or emergency departments (EDs) that are not currently reported on at a population level in the UK. From 1978 to 2002 data on injury occurrence was captured from a sample of EDs by the Home and Leisure Accident Surveillance System (HASS & LASS) but these data are now more than 10 years out of date, are no longer collected and are not available via the interactive online portal.

Given the importance of injury in children in terms of the short and long term morbidity and mortality, we have used data from a nationally representative primary care database to estimate injury rates, the disease burden in terms of numbers of children injured and estimates of the number of excess injuries that are attributable to socio-economic deprivation.

Methods

Study design and data source

We conducted a cohort study using prospectively-collected health data from 495 General Practices from across the UK (i.e. England, Scotland, Wales and Northern Ireland) that contribute to The Health Improvement Network (THIN) research database. THIN includes all health information reported to primary care, including symptoms, diagnoses and treatments which are encoded into the medical record using Read codes where diagnoses are based on the International Classification of Diseases version 10 (ICD10). In the UK the general practitioner (primary care physician or family doctor) holds electronic health records for their patients and these records contain information about primary care consultations and importantly, other types of healthcare utilisation such as hospital admission into secondary and tertiary care, thus providing a comprehensive source of health information. Practices that contribute to THIN are broadly representative of all general practices in the UK in terms of age and sex of patients, practice size, geographical distribution and data quality, [18], are thought to be complete enough for research, [19] and acceptable outcomes from regular data quality checks and audits are a condition of participation in the network. In addition, primary care data have been shown to be a reliable source of medical information for a range of health issues, [20].

We used individual medical records from an open cohort of 979,383 children born between the 1st of January 1990 and the 31st of December 2009 who were registered with a THIN general practice before the age of 5 years. Children entered the cohort i.e. medical records were included from the latest date of when the practice started contributing data to THIN, when the practice had acceptable mortality data, the registration of the child with the practice or birth if the child was registered with the practice within 30 days of birth. Follow up ended at the earliest date of the most recent data collection from practices, when the child transferred out of the practice, died, or the day before their 5th birthday. In the UK, records are automatically created when a new born baby is registered with a GP for the first time and records for existing patients are automatically transferred between practices if patients register with a new GP and are not reliant therefore on patients requesting that records are transferred. However we undertook a sensitivity analysis, restricting the analysis to participants with a minimum of 6 months person time in order to ensure that the incidence patterns we found were not biased by injured participants being more or less likely to register or transfer in or out of a practice and therefore contribute more or less person time to the study.

Outcome; injury types

We studied the three most common types of medically attended injury incurred by children under the age of 5 internationally, [1]: fractures (any site or severity), burns (any site or severity and including scalds and flame burns) and poisonings (including those from medicinal and non-medicinal products/sources). Incident injuries in children's records were defined by the presence of a diagnosis or treatment Read code in the medical record using comprehensive code lists for each injury type (available on request from authors). If a child had more than one injury code of the same type (e.g. Read codes for fracture at age 2 and again at age 4 years) both incident injuries were included. As some children had multiple Read code entries for the same injury type in close succession, we only considered new injury events as those with an interval of over 30 days between code entries to signify a new poisoning or burn event and over 100 days for a new fracture event. This was based on the analysis of Read code entry whereby intervals between children's first and subsequent codes were plotted using a histogram and the point at which the curve levelled out was selected as the end of the event window. However, we also conducted a sensitivity analysis varying this window to over 90 days for poisonings, 90 days for burns and 300 days for fractures to determine the impact of potential overestimation of our initial event numbers.

Exposure; socio-economic deprivation

Socio-economic deprivation was measured using the Townsend Index of material deprivation, in quintiles. This is an area-based composite score comprising measures of employment, car ownership, home ownership and overcrowding (i.e. number of adults per room) in an area of 400–600 households, [21]. Before general practices release their data to THIN, each patient is assigned a quintile of the Townsend index based on their home postcode and information from the 2001 UK census. This maintains patient anonymity and ensures that the patient's quintile is representative of their relative socio-economic position at national level. The most recent home address at the time of data extraction is used to assign the index.

Covariates

We assessed variation in injury by sex, age, calendar period, and socio-economic deprivation. Child age was divided into year intervals from birth, because of the known changes in risk of injury at different ages, [4,22] and calendar time was divided into 5-year periods.

Statistical methods

We calculated incidence rates (per 10,000 person years (PY)) and incidence rate ratios (IRR) using Poisson regression with a robust variance estimator for fractures, burns and poisonings. We mutually adjusted for sex, age, socio-economic deprivation and calendar period to provide adjusted incidence rate ratios (aIRR).

To assess whether deprivation and injury incidence rates varied over time we added terms for an interaction between deprivation quintile and calendar period to the models and tested statistical significance using a likelihood ratio test (LRT) with a p value smaller than 0.05 taken as statistically significant. In addition, we calculated adjusted injury IRRs between the most versus least socio-economically deprived groups at the start (1990–1994) and end (2005–2009) of the study period and conducted a test for trend (also using the LRT) for yearly incidence rate changes within Townsend quintiles.

To estimate the total burden of injuries in the UK in numbers we applied each year's incidence rates (1990–2009) to the mid-year UK population estimates (1990–2009), [23], giving an annual number of injuries for each injury type and then summed these to produce a total estimate of injuries over the entire study and also for each 5-year study period. To assess how the burden had changed over time we subtracted the total number of injuries in the 1990–1994 period from the total number of injuries in the 2005–2009 period for each injury type. In addition, we estimated the excess incidence of injuries in the study population that could be attributed to deprivation using the population attributable risk calculation described by Steenland and Armstrong which takes account of different levels of deprivation exposure (i.e. the proportion of children in each quintile) [24]. In this calculation, the (IRR-1/IRR) is calculated for each of the top four quintiles of deprivation compared with the least deprived (bottom) quintile and this is then multiplied by the proportion of children in the study in that quintile of deprivation. These are then summed to give the final attributable risk fraction.

Ethical approval

We used The Health Improvement Network (THIN) primary care database for this research. THIN data collection is undertaken by Cegedim Strategic Data and this has been approved by the UK South-East Multicentre Research Ethics Committee (SE-MREC). There is a standard process for managing ethical approval of individual studies that use these data which is managed by Cegedim's THIN Scientific Review Committee (SRC). A research protocol was submitted to the SRC and the protocol was approved in October 2009 (SRC Reference Number: 09–011). Patient informed consent is not required under this agreement nor is further additional ethics approvals from either the National Health Service ethics committees or from The University of Nottingham.

Results

Overall incidence rates

The study cohort comprised 979,383 children with a median study follow up time of 2.68 years (when they were under age 5). Fractures were the most common injury type; 20,804 fractures were incurred by 20,038 children (2% of the cohort), 15,880 burns were incurred by 15,286 children (1.5% of the cohort) and 10,155 poisonings were incurred by 9,772 children (1% of the cohort), all before the age of 5 (Table 1).

During the entire study period (1990–2009) the incidence of fractures was 75.8/10,000 PY (95% confidence interval 74.8–76.9), burn incidence was 57.9/10,000 PY (57.0–58.9) and poisoning incidence was 37.3/10,000 PY (36.5–38.0) (Table 2).

Incidence by age and sex

For each injury type boys experienced a higher rate of injury than girls (aIRR 1.09 (95% confidence interval 1.06–1.12) for fractures, 1.28 (1.24–1.33) for burns and 1.10 (1.06–1.14) for poisonings (Table 3)). Burns were most common at age 1 and poisonings at age 2, whereas fractures continued to increase with age (Tables 2 and 3).

Incidence by socio-economic deprivation

Rates for all injury types increased with increasing socio-economic deprivation (Table 2 and Figure 1, aIRR test for trend p<0.001 for each type). This gradient was steepest for burn injury with an absolute rate difference between children in the most versus the least deprived quintile of deprivation of 41.7/10,000 PY (aIRR comparing the most versus the least deprived quintile 1.94, 1.85–2.04). For poisoning there was a difference of 20.2/10,000 PY (aIRR 1.72, 1.61–1.84) and for fracture injury the absolute rate difference was only 7.0/10,000 PY (aIRR 1.11, 1.06–1.16). These gradients remained even when we restricted the analyses to participants with a minimum of 6 months person time.

However, the magnitude of this health inequality gap was not consistent over time within the study, particularly for burns and poisonings (test for interaction between calendar year and deprivation p = 0.29 for fracture, p = 0.01 for burn and p = 0.03 for poisoning) (Figure 1). For burns, in the period 1990–1994 there were 73.4/10,000 PY more injuries in the most deprived areas compared to the least (aIRR 2.22, 1.91–2.58) and this had fallen by 56% to 32.4/10,000 PY by the last study period, 2005–2009 (aIRR 1.79, 1.63–1.96). For poisonings, the absolute rate difference fell by 33% from 24.2/10,000 PY (adjusted IRR 1.51, 1.28–1.83) in 1990–1994 to 16.3/10,000 PY (adjusted IRR 1.75, 1.55–1.99) in 2005–2009 and for fractures fell by 32% from 12.1/10,000 PY (adjusted IRR 1.19, 1.00–1.41) to 8.24/10,000 PY (adjusted IRR1.13, 1.06–1.23).

Incidence by calendar period

There was a statistically significant increase in fracture incidence rates over time (test for trend p<0.001) with an absolute rate increase of 12.0/10,000 PY from the earliest period (1990–1994) to the latest period (2005–2009). Conversely, burn and poisoning incidence rates significantly decreased over time (test for trend p<0.001 for both burn and poisonings) with an absolute rate reduction of 39.2/10,000 for burn injuries and 25.4/10,000 for poisoning injuries.

Sensitivity analysis

When we used a more conservative approach to defining a new injury event by increasing the gap between Read code entries for the same injury type to over 90 days for poisonings, 90 days for burns and 300 days for fractures, the number of events reduced to 20,386 fractures, 15,658 burns and 10,103 poisonings. Therefore, this still captured the vast majority of events in our original analysis (97.9%, 98.6% and 99.9% of fractures, burns and poisonings respectively) indicating that most were likely to be true independent events. When we repeated all analyses of injury variation by age, sex, socio-economic status and calendar period our findings were almost identical to the original analyses.

Annual UK estimates of medically attended fractures, burns and poisonings

Using UK national population estimates, [23], we calculated that there were 519,109 fractures, 471,519 burns and 284,606 poisoning events in under-5s across the UK during the study period. However, as described above, the incidence rates for fractures increased and for burns and poisonings decreased over the study period. Therefore we estimated that in the period 2005–2009 there were an additional 34,749 fractures, 79,251 fewer burns and 31,754 fewer poisonings when compared to the earliest study period (1990–1994).

Table 1. Frequency of injury types in the study population (N = 979,383).

	Fractures	Burns	Poisonings
Number of children with no injury	959,472	964,176	969,611
Number of children with at least one injury (% of all children)	19,911 (2.03%)	15,207 (1.57%)	9,772 (1.00%)
Total number of injuries	20,668	15,796	10,155
Number of injuries before age 5, per child (% of injured children)			
1	19,206 (96.4%)	14,649 (96.3%)	9,417 (96.4%)
2	661 (3.3%)	528 (3.5%)	335 (3.4%)
≥3	44 (0.3%)	30 (0.2%)	20 (0.2%)

The population attributable risk

By calculating the attributable risk fraction, which assumes a causal relationship between deprivation and injury, we estimate that 3% of fractures, 30% of burns and 28% of poisonings could be attributed to deprivation. This means that per year 876 fractures, 5,485 burns and 3,034 poisonings could potentially be avoided if all children experienced the injury rates of those in the most affluent quintile of the population.

Discussion

The incidence of burns and poisonings in young children has decreased substantially over the past 20 years, whereas the incidence of factures has increased to a smaller, but still important extent. However, despite these encouraging changes, important health inequalities have persisted over time, whereby children in deprived areas continue to experience significantly more injuries than children in more affluent areas. By calculating the population attributable risk we estimate that annually, there are an additional 9,395 medically-attended injuries in children under 5 that potentially, could be avoided if all children experienced the injury rates of those in the most affluent areas of the UK. It may be possible therefore to reduce injury rates even further by targeting interventions at those children in the most socio-economically deprived areas.

Strengths and weaknesses of the study

As far as we are aware, this is the first study to estimate population-based incidence rates for the most common medically-attended childhood injuries that is not from self-reports of injury or a single source of presentation such as the emergency department or hospital admissions. Our cohort of nearly 1 million children is also the largest UK study to quantify injury-related health inequalities and how these have changed over time. Data show that THIN practice populations are broadly representative of the UK population in terms of demographics, disease prevalence and death rates, [18] and since in the UK approximately 98% of the population is registered with a GP [25] we believe that our study is generalizable to the wider UK population.

One potential explanation for our results is that participants from different socioeconomic backgrounds have different health seeking behaviour, resulting in injury ascertainment biases. For example, it is possible that people from lower socio-economic groups are more likely to register with a GP when an injury occurs, potentially inflating the incidence of injury in these groups. Whilst we cannot rule this out, only 0.4% of poisonings, 0.7% of burns and 0.8% of fractures were recorded within a week of registration with the GP practice. We did find that people from lower socio-economic groups contributed less person time to the study but when we restricted the analyses to people with at least 6 months of person time we found the same socio-economic gradients. This suggests that our results are not wholly explained by different patterns of health seeking behaviour from people in different socio-economic groups.

As with most studies using routinely-collected and medically-coded data, it is possible that some injuries have not been included because they were not Read-coded in the medical record. This may have led to underestimates of the crude incidence rates. However, there is little evidence to suggest that GP recording of injury using Read codes (rather than free text for example) is differentially influenced by a patient's socio-economic status and GPs do not have access to patients' Townsend scores which are added for research purposes when the data are downloaded from the practice.

We have estimated all incident injuries in children under the age of 5, however it is possible that we have misclassified new incident injuries as existing injuries and vice versa, under or overestimating the incidence rates. However the incidence rates we have presented are similar to those expected from other studies (see below) and our findings relating to health inequality gradients were robust when we undertook sensitivity analyses, changing the definition of new incident events. It is unlikely therefore that the health inequality patterns that we identified have been substantially affected by the way injury events have been defined.

A strength of this study was the use of an area-based measure of deprivation. Whilst this does not necessarily indicate an individual family's economic wealth it does provide a more comprehensive measure of the environment that the family is exposed to which has been shown to be important [26]. We did not have access to individual-level socio-economic data however, it is likely that decisions to commission injury prevention efforts would be made at an area level (e.g. Clinical Commissioning Group area, local authority wards or districts) and our study would support decisions to fund prevention in the most deprived localities.

Comparison with other studies

Injury incidence rates. Our data are consistent with previous studies. The incidence of fracture (75.8/10,000 person years across the 20 year study period) that we derived is comparable to data from European studies between 1988–2005 showing rates of fracture for children under five of between 50–100/10,000 person years,[27–29]. Likewise, our estimate of poisoning incidence (37.3/10,000 person years) is consistent with recent studies of ED attendances from high income countries such as Franklin et al who reported a poisoning incidence rate for 0–5 year olds in the USA in 2004 of 42.9/10,000, [30] and Xiang et al

Table 2. Incidence rates of injury types by socio-demographic characteristics.

	Person years (10,000 years)	Fractures		Burns		Poisonings	
		Frequency	Incidence rate (95% confidence interval) per 10,000 person years	Frequency	Incidence rate (95% confidence interval) per 10,000 person years	Frequency	Incidence rate (95% confidence interval) per 10,000 person years
Overall	272.5	20,668	75.8 (74.8–76.9)	15,796	57.9 (57.0–58.7)	10,155	37.3 (36.5–38.0)
Sex							
Female	132.7	9,615	72.5 (71.0–73.9)	6,702	50.5 (49.3–51.7)	4,703	35.4 (34.4–36.5)
Male	139.9	11,053	79.0 (77.5–80.5)	9,094	65.0 (63.7–66.3)	5,452	39.0 (37.9–40.0)
Age (years)							
<1 year	53.2	1,488	27.9 (26.5–29.4)	2,989	56.1 (54.1–58.1)	710	13.3 (12.4–14.3)
1	56.7	4,175	73.6 (71.4–75.9)	6,486	114.4 (111.6–117.2)	3,184	56.2 (54.2–58.1)
2	55.6	4,847	87.2 (84.8–89.7)	3,284	59.1 (57.1–61.1)	3,605	64.9 (62.8–67.0)
3	54.2	4,884	90.0 (87.5–92.6)	1,810	33.4 (31.8–34.9)	1,821	33.6 (32.1–35.1)
4	52.8	5,274	99.9 (97.3–102.7)	1,227	23.2 (22.0–24.6)	835	15.8 (14.8–16.9)
Socio-economic deprivation (Townsend Quintile)							
1 (least deprived)	65.5	4,868	74.3 (72.2–76.4)	2,807	42.8 (41.3–44.7)	1,852	28.3 (27.0–29.6)
2	52.2	3,901	74.7 (72.4–77.1)	2,461	47.1 (45.3–49.0)	1,766	33.8 (32.3–35.4)
3	51.6	3,879	75.1 (72.8–77.5)	2,996	58.0 (56.0–60.1)	2,035	39.4 (37.7–41.1)
4	48.5	3,783	78.0 (75.5–80.5)	3,436	70.8 (68.5–73.2)	2,180	44.9 (43.1–46.9)
5 (most deprived)	36.4	2,956	81.3 (78.4–84.2)	3,075	84.5 (81.6–87.6)	1,763	48.5 (46.2–50.8)
missing	18.3	1,281	70.0 (66.2–73.9)	1,021	55.8 (52.5–59.3)	559	30.5 (28.1–33.2)
Calendar Period							
1990–1994	21.2	1,431	67.4 (64.0–71.0)	1,914	90.2 (86.3–94.3)	1,177	55.5 (52.4–58.7)
1995–1999	62.3	4,701	75.4 (73.3–77.6)	3,740	60.0 (58.1–62.0)	2,779	44.6 (43.0–46.3)
2000–2004	89.4	6,621	74.0 (72.3–75.8)	5,061	56.6 (55.1–58.2)	3,198	35.8 (34.5–37.0)
2005–2009	99.6	7,915	79.4 (77.7–81.2)	5,081	51.0 (49.6–52.4)	3,001	30.1 (29.1–31.2)

Table 3. Unadjusted and adjusted incidence rate ratios for each injury type.

	Fractures		Burns		Poisonings	
	Incidence rate ratio (95% confidence interval)		Incidence rate ratio (95% confidence interval)		Incidence rate ratio (95% confidence interval)	
	Unadjusted	Adjusted[+]	Unadjusted	Adjusted[+]	Unadjusted	Adjusted[+]
Sex						
Female	1.00	1.00	1.00	1.00	1.00	1.00
Male	1.09 (1.06–1.12)	1.09 (1.06–0.12)	1.29 (1.25–1.33)	1.28 (0.24–0.33)	1.10 (1.06–1.14)	1.10 (1.06–1.14)
Age (years)*						
<1 year	1.00	1.00	1.00	1.00	1.00	1.00
1	2.64 (2.48–2.80)	2.64 (2.49–2.80)	2.04 (1.95–2.13)	2.06 (1.97–2.15)	4.21 (3.89–4.57)	4.25 (3.92–4.61)
2	3.12 (2.95–3.31)	3.13 (2.96–3.32)	1.05 (1.00–1.11)	1.07 (1.02–1.13)	4.87 (4.49–5.28)	4.97 (4.58–5.39)
3	3.22 (3.04–3.42)	3.24 (3.06–3.43)	0.59 (0.56–0.63)	0.61 (0.58–0.65)	2.52 (2.31–2.75)	2.60 (2.39–2.84)
4	3.58 (3.38–3.79)	3.60 (3.40–3.82)	0.41 (0.39–0.44)	0.43 (0.40–0.46)	1.19 (1.07–1.31)	1.25 (1.13–1.38)
Socio-economic group* (Townsend Quintile)						
1 (least)	1.00	1.00	1.00	1.00	1.00	1.00
2	1.01 (0.96–1.05)	1.01 (0.97–1.05)	1.10 (1.04–1.16)	1.10 (1.04–0.16)	1.20 (1.12–1.28)	1.20 (1.13–1.28)
3	1.01 (0.97–1.05)	1.02 (0.98–1.06)	1.35 (1.29–1.42)	1.35 (1.28–1.42)	1.39 (1.31–1.48)	1.40 (1.32–1.50)
4	1.05 (1.01–1.09)	1.06 (1.02–1.11)	1.65 (1.57–1.74)	1.64 (1.56–1.72)	1.59 (1.49–1.69)	1.60 (1.51–1.70)
5 (most)	1.10 (1.04–1.14)	1.11 (1.06–1.16)	1.97 (1.87–2.08)	1.94 (1.85–2.04)	1.71 (1.61–1.83)	1.72 (1.61–1.84)
missing	0.94 (0.88–1.00)	0.96 (0.90–1.02)	1.30 (1.21–1.40)	1.25 (1.17–1.35)	1.08 (0.98–1.19)	1.07 (0.97–1.17)
Calendar Period*						
1990–1994	1.00	1.00	1.00	1.00	1.00	1.00
1995–1999	1.12 (1.05–1.19)	0.95 (0.90–1.01)	0.66 (0.63–0.70)	0.81 (0.77–0.86)	0.80 (0.75–0.86)	0.85 (0.80–0.91)
2000–2004	1.10 (1.04–1.16)	0.93 (0.88–0.99)	0.63 (0.59–0.66)	0.77 (0.73–0.81)	0.64 (0.60–0.69)	0.69 (0.64–0.74)
2005–2009	1.18 (1.11–1.25)	1.01 (0.96–1.07)	0.56 (0.54–0.60)	0.67 (0.63–0.71)	0.54 (0.51–0.58)	0.57 (0.53–0.61)

*Likelihood ratio test for trend p<0.001 for fracture, burn and injury.
[+]Mutually adjusted for sex, age, socio-economic deprivation and calendar period.

who reported a drug-poisoning incidence rate for 0–5 year olds of 25.5/10,000 in the USA, [31]. Few studies have described the incidence of burn injury in children at the population level in high income countries. Of the studies that have been published, most describe either fatalities or the incidence of severe burns that require inpatient admission whereas our study includes both primary and secondary care attended injuries. Our burn incidence rate of 57.9/10,000 person years is therefore much higher than such reports. For example, Vloemans et al reported an incidence of 16.3/10,000 admissions of 0–4 year olds to specialist burn centres in 2000–2007, [32] and Alaghehbandan et al reported a rate of 2.6/10,000 admissions for children aged 2–4 in Canada in 2012, [33].

Health inequalities. We detected a socio-economic gradient for fractures that differs from previous studies that have reported little or no association between fracture and deprivation, [4,5,34]. It may be that this is due to our very large study size and increased power to detect small differences between socio-economic groups. Descriptions of poisonings and burns being associated with increased deprivation are more consistent in the literature and our incidence rate ratios are similar to those reported previously. For example we reported a 72% increase in incidence of poisoning in the most compared to the least deprived areas, similar to the incidence rate ratio found by Xiang et al of 1.63 (drug-related poisonings for all ages), [31]. We found that across the study period, children in the most deprived areas were nearly twice as

likely to have a burn injury compared to the most affluent areas. Other studies have shown a similar gradient. For example Hippisley-Cox et al showed that children under 15 in the most deprived areas in the East Midlands region of the UK were over three times more likely to have a hospital admission due to a burn or scald, [14] and Mulvaney et al showed that in 2004 for all ages, people in the most deprived quartile of areas were over 70% more likely to have a fire-related injury, [6].

Public health implications

We have shown that despite large decreases in the incidence of burns and poisonings in young children since 1990, substantial inequalities persist between social groups in the UK. In addition, the incidence of fractures is increasing and smaller, yet important inequalities in fracture incidence exist. We estimate that up to 30% of burns and poisonings and 3% of fractures could be avoided if injury prevention interventions successfully reduced injury rates in the poorest areas to levels seen in the most affluent areas. This could result in an estimated 9,395 fewer medically-attended injuries per year across the UK.

A range of injury prevention interventions have been identified to reduce the types of health inequality that we have shown. The National Institute for Health and Care Excellence (NICE) recommends that safety assessments are undertaken in the most vulnerable households and that where appropriate, safety advice is given and equipment is provided and fitted by professionals to help

A

Fractures

B

Burns

C

Poisonings

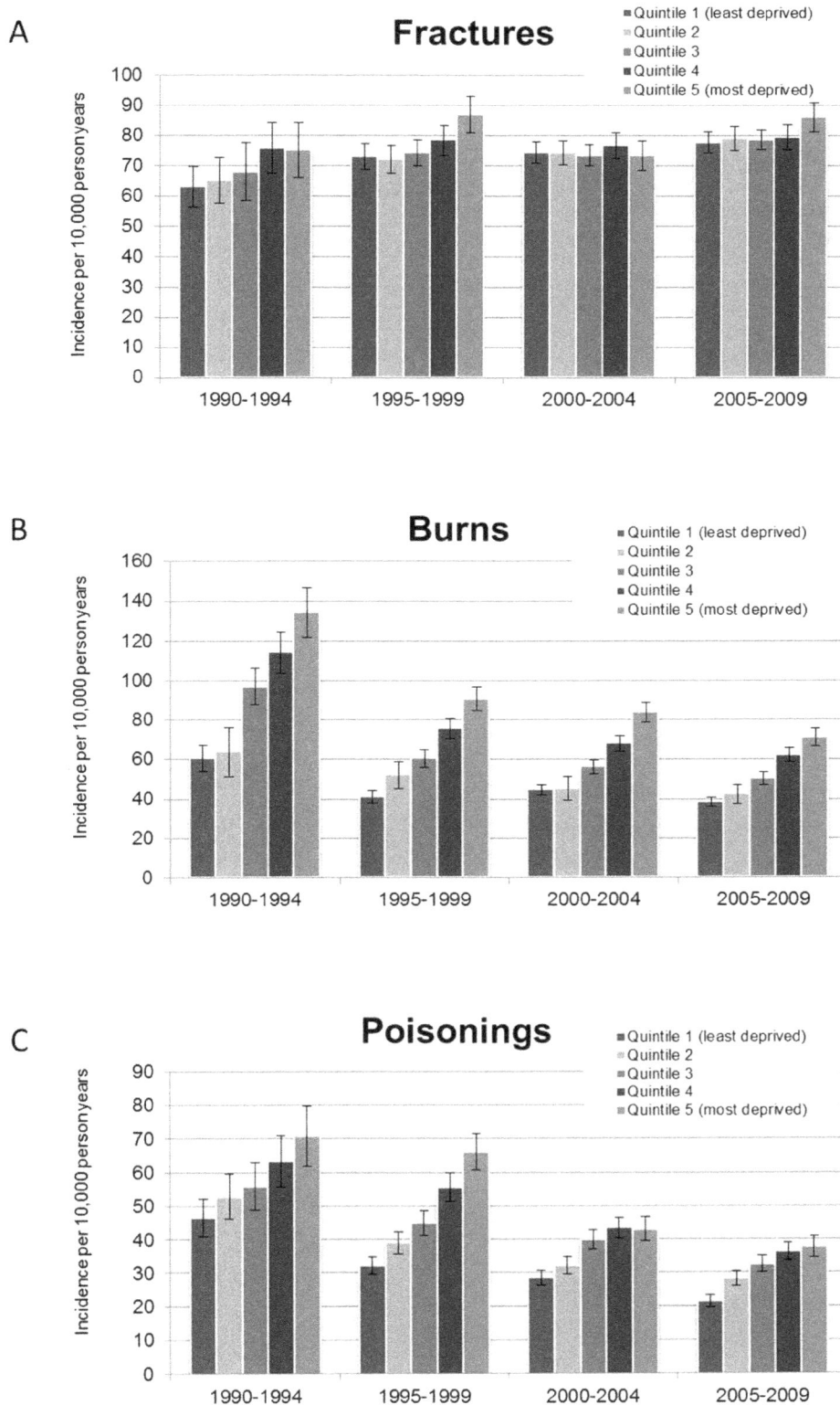

Figure 1. Incidence of fractures (A), burns (B) and poisonings (C) in 5-year periods. Columns represent each quintile of deprivation whereby 1 is the least deprived quintile and 5 is the most deprived quintile.

prevent injury occurring in young children, [35]. In the US the 'Protect the ones you love' initiative has given rise to a multi-

faceted national action plan for child injury prevention that includes elements of education, enforcement and environmental changes (so called 3E's) that can be targeted at the highest risk neighbourhoods and families.

The reduction of inequalities in health, including injuries, is a matter of social justice and international organisations such as the WHO and UNICEF have shown their commitment to reducing these inequalities through the Parma declaration 2010, [36] and the World report on child injury prevention 2012, [1]. In England, Clinical Commissioning Groups and Local Authorities have responsibilities to reduce health inequalities and need to follow NICE guidance to achieve continued reductions in injury incidence and greater equity across social groups. Further to this, policy makers should include the reduction of injury-related health inequalities as an outcome measure in itself, rather than focusing on injury rates alone. In doing this, local health commissioners/

decision makers are more likely to monitor and act upon health inequalities as recommended by NICE. An example of this is the Public Health Outcomes Framework in England which includes the reduction of injuries in young people as one of its indicators but this is measured by hospital admission rates, with no emphasis on the reduction of the health inequality gradient.

Author Contributions

Conceived and designed the experiments: EO DK JW LJT. Performed the experiments: EO. Analyzed the data: EO DK JW LJT. Contributed reagents/materials/analysis tools: LJT. Contributed to the writing of the manuscript: EO DK JW LJT.

References

1. Peden M, Oyegbite K, Ozanne-Smith J, Hyder A, Branche C, et al. (2008) World Report on child injury prevention. World health Organisation, Unicef.
2. Statistics OfN (2012) Death registration summary tables - England and Wales, 2011 (final). Part of the Death Registrations summary tables.
3. Edwards P, Roberts I, Green J, Lutchmun S (2006) Deaths from injury in children and employment status in family: analysis of trends in class specific death rates. BMJ 333: 119.
4. Orton E, Kendrick D, West J, Tata LJ (2012) Independent risk factors for injury in pre-school children: three population-based nested case-control studies using routine primary care data. PLoS One 7: e35193.
5. Lyons R, Delahunty A, McCabe M, Allen H, Nash P (2000) Incidence of childhood fractures in affluent and deprived areas: population based study. British Medical Journal 320: 149–149.
6. Mulvaney C, Kendrick D, Towner E, Brussoni M, Hayes M, et al. (2009) Fatal and non-fatal fire injuries in England 1995–2004: time trends and inequalities by age, sex and area deprivation. J Public Health (Oxf) 31: 154–161.
7. Kendrick D, Mulvaney C, Watson M (2009) Does targeting injury prevention towards families in disadvantaged areas reduce inequalities in safety practices? Health Educ Res 24: 32–41.
8. Roberts I, Power C (1996) Does the decline in child injury mortality vary by social class? A comparison of class specific mortality in 1981 and 1991. BMJ 313: 784–786.
9. Brown GW, Davidson S (1978) Social class, psychiatric disorder of mother, and accidents to children. Lancet 1: 378–381.
10. Haynes R, Jones AP, Reading R, Daras K, Emond A (2008) Neighbourhood variations in child accidents and related child and maternal characteristics: does area definition make a difference? Health Place 14: 693–701.
11. Reading R, Jones A, Haynes R, Daras K, Emond A (2008) Individual factors explain neighbourhood variations in accidents to children under 5 years of age. Soc Sci Med 67: 915–927.
12. Kendrick D, Marsh P (2001) How useful are sociodemographic characteristics in identifying children at risk of unintentional injury? Public Health 115: 103–107.
13. Pomerantz WJ, Dowd MD, Buncher CR (2001) Relationship between socioeconomic factors and severe childhood injuries. J Urban Health 78: 141–151.
14. Hippisley-Cox J, Groom L, Kendrick D, Coupland C, Webber E, et al. (2002) Cross sectional survey of socioeconomic variations in severity and mechanism of childhood injuries in Trent 1992–7. BMJ 324: 1132.
15. Office. TS (2012) Health and Social Care Act 2012. In: Government U, editor. Chapter 7.
16. (2012) Public Health Outcomes Framework. In: Health. Do, editor: Crown Copyright.
17. Parliament E (2008) Regulation on Community statistics on public health and health and safety at work. In: Parliament E, editor. OJ L 354/70. Official Journal of the European Union.
18. Blak BT, Thompson M, Dattani H, Bourke A (2011) Generalisability of The Health Improvement Network (THIN) database: demographics, chronic disease prevalence and mortality rates. Inform Prim Care 19: 251–255.

19. Bourke A, Dattani H, Robinson M (2004) Feasibility study and methodology to create a quality-evaluated database of primary care data. Inform Prim Care 12: 171–177.
20. Herrett EL, Thomas SL, Smeeth L (2011) Validity of diagnoses in the general practice research database. Br J Gen Pract 61: 438–439.
21. Townsend P, Phillimore P, Beattie A (1988) Health and deprivation: inequality and the North. London: Croom Helm.
22. MacInnes K, Stone DH (2008) Stages of development and injury: an epidemiological survey of young children presenting to an emergency department. BMC Public Health 8: 120.
23. Statistics. OfN All releases of Population Estimates for UK, England and Wales, Scotland and Northern Ireland.
24. Steenland K, Armstrong B (2006) An overview of methods for calculating the burden of disease due to specific risk factors. Epidemiology 17: 512–519.
25. Centre. HaSCI (2012) Attribution Data Set GP-Registered Populations 2010.
26. Roberts I, Marshall R, Norton R, Borman B (1992) An area analysis of child injury morbidity in Auckland. Journal of Paediatrics and Child Health 28: 438–441.
27. Cooper C, Dennison EM, Leufkens HG, Bishop N, van Staa TP (2004) Epidemiology of childhood fractures in Britain: a study using the general practice research database. J Bone Miner Res 19: 1976–1981.
28. Mayranpaa MK, Makitie O, Kallio PE (2010) Decreasing incidence and changing pattern of childhood fractures: A population-based study.[Erratum appears in J Bone Miner Res. 2011 Feb;26(2): 439]. Journal of Bone & Mineral Research 25: 2752–2759.
29. Rennie L, Court-Brown CM, Mok JY, Beattie TF (2007) The epidemiology of fractures in children. Injury 38: 913–922.
30. Franklin RL, Rodgers GB (2008) Unintentional Child Poisonings Treated in United States Hospital Emergency Departments: National Estimates of Incident Cases, Population-Based Poisoning Rates, and Product Involvement. Pediatrics 122: 1244–1251.
31. Xiang Y, Zhao W, Xiang H, Smith GA (2012) ED visits for drug-related poisoning in the United States, 2007. Am J Emerg Med 30: 293–301.
32. Vloemans AF, Dokter J, van Baar ME, Nijhuis I, Beerthuizen GI, et al. (2011) Epidemiology of children admitted to the Dutch burn centres. Changes in referral influence admittance rates in burn centres. Burns 37: 1161–1167.
33. Alaghehbandan R, Sikdar KC, Gladney N, MacDonald D, Collins KD (2012) Epidemiology of severe burn among children in Newfoundland and Labrador, Canada. Burns 38: 136–140.
34. Stark AD, Bennet GC, Stone DH, Christi P (2002) Association between childhood fractures and poverty: population based study. British Medical Journal 324: 457.
35. NICE (2010) Strategies to prevent unintentional injuries among under-15s.
36. Region WHOE (2010) Declaration on Environment and Health. 5th Ministerial Conference on Environment and Health, Parma, Italy.

20

A Study on Genetic Variants of Fibroblast Growth Factor Receptor 2 (*FGFR2*) and the Risk of Breast Cancer from North India

Sarah Siddiqui[1], Shilpi Chattopadhyay[1], Md. Salman Akhtar[1], Mohammad Zeeshan Najm[1], S. V. S. Deo[2], N. K. Shukla[2], Syed Akhtar Husain[1]*

1 Department of Biotechnology, Jamia Millia Islamia, New Delhi, India, 2 Department of Surgical Oncology, All India Institute of Medical Sciences, New Delhi, India

Abstract

Genome-Wide Association Studies (GWAS) have identified Fibroblast growth factor receptor 2 (*FGFR2*) as a candidate gene for breast cancer with single nucleotide polymorphisms (SNPs) located in intron 2 region as the susceptibility loci strongly associated with the risk. However, replicate studies have often failed to extrapolate the association to diverse ethnic regions. This hints towards the existing heterogeneity among different populations, arising due to differential linkage disequilibrium (LD) structures and frequencies of SNPs within the associated regions of the genome. It is therefore important to revisit the previously linked candidates in varied population groups to unravel the extent of heterogeneity. In an attempt to investigate the role of *FGFR2* polymorphisms in susceptibility to the risk of breast cancer among North Indian women, we genotyped rs2981582, rs1219648, rs2981578 and rs7895676 polymorphisms in 368 breast cancer patients and 484 healthy controls by Polymerase chain reaction-Restriction fragment length polymorphism (PCR-RFLP) assay. We observed a statistically significant association with breast cancer risk for all the four genetic variants ($P<0.05$). In per-allele model for rs2981582, rs1219648, rs7895676 and in dominant model for rs2981578, association remained significant after bonferroni correction ($P<0.0125$). On performing stratified analysis, significant correlations with various clinicopathological as well as environmental and lifestyle characteristics were observed. It was evident that rs1219648 and rs2981578 interacted with exogenous hormone use and advanced clinical stage III (after Bonferroni correction, $P<0.000694$), respectively. Furthermore, combined analysis on these four loci revealed that compared to women with 0–1 risk loci, those with 2–4 risk loci had increased risk (OR = 1.645, 95%CI = 1.152–2.347, $P=0.006$). In haplotype analysis, for rs2981578, rs2981582 and rs1219648, risk haplotype (GTG) was associated with a significantly increased risk compared to the common (ACA) haplotype (OR = 1.365, 95% CI = 1.086–1.717, $P=0.008$). Our results suggest that intron 2 SNPs of *FGFR2* may contribute to genetic susceptibility of breast cancer in North India population.

Editor: Nancy Lan Guo, West Virginia University, United States of America

Funding: Financial support for the production of the manuscript was provided by University Grants Commission (UGC) to Department of Biotechnology, Jamia Millia Islamia and Council of Scientific and Industrial Research (CSIR) to S. Siddiqui as scholarship under Grant No. File No. 09/466(0127)/2010-EMR-I. UGC (http://www.ugc.ac.in/) CSIR (http://csirhrdg.res.in/). The funders had no role in study design, data collection and analysis, decision to publish, or preparation of the manuscript.

Competing Interests: The authors have declared that no competing interests exist.

* Email: akhtarhusain2000@yahoo.com

Introduction

Worldwide, breast cancer is the most commonly diagnosed cancer and the leading cause of cancer mortality among women [1]. Asian countries have witnessed greatest increase of the globally rising breast cancer burden during the last several decades [2–6]. A similar trend has been observed in India [7–10] with a reported 0.5–2% per annum rise in incidence across all regions and in all age groups, particularly in younger age groups (<45 years) [11]. Further, it is predicted that breast cancer cases would increase by 26%, majorly in developing countries, by 2020 [12].

Breast carcinogenesis involves a complex combination of genetic, environmental as well as lifestyle factors. Inherited susceptibility makes an important contribution to breast cancer development and the risk is around two times more in first degree relatives of women with the disease [13]. Rare mutations in several high-penetrance genes like BReast CAncer genes (*BRCA1*, *BRCA2*) account for less than 25% of the familial breast cancer risk, and less than 5% of the overall risk [14,15]. Therefore, common variants present in other low penetrance genes may be more imperative and contribute to breast cancer along with lifestyle and environmental factors [16]. However, all of the common low risk variants described so far collectively account for <10% of the familial risk of breast cancer [17–25], leaving ample room for uncovering additional variants that confer risk of this disease and account for the genetic basis of the remaining major breast cancer fraction. Single nucleotide polymorphisms are the most common type of germline variations present in at least 1% of a population [26]. The effect of an individual SNP is usually small, but combinations of relevant SNPs across the genome may additively contribute to higher risk in a polygenic model [27]. Though supposed to be functionally insignificant, current evidence emphasizes their predominantly unexplored functional relevance [28–30].

Fibroblast Growth Factor Receptor 2 (FGFR2) belongs to the FGFR family of tyrosine kinase receptors and contributes to the process of tumorigenesis through cell growth, invasiveness, motility and angiogenesis [31]. It plays an important role during mammary gland development [32] and aberrant FGF signaling has been associated with the pathogenesis of multiple types of cancer [33–36]. FGFR2 overexpression has been observed in breast cancer cell lines and breast tumor tissues [37–38]. Human *FGFR2* gene, is located at chromosome 10q26, and contains 22 exons [39]. Two large Genome-Wide Association Studies (GWAS) have identified intron 2 SNPs of *FGFR2* to be associated with breast cancer risk, rs2981582 and rs1219648 were the most strongly associated marker SNPs in the two studies respectively [17,18]. Association of these variants with breast cancer has been evaluated in different ethnic regions with inconsistent findings [40–54]. Recent meta-analysis suggests their association with breast cancer risk in Caucasian and East Asian populations [55]. Both rs2981582 and rs1219648 fell in a 25 kb linkage disequilibrium (LD) block within intron 2 region of *FGFR2* [17,18]. Multiple haplotypes carrying the minor allele of rs2981582 were found to be associated with the risk in haplotype analysis [17]. Six polymorphisms including rs7895676 and rs2981578 were identified as potentially causal for breast cancer, with rs7895676 exhibiting strongest association in the combined analysis of European and Asian datasets [17]. Further analysis by Meyer et al. [56] support their functional relevance in relation to breast cancer risk. However, the association of rs2981578 and rs7895676 with breast cancer susceptibility still remains inconclusive [49–52,57].

Wide variations in genetic architecture, including differential allele frequencies of SNPs and differently evolved LD structure for the GWAS-identified genetic variants reflect differences among ethnicities and may contribute to disparities in the incidence and characteristics of breast cancer. Thus, variants identified in one study may not have the same impact on risk in other populations. Therefore, there is a need to replicate previously associated loci in multiple populations worldwide. This will help in determining the genetic heterogeneity among different population groups for these loci, particularly in India, which witnesses a rapidly rising breast cancer burden but relatively fewer studies to identify the common breast cancer associated variations. Such studies will assist in evaluating the generalizability of initial findings and to identify the causal variants. Therefore, we tried to assess the impact of *FGFR2* intron 2 polymorphisms (rs2981582, rs1219648, rs2981578 and rs7895676) on sporadic breast cancer and determined their association with the risk for North Indian women in a case control approach, including combined effect of these variants, LD structure measurement, haplotype analysis, as well as relation with patients' clinical, environmental and lifestyle characteristics. We observed significant association of these variants with breast cancer susceptibility for North Indian women.

Materials and Methods

Ethics Statement

The study was approved by Institution Ethics Committee of All India Institute of Medical Sciences (AIIMS), New Delhi and the Institutional Human Ethical Committee of Jamia Millia Islamia, New Delhi. All the participants provided their written informed consent to be included in the study.

Study subjects and specimen collection

This hospital-based case control study included a total of 852 genetically unrelated women subjects of North Indian ethnicity comprising 368 sporadic breast cancer cases and 484 healthy controls. Controls were frequency- matched to cases on age (±2 years) and geographical location. The study participation response rates for cases and controls were 88.46% and 81.07%, respectively. All breast cancer cases (aged 24–80 years) were newly diagnosed, histopathologically confirmed with primary breast cancer and were recruited from the Department of Surgical Oncology, AIIMS. Classification of breast cancer has been done according to TNM staging system by American Joint Committee on Cancer (AJCC) and Nottingham grading system for histological grading. Exclusion criteria included in the study were reported previous cancer history, metastasized cancer from other organs and previous exposure to radiotherapy or chemotherapy.

Detailed information on clinical profiles for cases and controls were collected from their medical records and are presented in Table S1. Included were tumor characteristics [age at diagnosis, tumor size, lymph node (LN) involvement, clinical stage, histological grade, estrogen receptor (ER) status, progesterone receptor (PR) status and human epidermal growth factor receptor 2 (HER2) status], reproductive history [including age at menarche, menopausal status, age at menopause, parity, age at first live birth and status of breastfeeding] as well as several demographic, lifestyle and environmental factors [Exogenous hormone use for purposes like contraception/infertility treatment/hormone replacement therapy (yes: for >6 months/No: for ≤6 months), BMI (Basal metabolic index, calculated as weight divided by squared height, kg/m^2), geographical location, education level and economic independence (employed/unemployed)].

Extraction of genomic DNA

Participating women provided 3–5 ml of venous blood samples used for isolating genomic DNA based on standard phenol–chloroform extraction method [58]. DNA samples were stored at −80°C until used for further analysis.

SNP selection and Genotype analysis

Previously reported *FGFR2* SNPs showing association with breast cancer in one or more GWAS and candidate gene studies including the two proposed functional variants (rs2981582C/T, rs1219648A/G, rs2981578A/G, rs7895676T/C) [17,18,40–52,56] were selected for genotyping. All the four SNPs were analyzed using the Polymerase chain reaction-restriction fragment length polymorphism (PCR-RFLP) assay. Details of selected SNPs, primer sequences used for PCR, sizes of the PCR products, restriction endonucleases (New England Biolabs, USA) used for digestion and their recognition sequences, as well as size of various digested fragments obtained distinguishing different genotypes for all the four SNPs are described in Table 1 and Table S2. For all the SNPs, restriction digested fragments were subjected to analysis by 2–3.5% agarose gel electrophoresis. In order to validate the data generated by PCR-RFLP assay method, 5% of randomly selected samples were directly sequenced. DNA sequencing was carried out at Xcelris Labs Ltd., India. The quality of genotyping was assessed by re-genotyping 10% of randomly selected samples; no discrepancy in the replicate genotyping could be obtained.

Statistical analysis

To compare the overall distribution of genotypes between patients and healthy controls 3×2 Chi-square (χ2) test was performed. Hardy–Weinberg equilibrium (HWE) was evaluated

Table 1. Primers used for genotyping *FGFR2* SNPs.

FGFR2 SNPs	Primer Sequences	PCR product length (base pairs)	Restriction endonucleases used	Genotype (size of digested fragments in base pairs)
rs2981582	F 5'CGTGAGCCAAGCCTCTACTT3'			CC (140, 84, 38)
	R 5'TAAGTGTGCTGTTCATTCA3'	262	AciI	CT (178, 140, 84, 38)
				TT (178, 84)
rs1219648	F 5'ATGGTACCGGTTTCCCAA3'			AA (180)
	R 5'TGTGATTTGTATGTGGTAG3'	180	BspQI	AG (180, 106, 74)
				GG (106, 74)
rs2981578	F 5'CCCAGAAAGCCTACATTCGT3'			AA (330)
	R 5'CAGGACCCAAGGAAGGCAG3'	330	AciI	AG (330, 182, 148)
				GG (182, 148)
rs7895676	F 5'AGGTGCGGTGGCTCATGTCTGTA3'			TT (292, 54)
	R 5'CTGACTTCAATGGCGGGACTCCAT3'	346	DpnII	CT (292, 175, 117, 54)
				CC (175, 117, 54)

by a goodness-of-fit $\chi 2$ test. For estimating associations between individual genotypes and breast cancer risk, and for cumulative risk analysis, odds ratios (ORs) and their 95% confidence intervals (CIs) were computed using unconditional logistic regression analysis with adjustment for age. One-way ANOVA (Analysis of variance) was carried out for estimating the contribution of different number of risk loci to breast cancer risk. These statistical analysis were performed using Statistical Package for the Social Sciences, version 17 (SPSS Inc., Chicago, IL, USA) and $P<0.05$ was considered statistically significant. Further, all P-values were corrected for multiple comparisons according to Bonferroni method. LD pattern and population haplotype frequencies for the SNPs were estimated using HaploView v4.2 [59]. Fisher's exact test was performed for determining the association of haplotypes with diseased condition.

Results

Results of genotype analysis on the four selected *FGFR2* intronic variants (rs2981582C/T, rs1219648A/G, rs2981578A/G, and rs7895676T/C) were available from 368 breast cancer cases/484 healthy controls and a notably significant association with breast cancer susceptibility was observed.

Hardy–Weinberg equilibrium testing

The observed genotype frequencies were found to be in agreement ($\chi 2$ test, $P>0.05$) with Hardy–Weinberg equilibrium in both cases ($P = 0.545$, 0.261, 0.347 and 0.832) and controls ($P = 0.526$, 0.569, 0.278 and 0.467) for the SNPs rs2981582, rs1219648, rs2981578 and rs7895676 respectively.

FGFR2 SNPs and overall breast cancer risk

Distribution of genotype and allele frequencies of the four *FGFR2* SNPs in breast cancer cases and controls are shown in Table 2. Chi-square test depicted a significant association for the four *FGFR2* variants with overall breast cancer risk ($P<0.05$). Logistic regression analysis (age adjusted) further confirmed this association which remained significant in per-allele model for rs2981582/T, rs1219648/G, rs7895676/C and in dominant model for rs2981578 (AG+GG) even after Bonferroni correction ($P<0.0125$).

To evaluate the cumulative risk for these SNPs, we categorized study subjects as carrying 0 risk loci, 1 risk loci, 2 risk loci, 3 risk loci and 4 risk loci (risk loci represents presence of risk allele at SNP position). For determining the contribution of different risk loci overall as well as in four different trio combinations of these SNPs, logistic regression and one-way ANOVA tests were performed (Table 3). Logistic regression analysis revealed a significantly higher risk in carriers with 2–4 risk loci (aOR = 1.645, 95%CI = 1.152–2.347, $P = 0.006$) compared to those with 0–1 risk loci. Further a progressively increased risk was noted from 1 risk loci (aOR = 1.600, 95%CI = 0.754–3.394) to 2 risk loci (aOR = 1.786, 95%CI = 1.076–2.964) to 3–4 risk loci (aOR = 1.855, 95%CI = 1.230–2.799) in comparison to 0 risk loci (Table S3). ANOVA determined significant ($P<0.05$) differences in the contribution of various risk loci to diseased condition for the four SNPs taken together as well as in different combinations (^cP values in Table 3). Moreover, logistic regression analysis revealed significant contribution of only two SNP combinations for breast cancer risk considering dichotomized 2–3 risk loci compared to 0–1 risk loci, including ABD (rs7895676, rs2981578 and rs1219648; aOR = 1.622, 95%CI = 1.150–2.289, $P = 0.006$), and BCD (rs2981578, rs2981582 and rs1219648; aOR = 1.431, 95%CI = 1.065–1.923, $P = 0.018$). On conducting multiple comparison analysis in ANOVA, similar trends were observed (Table S3, Table S4). Significant association with the risk was noted for 2 risk loci ($P = 0.026$) and 4 risk loci ($P = 0.002$) compared to 0 risk loci. Also for the four different SNP combinations, significant P values for all the risk loci were observed for combination BCD (^bP values in Table 3) indicating its predominant contribution towards risk.

FGFR2 SNPs and clinicopathological characteristics

Further we analyzed association of these variants with various clinicopathological characteristics including several reproductive and environmental risk factors of breast cancer in a stratified analytical approach (Table 4) The corrected P value cut-off after bonferroni correction was set as ($P<0.000694$).

For *rs2981582(C/T)/FGFR2*, genotype CT vs. CC (vs. = in comparison to) and combined CT+TT vs. CC significantly correlated with premenopausal status ($P = 0.024$, 0.046 respectively). T allele displayed stronger association with ER-positive women (TT vs. CC, $P = 0.001$; CT+TT vs. CC, $P = 0.012$) and

Table 2. Genotype and allele frequencies of *FGFR2* polymorphisms in sporadic breast cancer cases and controls.

Genotypes	Cases (N = 368)	Controls (N = 484)	[a]P	[b]P	aOR (95% CI)
FGFR2 (rs2981582)					
CC	144 (39.13%)	226 (46.69%)		-	1.000 (referent)
CT	168 (45.65%)	205 (42.36%)		0.084	1.300 (0.965–1.752)
TT	56 (15.22%)	53 (10.95%)	0.045	0.022	1.668 (1.078–2.582)
CC vs. CT+TT				0.025	1.379 (1.042–1.824)
C (%)	61.96	67.87		-	1.000 (referent)
T (%)	38.04	32.13		0.011*	1.297 (1.061–1.586)
FGFR2 (rs1219648)					
AA	110 (29.89%)	183 (37.81%)		-	1.000 (referent)
AG	192 (52.17%)	234 (48.35%)		0.042	1.375 (1.012–1.867)
GG	66 (17.93%)	67 (13.84%)	0.036	0.019	1.644 (1.084–2.495)
AA vs. AG+GG				0.015	1.435 (1.073–1.920)
A (%)	55.98	61.98		-	1.000 (referent)
G (%)	44.02	38.02		0.012*	1.282 (1.055–1.558)
FGFR2 (rs2981578)					
AA	54 (14.67%)	105 (21.69%)		-	1.000 (referent)
AG	185 (50.27%)	228 (47.11%)		0.019	1.581 (1.079–2.315)
GG	129 (34.05%)	151 (31.20%)	0.033	0.014	1.661 (1.108–2.489)
AA vs. AG+GG				0.009*	1.613 (1.124–2.314)
A (%)	39.81	45.25		-	1.000 (referent)
G (%)	60.19	54.75		0.025	1.249 (1.029–1.518)
FGFR2 (rs7895676)					
TT	71 (19.29%)	124 (25.62%)		-	1.000 (referent)
TC	179 (48.64%)	234 (48.35%)		0.097	1.349 (0.947–1.923)
CC	118 (32.07%)	126 (26.03%)	0.043	0.011*	1.649 (1.119–2.431)
TT vs. TC+CC				0.027	1.455 (1.044–2.029)
T (%)	43.61	49.79		-	1.000 (referent)
C (%)	56.39	50.21		0.011*	1.282 (1.058–1.555)

*P<0.0125, P values significant after Bonferroni correction.
OR odds ratio, CI confidence interval.
[a]P value for 3×2 χ2 test of comparison of overall genotype frequencies between cases and controls.
[b]P value and corresponding age-adjusted OR (aOR) with 95% CIs [aOR (95% CI)] for comparison of genotype frequencies between cases and controls by logistic regression analysis (age is not adjusted in allele frequency comparisons).

with PR-positive women (CT vs. CC, *P* = 0.035; CT+TT vs. CC, *P* = 0.024). Association with histologically less malignant grade I+II (TT vs. CC, *P* = 0.026), early age at menarche (CT+TT vs. CC, *P* = 0.040) and employed status (CT vs. CC, *P* = 0.003) was also observed.

For *rs1219648 (A/G)/FGFR2*, AG genotype presented a significantly higher distribution in premenopausal patients exhibiting higher risk (AG vs. AA, *P* = 0.035). Furthermore, G-carriers were more significantly linked to tumors with ER-positive status (GG vs. AA, *P* = 0.016), LN positive status (AG vs. AA, *P* = 0.001; AG+GG vs. AA, *P* = 0.004), and more malignant histological grade III (AG vs. AA, *P* = 0.019; AG+GG vs. AA, *P* = 0.018). Also, interaction of the risk allele with positive breastfeeding status (AG vs. AA, *P* = 0.037) and strongly with exogenous hormone exposure (GG vs. AA, *P* = 0.0001; AG+GG vs. AA, *P* = 0.004) was noted.

For *rs2981578 (A/G)/FGFR2*, G allele carriers were more likely to bear tumors of greater aggressiveness with advanced clinical stage III+IV (AG vs. AA, *P* = 0.0001; AG+GG vs. AA,

P = 0.002) and LN metastasis (AG vs. AA, *P* = 0.046). Association with late age at menarche (GG vs. AA, *P* = 0.011) and parous status (GG vs. AA, *P* = 0.033) was also observed.

For *rs7895676 (T/C)/FGFR2*, TC genotype exhibited significantly greater risk in PR-positive women (TC vs. TT, *P* = 0.019). Further association of the risk allele with LN-positive status (TC vs. TT, *P* = 0.002; TC+CC vs. TT, *P* = 0.013), pathologically less malignant grade I+II tumors (CC vs. TT, *P* = 0.014; TC+CC vs. TT, *P* = 0.027) and with negative breastfeeding status (CC vs. TT, *P* = 0.006; TC+CC vs. TT, *P* = 0.048) was evidenced.

Linkage Disequilibrium (LD) and Haplotype analysis

Setting measure of high LD between two genetic markers cut off to a value $r^2 \geq 0.80$, $D' = 1$, in control group of our study population, the four studied SNPs were found to be in moderate to weak LD (pair wise r^2 value range from 0.175–0.680, D' value range from 0.610–0.938, Figure S1). Haplotype frequencies were estimated for the four SNPs taken together as well as for different combinations of SNPs taken three and two at a time using

Table 3. Estimated risk of combined *FGFR2* SNPs (rs7895676, rs2981578, rs2981582 and rs1219648).

SNP Combi-nations	No. of risk loci	No. of risk loci (dichotomized)	No. of cases (%)	No. of controls (%)	aOR (95% CI)	[a]P value	[b]P value	[c]P value
[d]ABCD	0						-	
	1	0–1	56 (15.22)	110 (22.73)	1.000 (Referent)		0.234	
	2						0.026	
	3						0.115	
	4	2–4	312 (84.78)	374 (77.27)	1.645 (1.152–2.347)	0.006	0.002	0.037
ABC	0						-	
	1	0–1	69 (18.75)	116 (23.97)	1.000 (Referent)		0.013	
	2						0.086	
	3	2–3	299 (81.25)	368 (76.03)	1.375 (0.982–1.925)	0.064	0.002	0.007
BCD	0						-	
	1	0–1	105 (28.53)	175 (36.16)	1.000 (Referent)		0.027	
	2						0.002	
	3	2–3	263 (71.47)	309 (63.84)	1.431 (1.065–1.923)	0.018	0.003	0.011
ABD	0						-	
	1	0–1	62 (16.85)	119 (24.59)	1.000 (Referent)		0.250	
	2						0.006	
	3	2–3	306 (83.15)	365 (75.41)	1.622 (1.150–2.289)	0.006	0.006	0.028
ACD	0						-	
	1	0–1	112 (30.43)	177 (36.57)	1.000 (Referent)		0.148	
	2						0.572	
	3	2–3	256 (69.57)	307 (63.43)	1.329 (0.992–1.780)	0.056	0.006	0.029

OR odds ratio, *CI* confidence interval.

[a]P value and corresponding age-adjusted OR (aOR) with 95% CIs for combined risk analysis by logistic regression test.

[b]P value for association of different number of risk loci with breast cancer risk in comparison to 0 risk loci by one-way ANOVA analysis displaying multiple comparisons output.

[c]P value <0.05 represents significant difference between contribution of different number of risk loci to breast cancer risk.

[d]A = rs7895676, B = rs2981578, C = rs2981582 and D = rs1219648.

Table 4. Association of *FGFR2* rs2981582, rs1219648, rs2981578 and rs7895676 SNPs with clinicopathological, life style and environmental characteristics of breast cancer patients from North India.

Character-istic	FGFR2 rs2981582 Genotype (n)	aOR (95% CI)	P value	FGFR2 rs1219648 Genotype (n)	aOR (95% CI)	P value	FGFR2 rs2981578 Genotype (n)	aOR (95% CI)	P value	FGFR2 rs7895676 Genotype (n)	aOR (95% CI)	P value
Menopausal Status	CC (51/93)	1.000		AA (41/69)	1.000		AA (21/33)	1.000		TT (31/40)	1.000	0.660
	CT (79/89)	0.236 (0.067-0.827)	0.024	AG (88/104)	0.251(0.069-.909)	0.035	AG (74/111)	1.733 (0.418-7.191)	0.449	TC (77/102)	0.753 (0.212-2.669)	0.660
Pre/Post	TT (25/31)	0.671 (0.178-2.535)	0.557	GG (26/40)	1.128 (0.327-3.898)	0.849	GG (60/69)	0.559 (0.109-2.857)	0.485	CC (47/71)	0.800 (0.208-3.070)	0.745
	CT+TT (104/120)	0.349 (0.124-0.980)	0.046	AG+GG (114/144)	0.470 (0.168-1.316)	0.151	AG+GG (134/180)	1.137 (0.289-4.476)	0.855	TC+CC (124/173)	0.772 (0.242-2.468)	0.663
Age at Menopause	CC (39/54)	1.0000		AA (34/35)	1.000		AA (19/14)	1.000		TT (22/18)	1.000	
	CT (42/47)	0.615 (0.327-1.157)	0.132	AG (50/54)	0.852 (0.451-1.607)	0.620	AG (50/61)	1.819 (0.802-4.123)	0.152	TC (49/53)	1.121 (0.510-2.460)	0.777
(years)	TT (17/14)	0.640 (0.267-1.534)	0.317	GG (14/26)	1.009 (0.382-2.666)	0.985	GG (29/40)	1.895 (0.791-4.539)	0.151	CC (27/44)	1.896 (0.824-4.365)	0.133
≤49/≥50	CT+TT (59/61)	0.622 (0.347-1.113)	0.109	AG+GG (64/80)	0.883 (0.485-1.608)	0.685	AG+GG (79/101)	1.848 (0.846-4.035)	0.123	TC+CC (76/97)	1.397 (0.669-2.919)	0.374
ER Status	CC (56/88)	1.000		AA (46/64)	1.000		AA (24/30)	1.000		TT (37/34)	1.000	
Positive/	CT (81/87)	1.448 (0.905-2.317)	0.122	AG (86/106)	1.062 (0.650-1.733)	0.811	AG (93/92)	1.333 (0.711-2.498)	0.370	TC (78/101)	0.677 (0.382-1.200)	0.182
Negative	TT (35/21)	3.123 (1.621-6.018)	0.001	GG (40/26)	2.183 (1.155-4.127)	0.016	GG (55/74)	1.024 (0.530-1.977)	0.944	CC (57/61)	0.871 (0.475-1.596)	0.655
	CT+TT (116/108)	1.761 (1.135-2.732)	0.012	AG+GG (126/132)	1.285 (0.808-2.042)	0.290	AG+GG (148/166)	1.196 (0.657-2.177)	0.558	TC+CC (135/162)	0.751 (0.439-1.284)	0.296
PR Status	CC (59/85)	1.000		AA (48/62)	1.000		AA (25/29)	1.000		TT (29/42)	1.000	
Positive/	CT (91/77)	1.642 (1.035-2.606)	0.035	AG (102/90)	1.401 (0.863-2.272)	0.172	AG (86/99)	1.065 (0.571-1.984)	0.844	TC (101/78)	1.990 (1.118-3.544)	0.019
Negative	TT (29/27)	1.652 (0.874-3.121)	0.122	GG (29/37)	0.965 (0.516-1.805)	0.910	GG (68/61)	1.424 (0.742-2.732)	0.288	CC (49/69)	1.119 (0.606-2.064)	0.719
	CT+TT (120/104)	1.645 (1.067-2.535)	0.024	AG+GG (131/127)	1.270 (0.802-2.010)	0.308	AG+GG (154/160)	1.200 (0.663-2.170)	0.547	TC+CC (150/147)	1.573 (0.915-2.703)	0.101
HER 2 Status	CC (65/79)	1.000		AA (59/51)	1.000		AA (22/32)	1.000		TT (31/40)	1.000	
Tus	CT (86/82)	1.333 (0.841-2.113)	0.222	AG (88/104)	0.772 (0.476-1.253)	0.295	AG (95/90)	1.659 (0.884-3.115)	0.115	TC (91/88)	1.357 (0.765-2.406)	0.297
Positive/	TT (23/33)	0.814 (0.427-1.551)	0.532	GG (27/39)	0.595 (0.317-1.119)	0.107	GG (57/72)	1.173 (0.607-2.267)	0.635	CC (52/66)	0.983 (0.534-1.808)	0.955
Negative	CT+TT (109/115)	1.176 (0.765-1.808)	0.461	AG+GG (115/143)	0.722 (0.456-1.143)	0.164	AG+GG (152/162)	1.438 (0.790-2.619)	0.235	TC+CC (143/154)	1.190 (0.694-2.038)	0.527
Tumor size	CC(102/42)	1.000		AA (74/36)	1.000		AA (37/17)	1.000		TT (55/16)	1.000	

Table 4. Cont.

Characteristic	FGFR2 rs2981582 Genotype (n)	aOR (95% CI)	P value	FGFR2 rs1219648 Genotype (n)	aOR (95% CI)	P value	FGFR2 rs2981578 Genotype (n)	aOR (95% CI)	P value	FGFR2 rs7895676 Genotype (n)	aOR (95% CI)	P value
(cm)	CT (130/38)	1.500 (0.889–2.532)	0.129	AG (144/48)	1.574 (0.926–2.676)	0.094	AG (141/44)	1.612 (0.818–3.180)	0.168	TC (134/45)	0.880 (0.451–1.717)	0.708
>2/≤2	TT (37/19)	0.772 (0.391–1.524)	0.456	GG (51/15)	1.664 (0.818–3.386)	0.160	GG (91/38)	1.169 (0.581–2.353)	0.661	CC (80/38)	0.597 (0.300–1.191)	0.143
	CT+TT (167/57)	1.247 (0.773–2.011)	0.366	AG+GG (195/63)	1.597 (0.967–2.638)	0.068	AG+GG (232/82)	1.404 (0.742–2.658)	0.297	TC+CC (214/83)	0.746 (0.399–1.395)	0.359
Lymph node Status	CC (85/59)	1.000		AA (56/54)	1.000		AA (28/26)	1.000		TT (34/37)	1.000	
	CT (108/60)	1.359 (0.846–2.185)	0.205	AG (132/60)	2.360 (1.424–3.910)	0.001	AG (124/61)	1.904 (1.012–3.581)	0.046	TC (123/56)	2.521 (1.402–4.532)	0.002
Positive/	TT (32/24)	0.888 (0.463–1.702)	0.721	GG (37/29)	1.275 (0.677–2.400)	0.452	GG (73/56)	1.185 (0.616–2.281)	0.610	CC (68/50)	1.434 (0.778–2.642)	0.248
Negative	CT+TT (140/84)	1.218 (0.783–1.893)	0.382	AG+GG (169/89)	1.986 (1.239–3.185)	0.004	AG+GG (197/117)	1.558 (0.858–2.827)	0.145	TC+CC (191/106)	1.984 (1.154–3.413)	0.013
Clinical	CC (86/58)	1.000		AA (58/52)	1.000		AA (19/35)	1.000		TT (43/28)	1.000	
Stage	CT (88/80)	0.783 (0.491–1.248)	0.303	AG (111/81)	1.307 (0.799–2.137)	0.287	AG (120/65)	3.588 (1.851–6.955)	0.0001	TC (102/77)	0.911 (0.507–1.639)	0.756
III+IV/I+II	TT (29/27)	0.629 (0.327–1.212)	0.166	GG (34/32)	0.936 (0.496–1.767)	0.839	GG (64/65)	1.829 (0.923–3.624)	0.083	CC (58/60)	0.614 (0.329–1.145)	0.125
	CT+TT (117/107)	0.741 (0.479–1.148)	0.180	AG+GG (145/113)	1.197 (0.751–1.908)	0.450	AG+GG (184/130)	2.698 (1.442–5.051)	0.002	TC+CC (160/137)	0.776 (0.447–1.349)	0.369
Histologic-al grade	CC (32/93)	1.000		AA (12/87)	1.000		AA (8/39)	1.000		TT (17/43)	1.000	
	CT (27/112)	0.717 (0.396–1.299)	0.273	AG (38/118)	2.378 (1.152–4.907)	0.019	AG (36/126)	1.309 (0.551–3.113)	0.542	TC (32/122)	0.540 (0.264–1.107)	0.092
III/I+II	TT (4/48)	0.282 (0.093–0.857)	0.026	GG (13/48)	2.170 (0.904–5.210)	0.083	GG (19/88)	1.069 (0.421–2.715)	0.888	CC (14/88)	0.351 (0.152–0.807)	0.014
	CT+TT (31/160)	0.594 (0.337–1.046)	0.071	AG+GG (51/166)	2.318 (1.155–4.649)	0.018	AG+GG (55/214)	1.216 (0.526–2.811)	0.647	TC+CC (46/210)	0.464 (0.235–0.916)	0.027
Age at	CC (106/38)	1.000		AA (79/31)	1.000		AA (31/23)	1.000		TT (52/19)	1.000	
Menarche	CT (108/60)	0.624 (0.379–1.027)	0.064	AG (123/69)	0.683 (0.406–1.150)	0.151	AG (120/65)	1.447 (0.771–2.716)	0.250	TC (117/62)	0.669 (0.358–1.250)	0.207
(years)	TT (34/22)	0.582 (0.299–1.134)	0.112	GG (46/20)	0.911 (0.462–1.795)	0.787	GG (97/32)	2.432 (1.227–4.821)	0.011	CC (79/39)	0.738 (0.380–1.432)	0.370
>12/≤12	CT+TT (142/82)	0.613 (0.384–0.978)	0.040	AG+GG (169/89)	0.736 (0.447–1.209)	0.226	AG+GG (217/97)	1.769 (0.969–3.227)	0.063	TC+CC (196/101)	0.696 (0.385–1.259)	0.231
Age at first	CC (25/115)	1.000		AA (16/92)	1.000		AA (7/43)	1.000		TT (16/52)	1.000	
live birth	CT (25/134)	0.979 (0.521–1.840)	0.947	AG (34/151)	1.531 (0.782–2.997)	0.215	AG (39/136)	1.790 (0.728–4.399)	0.205	TC (30/141)	0.762 (0.370–1.566)	0.459

Table 4. Cont.

Character-istic	FGFR2 rs2981582 Genotype (n)	aOR (95% CI)	P value	FGFR2 rs1219648 Genotype (n)	aOR (95% CI)	P value	FGFR2 rs2981578 Genotype (n)	aOR (95% CI)	P value	FGFR2 rs7895676 Genotype (n)	aOR (95% CI)	P value
(years)	TT (13/41)	1.313 (0.599–2.879)	0.496	GG (13/47)	1.672 (0.723–3.868)	0.230	GG (17/111)	0.904 (0.342–2.388)	0.838	CC (17/97)	0.558 (0.253–1.229)	0.147
>29/≤29	CT+TT (38/175)	1.072 (0.602–1.909)	0.812	AG+GG (47/198)	1.568 (0.827–2.973)	0.169	AG+GG (56/247)	1.380 (0.577–3.302)	0.469	TC+CC (47/238)	0.671 (0.343–1.315)	0.246
BMI	CC (41/93)	1.000		AA (26/78)	1.000		AA (11/36)	1.000		TT (27/41)	1.000	
(kg/m²)	CT (53/107)	1.071 (0.642–1.785)	0.794	AG (61/121)	1.462 (0.837–2.553)	0.182	AG (50/121)	1.209 (0.555–2.633)	0.632	TC (50/115)	0.627 (0.338–1.165)	0.140
≥25/<25	TT (14/37)	0.819 (0.388–1.729)	0.600	GG (21/38)	1.628 (0.795–3.334)	0.183	GG (47/80)	1.783 (0.808–3.932)	0.152	CC (31/81)	0.562 (0.289–1.093)	0.090
	CT+TT (67/144)	1.005 (0.620–1.627)	0.985	AG+GG (82/159)	1.502 (0.881–2.560)	0.135	AG+GG (97/201)	1.437 (0.684–3.019)	0.339	TC+CC (81/196)	0.600 (0.336–1.070)	0.083
Parity	CC (140/4)	1.000		AA (108/2)	1.000		AA (50/4)	1.000		TT (68/3)	1.000	
Parous/Nu-	CT (159/9)	0.460 (0.131–1.619)	0.227	AG (185/7)	0.455 (0.090–2.297)	0.340	AG (175/10)	1.396 (0.392–4.974)	0.607	TC (171/8)	0.694 (0.165–2.924)	0.618
Liparous	TT (54/2)	1.155 (0.192–6.934)	0.875	GG (60/6)	0.200 (0.038–1.058)	0.058	GG (128/1)	11.886 (1.22–115.4)	0.033	CC (114/4)	1.028 (0.210–5.030)	0.972
	CT+TT (213/11)	0.586 (0.176–1.948)	0.383	AG+GG (245/13)	0.336 (0.072–1.558)	0.163	AG+GG (303/11)	2.311 (0.669–7.990)	0.186	TC+CC (285/12)	0.810 (0.207–3.168)	0.762
Breastfeed-	CC (126/18)	1.000		AA (97/13)	1.000		AA (48/6)	1.000		TT (68/3)	1.000	
ing	CT (155/13)	1.764 (0.807–3.857)	0.155	AG (183/9)	2.623 (1.060–6.488)	0.037	AG (169/16)	1.271 (0.458–3.527)	0.645	TC (167/12)	0.489 (0.129–1.861)	0.294
Yes/No	TT (51/5)	2.040 (0.687–6.056)	0.199	GG (52/14)	0.521 (0.222–1.223)	0.134	GG (115/14)	1.088 (0.384–3.085)	0.874	CC (97/21)	0.164 (0.045–0.602)	0.006
	CT+TT (206/18)	1.838 (0.894–3.779)	0.098	AG+GG (235/23)	1.340 (0.638–2.813)	0.440	AG+GG (284/30)	1.186 (0.456–3.084)	0.727	TC+CC (264/33)	0.283 (0.081–0.987)	0.048
Education	CC (77/65)	1.000		AA (51/58)	1.000		AA (31/23)	1.000		TT (44/27)	1.000	
Level	CT (91/72)	1.070 (0.676–1.694)	0.772	AG (103/85)	1.323 (0.817–2.143)	0.255	AG (102/81)	0.964 (0.518–1.792)	0.907	TC (88/84)	0.677 (0.381–1.204)	0.184
(years)	TT (24/32)	0.580 (0.306–1.101)	0.096	GG (38/26)	1.558 (0.830–2.926)	0.168	GG (59/65)	0.676 (0.352–1.297)	0.239	CC (60/58)	0.669 (0.365–1.227)	0.194
>12/≤12	CT+TT (115/104)	0.914 (0.596–1.402)	0.680	AG+GG (141/111)	1.381 (0.874–2.182)	0.167	AG+GG (161/146)	0.835 (0.463–1.506)	0.549	TC+CC (148/142)	0.674 (0.393–1.156)	0.152
Exogenous	CC (18/119)	1.000		AA (7/101)	1.000		AA (9/41)	1.000		TT (16/53)	1.000	
Hormone	CT (22/144)	1.037 (0.524–2.052)	0.916	AG (25/161)	2.333 (0.959–5.678)	0.062	AG (29/149)	0.947 (0.407–2.201)	0.899	TC (21/149)	0.503 (0.240–1.056)	0.069
Use	TT (13/40)	2.067 (0.910–4.696)	0.083	GG (21/41)	7.618 (2.972–19.53)	0.0001	GG (15/113)	0.636 (0.254–1.591)	0.333	CC (16/101)	0.553 (0.253–1.208)	0.137

Table 4. Cont.

Character-istic	FGFR2 rs2981582			FGFR2 rs1219648			FGFR2 rs2981578			FGFR2 rs7895676		
	Genotype (n)	aOR (95% CI)	P value	Genotype (n)	aOR (95% CI)	P value	Genotype (n)	aOR (95% CI)	P value	Genotype (n)	aOR (95% CI)	P value
Yes/No	CT+TT (35/184)	1.280 (0.686–2.388)	0.438	AG+GG (46/202)	3.473 (1.492–8.081)	0.004	AG+GG (44/262)	0.811 (0.362–1.817)	0.610	TC+CC (37/250)	0.524 (0.267–1.028)	0.060
Place of	CC (76/68)	1.000		AA (59/51)	1.000		AA (33/21)	1.000		TT (37/34)	1.000	
residence	CT (97/71)	1.185 (0.753–1.867)	0.463	AG (114/78)	1.254 (0.776–2.026)	0.355	AG (107/78)	0.892 (0.478–1.666)	0.720	TC (107/72)	1.373 (0.781–2.413)	0.271
Urban/Ru-	TT (34/22)	1.377 (0.727–2.608)	0.326	GG (34/32)	0.891 (0.482–1.649)	0.714	GG (67/62)	0.692 (0.361–1.328)	0.268	CC (63/55)	1.068 (0.588–1.939)	0.830
Ral	CT+TT (131/93)	1.231 (0.805–1.884)	0.338	AG+GG (148/110)	1.145 (0.727–1.802)	0.560	AG+GG (174/140)	0.803 (0.443–1.456)	0.470	TC+CC (170/127)	1.238 (0.730–2.100)	0.429
Economic	CC (66/73)	1.000		AA (49/54)	1.000		AA (19/31)	1.000		TT (33/36)	1.000	
independe-	CT (105/57)	2.036 (1.273–3.256)	0.003	AG (102/80)	1.395 (0.849–2.291)	0.189	AG (98/79)	0.713 (0.361–1.410)	0.331	TC (88/80)	1.206 (0.676–2.154)	0.526
Nce	TT (17/32)	0.557 (0.279–1.112)	0.097	GG (37/28)	1.420 (0.757–2.665)	0.275	GG (71/52)	0.540 (0.265–1.097)	0.088	CC (67/46)	1.637 (0.888–3.017)	0.114
Employed/ Unemploy-ed	CT+TT (122/89)	1.495 (0.968–2.309)	0.070	AG+GG (139/108)	1.402 (0.877–2.242)	0.158	AG+GG (169/131)	0.636 (0.331–1.219)	0.173	TC+CC (155/126)	1.374 (0.800–2.361)	0.250

$P < 0.000694$, P values significant after Bonferroni correction.

aOR age-adjusted odds ratio, CI confidence interval.

P value and corresponding age-adjusted OR (aOR) with 95% CIs [aOR (95% CI)] by logistic regression analysis.

Table 5. Frequencies of inferred haplotypes of *FGFR2* SNPs rs7895676, rs2981578, rs2981582 and rs1219648 in breast cancer cases and controls.

SNP combinations	[a]Haplotype	Cases (N = 368)	Controls (N = 484)	OR (95% CI)	[b]P value
[c]ABCD	TACA	0.362	0.405	1.000 (referent)	
	CGTG	0.329	0.265	1.388 (1.097–1.755)	0.007
	Others	0.309	0.330	1.053 (0.836–1.326)	0.681
ABC	TAC	0.359	0.402	1.000 (referent)	
	CGT	0.340	0.267	1.422 (1.126–1.797)	0.004
	Others	0.301	0.331	1.022 (0.811–1.289)	0.859
BCD	ACA	0.370	0.427	1.000 (referent)	
	GTG	0.340	0.287	1.365 (1.086–1.717)	0.008
	Others	0.290	0.286	1.173 (0.927–1.484)	0.187
ABD	TAA	0.365	0.405	1.000 (referent)	
	CGG	0.386	0.327	1.306 (1.045–1.632)	0.020
	Others	0.249	0.268	1.030 (0.806–1.315)	0.851
ACD	TCA	0.388	0.433	1.000 (referent)	
	CTG	0.337	0.260	1.442 (1.144–1.816)	0.002
	Others	0.275	0.307	0.996 (0.789–1.259)	1.000

OR odds ratio, *CI* confidence interval.
[a]Haplotype In the order of *FGFR2* SNPs rs7895676, rs2981578, rs2981582, rs1219648.
[b]P value and corresponding OR with 95% CI for Fisher's exact test.
[c]A = rs7895676, B = rs2981578, C = rs2981582 and D = rs1219648.
Others Include haplotypes that had a frequency <10%.

Haploview and the association with the risk was determined by applying Fisher's exact test (Table 5, Table S5). Increased risk for the haplotype having only risk alleles compared to the one having only common alleles was observed for all the possible combinations ($P<0.05$). However, contrary to the combined risk analysis, predominant contribution towards the risk in terms of higher odds ratio was observed for trio combinations ABC (rs7895676, rs2981578 and rs2981582; OR = 1.422, 95%CI = 1.126–1.797, $P = 0.004$) and ACD (rs7895676, rs2981582 and rs1219648; OR = 1.442, 95%CI = 1.144–1.816, $P = 0.002$). However, SNP combination BCD (rs2981578, rs2981582 and rs1219648), seems to be relevant as pair wise D$'$>0.80 for these three SNPs (Figure S1) and carriers of GTG (carrying only risk alleles) haplotype had a significantly greater risk compared to ACA (carrying only wild-type alleles) haplotype, (OR = 1.365, 95%CI = 1.086–1.717, $P = 0.008$). While among duo SNP combinations, AC (rs7895676 and rs2981582) displayed highest odds ratio (OR = 1.449, 95%CI = 1.153–1.822, $P = 0.002$), Table S5.

Discussion

In this case–control study of sporadic breast cancer in North Indian women we found that the variant genotypes rs2981582C/T, rs1219648A/G, rs2981578A/G and rs7895676T/C of *FGFR2* were all significantly associated with increased breast cancer risk. Recent identification of these intron 2 SNPs [17,18] has drawn substantial attention towards *FGFR2* as a candidate gene for breast cancer. At present, much effort is focussed into targeting additional genetic alterations that drive breast cancer and *FGFR2* which has been implicated in different types of human malignancies, including breast cancer [33–36], is a likely candidate.

Since a previous report from South India [60] did not succeed in replicating the association of the studied *FGFR2* variant with breast cancer, as was observed in Europeans and other Asian populations [17,46,47], it was relevant to revisit the region along with other SNPs from the same LD block. The purpose of our study was to unravel any heterogeneity in association between population groups. Such differences reflect the variations among distinct geographic areas and ethnicity, and accentuate the necessity of characterizing breast cancer susceptibility genes among ethnic groups.

Present study reports significant association of rs2981582 and rs1219648 with breast cancer, consistent with previous observations from two Asian studies by Liang et al. [46] and Kawase et al. [47]. T allele of rs2981582 has been linked with an increased activity of *FGFR2* and it has been shown that haplotype marked by this allele associates with a higher level of *FGFR2* transcription both in breast cancer cell lines and tumors [56]. We observed an association of risk allele at rs2981582 and rs1219648 loci with breast cancer in premenopausal women, similar to some previous studies revealing the association of these variants with breast cancer risk in younger women [43–46]. We also observed rs2981582 T allele and rs1219648 G allele association with ER-positive than ER-negative tumors and further association with PR-positive than PR-negative tumors for rs2981582. Such findings of association with reproductive hormones are supported by several earlier studies showing that *FGFR2* variants contribute to breast cancer and confer their effect primarily in ER-positive and PR-positive tumor subtypes [42,44,46,60,61]. Also, higher levels of FGFR2 expression have been reported in ER-positive than ER-negative cell lines and tumors [62–64]. It is well known that elevated level of endogenous sex hormones, particularly estrogens, may increase breast cancer risk [65] and further, in premenopausal women exposure of endogenous serum estrogen is much higher as compared to post-menopausal women [66]. For rs2981582, we also observed an association of T allele with lower grade tumors, in accordance with a previous study by Garcia-Closas et al. [61]; with an early age at menarche (≤12 years), an observation previously reported by Kawase et al. [47]; and with employed status. Early onset of menarche is considered a breast cancer risk factor [67,68] as early onset of menarche leads to early exposure of endogenous sex hormones and can induce proliferation of breast cells [67]. A significant proportion of breast cancer in India has been attributed to greater urbanization and changing life styles. Higher education and increased income have been shown to be as risk factors of breast cancer [69,70].

For rs1219648, we observed a strong association of G allele with more invasive tumors with higher chance of LN metastasis, consistent with a previous report from China [54], and with clinically advanced stage, suggesting its association with disease aggressiveness. Moreover, we observed a very strong association of the risk allele with the use of exogenous hormones (either as contraceptives/infertility treatment/hormone replacement therapy), this is in somewhat contradiction to a previous report by Rebbeck et al. [53], where never users of combined hormone replacement therapy (CHRT) with the risk allele were at higher risk. Further, association with positive breastfeeding status was also observed. Exogenous hormone exposure and breastfeeding have been described as important factors predictive of breast cancer risk [71].

Breast cancer tends to be diagnosed at an earlier age in developing countries than in European and American populations and a rapid rate of increase in incidence has been observed before menopause [72]. Moreover, it has also been reported that premenopausal women constitute about 50% of all the breast cancer patients in India [6]. Thus, results from our study demonstrating the association of rs2981582 and rs1219648 with premenopausal status suggest the importance of investigating these two SNPs in Indian context. Moreover, restriction of the risk conferred by FGFR2 variants to ER-positive and PR-positive tumors suggests that these SNPs affect the reproductive hormone-related pathway in the development of breast cancer in North Indian women. But these observations need to be confirmed in larger sample size studies from our population.

Recently done analysis by Meyer et al. have shown that two FGFR2 SNPs rs2981578 and rs7895676 within intron 2 region alter the DNA binding affinity of transcription factors octamer-binding transcription factor 1 (Oct-1)/runt-related transcription factor 2 (Runx2) and CCAAT/enhancer binding protein β (C/EBPβ) respectively, resulting in an increased FGFR2 gene expression both in cell lines and in breast tissues in patients homozygous for the risk allele as compared to those homozygous for the wild type allele [56]. These 2 SNPs are located in the same LD block of interest identified by GWAS [17,18]. Role of these as breast cancer susceptibility variants is not yet established. In our study we observed a significant association of G allele of rs2981578 with breast cancer risk which is in accordance with a previous African American study [49] and a Chinese study [52]. We also observed an association of G allele with LN-positive status and with advanced clinical stage suggesting that the risk allele might relate to a more aggressive form of breast cancer. Further, association with parous status was observed. For rs7895676, we observed significant association of C allele with breast cancer risk, consistent with an earlier study by Boyarskikh et al. [50]. We further observed association of C allele with PR-positive, LN-positive, less malignant grade I+II tumors and negative breastfeeding status. Both parity and breastfeeding have been described as important factors linked to breast cancer risk [71]. Moreover, nulliparity and negative breastfeeding status have been linked with increased risk for breast cancer in Indian population [73,74].

Association with exogenous hormone exposure and higher stage for SNPs rs1219648 and rs2981578 respectively, achieved statistical significance even after Bonferroni correction (P< 0.000694), while other clinical features lost statistical significance, suggesting the importance of these SNPs in sub-categorized breast cancers in our population. But these observations need to be confirmed in further studies with larger sample size, to rule out false positive results and to establish intron 2 FGFR2 SNPs as breast cancer susceptibility loci.

On conducting combined risk analysis in our study population of North Indian women relative risk of developing breast cancer is found to be elevated by around 65% for women carrying 2–4 risk loci as compared to the remaining groups carrying 0–1 risk loci (aOR = 1.645, 95%CI = 1.152–2.347). Moreover a progressively augmented risk with increasing number of risk loci was also noted demonstrating that a combination of these variants cumulatively increases risk (Table S3). In haplotype analysis, the FGFR2 rs2981578 G/rs2981582 T/rs1219648 G haplotype was associated with a significantly increased breast cancer risk compared with the rs2981578A/rs2981582 C/rs1219648 A haplotype. Our findings on combinatorial effect of these loci and haplotype analysis are to several extent similar to previous studies [44–46,51,75], though they included only 2 or 3 FGFR2 variants we are reporting here. Although, the tendency to increase breast cancer risk was significant across all the four SNPs tested, but the LD pattern between the four FGFR2 variants in our North Indian population was weak to moderate only, in contrast to Europeans, but resembling other Asian populations [17,46,47,75], indicating a fairly independent risk effect of each locus in our population, but the results warrant screening in larger sample sets. Moreover, we also observed significant differences in the contribution of different number of risk loci as well as different combinations of SNPs both in combined risk analysis as well as haplotype analysis, which resulted in varied extent of involvement towards risk.

To the best of our knowledge, we are reporting for the first time, a case control study on these four intronic FGFR2 variants taken together along with LD measurement, haplotype analysis and stratified analysis for possible correlation with patients' clinical parameters in susceptibility to breast cancer.

Location of these FGFR2 variants in intronic region suggests the probable explanation for their association with the risk through differential expression. Aberrant expression of alternatively spliced isoforms of FGFR2 has been shown to activate signal transduction leading to transformation in breast cancer cells [76]. Variable expression of FGFR2 in relation to intron 2 SNPs has been supported by the analysis carried out by Meyer et al. [56] and Huijts et al. [77]. Further, FGFR2 intron 2 shows a high degree of conservation in mammals, and number of conserved putative transcription-factor binding sites have been identified in it [17,78], some of which lie in close proximity to the significant SNPs. However, the exact mechanism of how these SNPs affect FGFR2 upregulation remains unclear.

Besides SNPs, other features of FGFR2 could be targeted in search for newer and efficient biomarkers in the future. Several altered FGFR2 characteristics have been linked with breast tumorigenesis and have shown promising results in studies on breast cancer cell lines and tumors, like amplification and over-expression, mutations, alternative splicing and isoform switching [33–38,62,76,79–83]. Though, none of them has reached the clinical phase as yet and there are many hurdles to be overcome, there is enough encouraging evidence suggesting that targeting FGFR2 along with other FGFRs in certain subtypes of breast cancer could be a valuable approach in the future [84–88].

In conclusion, our study revealed a significant association of FGFR2 intron 2 SNPs with breast cancer risk, as well as their interaction with various clinical parameters revealing their contribution to breast cancer susceptibility among North Indian women. Although, findings of the present study by themselves are unlikely to have any immediate clinical implications, however, such studies may play a key role in elucidating the biological mechanism that underline breast tumor heterogeneity, which may ultimately lead to improved treatment and prevention. These findings suggest that genetic variants of *FGFR2* might be used as candidate potential biomarkers for breast cancer risk. Further epidemiological and experimental studies of larger data sets along with sub-categorization by clinical parameters and expression studies are warranted to explore and confirm the role of these variants in increasing breast cancer risk, particularly from India, that will help us better understand the genetic heterogeneity in complex diseases like breast cancer.

Acknowledgments

The authors thank all the patients who participated in this study and acknowledge the efforts and contribution of the doctors, nurses, and hospital administration staff of AIIMS and all the support staff of Jamia Millia Islamia who made this study possible.

Author Contributions

Conceived and designed the experiments: SS SAH. Performed the experiments: SS. Analyzed the data: SS SAH. Contributed reagents/materials/analysis tools: SC MSA MZN. Wrote the paper: SS SAH. Diagnosed the patients and provided biological samples for the study: SVSD NKS.

References

1. Jemal A, Bray F, Center MM, Ferlay J, Ward E, et al. (2011) Global cancer statistics. CA Cancer J Clin 61(2): 69–90.
2. Hortobagyi GN, Garza SJ, Pritchard K, Amadori D, Haidinger R, et al. (2005) The global breast cancer burden: variations in epidemiology and survival. Clin Breast Cancer 6: 391–401.
3. Anderson BO, Jakesz R (2008) Breast cancer issues in developing countries: an overview of the breast health global initiative. World J Surg 32: 2579–85.
4. Porter P (2008) Westernizing women's risks? Breast cancer in lower-income countries. N Engl J Med 358: 213–6.
5. Green M, Raina V (2008) Epidemiology, screening and diagnosis of breast cancer in the Asia–Pacific region: current perspectives and important considerations. Asia Pac J Clin Oncol 4: 5–13.
6. Agarwal G, Pradeep PV, Aggarwal V, Yip CH, Cheung PS (2007) Spectrum of breast cancer in Asian women. World J Surg 31: 1031–40.
7. Leong SPL, Shen ZZ, Liu TJ, Agarwal G, Tajima T, et al. (2010) Is breast cancer the same disease in Asian and Western countries? World J Surg 34(10): 2308–24.
8. Takiar R, Srivastav A (2008) Time trend in breast and cervix cancer of women in India - (1990–2003). Asian Pac J Cancer Prev 9(4): 777–80.
9. Yeole BB (2008) Trends in cancer incidence in female breast, cervix uteri, corpus uteri, and ovary in India. Asian Pac J Cancer Prev 9(1): 119–22.
10. Nandakumar A, Ramnath T, Chaturvedi M (2010) The magnitude of cancer breast in India: a summary. Indian J Surg Oncol 1(1): 8–9.
11. Murthy NS, Agarwal UK, Chaudhry K, Saxena S (2007) A study on time trends in incidence of breast cancer –Indian scenario. Eur J Cancer Care 16: 185–6.
12. Breast cancer in developing countries (2009) Lancet 374(9701): 1567.
13. Collaborative Group on Hormonal Factors in Breast Cancer (2002) Breast cancer and breastfeeding: collaborative reanalysis of individual data from 47 epidemiological studies in 30 countries, including 50302 women with breast cancer and 96973 women without the disease. Lancet 360: 187–195.
14. Stratton MR, Rahman N (2008) The emerging landscape of breast cancer susceptibility. Nat Genet 40: 17–22.
15. Antoniou AC, Pharoah PD, McMullan G, Day NE, Ponder BA, et al. (2001) Evidence for further breast cancer susceptibility genes in addition to *BRCA1* and *BRCA2* in a population-based study. Genet Epidemiol 21: 1–18.
16. Chen YC, Hunter DJ (2005) Molecular epidemiology of cancer. CA Cancer J Clin 55(1): 45–54. quiz7.
17. Easton DF, Pooley KA, Dunning AM, Pharoah PD, Thompson D, et al. (2007) Genome-wide association study identifies novel breast cancer susceptibility loci. Nature 447(7148): 1087–1093.
18. Hunter DJ, Kraft P, Jacobs KB, Cox DG, Yeager M, et al. (2007) A genome-wide association study identifies alleles in *FGFR2* associated with risk of sporadic postmenopausal breast cancer. Nat Genet 39(7): 870–874.
19. Ahmed S, Thomas G, Ghoussaini M, Healey CS, Humphreys MK, et al. (2009) Newly discovered breast cancer susceptibility loci on 3p24 and 17q23.2. Nat Genet 41: 585–590.
20. Turnbull C, Rahman N (2008) Genetic predisposition to breast cancer: past, present, and future. Annu Rev Genomics Hum Genet 9: 321–345.
21. Turnbull C, Ahmed S, Morrison J, Pernet D, Renwick A, et al. (2010) Genomewide association study identifies five new breast cancer susceptibility loci. Nat Genet 42: 504–507.
22. Stacey SN, Manolescu A, Sulem P, Rafnar T, Gudmundsson J, et al. (2007) Common variants on chromosomes 2q35 and 16q12 confer susceptibility to estrogen receptor-positive breast cancer. Nat Genet 39: 865–869.
23. Ghoussaini M, Pharoah PD (2009) Polygenic susceptibility to breast cancer: current state-of-the-art. Future Oncol 5: 689–701.
24. Ghoussaini M, Fletcher O, Michailidou K, Turnbull C, Schmidt MK, et al. (2012) Genome-wide association analysis identifies three new breast cancer susceptibility loci. Nat Genet 44: 312–318.
25. Thomas G, Jacobs KB, Kraft P, Yeager M, Wacholder S, et al. (2009) A multistage genome-wide association study in breast cancer identifies two new risk alleles at 1p11.2 and 14q24.1 (RAD51L1). Nat Genet 41: 579–584.
26. Taylor JG, Choi EH, Foster CB, Chanock SJ (2001) Using genetic variation to study human disease. Trends Mol Med 7(11): 507–12.
27. Pharoah PD, Antoniou A, Bobrow M, Zimmern RL, Easton DF, et al. (2002) Polygenic susceptibility to breast cancer and implications for prevention. Nat Genet 31: 33–36.
28. Collins FS, Guyer MS, Charkravarti A (1997) Variations on a theme: cataloguing human DNA sequence variation. Science 278: 1580–1581.
29. Chakravarti A (1998) It's raining SNPs, hallelujah! Nat Genet 19: 216–217.
30. Mehrian-Shai R, Reichardt JK (2004) A renaissance of "biochemical genetics"? SNPs, haplotypes, function, and complex diseases. Mol Genet Metab 83: 47–50.
31. Wesche J, Haglund K, Haugsten EM (2011) Fibroblast growth factors and their receptors in cancer. Biochem J 437: 199–213.
32. Dillon C, Spencer-Dene B, Dickson C (2004) A crucial role for fibroblast growth factor signaling in embryonic mammary gland development. J Mammary Gland Biol Neoplasia 9: 207–215.
33. Turner N, Grose R (2010) Fibroblast growth factor signalling: from development to cancer. Nat Rev Cancer 10: 116–129.
34. Katoh M (2008) Cancer genomics and genetics of *FGFR2*. Int J Oncol 33: 233–237.
35. Jang JH, Shin KH, Park JG (2001) Mutations in *FGFR2* and *FGFR3* genes associated with human gastric and colorectal cancers. Cancer Res 61: 3541–3543.
36. Pollock PM, Gartside MG, Dejeza LC, Powell MA, Mallon MA, et al. (2007) Frequent activating *FGFR2* mutations in endometrial carcinomas parallel

germline mutations associated with craniosynostosis and skeletal dysplasia syndromes. Oncogene 26: 7158–7162.

37. Penault-Llorca F, Bertucci F, Ade'laïde J, Parc P, Coulier F, et al. (2000) Characterization of fibroblast growth factor receptor 2 overexpression in the human breast cancer cell line SUM-52PE. Breast Cancer Res 2: 311–320.

38. Adnane J, Gaudray P, Dionne CA, Crumley G, Jaye M, et al. (1991) BEK and FLG, two receptors to members of the FGF family, are amplified in subsets of human breast cancers. Oncogene 6: 659–63.

39. Ingersoll RG, Paznekas WA, Tran AK, Scott AF, Jiang G, et al. (2001) Fibroblast growth factor receptor 2 (FGFR2): genomic sequence and variations. Cytogenet Cell Genet 94: 121–126.

40. Huijts PEA, Vreeswijk MPG, Kroeze-Jansema KHG, Jacobi CE, Seynaeve C, et al. (2007) Clinical correlates of low-risk variants in FGFR2, TNRC9, MAP3K1, LSP1 and 8q24 in a dutch cohort of incident breast cancer cases. Breast Cancer Res 9: R78.

41. Raskin L, Pinchev M, Arad C, Lejbkowicz F, Tamir A, et al. (2008) FGFR2 is a breast cancer susceptibility gene in Jewish and Arab Israeli populations. Cancer Epidemiol Biomarkers Prev 17: 1060–1065.

42. Hemminki K, Müller-Myhsok B, Lichtner P, Engel C, Chen B, et al. (2010) Low-risk variants FGFR2, TNRC9 and LSP1 in german familial breast cancer patients. Int J Cancer 126: 2858–2862.

43. Barnholtz-Sloan JS, Shetty PB, Guan X, Nyante SJ, Luo J, et al. (2010) FGFR2 and other loci identified in genome-wide association studies are associated with breast cancer in african-american and younger women. Carcinogenesis 31: 1417–1423.

44. Fu F, Wang C, Huang M, Song C, Lin S, et al. (2012) Polymorphisms in second intron of the FGFR2 gene are associated with the risk of early-onset breast cancer in Chinese Han women. Tohoku J Exp Med 226: 221–229.

45. Jara L, Gonzalez-Hormazabal P, Cercen~o K, Di Capua GA, Reyes JM, et al. (2013) Genetic variants in FGFR2 and MAP3K1 are associated with the risk of familial and early-onset breast cancer in a South- American population. Breast Cancer Res Treat 137: 559–569.

46. Liang J, Chen P, Hu Z, Zhou X, Chen L, et al. (2008) Genetic variants in fibroblast growth factor receptor 2 (FGFR2) contribute to susceptibility of breast cancer in Chinese women. Carcinogenesis 29: 2341–2346.

47. Kawase T, Matsuo K, Suzuki T, Hiraki A, Watanabe M, et al. (2009) FGFR2 intronic polymorphisms interact with reproductive risk factors of breast cancer: Results of a case control study in Japan. Int J Cancer 125: 1946–1952.

48. Long J, Zhang B, Signorello LB, Cai Q, Halverson SD, et al. (2013) Evaluating Genome-Wide Association Study-Identified Breast Cancer Risk Variants in African-American Women. PLoS ONE 8(4): e58350.

49. Udler MS, Meyer KB, Pooley KA, Karlins E, Struewing JP, et al. (2009) FGFR2 variants and breast cancer risk: fine-scale mapping using African American studies and analysis of chromatin conformation. Hum Mol Genet 18(9): 1692–1703.

50. Zheng W, Cai Q, Signorello LB, Long J, Hargreaves MK, et al. (2009) Evaluation of 11 breast cancer susceptibility loci in African-American women. Cancer Epidemiol Biomarkers Prev 18: 2761–2764.

51. Hao D, Zheng Y, Ogundiran TO, Adebamowo C, Nathanson KL, et al. (2012) Evaluation of 19 susceptibility loci of breast cancer in women of African ancestry. Carcinogenesis 33: 835–840.

52. Chen F, Lv M, Xue Y, Zhou J, Hu F, et al. (2012) Genetic variants of fibroblast growth factor receptor 2 (FGFR2) are associated with breast cancer risk in Chinese women of the Han nationality. Immunogenetics 64: 71–76.

53. Rebbeck TR, DeMichele A, Tran TV, Panossian S, Bunin GR, et al. (2009) Hormone-dependent effects of FGFR2 and MAP3K1 in breast cancer susceptibility in a population-based sample of post-menopausal African-American and European-American women. Carcinogenesis 30: 269–274.

54. Chen XH, Li ZQ, Chen Y, Feng YM (2011) Risk of aggressive breast cancer in women of Han nationality carrying TGFB1 rs1982073 C allele and FGFR2 rs1219648 G allele in North China. Breast Cancer Res Treat 125: 575–582.

55. Wang H, Yang Z, Zhang H (2013) Assessing interactions between the associations of fibroblast growth factor receptor 2 common genetic variants and hormone receptor status with breast cancer risk. Breast Cancer Res Treat 137: 511–522.

56. Meyer KB, Maia A, O'Reilly M, Teschendorff AE, Chin S, et al. (2008) Allele-specific up-regulation of FGFR2 increases susceptibility to breast cancer. PLoS Biol 6: e108.

57. Boyarskikh UA, Zarubina NA, Biltueva JA, Sinkina TV, Voronina EN, et al. (2009) Association of FGFR2 gene polymorphisms with the risk of breast cancer in population of West Siberia. European Journal of Human Genetics 17: 1688–1591.

58. Sambrook J, Russell DW (2001) Molecular cloning: a laboratory manual. Cold Spring Harbor Laboratory Press, Cold Spring Harbor.

59. Barrett JC, Fry B, Maller J, Daly MJ (2005) Haploview: analysis and visualization of LD and haplotype maps. Bioinformatics 21: 263–265.

60. Samson M, Rama R, Swaminathan R, Sridevi V, Nancy KN, et al. (2009) CYP17 (T-34C), CYP19 (Trp39Arg), and FGFR2 (C-906T) Polymorphisms and the Risk of Breast Cancer in South Indian Women. Asian Pacific J Cancer Prev 10: 111–114.

61. Garcia-Closas M, Hall P, Nevanlinna H, Pooley K, Morrison J, et al. (2008) Heterogeneity of breast cancer associations with five susceptibility loci by clinical and pathological characteristics. PLoS Genet 4(4): e1000054.

62. Luqmani YA, Graham M, Coombes RC (1992) Expression of basic fibroblast growth factor, FGFR1 and FGFR2 in normal and malignant human breast, and comparison with other normal tissues. Br J Cancer 66: 273–80.

63. Tozlu S, Girault I, Vacher S, Vendrell J, Andrieu C, et al. (2006) Identification of novel genes that co-cluster with estrogen receptor alpha in breast tumor biopsy specimens, using a largescale real-time reverse transcription-PCR approach. Endocr Relat Cancer 13: 1109–1120.

64. Zang XP, Pento JT (2002) Keratinocyte growth factor-induced motility of breast cancer cells. Clin Exp Metastasis 18: 573–580.

65. Key T, Appleby P, Barnes I, Reeves G (2002) Endogenous sex hormones and breast cancer in postmenopausal women: reanalysis of nine prospective studies. J. Natl Cancer Inst 94: 606–616.

66. Clemons M, Goss P (2001) Estrogen and the risk of breast cancer. N Engl J Med 344: 276–285.

67. Clavel-Chapelon F, E3N-EPIC Group1 (2002) Differential effects of reproductive factors on the risk of pre- and postmenopausal breast cancer. Results from a large cohort of French women. Br J Cancer 86: 723–727.

68. Gao YT, Shu XO, Dai Q, Potter JD, Brinton LA, et al. (2000) Association of menstrual and reproductive factors with breast cancer risk: results from the Shanghai Breast Cancer Study. Int J Cancer 87: 295–300.

69. Madigan MP, Zeigler RG, Benichou J, Byrne C, Hoover RN (1995) Proportion of breast cancer cases in the United States explained by well-established risk factors. J Natl Cancer Inst 87: 1681–1685.

70. Tavani A, Gallus S, La Vecchia C, Negri E, Montella M, et al. (1999) Risk factors for breast cancer in women under 40 years. Eur J Cancer 35: 1361–7.

71. Key TJ, Verkasalo PK, Banks E (2001) Epidemiology of breast cancer. Lancet Oncol 2(3): 133–40.

72. Bray F, McCarron P, Parkin DM (2004) The changing global patterns of female breast cancer incidence and mortality. Breast Cancer Res 6: 229–239.

73. Rao DN, Ganesh B, Desai PB (1994) Role of reproductive factors in breast cancer in a low-risk area: a case-control study. Br J Cancer 70: 129–32.

74. Gajalakshmi V, Mathew A, Brennan P, Rajan B, Kanimozhi V, et al. (2009) Breast feeding and breast cancer risk in India: a multicenter case-control study. Int J Cancer 125: 662–5.

75. Chan M, Ji SM, Liaw CS, Yap YS, Law HY, et al. (2012) Association of common genetic variants with breast cancer risk and clinicopathological characteristics in a Chinese population. Breast Cancer Res Treat 136(1): 209–20.

76. Moffa AB, Tannheimer SL, Ethier SP (2004) Transforming potential of alternatively spliced variants of fibroblast growth factor receptor 2 in human mammary epithelial cells. Mol Cancer Res 2: 643.

77. Huijts PEA, Dongen MV, de Goeij MCM, Moolenbroek AJV, Blanken F, et al. (2011) Allele-specific regulation of FGFR2 expression is cell type-dependent and may increase breast cancer risk through a paracrine stimulus involving FGF10. Cancer Research 13: R72.

78. Carroll JS, Meyer CA, Song J, Li W, Geistlinger TR, et al. (2006) Genome-wide analysis of estrogen receptor binding sites. Nat Genet 38: 1289–1297.

79. Haugsten EM, Wiedlocha A, Olsnes S, Wesche J (2010) Roles of Fibroblast Growth Factor Receptors in Carcinogenesis. Mol Cancer Res 8: 1439–1452.

80. Turner N, Lambros MB, Horlings HM, Pearson A, Sharpe R, et al. (2010) Integrative molecular profiling of triple negative breast cancers identifies amplicon drivers and potential therapeutic targets. Oncogene 29: 2013–23.

81. Cha JY, Lambert QT, Reuther GW, Der CJ (2008) Involvement of fibroblast growth factor receptor 2 isoform switching in mammary oncogenesis. Mol Cancer Res 6: 435–45.

82. Tannheimer SL, Rehemtulla A, Ethier SP (2000) Characterization of fibroblast growth factor receptor 2 overexpression in the human breast cancer cell line SUM-52PE. Breast Cancer Res 2000 2: 311–20.

83. Moffa AB, Ethier SP (2007) Differential signal transduction of alternatively spliced FGFR2 variants expressed in human mammary epithelial cells. J Cell Physiol 210: 720–731.

84. Brooks N, Kilgour E, Smith PD (2012) Molecular Pathways: Fibroblast Growth Factor Signaling: A New Therapeutic Opportunity in Cancer. Clin Cancer Res 18: 1855–1862.

85. Hynes NE, Dey JH (2010) Potential for Targeting the Fibroblast Growth Factor Receptors in Breast Cancer Cancer Res 70: 5199–5202.

86. Zhao WM, Wang L, Park H, Chhim S, Tanphanich M, et al. (2010) Monoclonal antibodies to fibroblast growth factor receptor 2 effectively inhibit growth of gastric tumor xenografts. Clin Cancer Res 16: 5750–8.

87. Bai A, Meetze K, Vo NY, Kollipara S, Mazsa EK, et al. (2010) GP369, an FGFR2-IIIb-specific antibody, exhibits potent antitumor activity against human cancers driven by activated FGFR2 signaling. Cancer Res 70: 7630–9.

88. Koziczak M, Holbro T, Hynes NE (2004) Blocking of FGFR signaling inhibits breast cancer cell proliferation through downregulation of D-type cyclins. Oncogene 23: 3501–8.

21

Iron Status and Reproduction in US Women: National Health and Nutrition Examination Survey, 1999-2006

Elizabeth M. Miller*

Department of Anthropology, University of South Florida, Tampa, Florida, United States of America

Abstract

Women experience significant changes in iron status throughout their reproductive lifespans. While this is evident in regions with high rates of malnutrition and infectious disease, the extent of reproductive-related changes is less well known in countries with low rates of iron deficiency anemia, such as the United States. The goal of this study is determine the relationship between women's reproductive variables (pregnancy, parity, currently breastfeeding, regular menstruation, hormonal contraceptive use, and age at menarche) and iron status (hemoglobin, ferritin, transferrin receptor, and % transferrin saturation) using an anthropological framework for interpreting the results. Data from women aged 18–49 were taken from the 1999–2006 US NHANES, a nationally representative cross-sectional sample of US women. Using multiple imputation and complex survey statistics, women's reproductive variables were regressed against indicators of iron status. Pregnant women had significantly poorer iron status, by most indicators, than non-pregnant women. All biomarkers demonstrated significantly lower iron levels with increasing parity. Women who were having regular periods had iron indicators that suggested decreased iron levels, while women who used hormonal contraceptives had iron indicators that suggested increased iron levels. Despite relatively good iron status and widespread availability of iron-rich foods in the US, women still exhibit patterns of iron depletion across several reproductive variables of interest. These results contribute to an ecological approach to iron status that seeks to understand variation in iron status, with the hopes that appropriate, population-specific recommendations can be developed to improve women's health.

Editor: James F. Collins, University of Florida, United States of America

Funding: This author has no support or funding to report.

Competing Interests: The author has declared that no competing interests exist.

* Email: emm3@usf.edu

Introduction

Globally, reproductively-active women are at risk of iron-deficiency anemia, which causes significant morbidity and mortality [1,2]. The effects of low iron in women can have broad global effects on their physical and cognitive capabilities as well as specific effects on perinatal outcomes and infant health [3,4]. During pregnancy, iron is allocated to the fetus to a high degree, particularly in the later trimesters [5,6]. This can lead to maternal and fetal iron deficiency anemia, particularly in women with poor iron status pre-pregnancy [4,7–9]. There is also evidence that this can affect women across their reproductive careers: a growing body of literature suggests that increasing parity is associated with decreased indicators of iron status and greater likelihood of iron-deficiency anemia [10–14]. While pregnancy depletes maternal iron stores, after birth women have relatively low iron needs that allows for repletion of iron stores before the next pregnancy [14]. When inter-birth intervals are short or when dietary iron is insufficient, parity-related maternal iron depletion can result [14,15].

Iron status has also been implicated in other aspects of women's reproduction, mainly attributed to the loss of iron via menstrual blood. Menstrual blood loss has been associated with poorer indicators of iron status [16–18], although this perspective is controversial [19]. Fittingly, the use of hormonal contraceptive, which is generally associated with lighter menstrual periods, is associated with better indicators of iron status than in women who do not use hormonal contraceptives [10,17]. Breastfeeding is also associated with lower dietary iron needs [20,21] due to low levels of iron in breast milk and lactational amenorrhea [22–25], particularly in undernourished populations.

The National Health and Nutrition Examination Survey (NHANES) offers a unique opportunity to investigate markers of iron status across a broad cross-section of reproductive-aged US women. Compared to the global population, the United States has low rates of iron-deficiency anemia; however, it does appear that reproduction-related iron depletion can occur, particularly in pregnant women [26] and African American women [12]. This study will investigate the relationship between reproductive variables and markers of iron status using a biological anthropology framework. Specifically, it will explore how pregnancy, parity, breastfeeding, menstruation, hormonal contraceptive use, and menarche are associated with four indicators of iron status:

Table 1. Weighted descriptive statistics for study variables for women aged 18–49 who participated in the NHANES physical examination during 1999–2006, before and after multiple imputation of missing values.

		Pre-imputed weighted descriptive statistics			Imputed weighted descriptive statistics[a]		
		Mean or %	SE	n	Mean or %	SE	95% CI
Iron Status	Hemoglobin (g/dL)	13.50	0.37	6225	13.50	0.036	13.43, 13.57
	Ferritin (ng/mL)	57.84	1.03	6162	57.72	1.05	55.67, 59.78
	% Transferrin saturation	3.57	0.037	2824	3.70	0.042	3.61, 3.78
	Transferrin receptor (mg/L)[b]	22.60	0.19	6153	22.58	1.18	22.22, 22.94
Reproductive Status	% Pregnant	6.43	0.32	6463	6.52	0.32	5.89, 7.16
	Parity	1.54	0.028	5616	1.53	0.027	1.47, 1.58
	% Currently breastfeeding	2.01	0.34	5107	1.90	0.33	1.26, 2.53
	% Currently using hormonal contraceptive	16.02	0.84	5608	15.86	0.78	14.33, 17.39
	% Ever used hormonal contraceptive	77.46	0.86	5942	77.00	0.87	75.28, 78.70
	% Had regular periods in past year	72.40	0.83	5947	72.58	0.84	70.92, 74.23
	Age at menarche (years)	12.60	0.028	5854	12.60	0.027	12.55, 12.65
Covariates	% Hispanic	15.47	0.13	6603	15.47	0.13	–[c]
	% Non-Hispanic black	13.48	0.11	6603	13.48	0.11	–[c]
	% Non-Hispanic white	65.45	0.10	6603	65.45	0.10	–[c]
	% Other	5.60	0.045	6603	5.60	0.045	–[c]
	BMI (kg/m²)	27.86	0.16	6468	27.87	0.16	27.56, 28.19
	CRP (g/L)	0.47	0.014	6173	0.47	0.014	0.44, 0.50
	Age (years)	33.99	0.17	6603	33.99	0.17	–[c]
	Dietary iron intake (mg)	13.73	0.14	6252	13.73	0.14	13.46, 14.00

[a]All n = 6603 (except transferrin receptor).
[b]The n for the imputed mean for transferrin receptor is 3295; based on 2003–2006 survey years only.
[c]All variables were available in original data set, so no 95% CI were generated by PROC MIANALYZE.

hemoglobin, ferritin, transferrin receptor, and percent transferrin saturation. This research will test the following hypotheses:

1) Women will show differences in iron status depending on their current and past reproductive history. This hypothesis leads to three predictions: a) Pregnant women will have lower iron status than women who are not pregnant; b) Women who are currently breastfeeding will have iron indicators that indicate post-pregnancy iron recovery; and c) Increasing parity (reproductive history) will be negatively associated with indicators of iron status.

2) Women will experience short- and long-term effects of menstruation on iron status. This hypothesis leads to two predictions: a) Regularly menstruating women will have iron indicators that indicate lower iron status; and b) Earlier age at menarche will be associated with lower iron status.

The US NHANES offers an opportunity to examine several indicators of iron status in reproductive-aged women. Hemoglobin, an iron-containing oxygen carrier protein in red blood cells, is the most common iron indicator used to diagnose anemia. Low hemoglobin is diagnostic of anemia (the lowered ability of the blood to carry oxygen) but cannot necessarily distinguish between iron deficiency anemia and other causes of anemia. Serum ferritin, an iron storage protein, correlates well with global iron stores (except in the presence of inflammation). Low serum ferritin is especially useful in distinguishing between iron deficiency anemia and other forms of anemia [27]. Percent transferrin saturation is the percent iron bound to transferrin (an iron carrier protein), and is also a measure of iron deficiency. Finally, serum transferrin receptor binds to transferrin in order to transfer iron into cells. Transferrin receptor increases during iron deficiency as the body's tissues attempt to increase intercellular iron concentration, and can be used to distinguish iron deficiency anemia from other forms of anemia even when inflammation is present. These four measurements offer similar, but slightly different, perspectives on iron status and can provide insight into the dynamics of iron physiology in reproductive-aged women.

Subjects and Methods

Ethics statement

This study was originally approved by the National Center for Health Statistics Research Ethics Review Board, and participants underwent informed consent before data collection. Because the current study is a secondary analysis of de-identified data, the University of South Florida Institutional Review Board determined that this research is not human subjects research and thus not subject to review.

Sample design

The NHANES is a US-representative survey conducted by the Centers for Disease Control and Prevention (CDC), which has been collecting data on a two-year continuous basis since 1999. The goal of the NHANES is to collect health and nutrition-related data on the general US population. NHANES uses a complex sample design in which participants are weighted according to geographic and census information, and certain groups (such as pregnant women) are oversampled for analytical purposes [28]. Adding to the complexity of the data, not all NHANES participants who took part in the interview decided to take part in the physical examination. There are also considerable missing data, particularly in the reproductive health questionnaire. Although 6603 women between the ages of 18 and 49 participated

in the physical examination between 1999 and 2006, rates of missing data were fairly high (see Table 1). Therefore, the current study uses a multiple imputation method to correct for missing responses and increase available sample size.

Variable selection

Iron status. NHANES 1999–2006 has multiple variables relating to iron status. Information relating to laboratory analysis of iron status variables are available in the NHANES documentation on the CDC website. All continuous variables were left as untransformed linear variables for analysis.

Found in red blood cells, hemoglobin is the main oxygen-transporting protein in the body. Each hemoglobin molecule contains one iron ion. Around 70% of the body's iron is located in hemoglobin. Hemoglobin levels are used to diagnose iron-deficiency anemia, with values of <12–12.5 g/dL generally considered anemic in women [29], although can vary by pregnancy status [3]. In the NHANES, hemoglobin was measured as part of the complete blood count using the Coulter HMX Hematology Analyzer [30–33]. Hemoglobin levels (g/dL) are available for all children and adults who completed the physical examination [30–33].

Ferritin is an iron-storage protein that is indirectly used as a measure of iron levels in the body. Ferritin levels of <12 ng/mL are considered indicative of iron deficiency [29]. Ferritin levels (ng/mL) are available for all adults and children from survey years 1999–2002 and in reproductive aged-women (12–49 years) in survey years 2003–2006 [30–33]. Two different assays were used to measure ferritin across data years: in years 1999–2003 BioRad Laboratories' two-site immunoradiometric assay kit was used, while in 2004 and later years the Roche/Hitachi immunoturbidity assay was used. The Roche/Hitachi method gives a higher ferritin estimate than the BioRad assay, and must be normalized using a derived piecewise linear equation [34]. While the 2003 data were normalized to the 2004 data prior to release, investigators that use the 1999–2002 data with later releases, including the current study, must adjust the earlier values using provided equations [34]. Ferritin levels are increased during acute-phase inflammation [35], so C-reactive protein (CRP) should be included in multivariate models as a control variable.

Transferrin receptor is a carrier protein for transferrin, providing transportation for iron into cells and helping maintain iron homeostasis in the body. Transferrin receptor is upregulated in the case of low body iron in order to help maintain intracellular iron levels, and is frequently elevated in pregnancy [36–38]. Previous research has indicated that the cutoff for iron deficiency for transferrin receptor in reproductive-aged women is > 5.33 mg/L [39]. In the NHANES, serum transferrin receptor was measured via immunoturbidity assay using Roche kits on the Hitachi Mod P clinical analyzer [32,33]. Serum transferrin receptor (mg/L) was available for all women aged 12–49 years in survey years 2003–2006, but was only available for pregnant women in survey years 1999–2002 [30–33]. While multiple imputation would theoretically replace the missing data in the earlier survey years, in practice multiple imputation of all 8 years lead to biased data and models that would not converge. Therefore, the decision was made to perform analyses on transferrin receptor for 2003–2006 only, and impute the missing data only in those years.

Percent transferrin saturation is a measure of the total body iron that is bound to transferrin, which is a blood protein that binds to and controls the release of the body's iron. Percent transferrin saturation was calculated using the formula: serum iron/total iron-binding capacity x 100%. Serum iron and total iron-binding capacity were measured using automated AAII-25 colorimetric method modified to be performed on the Alpkem Flow Solutions 3000 system [30–33]. Percent transferrin saturation was available in 1999–2000 for men and women of all ages and in 2001–2006 for women between the ages of 12 and 59 years [30–33]. Percent transferrin saturation is considered deficient when values fall below 16% [29].

Reproductive history variables. Reproduction-related variables are available for all women above the age of 12 in the reproductive health questionnaire. Some reproductive variables were constructed using more than one variable in order to accurately represent the survey methods and the population's response. For all constructed reproductive variables, respondents with missing values for both questions were left missing.

Pregnancy status was determined by the results of the urine pregnancy test. A continuous parity variable was constructed based on a combined variable, first by using a variable that asks if women had ever been pregnant and for those that said yes, using the number of reported live births. Women who had no pregnancies were reported to have a parity of 0; for all others, the reported live births were used as their parity value.

A dichotomous variable for currently breastfeeding women was created using three variables: First, women who reported never being pregnant were coded as not currently breastfeeding. Second, women who had given birth within the past two years were asked if they were currently breastfeeding; those that said yes were coded as currently breastfeeding and those that said no were coded as not currently breastfeeding. Finally, women who had reported giving birth 2 or more years ago were coded as not currently breastfeeding (the NHANES survey made the assumption during data collection that women 2 or more years post birth were not currently breastfeeding).

Two dichotomous variables for hormonal contraceptive use were created: one, for current use of hormonal contraception, and two, for using hormonal contraception at any point during the life span.

Reported having regular menstrual periods over the previous 12 months was included as a dichotomous variable. To assess the long-term effects of menstrual history, recalled age at menarche was included as a continuous variable.

Control variables. Regression analyses were controlled for the following variables: Age, CRP level, body mass index (BMI), survey year, ethnicity, dietary iron intake from 24-hour recall, and household income. Age, BMI, CRP, and dietary iron intake were included as continuous variables. Yearly household income was coded as dummy variables in $5000 increments, up to $75,000+. Ethnicity was coded as dummy variables for Hispanic (including Mexican Americans), non-Hispanic black and other, with non-Hispanic white as the reference category. Survey year for each two-year data-release period was included as dummy variables.

Eight-year examination sample weights were calculated using the 4-year weight for survey years 1999–2002 and two-year weights for 2003-2004 and 2005–2006. The 4-year weights were multiplied by ½ and the 2-year weights were multiplied by ¼ to create the 8-year weight variable. To create the 4-year weights for the transferrin receptor models for 2003–2004 and 2005–2006, the 2-year examination sample weights were multiplied by ½ [28].

Statistical methods

Excluding individuals who have missing values from analysis can lead to biased results [40,41]. Multiple imputation (MI) is a statistical method for replacing missing variables in a data set. Imputation models use a probability model on both complete and missing data in a set to generate likely variables for missing values.

In multiple imputation, several imputed data sets are generated, and the desired statistical analysis is performed on each one. After analysis, the results from each imputed set are averaged across variables to help control for the variance introduced by the imputation process [40,41].

Multiple imputation proceeds through three steps: 1) the generation of the MI data sets, which generates likely values for missing variables based on available data; 2) complex survey regression analyses based on the MI data sets; and 3) the synthesis of the imputed data sets and regression analyses, which combines the imputed results and reports the variability introduced by the imputation process [41,42]. The MI process was performed in SAS 9.3 (SAS Institute, Inc., Cary, North Carolina). Statistical significance was assessed at $\alpha = 0.05$ (two-sided).

The multiple imputation of data sets was performed using PROC MI in SAS. In SAS, PROC MI uses a Markov chain Monte Carlo method that assumes arbitrary missing data and multivariate normality. Standard usage of MI data sets suggests that at least 5 imputed data sets should be used, although this number may be higher for data sets with more missing data [43]. Due to the high levels of missing values for some variables in the data set, $n = 50$ imputations were performed in this analysis. For 50 imputations, reliability estimates for each variable were above 95%. All variables mentioned above were included in the imputation analysis, but income variables were dropped from regression analysis because they were not statistically significant and had no biological rationale for being included as a control variable.

A special mention should be made of dichotomous variables in MI procedures. Imputed dichotomous variables are not dichotomous themselves, but instead range as a proportion between 0 and 1. Some practitioners round the imputed fractions to the nearest 0 or 1; however, this practice leads to biased estimates of these variables [44]. Analysis of a variety of methods for handling dichotomous variables suggests that for the majority of cases, imputed fractions should be left alone for regression analysis [45]. Therefore, imputed dichotomous variables in this study were left as-is for analysis.

Analysis of imputed data sets was performed using PROC SURVEYMEANS for descriptive statistics and PROC SURVEYREG for linear regression. All survey analyses (descriptive and regression) were adjusted using NHANES-provided variables for strata and cluster, and the adjusted 8-year sample weight described above (or the 4-year sample weight for the transferrin receptor model). The imputed data sets were added to the model as part of the domain statement. This allows the analyses to be performed on each imputed data set.

For the PROC SURVEYREG analyses, four models were run with each iron biomarker (hemoglobin, ferritin, transferrin receptor, and % transferring saturation) as dependent variables. Independent variables for each model were as follows: current pregnancy, parity, currently breastfeeding, currently using contraceptive pills, ever used contraceptive pills, having regular periods in the past 12 months, and age at menarche. All models were adjusted for ethnicity (with white ethnicity as the reference variable), survey release years (with 1999–2000 as the reference variable except the transferrin receptor model, which used 2003–2004 as the reference variable), BMI, CRP, age, and 24-hour recall of dietary iron intake.

To complement MI analysis, it is recommended that an analysis of all complete cases (cases with no missing data) be performed in order to assess potential areas of bias, either in the complete case or in the multiple imputation [46]. In this study, complete case analyses were performed for each model using PROC SUR-

VEYREG and was adjusted for examination weight, strata, and cluster as described above. The subdomain for this analysis was female exam participants ages 18–49. Descriptive statistics for the non-imputed, original data were performed using PROC SURVEYMEANS and the parameters described above.

The final step was performed using PROC MIANALYSIS. This procedure synthesizes the results of the 50 imputed data sets, providing summary means and adjusted variances for PROC SURVEYMEANS, and summary parameter estimates and adjusted variances for the results of PROCSURVEYREG. This method also provides 95% confidence intervals for means and parameter estimates. Using these three steps, results are adjusted for both the multiple imputation process and the complex survey design of NHANES.

Results

Descriptive statistics were performed on both the original data sets and the imputed data sets using PROC SURVEYMEANS, to adjust for the complex survey design (Table 1). The percent missing data, derived from the total number of eligible women ($n = 6603$), ranged from 0% to 32.7% depending on the variable of interest. Graphs of the weighted association between iron biomarkers and pregnancy are found in Figure 1 and iron biomarkers and parity in Figure 2. Hemoglobin, ferritin, and % transferrin saturation declined with increasing parity and was also reduced in pregnant women. Transferrin receptor increased with increasing parity, and was higher in non-pregnant women compared to pregnant women. Table 2 shows the percentage of women who fall below the cutoff value for each iron biomarker, as well as the percentage of women considered iron deficient, as defined by having two out of three values of hemoglobin, ferritin, and % transferrin saturation below their respective cutoff values [47].

Complete case results (estimates and p-values) for survey regression for the four models is found in Table 3. In general, there were between 60–65% complete cases for each model out of the eligible women in the study population. Results do not appear to differ significantly between the complete case results and the imputed results, reported in Table 4.

Imputed estimates, 95% confidence intervals, and p-values for each of the four models (analyzed using imputed values and PROC SURVEYREG) can be found in Table 4. In the hemoglobin model, there was a significant negative association between pregnancy and hemoglobin, parity and hemoglobin, and having regular periods and hemoglobin. In addition, white American women had significantly higher hemoglobin than all other ethnicities.

In the ferritin model, ferritin was significantly negatively associated with pregnancy, parity, and having regular periods. Ferritin was significantly positively associated with taking hormonal contraceptive. Several covariates were also statistically significant. Hispanic women had significantly lower ferritin levels while women whose ethnicity was given as "other" had significantly higher ferritin levels. Ferritin was also significantly positively associated with current age and CRP level.

Transferrin receptor levels were significantly positively associated with having regular menstrual periods and parity. Transferrin receptor was negatively associated with pregnancy and taking hormonal contraceptive pills. Transferrin receptor levels were also significantly higher in non-Hispanic black women and in women with higher BMIs.

Percent transferrin saturation was significantly negatively associated with parity and having regular menstrual periods.

Hispanic and non-Hispanic black women had significantly lower % transferrin saturation than white women. Finally, % transferrin saturation was significantly negatively associated with BMI and CRP.

Discussion

Pregnancy had a clear effect on some, but not all, of the iron status measures. Pregnancy was associated with lower levels of hemoglobin and ferritin, indicating that iron availability to red blood cells and iron storage is compromised during pregnancy. This is a typical finding for pregnant women, as the fetus's high iron needs depletes mothers' iron stores, particularly as pregnancy progresses. Similarly, % transferrin saturation was lower in pregnant women than non-pregnant women, but not significantly so. Curiously, transferrin receptor levels were significantly lower in pregnant women compared to non-pregnant women. As transferrin receptor is usually higher under conditions of low body iron, this result is opposite of what would be predicted by previous literature [36,37]. However, it may be an expected result in the context of maternal-fetal iron transfer. Maternal physiology is hypothesized to negotiate the allocation of resources between maternal and fetal somatic needs, which may sometimes conflict with fetal interests [48,49]. In the case of maternal-fetal iron transfer, previous research suggests that fetal iron transfer has priority over maintaining maternal iron stores [50], and that fetal iron deficiency only occurs after maternal iron stores have been severely compromised [51,52]. The current results suggest that transferrin receptor may be downregulated during pregnancy in an attempt to allocate iron away from the mother's tissues and toward the fetus. These results hint at a pregnancy iron transfer system that depletes bodily iron during pregnancy in favor of fetal iron stores, supporting previous findings. However, more research is necessary to confirm the physiological mechanisms that may underlie such a mechanism.

There were no significant effects of breastfeeding on any iron status values. Unfortunately, analysis of this variable was hampered by the low rate of breastfeeding in US women: only 2% of women reported that they were currently breastfeeding. Replicating these findings in a population of women with higher breastfeeding rates would better test the hypothesis that the postpartum period is a time of iron repletion in reproducing women.

These results provide evidence that postpartum iron repletion is incomplete in US women, and has an additive negative effect with each child. Increasing parity was found to have a small but statistically significant impact on all indicators of iron status. These results replicate parity-related maternal iron depletion findings in developing countries with high rates of iron-deficiency anemia, albeit with smaller statistical estimates [14]. Despite the relatively good overall iron status of the US population, high-parity women are vulnerable to poor iron status. This effect may be particularly worrisome in high parity women who become pregnant [26].

The results show that having regular periods across the past 12 months is associated with lower iron stores than not having regular periods, and that taking hormonal contraceptive pills is associated with higher iron status. This seemingly points to the traditional view that menstrual blood loss directly affects iron status, and that contraception's protective effect is due to lighter menstrual periods while on the pill [16,17]. More recently, however, mouse models have demonstrated a direct relationship between estrogen and iron homeostasis [53,54]. Work on this relationship shows that that estrogen directly inhibits the expression of hepcidin, a liver-produced peptide hormone that inhibits iron intake across the gut

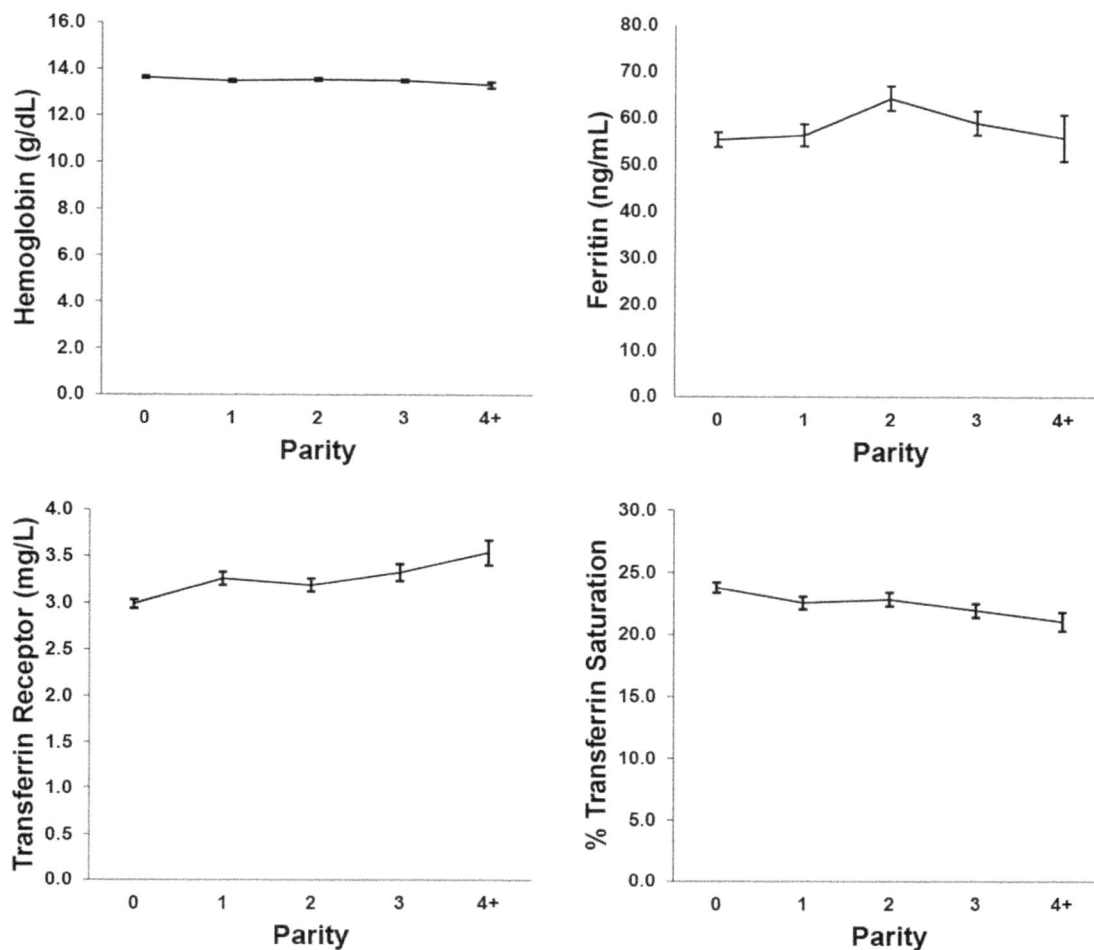

Figure 1. Weighted (unimputed) means and ±1 standard error of the mean for measures of iron status by pregnancy status.

and is a regulator of iron homeostasis in the body [55]. When estrogen is high, hepcidin is low and iron uptake into the body is increased. The authors proposed that this is a mechanism to regulate iron uptake across the menstrual cycle, and can explain the higher level of iron in women who take hormonal contraceptives [55].

Despite the immediate impact of having regular periods and using contraceptive pills on iron status, there appears to be no long-term effects: history of contraceptive pill use and age at menarche were not significantly associated with iron stores in this population. It could be hypothesized that menstruation-related iron loss should accumulate, particularly in a population who spends a high proportion of their reproductive careers menstruating [56]. However, these results call into question the idea that blood loss is the sole cause of altered iron stores in menstruating women. This perspective has also been advanced by Clancy et al. [19], who note that a thicker endometrium (and greater potential menstrual blood loss) is actually associated with higher hemoglobin in reproductive-aged Polish women. Contrary to established wisdom, their work shows menstruation is associated with better, not worse, iron status, and suggests that iron is a sensitive indicator of reproductive condition. Rather than assume that menstrual blood loss leads to anemia, a closer examination of the co-relationship between hepcidin, iron absorption, estrogen, and reproduction in women is warranted. It is more likely that

menstruation-related iron homeostasis is tightly regulated, even in women who continually menstruate throughout their reproductive career.

The results showed significantly different measures of iron status between ethnic groups in the US. Non-Hispanic white women had higher hemoglobin compared to other groups, Hispanic women had lower ferritin and % transferrin saturation compared to the reference group (non-Hispanic white women), and non-Hispanic black women had higher levels of transferrin receptor and lower % transferrin saturation compared to the reference group. These differences raise several questions. First, what is the normal range of variation in US women? Why does it vary between groups, and what are the factors that contribute to this reaction norm? Some researchers suggest a lower threshold for iron-deficiency anemia for African-American women [3], for example, but what drives this difference? Second, it also demonstrates that there may be no one picture of low iron status in women, and that each iron indicator may offer a slightly different interpretation of the physiological processes involved in the body's response to low iron. Further research would untangle the meaning of these different pathways, particularly in the context of women's reproduction. Finally, it is worth investigating population-specific reproductive outcomes due to poor iron status. There are well-known consequences of maternal iron-deficiency anemia, including preterm birth, low birth weight, increased maternal morbidity,

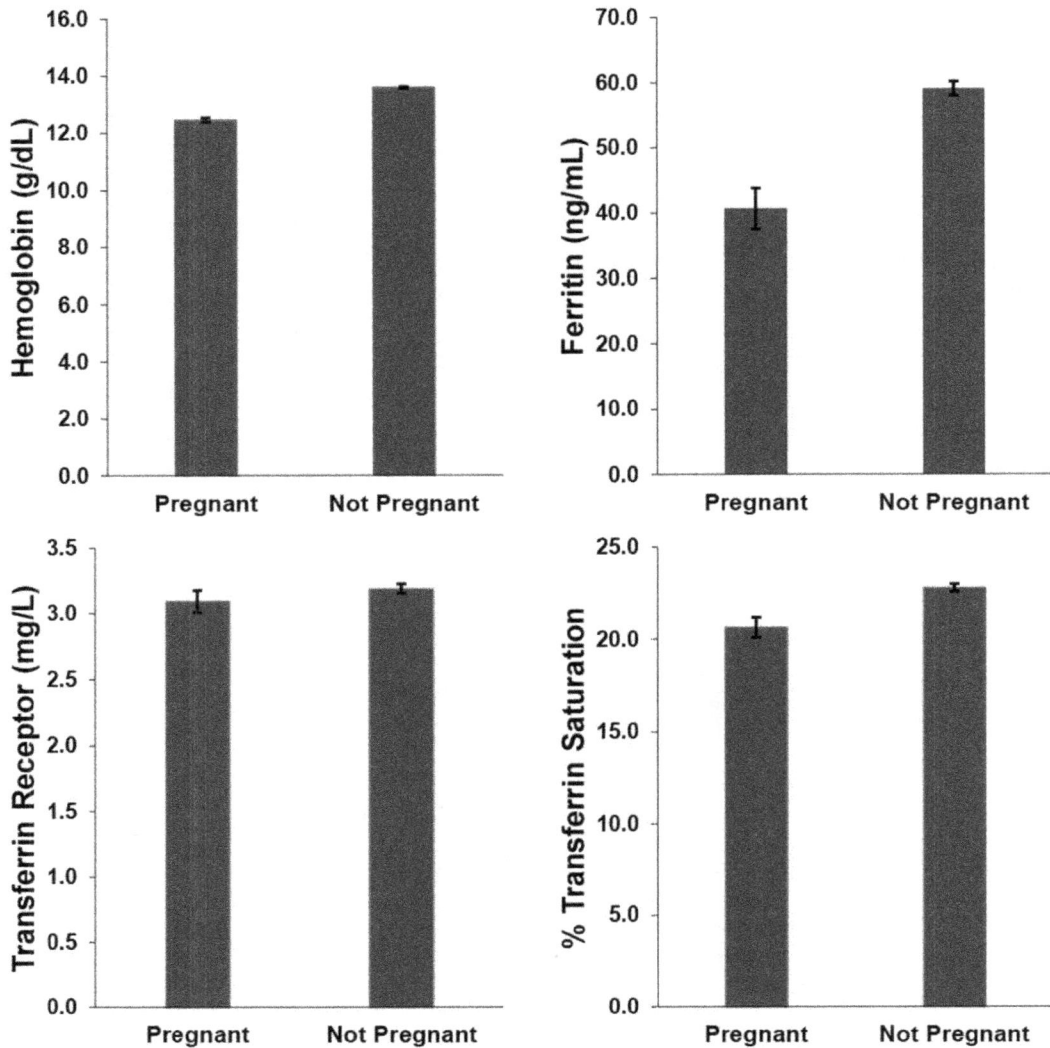

Figure 2. Weighted (unimputed) means and ±1 standard error of the mean for measures of iron status by parity.

increased risk of infant iron-deficiency, poor neurocognitive development in infants, and others [4,7]. However, meta-analyses indicate that most of these adverse outcomes (with the exception of pre-term birth) are not consistent across studies [57]. Rather than doubt the possibility of these adverse outcomes, an anthropological approach would instead posit that there may be ecological variation in the appearance of these outcomes. Instead, the question becomes: who do these adverse outcomes happen to, and why? Further work from an anthropological perspective may

Table 2. Non-imputed, weighted percentages of NHANES women who are below iron indicator cutoffs by pregnancy status (See Table 1 for number of non-missing values in each category).

	Non-pregnant women	Pregnant women
Hemoglobin (<12 g/dL)	6.9%	29.1%
Ferritin (<12 ng/mL)	10.9%	18.5%
Transferrin receptor (>5.33 mg/L)[a]	5.4%	5.7%
% Transferrin saturation (<16%)	29.7%	39.1%
% Iron deficient[b]	9.8%	25.4%

[a]Percentages based on 2003–2006 survey years only.
[b]Calculated based on percentage of women who had two of three values (hemoglobin, ferritin, and % transferrin saturation) below cutoff.

Table 3. Weighted estimates and p-values for complete case survey regression models of hemoglobin, ferritin, % transferrin saturation, and transferrin receptor as dependent variables, reproductive variables as independent variables, and ethnicity, survey release year, and other covariates as control variables.

		Hemoglobin $n=4255$ $R^2=0.15$		Ferritin $n=4252$ $R^2=0.071$		% Transferrin Saturation $n=4245$ $R^2=0.095$		Transferrin Receptor[a] $n=2019$ $R^2=0.099$	
		Estimate	p	Estimate	p	Estimate	p	Estimate	p
Reproductive Status	Currently pregnant	−1.02	<0.0001	−19.94	<0.0001	−0.58	0.48	−0.033	0.74
	Parity	−0.081	0.0003	−2.27	0.0026	−0.66	0.0002	0.047	0.17
	Currently breastfeeding	0.037	0.78	3.41	0.5687	−0.98	0.35	0.37	0.14
	Current birth control use	−0.034	0.59	9.97	0.0108	1.44	0.042	−0.33	0.0001
	Ever use birth control	0.026	0.69	−0.062	0.98	−0.042	0.95	−0.00070	0.99
	Having regular periods	−0.20	0.0032	−16.62	<0.0001	−1.22	0.067	0.013	0.93
	Age at menarche	−0.024	0.076	−0.65	0.3056	−0.070	0.59	−0.0051	0.74
Ethnicity[b]	Hispanic	−0.29	<0.0001	−4.09	0.0355	−1.49	0.016	−0.053	0.60
	Non-Hispanic black	−1.06	<0.0001	−0.022	0.9935	−2.84	<0.0001	0.54	<0.0001
	Other	−0.47	0.0004	7.73	0.0711	−1.85	0.034	0.29	0.12
Survey Release[c,d]	2001–2002	−0.033	0.70	−10.39	0.0011	−0.22	0.75	–	–
	2003–2004	0.14	0.11	2.61	0.4303	0.41	0.60	–	–
	2005–2006	0.094	0.28	0.14	0.9627	0.025	0.97	−0.25	0.0023
Other Covariates	BMI (kg/m²)	0.0018	0.55	0.11	0.5819	−0.27	<0.0001	0.029	0.0002
	CRP (g/L)	−0.087	0.0017	10.54	<0.0001	−2.34	<0.0001	0.053	0.18
	Age (years)	−0.00020	0.96	0.73	<0.0001	0.040	0.16	−0.00060	0.90
	Dietary iron intake (mg)	−0.00010	0.95	0.044	0.7448	−0.013	0.63	0.0043	0.32

[a]Transferrin receptor model is based on survey years 2003–2006 only.
[b]Reference category is white ethnicity.
[c]Reference category is survey release year 1999–2000 (hemoglobin, ferritin, and % transferrin saturation models).
[d]Reference category is survey release year 2003–2004 (transferrin receptor model only).

Table 4. Weighted estimates, 95% confidence intervals, and p-values for imputed survey regression models of hemoglobin, ferritin, % transferrin saturation, and transferrin receptor as dependent variables, reproductive variables as independent variables, and ethnicity, survey release year, and other covariates as control variables.

		Hemoglobin[a] $R^2 = 0.17$[c]			Ferritin[a] $R^2 = 0.12$[c]			% Transferrin Saturation[a] $R^2 = 0.093$[c]			Transferrin Receptor[b] $R^2 = 0.10$[c]		
		Estimate	95% CI	p	Estimate	95% CI	p	Estimate	95% CI	p	Estimate	95% CI	p
Reproductive Status	Currently pregnant	-1.12	-1.24, -0.99	<0.0001	-19.60	-27.03, -12.16	<0.0001	-0.58	-1.84, 0.67	0.36	-0.29	-0.51, -0.057	0.014
	Parity	-0.066	-0.10, -0.030	0.0003	-2.94	-4.55, -1.34	0.0003	-0.62	-0.90, -0.34	<0.0001	0.10	0.052, 0.15	<0.0001
	Currently breastfeeding	-0.076	-0.34, 0.19	0.57	-7.40	-21.12, 6.32	0.29	-0.95	-3.38, 1.48	0.44	0.37	-0.14, 0.88	0.15
	Current birth control use	-0.077	-0.20, 0.043	0.21	14.74	6.24, 23.23	0.0007	1.18	-0.084, 2.45	0.067	-0.40	-0.57, -0.23	<0.0001
	Ever use birth control	0.057	-0.056, 0.17	0.32	0.56	-4.36, 5.47	0.82	-0.0058	-1.08, 1.06	0.99	-0.059	-0.25, 0.13	0.55
	Having regular periods	-0.28	-0.37, -0.19	<0.0001	-32.25	-38.43, -26.08	<0.0001	-1.42	-2.34, -0.50	0.0025	0.29	0.068, 0.52	0.011
	Age at menarche	-0.012	-0.035, 0.011	0.29	-0.70	-1.91, 0.51	0.26	0.022	-0.20, 0.25	0.84	0.015	-0.024, 0.053	0.45
Ethnicity[d]	Hispanic	-0.25	-0.35, -0.14	<0.0001	-4.09	-7.92, -0.26	0.036	-1.59	-2.55, -0.63	0.0012	0.042	-0.13, 0.21	0.62
	Non-Hispanic black	-1.08	-1.17, -0.98	<0.0001	6.57	-0.27, 13.41	0.060	-2.53	-3.34, -1.73	<0.0001	0.91	0.68, 1.14	<0.0001
	Other	-0.31	-0.49, -0.13	0.0008	11.76	2.37, 21.16	0.014	-1.45	-2.89, -0.0058	0.049	0.086	-0.15, 0.33	0.48
Survey Release[e,f]	2001–2002	-0.0031	-0.18, 0.18	0.97	-6.80	-12.06, -1.53	0.012	-0.10	-1.17, 0.96	0.85	—	—	—
	2003–2004	0.21	0.057, 0.37	0.0077	9.38	4.95, 13.81	<0.0001	0.94	-0.20, 2.08	0.11	—	—	—
	2005–2006	0.11	-0.05, 0.28	0.17	3.11	-2.18, 8.40	0.25	0.054	-1.00, 1.11	0.92	-0.052	-0.21, 0.10	0.51
Other Covariates	BMI (kg/m²)	0.00064	-0.0043, 0.0056	0.80	0.23	-0.17, 0.62	0.26	-0.27	-0.31, -0.22	<0.0001	0.033	0.025, 0.042	<0.0001
	CRP (g/L)	-0.032	-0.082, 0.017	0.20	12.61	7.49, 17.73	<0.0001	-1.96	-2.43, -1.48	<0.0001	-0.016	-0.090, 0.057	0.66
	Age (years)	0.000067	-0.0050, 0.0052	0.98	1.16	0.90, 1.41	<0.0001	0.067	0.021, 0.11	0.0046	-0.0026	-0.012, 0.0065	0.58
	Dietary iron intake (mg)	-0.0017	-0.0062, 0.0028	0.45	-0.12	-0.37, 0.14	0.37	-0.024	-0.067, 0.019	0.27	0.0024	-0.0063, 0.011	0.59

[a]The n for the hemoglobin, ferritin, and % transferrin saturation model is 6603 (all years).
[b]The n for the transferrin receptor model is 3295 (survey years 2003–2006 only).
[c]Mean R^2 of 50 imputations.
[d]Reference category is white ethnicity.
[e]Reference category is survey release year 1999–2000 (hemoglobin, ferritin, and % transferrin saturation models).
[f]Reference category is survey release year 2003–2004 (transferrin receptor model only).

provide better insight into the ecology of iron use in women's reproduction.

One interesting finding in this study is that reported levels of dietary iron intake in the current study were not significantly associated with indicators of iron status in statistical analyses. Interestingly, the reported dietary intake of iron in this sample of women (13.73 mg/day) was lower than the recommended daily intake of 18 mg/day for reproductive-aged women; however, rates of iron deficiency were 9.8% in non-pregnant women and 25.4% in pregnant women (Table 2). These results show that while women in the US have clear reproductive-related changes in iron status, low iron is considerably less prevalent in non-pregnant women, despite their lower-than-recommended dietary intake.

When viewed through an anthropological framework, these results challenge current interpretations of the variation in women's reproduction in several ways. First, rather than use cut-off levels that determine iron deficiency, this study instead examined iron status as continuous variables, as is typical in biological anthropology. Therefore, these results do not make recommendations relating to supplementation or the avoidance of reproductive-related low iron in the US. Rather, they are intended to show associated patterns and to help identify potential future research areas of interest to both anthropologists and nutritional scientists. Second, although many of these results are statistically significant, they may not all be biologically significant. For example, the parity results, although significant, would require a large number of children in most cases to find a biologically meaningful effect. While this is uncommon among US women, populations with higher fertility rates should be advised of parity-related effects. Third, the results from this study challenge what is considered a "normal" iron status in US women. These results show evidence of reproduction-related changes in iron status in US women despite the widespread availability of iron-rich foods and supplements. Perhaps rather than viewing every case of low iron during pregnancy as a problem in need of correction, low iron should be viewed as a normal function of women's pregnancy, provided these women and their infants do not experience adverse outcomes [58,59]. This falls in line with other research that suggests that pregnant women should have lower cutoff thresholds for anemia, and that these cutoffs may vary by ethnicity [3]. Finally, these results highlight the contradictory nature of recommending supplementation while stating that some degree of low iron is normal in reproducing women. To reconcile the contradiction, it may be true that US women need iron supplementation during their pregnancy, but might not need the daily high doses of iron recommended by health officials. For example, a meta-analysis of the literature has found that intermittent iron supplementation prevents iron deficiency in pregnant women as well as daily supplementation, with fewer adverse effects [60]. The current results do suggest that certain situations may require more attention to risk factors that might require iron supplementation, such as very high parity women and non-white women. By incorporating some tolerance of low iron as "normal," and by understanding the ecological variation in iron status between populations, supplementation recommendations can help avoid under- and over-treating low iron in reproductive-aged women. These results can help point researchers to more specific iron supplementation recommendations for pregnant and non-pregnant women, both in the US and on the global stage.

There are several limitations to this study. First, these results are limited by the data collection. The NHANES was not specifically designed for a study of this nature, so data are limited and missing in many cases. This was partially corrected by means of multiple imputation, but the limitations on data between survey releases could not be statistically overcome, particularly in the case of transferrin receptor data. Similarly, there are limited types of questions available in the survey, and not all questions of interest could be asked using this data. For example, women's interbirth interval is a very important data point when considering the pregnancy-depletion/postpartum-repletion cycle and parity-related iron depletion. Despite these limitations, these results offer insight into the mechanisms of reproductive-related iron status in US women and suggest future research into the mechanisms of reproductive iron homeostasis.

Acknowledgments

The author would like to thank Kate Clancy and an anonymous reviewer for greatly improving this manuscript.

Author Contributions

Conceived and designed the experiments: EMM. Analyzed the data: EMM. Wrote the paper: EMM.

References

1. Balarajan Y, Ramakrishnan U, Özaltin E, Shankar AH, Subramanian SV (2011) Anaemia in low-income and middle-income countries. Lancet 378: 2123–2135.
2. Kassebaum NJ, Jasrasaria R, Johns N, Wulf S, Chou D, et al. (2013) A systematic analysis of global anaemia burden between 1990 and 2010. Lancet 381: S72.
3. Cao C, O'Brien KO (2013) Pregnancy and iron homeostasis: an update. Nutr Rev 71: 35–51.
4. Allen LH (2000) Anemia and iron deficiency: effects on pregnancy outcome. Am J Clin Nutr 71: 1280s–1284s.
5. Milman N (2006) Iron and pregnancy: A delicate balance. Ann Hematol 85: 559–565.
6. Bothwell TH (2000) Iron requirements in pregnancy and strategies to meet them. Am J Clin Nutr 72: 257S–264S.
7. Scholl TO (2005) Iron status during pregnancy: setting the stage for mother and infant. Am J Clin Nutr 81: 1218S–1222S.
8. Scholl TO, Reilly T (2000) Anemia, iron and pregnancy outcome. J Nutr 130: 443.
9. Allen LH (1997) Pregnancy and iron deficiency: Unresolved issues. Nutr Rev 55: 91–101.
10. Milman N, Kirchhoff M, JØrgensen T (1992) Iron status markers, serum ferritin and hemoglobin in 1359 Danish women in relation to menstruation, hormonal contraception, parity, and postmenopausal hormone treatment. Ann Hematol 65: 96–102.
11. Kessel E, Sastrawinata S, Mumford SD (1985) Correlates of fetal growth and survival. Acta Pædiatr 74: 120–127.
12. Chang S-C, O'Brien KO, Nathanson MS, Mancini J, Witter FR (2003) Hemoglobin concentrations influence birth outcomes in pregnant African-American adolescents. J Nutr 133: 2348–2355.
13. Desalegn S (1993) Prevalence of anaemia in pregnancy in Jima town, southwestern Ethiopia. Ethiop Med J 31: 251–258.
14. Miller EM (2010) Maternal hemoglobin depletion in a settled northern Kenyan pastoral population. Am J Hum Biol 22: 768–774.
15. Winkvist A, Rasmussen KM, Habicht JP (1992) A new definition of maternal depletion syndrome. Am J Public Health 82: 691–694.
16. Milman N, Clausen J, Byg KE (1998) Iron status in 268 Danish women aged 18–30 years: influence of menstruation, contraceptive method, and iron supplementation. Ann Hematol 77: 13–19.
17. Milman N, Rosdahl N, Lyhne N, Jørgensen T, Graudal N (1993) Iron status in Danish women aged 35–65 years: Relation to menstruation and method of contraception. Acta Obstetr et Gynecol Scand 72: 601–605.
18. Beard JL (2000) Iron requirements in adolescent females. J Nutr 130: 440.
19. Clancy KB, Nenko I, Jasienska G (2006) Menstruation does not cause anemia: endometrial thickness correlates positively with erythrocyte count and hemoglobin concentration in premenopausal women. Am J Hum Biol 18: 710–713.
20. Dewey KG (2004) Impact of breastfeeding on maternal nutritional status. Adv Exp Med Biol 554: 91–100.

21. Dewey KG, Cohen RJ (2007) Does birth spacing affect maternal or child nutritional status? A systematic literature review. Matern Child Nutr 3: 151–173.

22. Labbok MH (2001) Effects of breastfeeding on the mother. Ped Clin N Am 48: 143–158.

23. Fransson G-B, Lönnerdal B (1980) Iron in human milk. J Pediatr 96: 380–384.

24. Lonnerdal B (1984) Iron and breast milk. In: Stekel A, editor. Iron Nutrition in Infancy and Childhood. New York: Vevy/Raven Press. pp. 95–118.

25. Quinn EA (2014) Too much of a good thing: Evolutionary perspectives on infant formula fortification in the United States and its effects on infant health. Am J Hum Biol 26: 10–17.

26. Mei Z, Cogswell ME, Looker AC, Pfeiffer CM, Cusick SE, et al. (2011) Assessment of iron status in US pregnant women from the National Health and Nutrition Examination Survey (NHANES), 1999–2006. Am J Clin Nutr 93: 1312–1320.

27. Jacobs A, Miller F, Worwood M, Beamish M, Wardrop C (1972) Ferritin in the serum of normal subjects and patients with iron deficiency and iron overload. BMJ 4: 206.

28. CDC (2006) Analytic and reporting guidelines. The National Health and Nutrition Examination Survey (NHANES) Atlanta, GA: Center for Disease Control and Prevention.

29. Cook JD, Baynes RD, Skikne BS (1992) Iron deficiency and the measurement of iron status. Nutr Res Rev 5: 198–202.

30. National Center for Health Statistics. 1999–2000 National Health and Nutrition Examination Survey (NHANES). Available: http://wwwn.cdc.gov/nchs/nhanes/search/nhanes99_00.aspx. Accessed 2014 May 26.

31. National Center for Health Statistics. 2001–2002 National Health and Nutrition Examination Survey (NHANES). Available: http://www.cdc.gov/nchs/nhanes/nhanes01_02.htm. Accessed 2014 May 26.

32. National Center for Health Statistics. 2003–2004 National Health and Nutrition Examination Survey (NHANES). Available: http://www.cdc.gov/nchs/nhanes/nhanes03_04.htm. Accessed 2014 May 26.

33. National Center for Health Statistics. 2005–2006 National Health and Nutrition Examination Survey (NHANES). Available: http://www.cdc.gov/nchs/nhanes/nhanes05_06.htm. Accessed 2014 May 26.

34. CDC (2006) National Health and Nutrition Examination Survey. 2003–2004 Data documentation, codebook, and frequencies. Ferritin and transferrin receptor. Atlanta, GA: Center for Disease Control.

35. Thurnham DI, McCabe LD, Haldar S, Wieringa FT, Northrop-Clewes CA, et al. (2010) Adjusting plasma ferritin concentrations to remove the effects of subclinical inflammation in the assessment of iron deficiency: a meta-analysis. Am J Clin Nutr 92: 546–555.

36. Akesson A, Bjellerup P, Berglund M, Bremme K, Vahter M (1998) Serum transferrin receptor: a specific marker of iron deficiency in pregnancy. The American journal of clinical nutrition 68: 1241–1246.

37. Carriaga MT, Skikne BS, Finley B, Cutler B, Cook JD (1991) Serum transferrin receptor for the detection of iron deficiency in pregnancy. Am J Clin Nutr 54: 1077–1081.

38. Choi JW, Im MW, Pai SH (2000) Serum transferrin receptor concentrations during normal pregnancy. Clin Chem 46: 725–727.

39. Mei Z, Pfeiffer CM, Looker AC, Flores-Ayala RC, Lacher DA, et al. (2012) Serum soluble transferrin receptor concentrations in US preschool children and non-pregnant women of childbearing age from the National Health and Nutrition Examination Survey 2003–2010. Clin Chim Acta 413: 1479–1484.

40. Little RJ, Rubin DB (2002) Statistical analysis with missing data. New York, NY: Wiley.

41. Royston P (2004) Multiple imputation of missing values. Stata Journal 4: 227–241.

42. Berglund PA (2010) An introduction to multiple imputation of complex sample data using SAS v9.2. SAS Global Forum Proceedings Cary, NC: SAS Institute Inc.

43. Graham JW, Olchowski AE, Gilreath TD (2007) How many imputations are really needed? Some practical clarifications of multiple imputation theory. Prev Sci 8: 206–213.

44. Horton NJ, Lipsitz SR, Parzen M (2003) A potential for bias when rounding in multiple imputation. Am Stat 57: 229–232.

45. Allison PD (2005) Imputation of categorical variables with PROC MI. SAS Users Group International, 30th Meeting (SUGI 30): Citeseer.

46. Sterne JA, White IR, Carlin JB, Spratt M, Royston P, et al. (2009) Multiple imputation for missing data in epidemiological and clinical research: Potential and pitfalls. BMJ 338.

47. Looker AC, Dallman PR, Carroll MD, Gunter EW, Johnson CL (1997) Prevalence of iron deficiency in the United States. JAMA 277: 973–976.

48. Abrams ET, Meshnick SR (2009) Malaria during pregnancy in endemic areas: a lens for examining maternal-fetal conflict. Am J Hum Biol 21: 643–650.

49. Haig D (1993) Genetic conflicts in human pregnancy. Q Rev Biol 68: 495–532.

50. Van Santen S, de Mast Q, Luty AJF, Wiegerinck ET, Van der Ven AJAM, et al. (2011) Iron homeostasis in mother and child during placental malaria infection. Am J Trop Med Hygiene 84: 148–151.

51. McArdle HJ, Gambling L, Kennedy C (2014) Iron deficiency during pregnancy: the consequences for placental function and fetal outcome. Proc Nutr Soc 73: 9–15.

52. Gambling L, Lang C, McArdle HJ (2011) Fetal regulation of iron transport during pregnancy. Am J Clin Nutr: 1903S–1907S.

53. Ikeda Y, Tajima S, Izawa-Ishizawa Y, Kihira Y, Ishizawa K, et al. (2012) Estrogen regulates hepcidin expression via GPR30-BMP6-dependent signaling in hepatocytes. PLOS ONE 7: e40465.

54. Hou Y, Zhang S, Wang L, Li J, Qu G, et al. (2012) Estrogen regulates iron homeostasis through governing hepatic hepcidin expression via an estrogen response element. Gene 511: 398–403.

55. Yang Q, J J, Katz S, Abramson SB, Huang X (2012) 17β-Estradiol Inhibits Iron Hormone Hepcidin Through an Estrogen Responsive Element Half-Site. Endocrinology 153: 3170–3178.

56. Strassmann BI (1997) The biology of menstruation in Homo sapiens: Total lifetime menses, fecundity, and nonsynchrony in a natural-fertility population. Curr Anthropol 38: 123–129.

57. Xiong X, Buekens P, Alexander S, Demianczuk N, Wollast E (2000) Anemia during pregnancy and birth outcome: a meta-analysis. Am J Perinatol 17: 137–146.

58. Beaton GH (2000) Iron needs during pregnancy: do we need to rethink our targets? Am J Clin Nutr 72: 265S–271S.

59. Yip R (2000) Significance of an abnormally low or high hemoglobin concentration during pregnancy: special consideration of iron nutrition. Am J Clin Nutr 72: 272S–279S.

60. Pena-Rosas JP, De-Regil LM, Dowswell T, Viteri FE (2012) Intermittent oral iron supplementation during pregnancy. Cochrane Database Syst Rev 7: Cd009997.

22

A Physiologically-Motivated Compartment-Based Model of the Effect of Inhaled Hypertonic Saline on Mucociliary Clearance and Liquid Transport in Cystic Fibrosis

Matthew R. Markovetz[1], Timothy E. Corcoran[1,2,6], Landon W. Locke[2], Michael M. Myerburg[2], Joseph M. Pilewski[2], Robert S. Parker[1,3,4,5]*

1 Department of Chemical and Petroleum Engineering, Swanson School of Engineering, University of Pittsburgh, Pittsburgh, PA, United States of America, **2** Pulmonary Allergy and Critical Care Medicine, University of Pittsburgh, Pittsburgh, PA, United States of America, **3** McGowan Institute of Regenerative Medicine, University of Pittsburgh, Pittsburgh, PA, United States of America, **4** Clinical Research, Investigation, and Systems Modeling of Acute Illness (CRISMA) Laboratories, University of Pittsburgh, Pittsburgh, PA, United States of America, **5** University of Pittsburgh Cancer Institute, University of Pittsburgh, Pittsburgh, PA, United States of America, **6** Department of Bioengineering, Swanson School of Engineering, University of Pittsburgh, Pittsburgh, PA, United States of America

Abstract

Background: Cystic Fibrosis (CF) lung disease is characterized by liquid hyperabsorption, airway surface dehydration, and impaired mucociliary clearance (MCC). Herein, we present a compartment-based mathematical model of the airway that extends the resolution of functional imaging data.

Methods: Using functional imaging data to inform our model, we developed a system of mechanism-motivated ordinary differential equations to describe the mucociliary clearance and absorption of aerosolized radiolabeled particle and small molecules probes from human subjects with and without CF. We also utilized a novel imaging metric *in vitro* to gauge the fraction of airway epithelial cells that have functional ciliary activity.

Results: This model, and its incorporated kinetic rate parameters, captures the MCC and liquid dynamics of the hyperabsorptive state in CF airways and the mitigation of that state by hypertonic saline treatment.

Conclusions: We postulate, based on the model structure and its ability to capture clinical patient data, that patients with CF have regions of airway with diminished MCC function that can be recruited with hypertonic saline treatment. In so doing, this model structure not only makes a case for durable osmotic agents used in lung-region specific treatments, but also may provide a possible clinical endpoint, the fraction of functional ciliated airway.

Editor: Nades Palaniyar, The Hospital for Sick Children and The University of Toronto, Canada

Funding: MRM is supported by a Graduate Assistantships in Areas of National Need (GAANN) fellowship (U.S. Department of Education (www.ed.gov), P200A120195). The functional imaging project in [6] and TEC were supported by National Institutes of Health (www.nih.gov) R01HL108929. RSP acknowledges support of the B.P. America Faculty Fellowship in the Swanson School of Engineering. MMM acknowledges support from National Institutes of Health (www.nih.gov) RO1HL112862. Work performed in HBE cell cultures was supported by the NIH (www.nih.gov) P30DK072506 and the Cystic Fibrosis Foundation (www.cff.org) Research Development Program. The content is solely the responsibility of the authors and does not necessarily represent the official views of the National Heart, Lung, and Blood Institute or the National Institutes of Health. The funders had no role in study design, data collection and analysis, decision to publish, or preparation of the manuscript.

* Email: rparker@pitt.edu

Introduction

Cystic Fibrosis (CF) is an autosomal recessive disease that arises from a defect in the Cystic Fibrosis Transmembrane Conductance Regulator (CFTR) gene. CF affects multiple organ systems, with the most detrimental effects occurring in the lungs [1]. CFTR encodes an anion channel on epithelial surfaces, that is dysfunctional or absent from the CF epithelium. The associated loss of Cl^- and HCO_3^- secretion along with a tendency to hyperabsorb Na^+ through the epithelial sodium channel (ENaC) results in osmotic gradients that favor rapid absorption of the airway surface liquid (ASL) layer, leading to dehydrated airway mucus secretions and impaired mucociliary clearance (MCC) [2], [3]. The inability to clear pathogens via MCC leads to chronic infection, inflammation, airway damage, and premature respiratory failure.

Inhaled agents that reverse osmotic gradients in the airways are used to treat the ASL dehydration defect associated with CF. Hypertonic saline (HS) is one such osmotic agent that has been shown to increase both MCC and lung function in patients with CF [4], [5]. More recently CFTR modulators have been developed that substantially improve lung function in individuals with specific CFTR mutations [6].

Outcome measures and biomarkers that quantify the basic pathophysiology of CF lung disease are needed to allow for the rapid screening of new therapeutics for CF. Ideally, these screening methods seek to quantify the basic pathophysiology of CF lung disease. Mucociliary clearance scans, which quantify the clearance of a radiolabeled particulate from the lungs, are one such functional imaging method for studying outcomes in CF. We have expanded this method to include measuring the clearance of a radiolabeled small-molecule that can be absorbed as well as cleared via MCC. Similar techniques have been used in the past to resolve the individual components of lung clearance [7], [8]. Our *in vivo* method utilizes Technetium 99m sulfur colloid (Tc-SC) as the non-absorbable particle probe and Indium 111-DTPA (DTPA) as the small molecule probe. The probes are delivered together in a liquid aerosol. Figure 1 presents a schematic for pharmaceutical clearance from the airway epithelium. We assume that MCC clears the probes at similar rates and that the difference in their clearance rates is therefore associated with the absorption of the small molecule. Previous *in vitro* studies have demonstrated a relationship between DTPA and airway surface liquid absorption rates [9]. DTPA absorption is increased both *in vivo* in CF airways and *in vitro* in CF airway cell cultures [9], [10]. Decreases in DTPA absorption after osmotic therapies have also been demonstrated *in vitro* and *in vivo* [9], [10]. Thus, multi-probe methods provide measurements of both MCC and ASL absorption rates [10]. Successful CF therapies should restore ASL volume by correcting defective airway epithelial ion transport [11], [12]. The restoration of airway hydration should be rapidly detectable through these multi-probe imaging methods as decreased liquid absorption rates are reflected through slower absorption of DTPA and improvements in MCC cause increased Tc-SC clearance.

Herein we present a compartment-based model of particle and small molecule clearance from the human respiratory tract that uses functional imaging data to inform model structure and quantitate parameter values. Our goal in developing this model is to better resolve the specific physiological mechanisms that

contribute to the composite functional imaging result. We believe that these mechanism-specific measurements may provide more sensitive and specific evaluations of therapeutic efficacy than the currently used image-derived metrics. The challenge is to construct a mathematical representation of the physiology that can resolve the underlying mechanisms and their interactions.

There have been a number of compartment-based pharmacokinetic (PK) models for inhaled pharmaceuticals [13], [14], [15], [16], [17], but to our knowledge none have considered the PK behavior of the radiopharmaceuticals used for functional imaging from which our data originates, nor has anyone assessed absorption kinetics with the methodology we have employed. We hypothesize that by dividing the lung into a solely absorptive peripheral lung region and separate central lung region that has both absorptive and MCC capability, and by subdividing this central lung region into fractions with, and without, functional ciliated airway, we can reproduce the dynamics of simultaneous particle and small molecule probe clearance from the lung. We further hypothesize that (i) functional ciliated airway clears at the same rate in patients with CF and non-CF subjects; (ii) the fraction of functional ciliated airway (FFCA) is decreased in CF; and (iii) FFCA can be increased through inhalation of HS. Our models provide estimates of FFCA, MCC, and large airway and peripheral lung absorption, the latter of which we believe is related to liquid hyper-absorption in CF small airways. These measured parameters may substantially expand the utility of our functional imaging measurement by providing more mechanistic insight into lung physiology and response to therapeutic agents (a list of all abbreviations and their definition used in this work can be found in Table 1).

Results

Model Synthesis and Assumptions

Starting from the original model of Sakagami [15], we extend it structurally to account for the dynamics and kinetics observed in

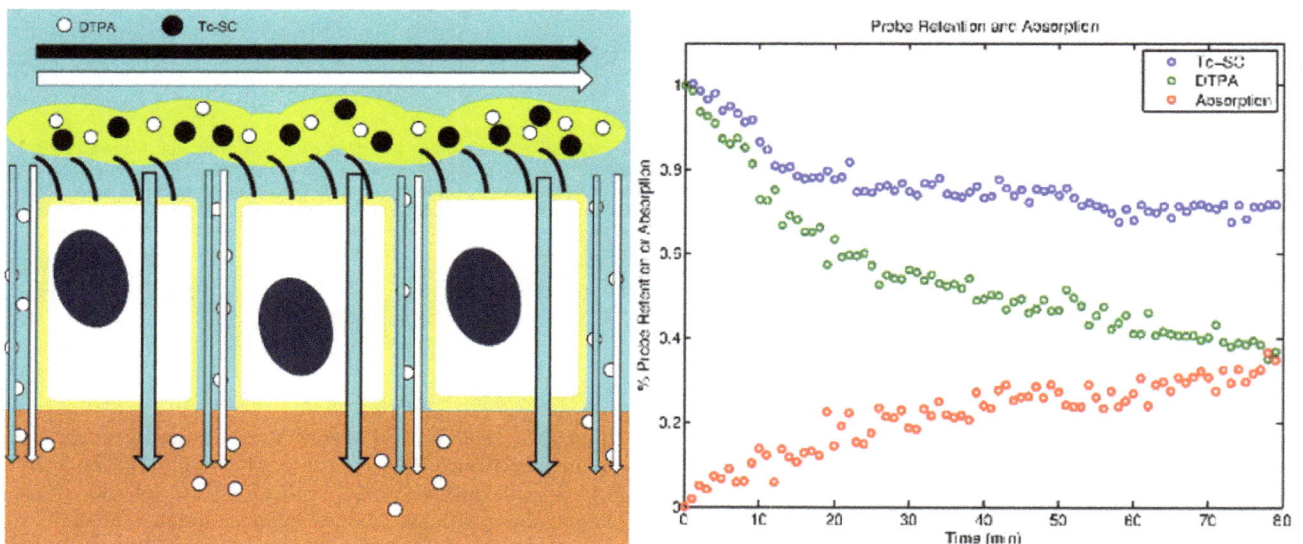

Figure 1. Left panel: schematic of transport routes in the airway epithelium. The black and white horizontal arrows represent mucociliary clearance of Tc-SC and DTPA, respectively. DTPA (downward white arrow) absorbs across the airway epithelium via the paracellular route. Water (downward blue arrow) also absorbs across the epithelium via the transcellular and paracellular route. Right panel: normalized Tc-SC (blue circles) and DTPA (green circles) retention curves with the difference between the respective datasets at each time point shown as absorption (red circles) in CF subject 8.

Table 1. Abbreviations and constants in the work presented herein.

Abbreviation	Description
AIC	Akaike Information Criterion; a Metric of Model Appropriateness
ASL	Airway Surface Liquid Layer
C	Imaging Region of Interest About the Central Lung; Analogous to L in Model
CF	Cystic Fibrosis
CFTR	Cystic Fibrosis Transmembrane Conductance Regulator
CI	Confidence Interval
DMEM	Dulbecco's Modified Eagle Medium
DTPA	Indium-111 Diethylene Triamine Pentaacetic Acid
ENaC	Epithelial Sodium Channel
FFCA	Fraction of Functional Ciliated Airway
HBE	Human Bronchial Epithelial (cell)
HS	Hypertonic Saline
IS	Isotonic Saline
k	Number of Free Parameters in Model
MCC	Mucociliary Clearance
N	Number of Data Points Analyzed for Model Fit
ODE	Ordinary Differential Equation
PK	Pharmacokinetic
Tc-SC	Technetium-99m Sulfur Colloid
W_i	Weighting Factor of the ith Element of the Dataset for AIC
y_i	i^{th} Value of Dataset
$\hat{y}_i$	i^{th} Value of Model Fit

the clinical data set. Founded on a basic understanding of lung anatomy and physiology, the lung structure can be lumped into two key dynamical structures as shown in Figure 2. Additional assumptions made in synthesizing this model are as follows:

- A fraction of the large airways (L), which are represented in the central (C) lung region of interest (ROI) [18], has functional MCC, with MCC in the remainder of L being non-functional. This allows the subdivision of L into two sub-compartments: L_F, which has functional MCC, and L_N, which has no functional MCC.
- The initial doses of the radiopharmaceuticals delivered to either the central (C_0) or peripheral (P_0) lung regions are described as the number of counts within C or in the area outside of C but within the whole lung ROI in the first image, respectively [10] (Figure S1 provides a visual representation of the C and P ROIs).
- 10% of inhaled radiopharmaceuticals were assumed to deposit in the trachea (T_0) [15]. However, neither counts in T nor the bloodstream (B) have a unique impact on the clearance of the Tc-SC and DTPA.
- MCC in the distal lung D, which contains small and intermediate-sized airways in addition to alveoli [18], is a slow process; given the 80-min timescale of our data this rate cannot be resolved with confidence. As a result, the MCC term from D to L, k_{DL}, is neglected.

The result of these assumptions is a three-compartment model for MCC in the lung wherein two compartments (D and L_N) are

absorptive and one compartment (L_F) has MCC in addition to absorptive clearance, as shown in Figure 2.

Model Equations

Equations modeling the transport of both of the probes are outlined below. The model parameters k_{LT}, k_{DB}, k_{LB} and FFCA, the fraction of L with functional MCC, were determined by nonlinear least-squares regression as described in **Methods**. For Tc-SC clearance, k_{DB} and k_{LB} are set equal to 0. The mathematical description of this model, written as ODEs representing the change in counts in each model compartment, is as follows (see Table 2 for full list of model abbreviations):

$$\frac{dD}{dt} = -k_{DB}D \tag{1}$$

$$\frac{dL_N}{dt} = -k_{LB}L_N \tag{2}$$

$$\frac{dL_F}{dt} = -k_{LB}L_F - k_{LT}L_F \tag{3}$$

$$\frac{dT}{dt} = k_{LT}L_F \tag{4}$$

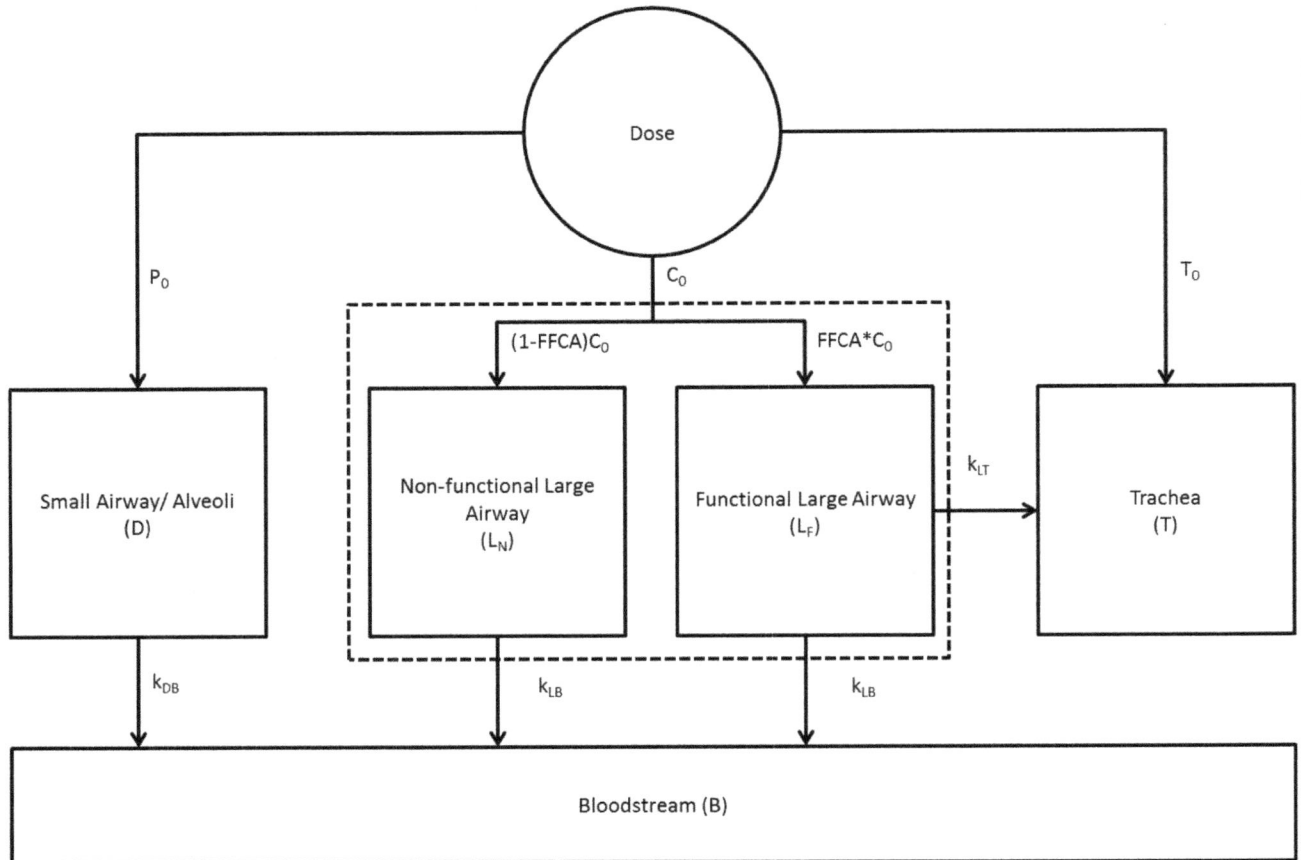

Figure 2. Schematic model structure describing the clearance of small molecule and particle probes from the lung. Initial depositions: T_0 = trachea, C_0 = central, P_0 = peripheral. See Table 1 for full list of model abbreviations.

$$\frac{dB}{dt} = k_{DB}D + k_{LB}(L_N + L_F) \qquad (5)$$

Model Fit and Predictions

The ability of our model to reproduce therapeutic response after the inhalation of hypertonic saline was studied using imaging data from patients with CF who inhaled isotonic saline (IS) and hypertonic saline on alternating study days [10]. Retention of Tc-SC, which is a metric of MCC, is shown with model fit for each patient group in Figure 3 [3]. Data from pediatric patients with CF and healthy controls who inhaled isotonic saline is also shown. The model captured the dynamics of MCC in all patient groups. The previously described increases in MCC associated with HS inhalation are apparent in the image-derived data and the model fits. However, as previously reported, no statistical differences in baseline MCC were detected between the CF IS, pediatric CF, and control groups [10].

DTPA is assumed to deposit in the same regions and clear by MCC at the same rate as Tc-SC; DTPA absorption is then captured by regressing the parameters k_{DB} and k_{LB}. Additionally, our previous studies have shown that the absorption of DTPA indicates changes in the absorption of ASL [9]. As such, the effect of hypertonic saline on liquid absorption, using DTPA as an

analog, is shown in Figure 4, along with the model fit for each group [10]. The model again captured the dynamics of absorption in all groups. Increased baseline rates of DTPA absorption are apparent in both adult and pediatric CF groups, as previously described [10].

Our model predicts that both Tc-SC retention and liquid absorption will follow trajectories within narrow envelopes based on the predicted upper and lower 95% confidence intervals (CIs) of the model parameters. These CI envelopes are derived using all possible combinations of the upper and lower 95% CIs and nominal values of the model parameters to generate the extreme values of model predictions. Figure 5 shows that predicted model trajectories lead to different final values of Tc-SC retention for all adult patient groups, with no overlap in trajectory envelopes of CF IS and non-CF groups for t>18 min and no overlap between non-CF and HS trajectories for t>27 min. In other words, the three adult patient subgroups have characteristically different total MCC behavior. Pediatric CF clearance trajectories closely resemble those of adult patients with CF, but are not shown for ease of interpretation. Patients with CF display less MCC than non-CF subjects, which appears to contradict our finding in [10]. However, the present work evaluates the entire time course of clearance, while the end of study value (t = 80 min) was used as the evaluation time point in [10]. By using the entire data sequence, particularly the dynamic response at short times, we are able to parametrically estimate and differentiate - with confidence - the MCC and absorption dynamics between patients with CF and

Table 2. Model parameters in the work presented herein.

Parameter	Description
B	Bloodstream Model Compartment (units counts)
C_0	Initial Counts in L (units counts)
D	Distal Lung Model Compartment (units counts)
FFCA	Free Parameter; Fraction of C_0 in L_F (units counts)
L	Large Airway Model Super-Compartment (units counts)
L_F	Sub-compartment of L with Functional MCC (units counts)
L_N	Sub-compartment of L without Functional MCC (units counts)
k_{DB}	Free Parameter; Rate Constant of Absorption in D (units min^{-1})
k_{DL}	Free Parameter (Unused in Final Model); Rate Constant of MCC from D to L (units min^{-1})
k_{LB}	Free Parameter; Rate Constant of Absorption in L (units min^{-1})
k_{LT}	Free Parameter; Rate Constant of MCC from L to T (units min^{-1})
P_0	Initial Counts in D (units counts)
T	Trachea Model Compartment (units counts)

non-CF subjects. These analyses also indicate that MCC function in patients with CF can be rescued by HS treatment, which caused total MCC to exceed that of non-CF subjects.

Figure 6 shows that the model-predicted trajectories for liquid absorption have no overlap for all t>0. Pediatric CF trajectories again resemble those of adult patients with CF, but are not shown. Patients with CF have higher absorption than non-CF subjects, which can be partially remediated by HS treatment. Combined, the results in Figures 5 and 6 indicate that HS has two distinct mechanisms of action, both rescuing MCC and ameliorating liquid hyperabsorption [4].

It has been proposed that the apparent increase of MCC following HS treatment occurs by increasing the rate at which MCC occurs [4], [19]. Our model suggests that the intrinsic rate of MCC is the same in all patient groups, and the rescue of MCC can be attributed to the recruitment of inactive portions of the airway. Figure 7A shows that the rate of MCC, k_{LT}, is not significantly different between all patient groups (p>0.05).

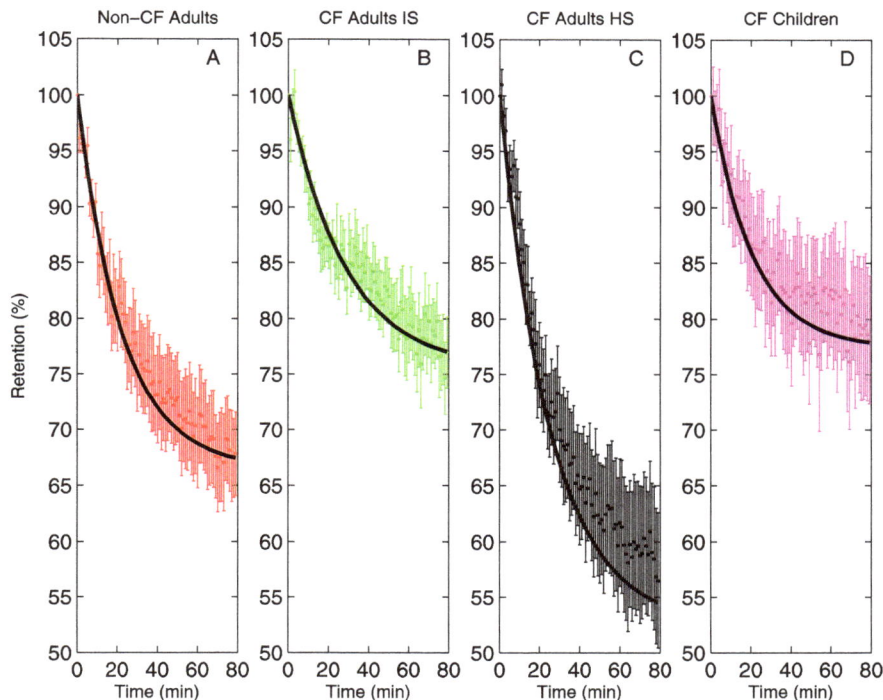

Figure 3. Tc-SC retention (mean ± SEM) vs. model fit (black line) for four patient subgroups. (A) Non-CF subjects (n = 9) (B) patients with CF (n = 12). (C) patients with CF after inhalation of hypertonic saline (n = 11). (D) Pediatric patients with CF. Data from [10].

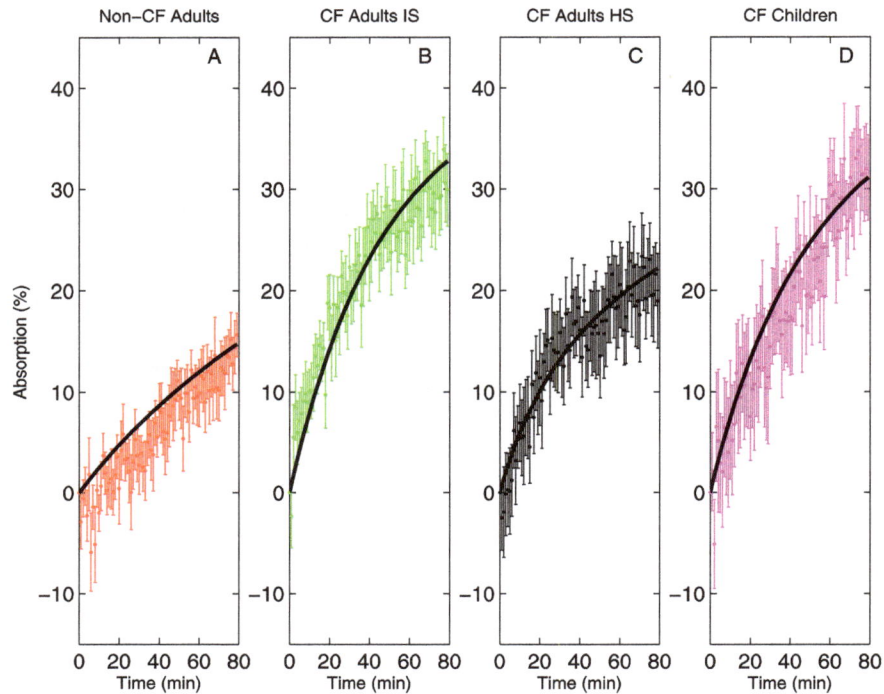

Figure 4. DTPA absorption (mean $\pm$ SEM) vs. model fit (line) for four patient subgroups. (A) Non-CF subjects (n = 9) (B) patients with CF (n = 12). (C) patients with CF after inhalation of hypertonic saline (n = 11). (D) Pediatric patients with CF. Data from [10].

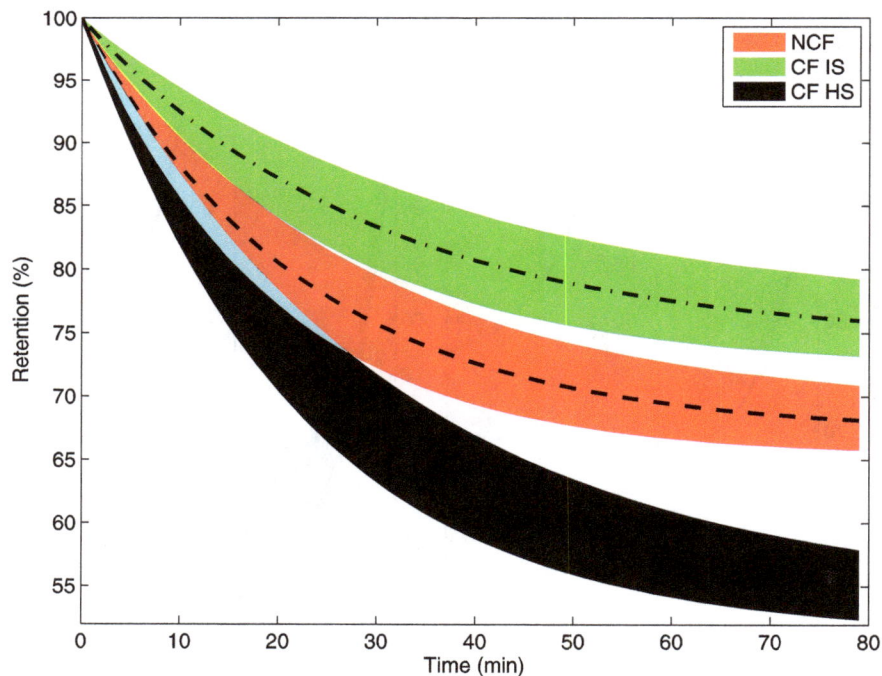

Figure 5. Estimated Tc-SC retention trajectories for three patient subgroups. Non-CF (red with dashed line), CF IS (green with dotted dashed line), CF HS (blue with line). Shaded envelope characterizes 95% confidence interval (CI) of retention prediction by the model. Pediatric CF subjects not shown due to overlap with adult CF.

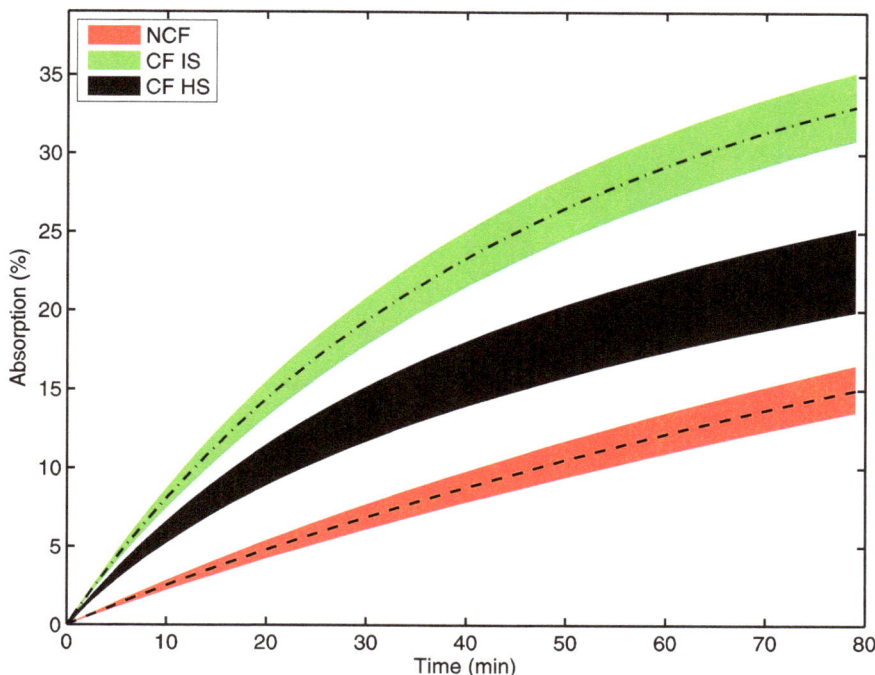

Figure 6. Estimated DTPA absorption trajectories for three groups. Non-CF (red with dashed line), CF IS (green with dotted dashed line), CF HS (blue with line). Shaded envelope characterizes 95% confidence interval (CI) of retention prediction by the model. Pediatric CF subjects not shown due to overlap with adult CF.

However, the parameter FFCA (Figure 7B), which describes the fractional area of large airways with functional MCC, is significantly lower in patients with CF versus non-CF subjects (p<0.05). Patients with CF given HS, however, show a significantly increased FFCA (p<0.05). This would support the concept of increased MCC, not through an intrinsic rate increase, but through an increase in the overall epithelial area contributing to MCC.

Our model also agrees with the previous reports that absorption, represented by k_{DB} and k_{LB} in our model, is increased in patients with CF vs. non-CF subjects (p<0.001 both parameters). The model demonstrates that HS inhalation decreases absorption in the peripheral lung (k_{DB}), which includes both small and intermediate sized airways and alveolar regions, more than IS inhalation (p<0.001). All model parameters are similar when comparing baseline measurements in the pediatric and adult CF IS groups (p = NS). Our parameters, as well as those of similar studies, are shown in Table 3.

In Vitro Evaluation of Model Prediction

In order to verify that hydration increases the fraction of functional ciliated area, we imaged CF HBE cultures (6 lines, n = 12) before and after addition of 10 μL of Dulbecco's Modified Eagle Media (DMEM) (Sigma-Aldrich, St. Louis, MO, USA), a liquid cell culture media, to the apical surface and again after a second addition of 10 μL of DMEM. We determined that hydration of HBE cells by addition of 10 μL significantly increases the fraction of functional ciliated area (p<0.0005) above baseline. No further increase in FFCA was observed following a second addition of 10 μL DMEM (p = NS), as shown in Figure 8A. CF HBE cells were imaged following apical addition of either 5 μL IS (n = 6) or HS (n = 6). A comparison of relative effect of IS and HS in CF HBE cells is shown in Figure 8B. Both IS and HS additions

increase functional area (p<0.05 and p<0.001, respectively). However, HS increases functional area significantly more than IS (p<0.01).

Discussion

The failure of the CF airway epithelium to secrete Cl^- and absorb Na^+ in a normal manner results in a net osmotic gradient that favors rapid absorption of liquid from the ASL, resulting in diminished MCC and an accumulation of dehydrated mucus in the airways. Nuclear imaging methods have been previously developed to measure MCC and have been used as biomarkers of therapeutic efficacy. A novel method that measures both MCC and ASL absorption has been explored more recently [10]. This method involves the inhalation of radiolabeled particle and small molecule probes (Tc-SC and DTPA, respectively). The difference between total DTPA clearance and Tc-SC clearance can be used to estimate the absorption of DTPA, and previous studies have demonstrated: (i) a positive and significant correlation between DTPA and ASL absorption rates [9]; (ii) DTPA absorption response to the use of osmotic therapies both *in vivo* and *in vitro* [10], [9].

We have developed a model that considers the basic mechanisms governing small molecule and particle probe clearance from physiologically distinct compartments of the lung. The combination of these mechanisms is reflected in the imaging result. Compartment or mechanism specific results provide additional insight into CF lung pathophysiology and therapeutic mechanisms of action. They may also provide more sensitive and accurate predictions of therapeutic efficacy than analyses of the composite imaging data as the compartmental description incorporates the inherent time-correlation of mass transport within the model structure.

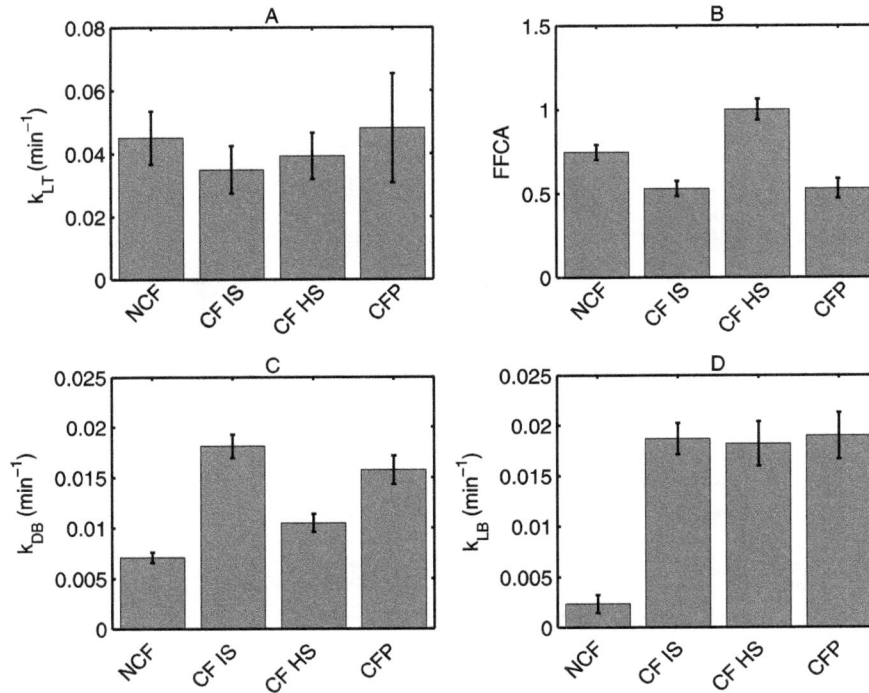

Figure 7. Least-squares solutions for model parameters are shown with 95% confidence intervals for four groups: Non-CF (NCF), CF HS, CF IS, and Pediatric CF (CFP). (A) MCC rate constant (k_{LT}) (min^{-1}). (B) Fraction (FFCA) of large airway with functional MCC. (C) Peripheral lung absorptive rate constant (k_{DB}) (min^{-1}). (D) Large airway absorptive rate constant (k_{LB}) (min^{-1}).

Model Structure Selection and Analysis

Our physically descriptive model includes central and peripheral lung compartments. The central zone includes large airways, intermediate and small airways, and alveoli while the peripheral zone includes only intermediate and small airways and alveoli [18], [20] (See Figure S1). The peripheral zone includes both smaller airways and alveoli in a single compartment. The model also includes compartments for the trachea and blood. As determined by Akaike Information Criterion (AIC) [21] analysis, a quantitative metric that weights the model accuracy (as measured by sum-squared error) against the cost of model complexity (quantified by the number of parameters in a model), the most appropriate model given the timeframe of our data assumed zero MCC from the peripheral compartment. Model rate constants describing MCC from the functional large airway compartment (k_{LT}), absorption from the small airway/alveolar

compartment (k_{DB}), large airway absorption (k_{LB}), and FFCA were fit to the data. The fixed mathematical structure of the model is able to capture the dynamics of both MCC and the absorption of DTPA in the lungs of all patient groups.

An alternative, and more highly parameterized, model than that shown in Figure 2 would include parameter k_{DL} as an MCC rate constant from compartment D to compartment L, in addition to MCC rate constant k_{LT} and absorption rate constants k_{DB} and k_{LB}. All kinetics were assumed to be first order. Furthermore, the initial dosing of probes was included using a free dosing parameter (C/P), representing the ratio of radiopharmaceutical doses delivered to the large airways and peripheral lung. Under the assumption that Technetium 99m-labeled Sulfur Colloid (Tc-SC) is not absorbed in any lung region, the MCC curve was found to be bi-exponential, as suggested previously [15]. However, regression and analysis of the model parameters via the MATLAB

Table 3. Pharmacokinetic Lung Clearance Parameter Values.

Study	$k_{LT}(min^{-1})$	$k_{DB}(min^{-1})$
NCF	0.0450 ± 0.0085	0.0071 ± 0.0005
CF HS	0.0393 ± 0.0073	0.0105 ± 0.0009
CF IS	0.0349 ± 0.0076	0.0181 ± 0.0012
CF Pediatric	0.0481 ± 0.0173	0.0157 ± 0.0014
Sakagami* [14]	0.022 ± 0.002	0.048 ± 0.003

Values from this study are shown with ± 95.
*PK model in isolated perfused rat lung. Three fluorescent markers used, but only the parameter values for sodium fluorescein (F-Na) are shown since $MW_{F-Na} = 376 Da \approx MW_{DTPA}$.

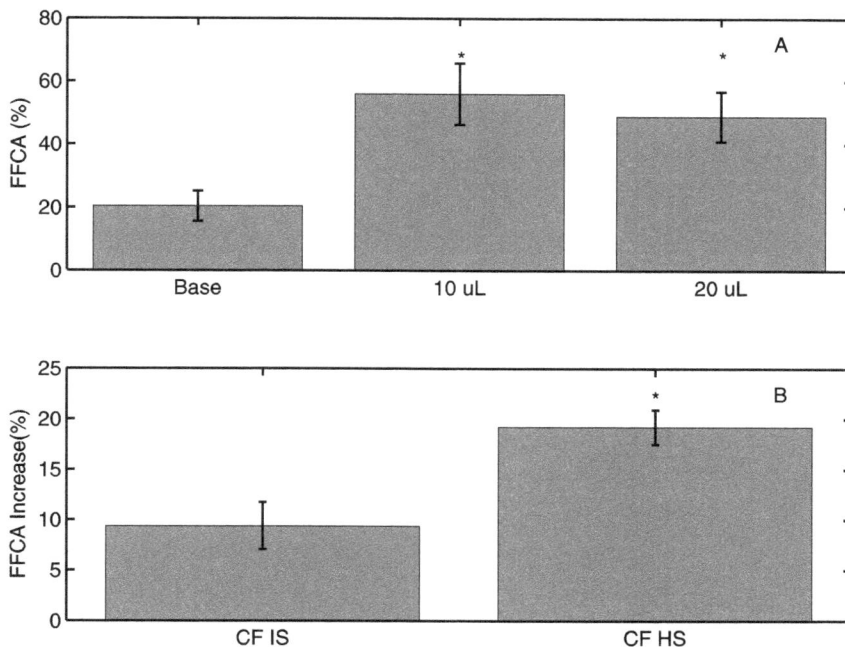

Figure 8. FFCA determined *in vitro* in CF HBE cells is shown $\pm$ SEM. (A) Activated area is significantly greater between 10 μL and baseline (* $p < 0.0005$) and 2×10 μL and baseline (* $p < 0.0005$). Activated area is not significantly greater between hydrated groups ($p > 0.05$). (B) A two-tailed t-test with unequal variances assumed reveals that the increase in active area induced by HS in cells is significantly greater than that of IS (* $p < 0.01$).

functions *lsqnonlin* (a nonlinear least-squares regression algorithm) and *nlparci* (an algorithm that computes confidence intervals on estimated parameters from the covariance matrix) yielded wide parameter confidence intervals, approximately ± 10 times the nominal parameter value. By eliminating k_{DL} the confidence intervals on parameter estimates are tightened dramatically (the worst case parameter CI from the model herein is k_{LB} in non-CF subjects which has CI's that are $\pm 39\%$ of the nominal value).

While a two-compartment model, like that proposed by Sakagami in [15], may be used to describe clearance, the parameters may not be able to be estimated with confidence if a physiological rate process captured by a parameter in the model is on the timescale of the experiment, or longer. The 80-minute functional imaging session inherently limits the confidence that can be derived for slower physiological processes. Therefore we hypothesized that the departure from monoexponential clearance seen in the retention curves could be explained by a non-zero steady state value for pharmaceutical retention. While this is aphysiologic over a period of days, an apparent non-zero baseline would manifest if a slow clearance process was occurring and data collection was short by comparison to the half-life of the clearance. This behavior can be realized in a number of ways in a kinetic model. In the present study, it is most easily incorporated by adding a new compartment that has no apparent MCC mechanism over the experimental timescale. Thus, while we believe that MCC in D can be observed on a longer timescale, we consider its mechanism to be practically unidentifiable (i.e. there is insufficient data to inform this parameter) over the timescale examined in the present work [22].

The model structure presented in Figure 2, and its grounding assumptions discussed in the **Results** section may fail to include mechanisms that could manifest on timescales longer than the 80 minute imaging period. To address the question of model appropriateness on the timescales of our data, we compared our model to the following alternative model structures with AIC as the basis for quantitative comparison:

Case 1. Exclude k_{LB}: DTPA absorption in L, represented by rate constant k_{LB}, is not appreciable over the 80-minute functional imaging timescale and should not be regressed to achieve model fit

Case 2. Include k_{DL}: MCC in D, represented by rate constant k_{DL}, is significant over the 80-minute functional imaging study timescale

The AIC values of each case above, in comparison to the model in Figure 2, are given in Table 4. These values demonstrate that the Figure 2 model displays the best combination of model fit and parsimony for the data set from [10]. Parsimony was especially important for model selection between the nominal case and Case 2, where the difference between AIC of the two cases was less than $\pm 1\%$. However, it is important to again note that there may in fact be clearance mechanisms from D, L_N, and L_F that are not accounted for in this model because of constraints on our ability to quantitatively resolve their effects with confidence over the timescale of imaging. This is illustrated graphically in Figure 9, where it is clear that we cannot confidently identify the parameter k_{DL} employed in Case 2 above.

Parametric Considerations

In non-CF subjects, FFCA is found to be <1. To our knowledge, the notion that not all of the surface of the conducting airways has functional cilia is a novel finding in humans. Hoegger *et al.* [23] recently report that even in the trachea, the most conductive airway, of newborn pigs without CF $\approx 70\%$ of particles clear in ten minutes and that those same particles are only actively moving $\approx 80\%$ of the time. While this timeframe is considerably shorter than the one in our study, it has been established that particles can be retained in the conducting airways of non-CF animals for a potentially significant amount of time. It would be reasonable to assume that particles deposited deeper in the

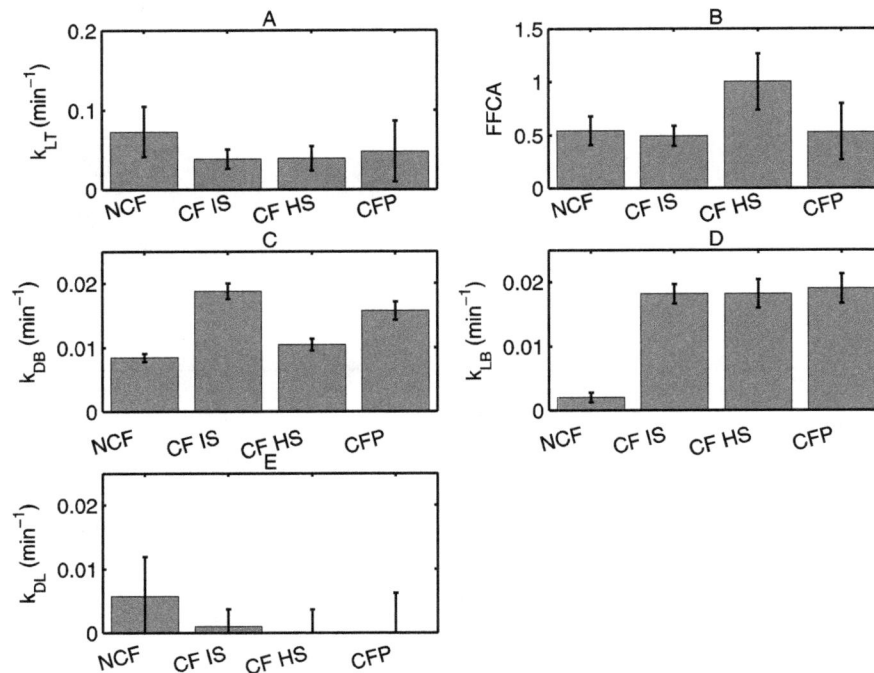

Figure 9. Least-squares solutions for model parameters in case 2 of Table 3 are shown for comparison to the selected model with 95% confidence intervals for four patient groups: Non-CF (NCF), CF HS, CF IS, and Pediatric CF (CP). (A) MCC rate constant (kLT) (min-1) reiterates that kLT is the same in all groups. (B) Fraction (FFCA) of large airway with functional MCC. (C) Peripheral lung absorptive rate constant (kDB) (min-1) and (D) large airway absorptive rate constant (kLB) are nearly identical to their analogs in the selected model. (E) MCC rate constant (kDL) (min-1) from D to L is clearly unidentifiable, and the nominal value is much smaller than kLT in each group. Confidence intervals are also widened in all parameters directly related to MCC.

airways, like those in our study, would be retained longer. Thus we have further reason to believe, in addition to the *in vitro* findings presented here, that our estimation of FFCA as a model parameter is grounded in realistic physiology.

Our model asserts that the rate of DTPA absorption (k_{DB}) is increased in the peripheral lung (small airway and alveoli) compartment of patients with CF as compared to non-CF subjects. Hypertonic saline slows this rate to nearly non-CF levels. Previous *in vitro* studies have related DTPA hyperabsorption to liquid hyperabsorption [9]. It is assumed that DTPA hyperabsorption occurs via a paracellular mechanism, driven by increased paracellular liquid absorption, as DTPA has no known transcellular route by which to absorb. Therefore, it is likely that our current result reflects the basic liquid absorption defect associated with CF. The aerosol delivery techniques utilized to deliver the radiopharmaceuticals targeted large and small airways through a specialized breathing pattern. Additionally, transient correction of

the absorption defect would be expected after administration of an inhaled osmotic therapy based on most current hypotheses of airway disease in CF [24]. However, we cannot completely exclude the possibility of alveolar effects that may be related to yet undocumented physiological differences between the alveolar regions of CF and non-CF lungs.

The rate at which DTPA absorbs in the large airways (k_{LB}) is similar to k_{DB} in the CF IS, CF pediatric and non-CF groups. However, while hypertonic saline decreases the value of k_{DB} in patients with CF, it has no significant effect on k_{LB}. MCC is the dominant clearance mode in the large airways in both IS and HS cases. We have shown *in vitro* that HS modulates the FFCA of the airway epithelium and have shown *in vivo* that increased MCC can be attained by modulating FFCA without requiring change in MCC rate. The two rate constants in the central region $(k_{LT}$ and $k_{LB})$ describe competing and correlated processes, whereas FFCA describes a more macroscopic phenomenon. Therefore, we would

Table 4. AIC Values for Various Model Structures.

	Model	Case 1	Case 2
NCF	−2546.28	−2535.65	−2543.38
CF HS	−2430.25	−2227.60	−2426.25
CF IS	−2775.62	−2287.07	−2775.57
CF Pediatric	−1858.37	−1597.47	−1854.37

The Akaike Information Criterion (AIC) is a metric for determining the most appropriate model for a system, where better fit is balanced against a penalty for overparameterization. Total AIC is shown as calculated from Equation 7 for all cases: 1) exclude k_{LB} from model structure; 2) include k_{PL} in model structure.

expect that a change in one rate constant in L would induce a corresponding change in the other. Between IS and HS days there is no change in k_{LT} (the dominant process), so we would not expect a change in k_{LB} either. However, due to the increase in FFCA, total MCC increases in the central lung after HS inhalation, which results in less DTPA being present and able to absorb in accordance with its unchanged rate constant. In effect, the underlying rate of DTPA absorption is unchanged, but an increase in total MCC as a result of increased FFCA leads to less DTPA being available for absorption and a smaller total quantity of DTPA absorbed in the CF HS case. In the case of D, however, we have assumed there is no competing, certainly no governing, MCC term in D. Thus, conditions affecting D must result changes in k_{DB}.

Study Limitations

A primary limitation of the functional imaging method utilized is its inability to uniquely discern airways and alveoli. Given the three dimensional nature of the lung architecture, small airways and alveoli are likely to be included in any zone analyzed via 2D imaging. The small sizes of these structures make them impossible to differentiate from each other through direct imaging, though other physiological measurements (such as 24 hr MCC) may help to differentiate their functional effects. The limited time scale of imaging (80 minutes) in the current study may have also limited assessment of small airway mucociliary clearance. Extended-duration imaging studies may yield additional data that can inform processes with slower rates and model parameters such as k_{DL}, which was excluded from the Figure 2 model on AIC grounds.

Physiological Implications

Our original study (see [10]) described significant differences in baseline whole lung DTPA absorption when comparing CF and healthy subjects. MCC was decreased in the CF groups, but not at statistically significant levels. In this study we find that MCC is decreased (in a statistically significant way) in the CF IS group for $t > 13$ minutes. The difference between these two findings arises from differences in the analysis tools used in this work versus the endpoint analysis performed in [10]. The confidence intervals presented here are around the parameters of the model, as opposed to being derived from statistical analysis of a final retention value, as in [10]. Our parameters govern the entire time-course of clearance, and thus are informed by the entire dynamic of the data given in [10]. The resulting confidence-interval-derived envelopes in Figures 5 and 6 capture the uncertainty of each physiologically descriptive parameter in the model. This is achieved by simulating the model at all possible combinations of upper and lower CIs for each parameter and determining the extreme values of model prediction at every time point. Hence, the CIs about our parameters are used to generate physiologically, as opposed to empirically, informed predictions of clearance behavior in each subject group population. The narrowness of our parameter CIs indicates confidence in the model parameter estimates (in that they are well informed from the dynamic data in [10]) and generates narrow prediction envelopes in each case, indicating a physiological difference in MCC dynamics between patients with CF and non-CF subjects that is not found via our previous endpoint-analysis methods.

Response to HS inhalation was apparent in terms of both decreased absorption and increased MCC as compared to IS inhalation. These trends are reflected in our modeled result. Our model suggests that the observed increase in MCC following HS inhalation is due to an increase in FFCA rather than an increase in MCC rate, and a detailed analysis of this hypothesis using the *in*

vivo imaging data is ongoing. The model also predicts that FFCA is reduced in patients with CF as compared to the healthy population. We used this prediction as a hypothesis about inducing a functional change *in vivo* that can be tested *in vitro*. To further elucidate this phenomenon, and validate that such behavior is possible, we performed *in vitro* studies with HBE cell cultures. A quantitative visual assay of ciliary movement demonstrated that a larger fraction of the cell culture surface was activated after the addition of hypertonic saline vs. isotonic saline.

Clinical Relevance

Some previous imaging studies have shown significant differences in whole lung MCC between CF and non-CF subjects [25], [26] while others have not [4]. By ascribing a fixed mathematical structure to our model, we constrained the clearance curves to a single family of dynamical forms, which allows for more sensitive comparisons between the dynamical, and also endpoint, behavior present from one patient group to another. This ultimately increases our confidence in the model assertion that MCC is decreased in patients with CF and can be increased by hypertonic saline inhalation and, subsequently, that our model offers a better tool than statistical models for use in clinically gauging MCC.

Applications of this model may include the design of dosing regimens for agents targeting changes in MCC and/or absorption. For example, the timeline of the effects associated with an osmotic therapy (correction of liquid absorption defects) could be assessed independently of the resulting secondary effects (recruitment of functional ciliated airway, large and small airway clearance). Dosing timed in accordance with the duration of the counter-absorptive effect may provide more continuous clearance from the lungs and patient benefit, though outcome assessment is beyond the scope of the model at present. The model could also be used to resolve the pharmacodynamics of medications with subtle, complex, or multiple therapeutic effects, to the degree that these agents impact MCC and absorption.

Conclusions

Our physiologically motivated compartmental model is able to reproduce the clearance behavior of both large particle (Tc-SC) and small molecule (DTPA) radiolabeled probes as informed by functional imaging data. The model asserts that liquid absorption rate is increased in the peripheral lung of patients with CF as compared to non-CF subjects, and that hypertonic saline will decrease the rate of absorption in patients with CF to near non-CF levels. Our model also attributes increased MCC induced by hypertonic saline treatment to an increase in airway surface area with functional ciliary clearance, as opposed to an increased rate of clearance. The physiology inherent to the model structure and parameterization allow for increased sensitivity in gauging the effects of hypertonic saline *in vivo* in a real-time manner. This model should, therefore, be extendable to other treatments, both present and future, that target the liquid hyperabsorption and MCC deficiency present in cystic fibrosis.

Materials and Methods

Functional Imaging Methods

Data from previously reported clinical imaging studies were utilized [10]. These studies included both adult (n = 12) and pediatric (n = 9) patients with CF and healthy controls (n = 9). Raw imagining data from this study can be found in Table S1. An aerosol based functional imaging technique that measures the clearance of two different radiopharmaceutical probes from the lungs over 80 minutes was used. Indium-111-labeled diethylene triamine pentaacetic acid (DTPA) is a small molecule probe (≈ 500 Da) that is cleared from the lung through both absorption and MCC while Technetium-99m-labeled sulfur colloid (Tc-SC) is a particle probe (≈ 300nm) that is cleared only by MCC. DTPA absorption is calculated by subtracting the Tc-SC clearance rate (MCC) from the total In-DTPA clearance rate. Both probes were mixed and delivered together via nebulizer in the same liquid aerosol. All patient studies were approved by the University of Pittsburgh Institutional Review Board (clinicaltrial.gov numbers NCT01223183 and NCT01486199).

The aerosolized probes were delivered simultaneously by nebulizer using a technique that deposited aerosol primarily in the airways [10]. Their clearance (normalized decrease in radioactive counts over time) was then independently assessed over 80 minutes using dynamic planar scintigraphy. Whole, peripheral and central lung zones were considered, where the central zone was defined as a rectangle with $\frac{1}{2}$ the height and width of the whole lung region of interest postioned along the medial lung border and centered vertically. At t = 10 minutes (11th imaging frame) subjects inhaled nebulized saline treatments for 10 minutes. Adult patients with CF inhaled 7% hypertonic saline (HS, n = 11) on one testing day and isotonic saline (IS) on the other. Control and pediatric CF subjects performed a single testing day with isotonic saline. Previous *in vitro* studies have demonstrated a relationship between DTPA and ASL absorption. Since DTPA has no known route for intracellular transport this relationship is presumably due to the contribution of paracellular liquid flows. Changes in DTPA absorption in response to osmotic therapies have previously been demonstrated both *in vitro* [9] and *in vivo* [10]. Analysis of the Tc-SC and DTPA retention curves as well as DTPA absorption plotted with a logarithmic ordinate showed that the data did not follow a monoexponential profile, which guided selection of the model structure and kinetics necessary to accurately reproduce the data.

Initial Model Structure

Sakagami [15] proposed a robust modeling scaffold for inhaled pharmaceuticals that takes into account the regional pharmacokinetic differences between the large conducting airways (L) and the distal lung (D), consisting of smaller airways and alveoli. Analysis of the corresponding system of compartment-based ordinary differential equations (ODEs) yielded a bi-exponential retention curve for Tc-SC as proposed by Byron [14]. However, this model structure could not be reconciled with the whole of the data used herein (see **Discussion**).

Model Parameter Estimation

Regression of model parameters, regardless of model structure, was performed sequentially as follows. Model parameters were estimated using nonlinear least-squares regression (via *lsqnonlin* in MATLAB, ©2013, The MathWorks, Natick, MA) between model predictions and experimental data. The experimental design allowed for sequential estimation of the MCC and absorption rate parameters as follows:

1. The parameters that govern MCC (k_{LT} and FFCA) were fit to the Tc-SC retention data.
2. The regressed MCC parameters were then fixed, and the absorption rate parameters (k_{DB} and k_{LB}) were fit to the absorption curve.
3. Parameter uncertainty was calculated using the *nlparci* function in MATLAB (©2013, The MathWorks, Natick, MA) to obtain confidence intervals on all model parameters.

Model Analysis

The assumptions above were tested individually, and in combination, for appropriateness using the Akaike Information Criterion (AIC). Akaike [21] originally proposed that model appropriateness could be assessed according to the equation:

$$AIC = (-2)ln(maximum\ likelihood) + 2k \qquad (6)$$

Where a Gaussian distribution represents the maximum likelihood of the data and k is the number of free parameters in the model. Thus, the model with the least value of AIC is deemed most appropriate in terms of model fit and parsimony. Yamaoka and colleagues [27] further elaborated on this information criterion by proposing that for a process with Gaussian error the AIC can found from the equation:

$$AIC = Nln(\sum_{i=1}^{N}((\hat{y}_i) - y_i)^2/N) + 2k \qquad (7)$$

Where $\hat{y}_i$ is the model fit and y_i is the data value at the ith image of our N = 80n set because there are 80 images per patient and n patients per study group.

In Vitro Assessment of Ciliary Activation

We developed an *in vitro* imaging assay to measure the fraction of the epithelium that has functional MCC in order to test our hypotheses that FFCA is decreased in CF and that hydration can recruit areas of otherwise non-functional cilia. Fully differentiated human bronchial epithelial (HBE) cell cultures were viewed using a phase-contrast objective (Nikon Eclipse TI). These cultures were derived from lungs removed at the time of lung transplantation and prepared using previously described methods approved by the University of Pittsburgh IRB [28]. A series of 10 images was taken of each culture that allowed for the determination of the change in pixel intensity between successive images in the stack. Ciliary beat can be observed under these conditions and is characterized by a change in light intensity measured by the camera. This change in light intensity can be translated to a change in pixel intensity in the images obtained when placed in sequence to form a movie of ciliary motion (see Figure S2 and Video S1). The average change in pixel intensity of all cultures was determined in both CF lines (n = 6) and a non-CF line. Average changes in the intensity of each pixel from 12 untreated cultures from the non-CF line were measured and the average change in intensity over all pixels was used as a baseline measurement of functional ciliary movement. Pixels in each stack with average change in intensity greater than the non-CF baseline were said to have functional ciliary movement. To test the effect of osmotic agents, 5 μL of either isotonic (300 mOsm) or hypertonic (600 mOsm) saline was added to the apical surface of cells prior to imaging (see Table S2 for data). To test for saturating effects of hydration, we sequentially added Dulbecco's Modified Eagle Medium (DMEM) from the basolateral bath to the apical surface of the cultures as follows: 10 μL of DMEM was added to the apical surface of the cells from the basolateral bath before the cells were imaged, and an additional 10 μL of basolateral DMEM was added to the apical surface prior to a second, identical, imaging routine (see Table S3 for data).

Supporting Information

Figure S1   Shown is the initial posterior frame of a Tc-SC imaging series. The dotted outline of the right lung is a tracing of the outline of the lung as it appears in a transmission scan. The filled in blue rectangle is the C ROI. The remaining lung ROI represents P.

Figure S2   A pseudo-color image of non-CF HBE cells under $10\times$ enhancement is shown. The viewing frame is identical to that in Video S1. Darker (more blue) regions show areas with lower average change in pixel intensity during Video S1 whereas lighter (more yellow) regions show areas with higher average change. In combination with Video S1 we show that regions that display little visible movement are more blue, and the regions with visible motion, particularly the hurricane regions, are more yellow.

Acknowledgments

The authors would like to thank Li Ang Zhang for his assistance in code development and Stefanie Brown for her assistance in maintaining the HBE cell lines used in this work.

Author Contributions

Conceived and designed the experiments: MRM TEC LWL MMM RSP. Performed the experiments: MRM TEC LWL. Analyzed the data: MRM TEC LWL MMM RSP. Contributed reagents/materials/analysis tools: MRM TEC LWL MMM JMP RSP. Wrote the paper: MRM TEC LWL MMM JMP RSP. Designed software used in analysis: MRM LWL MMM. Obtained permission for use of cell line: MMM JMP. Obtained informed consent of patients: MMM JMP.

References

1. O'Reilly R, Elphick HE (2013) Development, clinical utility, and place of ivacaftor in the treatment of cystic fibrosis. Drug Design, Development and Therapy 7: 929–37.
2. Boucher RC (2007) Cystic fibrosis: a disease of vulnerability to airway surface dehydration. Trends in Molecular Medicine 13: 231–40.
3. Corcoran TE, Thomas KM, Myerburg MM, Muthukrishnan A, Weber L, et al. (2010) Absorptive clearance of DTPA as an aerosol-based biomarker in the cystic fibrosis airway. The European Respiratory Journal 35: 781–6.
4. Donaldson SH, Bennett WD, Zeman KL, Knowles MR, Tarran R, et al. (2006) Mucus clearance and lung function in cystic fibrosis with hypertonic saline. The New England Journal of Medicine 354: 241–50.
5. Elkins MR, Robinson M, Rose BR, Harbour C, Moriarty CP, et al. (2006) A controlled trial of long-term inhaled hypertonic saline in patients with cystic fibrosis. New England Journal of Medicine 354: 229–240.
6. Accurso FJ, Rowe SM, Clancy J, Boyle MP, Dunitz JM, et al. (2010) Effect of vx-770 in persons with cystic fibrosis and the g551d-cftr mutation. New England Journal of Medicine 363: 1991–2003.
7. Bennett WD, Ilowite JS (1989) Dual pathway clearance of 99mtc-dtpa from the bronchial mucosa1~3. The American review of respiratory disease 139: 1132.
8. Ilowite JS, Bennett WD, Sheetz MS, Groth ML, Nierman DM (1989) Permeability of the bronchial mucosa to 99mtc-dtpa in asthma. American Review of Respiratory Disease 139: 1139–1143.
9. Corcoran TE, Thomas KM, Brown S, Myerburg MM, Locke LW, et al. (2013) Liquid hyper-absorption as a cause of increased DTPA clearance in the cystic fibrosis airway. EJNMMI research 3: 14.
10. Locke L, Myerburg M, Markovetz M, Parker R, Weber L, et al. (2014) Quantitative Imaging of Airway Liquid Absorption in Cystic Fibrosis. European Respiratory Journal: In Press.
11. Eckford PDW, Li C, Ramjeesingh M, Bear CE (2012) Cystic fibrosis transmembrane conductance regulator (CFTR) potentiator VX-770 (ivacaftor) opens the defective channel gate of mutant CFTR in a phosphorylation-dependent but ATP-independent manner. The Journal of Biological Chemistry 287: 36639–49.
12. Van Goor F, Hadida S, Grootenhuis PDJ, Burton B, Stack JH, et al. (2011) Correction of the F508del-CFTR protein processing defect in vitro by the investigational drug VX-809. Proceedings of the National Academy of Sciences of the United States of America 108: 18843–8.
13. Byron P, Patton J (1994) Drug delivery via the respiratory tract. Journal of Aerosol medicine 7: 49–75.
14. Sakagami M, Byron PR, Venitz J, Rypacek F (2002) Solute disposition in the rat lung in vivo and in vitro: determining regional absorption kinetics in the presence of mucociliary escalator. Journal of Pharmaceutical Sciences 91: 594–604.
15. Sakagami M (2006) In vivo, in vitro and ex vivo models to assess pulmonary absorption and disposition of inhaled therapeutics for systemic delivery. Advanced Drug Delivery Reviews 58: 1030–60.
16. Weber B, Hochhaus G (2013) A pharmacokinetic simulation tool for inhaled corticosteroids. The AAPS Journal 15: 159–71.
17. Sturm R (2012) An advanced stochastic model for mucociliary particle clearance in cystic fibrosis lungs. Journal of Thoracic Disease 4: 48–57.
18. Biddiscombe MF, Meah SN, Underwood SR, Usmani OS (2011) Comparing lung regions of interest in gamma scintigraphy for assessing inhaled therapeutic aerosol deposition. Journal of aerosol medicine and pulmonary drug delivery 24: 165–173.
19. Donaldson SH, Corcoran TE, Laube BL, Bennett WD (2007) Mucociliary clearance as an outcome measure for cystic fibrosis clinical research. Proceedings of the American Thoracic Society 4: 399–405.
20. Newman S, Bennett WD, Biddiscombe M, Devadason SG, Dolovich MB, et al. (2012) Standardization of techniques for using planar (2d) imaging for aerosol deposition assessment of orally inhaled products. Journal of aerosol medicine and pulmonary drug delivery 25: S–10.
21. Akaike H (1974) A new look at the statistical model identification. Automatic Control, IEEE Transactions on 19: 716–723.
22. Raue A, Kreutz C, Maiwald T, Bachmann J, Schilling M, et al. (2009) Structural and practical identifiability analysis of partially observed dynamical models by exploiting the profile likelihood. Bioinformatics (Oxford, England) 25: 1923–9.
23. Hoegger MJ, Fischer AJ, McMenimen JD, Ostedgaard LS, Tucker AJ, et al. (2014) Impaired mucus detachment disrupts mucociliary transport in a piglet model of cystic fibrosis. Science 345: 818–822.
24. Boucher R (2004) New concepts of the pathogenesis of cystic fibrosis lung disease. European Respiratory Journal 23: 146–158.
25. Regnis Ja, Robinson M, Bailey DL, Cook P, Hooper P, et al. (1994) Mucociliary clearance in patients with cystic fibrosis and in normal subjects. American Journal of Respiratory and Critical Care Medicine 150: 66–71.
26. Robinson M, Eberl S, Tomlinson C, Daviskas E, Regnis J, et al. (2000) Regional mucociliary clearance in patients with cystic fibrosis. Journal of Aerosol Medicine 13: 73–86.
27. Yamaoka K, Nakagawa T, Uno T (1978) Application of Akaike's information criterion (AIC) in the evaluation of linear pharmacokinetic equations. Journal of Pharmacokinetics and Biopharmaceutics 6: 165–75.
28. Myerburg MM, Harvey PR, Heidrich EM, Pilewski JM, Butterworth MB (2010) Acute regulation of the epithelial sodium channel in airway epithelia by proteases and trafficking. American Journal of Respiratory Cell and Molecular Biology 43: 712–9.

Permissions

All chapters in this book were first published in PLOS ONE, by The Public Library of Science; hereby published with permission under the Creative Commons Attribution License or equivalent. Every chapter published in this book has been scrutinized by our experts. Their significance has been extensively debated. The topics covered herein carry significant findings which will fuel the growth of the discipline. They may even be implemented as practical applications or may be referred to as a beginning point for another development.

The contributors of this book come from diverse backgrounds, making this book a truly international effort. This book will bring forth new frontiers with its revolutionizing research information and detailed analysis of the nascent developments around the world.

We would like to thank all the contributing authors for lending their expertise to make the book truly unique. They have played a crucial role in the development of this book. Without their invaluable contributions this book wouldn't have been possible. They have made vital efforts to compile up to date information on the varied aspects of this subject to make this book a valuable addition to the collection of many professionals and students.

This book was conceptualized with the vision of imparting up-to-date information and advanced data in this field. To ensure the same, a matchless editorial board was set up. Every individual on the board went through rigorous rounds of assessment to prove their worth. After which they invested a large part of their time researching and compiling the most relevant data for our readers.

The editorial board has been involved in producing this book since its inception. They have spent rigorous hours researching and exploring the diverse topics which have resulted in the successful publishing of this book. They have passed on their knowledge of decades through this book. To expedite this challenging task, the publisher supported the team at every step. A small team of assistant editors was also appointed to further simplify the editing procedure and attain best results for the readers.

Apart from the editorial board, the designing team has also invested a significant amount of their time in understanding the subject and creating the most relevant covers. They scrutinized every image to scout for the most suitable representation of the subject and create an appropriate cover for the book.

The publishing team has been an ardent support to the editorial, designing and production team. Their endless efforts to recruit the best for this project, has resulted in the accomplishment of this book. They are a veteran in the field of academics and their pool of knowledge is as vast as their experience in printing. Their expertise and guidance has proved useful at every step. Their uncompromising quality standards have made this book an exceptional effort. Their encouragement from time to time has been an inspiration for everyone.

The publisher and the editorial board hope that this book will prove to be a valuable piece of knowledge for researchers, students, practitioners and scholars across the globe.

List of Contributors

Chiara Horlin and Richard Parsons
School of Occupational Therapy & Social Work, CHIRI, Curtin University, Perth, Australia

Torbjorn Falkmer
School of Occupational Therapy & Social Work, CHIRI, Curtin University, Perth, Australia
Rehabilitation Medicine, Department of Medicine and Health Sciences (IMH), Faculty of Health Sciences, Linkö ping University & Pain and Rehabilitation Centre, Linkö ping, Sweden
School of Occupational Therapy, La Trobe University, Melbourne, VIC, Australia

Marita Falkmer
School of Occupational Therapy & Social Work, CHIRI, Curtin University, Perth, Australia
School of Education and Communication, CHILD Programme, Institute of Disability Research, Jönköping University, Jo¨nko¨ ping, Sweden

Matthew A. Albrecht
School of Psychology, CHIRI, Curtin University, Perth, Australia

Victoria Q. Tao, Yoyo W. Y. Chu, Gary T. K. Mok, Wanling Yang, So Lun Lee, Winnie W. Y. Tso and Yu-lung Lau
Department of Paediatrics and Adolescent Medicine, LKS Faculty of Medicine, The University of Hong Kong, Hong Kong Special Administrative Region, China

Kelvin Y. K. Chan and Anita S. Y. Kan
Department of Obstetrics and Gynecology, Queen Mary Hospital, Hong Kong Special Administrative Region, China

Tiong Y. Tan
Department of Paediatrics and Adolescent Medicine, LKS Faculty of Medicine, The University of Hong Kong, Hong Kong Special Administrative Region, China,
Victorian Clinical Genetics Service, Murdoch Children's Research Institute, Royal Children's Hospital, Department of Paediatrics, University of Melbourne, Melbourne, Australia

Brian H. Y. Chung
Department of Paediatrics and Adolescent Medicine, LKS Faculty of Medicine, The University of Hong Kong, Hong Kong Special Administrative Region, China,
Department of Obstetrics and Gynecology, LKS Faculty of Medicine, The University of Hong Kong, Hong Kong Special Administrative Region, China

Stefano Mattioli and Andrea Farioli
Department of Medical and Surgical Sciences (DIMEC), University of Bologna, Bologna, Italy

Patrizia Legittimo
Unit of Occupational Medicine, S.Orsola-Malpighi University Hospital, Bologna, Italy
Occupational and Environmental Epidemiology Unit, ISPO Cancer Prevention and Research Institute, Florence, Italy

Lucia Miligi and Alessandra Benvenuti
Occupational and Environmental Epidemiology Unit, ISPO Cancer Prevention and Research Institute, Florence, Italy

Alessandra Ranucci and Corrado Magnani
Cancer Epidemiology Unit - Department of Translational Medicine, CPO Piemonte and University of Eastern Piedmont, Novara, Italy

Alberto Salvan
Currently retired, IASI-CNR, Rome, Italy

Roberto Rondelli
Paediatric Oncology-Haematology "Lalla Sera`gnoli", Policlinico S.Orsola-Malpighi, Bologna, Italy

Wing Fai Tang, Elizabeth T. Lau and Mary H. Tang
Department of Obstetrics and Gynecology, LKS Faculty of Medicine, The University of Hong Kong, Hong Kong Special Administrative Region, China

Pranav K. Gandhi
Department of Pharmacy Practice, School of Pharmacy, South College, Knoxville, TN, United States of America

Lindsay A. Thompson and Sanjeev Y. Tuli
Department of Pediatrics, College of Medicine, University of Florida, Gainesville, FL, United States of America

Dennis A. Revicki
Outcomes Research, Evidera, Bethesda, MD, United States of America

Elizabeth Shenkman and I-Chan Huang
Department of Health Outcomes and Policy, College of Medicine, University of Florida, Gainesville, FL, United States of America
Department of Epidemiology and Cancer Control, St. Jude Children's Research Hospital, Memphis, TN, United States of America

Lidia Panico
Institut National d'Etudes De´mographiques, Paris, France

Beth Stuart
Faculty of Medicine, University of Southampton, Southampton, United Kingdom

Mel Bartley and Yvonne Kelly
International Centre for Lifecourse Studies, Department for Epidemiology and Population Health, University College London, London, United Kingdom

Shanti Raman
Department of Community Paediatrics, South Western Sydney Local Health District, Liverpool Hospital, Liverpool, New South Wales, Australia

Krishnamachari Srinivasan
Department of Psychiatry, St John's Medical College, Bangalore, India

Anura Kurpad
Department of Physiology, St John's Medical College, Bangalore, India

Husna Razee and Jan Ritchie
School of Public Health & Community Medicine, University of New South Wales, Sydney, New South Wales, Australia

Ian Hodgson
Independent Consultant, Bingley, United Kingdom

Mary L. Plummer
Independent Consultant, Dar es Salaam, Tanzania

Sarah N. Konopka and Edna Jonas
Center for Health Services, Management Sciences for Health, Arlington, Virginia, USA

Christopher J. Colvin
Centre for Infectious Disease Epidemiology and Research (CIDER), Division of Social and Behavioural Sciences, School of Public Health and Family Medicine, University of Cape Town, Cape Town, South Africa

Jennifer Albertini
United States Agency for International Development (USAID)/Africa Bureau, Washington, D.C., USA

Anouk Amzel
USAID/Bureau for Global Health (BGH)/Office of HIV/AIDS, Washington, D.C., USA,

Karen P. Fogg
USAID/BGH/Office of Health, Infectious Diseases, and Nutrition, Washington, D.C., USA

Malik Coulibaly, Elisabeth Thio and Issa Siribié
Projet MONOD ANRS 12206, Centre de Recherche Internationale pour la Santé , Site ANRS Burkina, Université de Ouagadougou, Ouagadougou, Burkina Faso

Nicolas Meda
Projet MONOD ANRS 12206, Centre de Recherche Internationale pour la Santé , Site ANRS Burkina, Université de Ouagadougou, Ouagadougou, Burkina Faso Centre Muraz, Bobo Dioulasso, Burkina Faso

Caroline Yonaba and Ludovic Kam
Service de Pédiatrie, CHU Yalgado Ouédraogo, Ouagadougou, Burkina Faso

Sylvie Ouedraogo, Fla Koueta and Diarra Ye
Service de Pédiatrie Médicale, CHU Charles de Gaulle, Ouagadougou, Burkina Faso

Malika Congo
Laboratoire de Bactériologie - Virologie CHU Yalgado Ouédraogo, Ouagadougou, Burkina Faso

Mamoudou Barry
Service de laboratoire, CHU Charles de Gaulle, Ouagadougou, Burkina Faso

Stéphane Blanche
Groupe hospitalier Necker- Enfants malades, Paris, France

Phillipe Van De Perre
Inserm U1058, Universite´ Montpellier 1, Montpellier, France

Valériane Leroy
Inserm, U897, Institut de SantéPublique, Epidémiologie et Développement (ISPED), Université de Bordeaux, Bordeaux, France

Narcisse Muganga
1 Kigali University Teaching Hospital, Department of Pediatrics, Kigali, Rwanda

Philippe R. Mutwa
Kigali University Teaching Hospital, Department of Pediatrics, Kigali, Rwanda
Department of Global Health and Amsterdam Institute for Global Health and
Development, Academic Medical Center, Amsterdam, The Netherlands

Kimberly R. Boer
Department of Global Health and Amsterdam Institute for Global Health and
Development, Academic Medical Center, Amsterdam, The Netherlands
Biomedical Research, Epidemiology Unit, Royal Tropical Institute, Amsterdam, The Netherlands

Brenda Asiimwe-Kateera, Joep M. A. Lange and Peter Reiss
Department of Global Health and Amsterdam Institute for Global Health and
Development, Academic Medical Center, Amsterdam, The Netherlands

Janneke van de Wijgert
Department of Global Health and Amsterdam Institute for Global Health and
Development, Academic Medical Center, Amsterdam, The Netherlands
Institute of Infection and Global Health, University of Liverpool, Liverpool, United of Kingdom Rinda Ubuzima, Kigali, Rwanda

Sibyl P. M. Geelen
Department of Global Health and Amsterdam Institute for Global Health and
Development, Academic Medical Center, Amsterdam, The Netherlands
Wilhelmina Children's Hospital, University Medical Centre Utrecht, Utrecht, The Netherlands

Diane Tuyishimire
Outpatients Clinic, Treatment and Research on HIV/AIDS Centre, Kigali, Rwanda

Anita Asiimwe
Ministry of Health of Rwanda, Kigali, Rwanda

Cui-ling Li, Kai Zhao, Omar Ibrahim Farah, Jiao-jiao Wang and
Hui-ping Zhang
Family Planning Research Institute, Tongji Medical College, Huazhong University of Science and Technology, Wuhan, Hubei, China

Hui Li
Department of Science and Technology Service, Hubei Provincial Population and Family Planning Commission, Wuhan, Hubei, China

Rong-ze Sun
Renmin Hospital of Wuhan University, Wuhan, Hubei, China

Bhim Gopal Dhoubhadel and Koya Ariyoshi
Department of Clinical Medicine, Institute of Tropical Medicine, Nagasaki University, Nagasaki, Japan
Graduate School of Biomedical Sciences, Nagasaki University, Nagasaki, Japan

Michio Yasunami and Motoi Suzuki
Department of Clinical Medicine, Institute of Tropical Medicine, Nagasaki University, Nagasaki, Japan

Hien Anh Thi Nguyen, Thu Huong Vu and Duc Anh Dang
Department of Bacteriology, National Institute of Hygiene and Epidemiology, Hanoi, Vietnam

Ai Thi Thuy Nguyen
Department of Microbiology, Khanh Hoa General Hospital, NhaTrang, Vietnam

Lay-Myint Yoshida
Department of Pediatric Infectious Diseases, Institute of Tropical Medicine, Nagasaki University, Nagasaki, Japan

Erica L. Pufall, Jeffrey W. Eaton, Laura Robertson and Simon Gregson
Department of Infectious Disease Epidemiology, Imperial College London, St. Mary's Campus, Norfolk Place, London, United Kingdom

Constance Nyamukapa
Department of Infectious Disease Epidemiology, Imperial College London, St. Mary's Campus, Norfolk Place, London, United Kingdom
Biomedical Research and Training Institute, Avondale, Harare, Zimbabwe

Reggie Mutsindiri, Godwin Chawira and Shungu Munyati
Biomedical Research and Training Institute, Avondale, Harare, Zimbabwe

Sharon Banschbach, Eileen Beckman, Kelli Howard, Erin Frank, Kelli Harmon and Patrick Lahni
Division of Critical Care Medicine, Cincinnati Children's Hospital Medical Center and Cincinnati Children's Research Foundation, Cincinnati, OH, United States of America

Sarah J. Atkinson
Division of Critical Care Medicine, Cincinnati Children's Hospital Medical Center and Cincinnati Children's Research Foundation, Cincinnati, OH, United States of America
Department of Surgery, University of Cincinnati, Cincinnati, OH, United States of America

Natalie Z. Cvijanovich
UCSF Benioff Children's Hospital Oakland, Oakland, CA, United States of America

Neal J. Thomas
Penn State Hershey Children's Hospital, Hershey, PA, United States of America

Geoffrey L. Allen
Children's Mercy Hospital, Kansas City, MO, United States of America

Nick Anas
Children's Hospital of Orange County, Orange, CA, United States of America

Michael T. Bigham
Akron Children's Hospital, Akron, OH, United States of America

Mark Hall
Nationwide Children's Hospital, Columbus, OH, United States of America

Robert J. Freishtat
Children's National Medical Center, Washington, DC, United States of America

Anita Sen
Morgan Stanley Children's Hospital, Columbia University Medical Center, New York, NY, United States of America

Keith Meyer
Miami Children's Hospital, Miami, FL, United States of America

Paul A. Checchia
Texas Children's Hospital, Houston, TX, United States of America

Thomas P. Shanley and Michael Quasney
C. S. Mott Children's Hospital at the University of Michigan, Ann Arbor, MI, United States of America

Jeffrey Nowak
Children's Hospital and Clinics of Minnesota, Minneapolis, MN, United States of America

Scott L. Weiss
The Children's Hospital of Philadelphia, Philadelphia, PA, United States of America

Christopher J. Lindsell
Department of Emergency Medicine, University of Cincinnati College of Medicine, Cincinnati, OH, United States of America

Hector R. Wong
Division of Critical Care Medicine, Cincinnati Children's Hospital Medical Center and Cincinnati Children's Research Foundation, Cincinnati, OH, United States of America
Department of Pediatrics, University of Cincinnati College of Medicine, Cincinnati, OH, United States of America

Ahmed S. Rahman, Mohammad Jyoti Raihan, Mohammad Mehedi Hasan and Tahmeed Ahmed
Centre for Nutrition and Food Security, International Centre for Diarrhoeal Diseases Research, Bangladesh (icddr,b), Dhaka, Bangladesh

Mohammad Rafiqul Islam
CCEB, School of Medicine and Public Health, University of Newcastle, Newcastle, Australia

Tracey P. Koehlmoos
Department of Health Administration and Policy, College of Health and Human Services, George Mason University, Fairfax, Virginia, United States of America

Charles P. Larson
Department of Pediatrics, University of British Columbia and Centre for International Child Health, BC Children's Hospital, Vancouver, British Columbia, Canada

Jeffrey D. Galley
Division of Biosciences, College of Dentistry, Ohio State University, Columbus, Ohio, United States of America

Michael Bailey
Division of Biosciences, College of Dentistry, Ohio State University, Columbus, Ohio, United States of America
The Institute for Behavioral Medicine Research, The Ohio State University Wexner Medical Center, Columbus, Ohio, United States of America

Claire Kamp Dush and Sarah Schoppe-Sullivan
Department of Human Science, The Ohio State University, Columbus, Ohio, United States of America,

Lisa M. Christian
The Institute for Behavioral Medicine Research, The Ohio State University Wexner Medical Center, Columbus, Ohio, United States of America
Department of Psychiatry, The Ohio State University Wexner Medical Center, Columbus, Ohio, United States of America
Department of Obstetrics and Gynecology, The Ohio State University Wexner Medical Center, Columbus, Ohio, United States of America
Psychology, The Ohio State University, Columbus, Ohio, United States of America

Tong Gong, Cecilia Lundholm, Gustaf Rejnö, Niklas Långström
Department of Medical Epidemiology and Biostatistics, Karolinska Institutet, Stockholm, Sweden

Carina Mood
Swedish Institute for Social Research, Stockholm University, Stockholm, Sweden

Catarina Almqvist
Department of Medical Epidemiology and Biostatistics, Karolinska Institutet, Stockholm, Sweden
Astrid Lindgren Children's Hospital, Lung and Allergy Unit, Karolinska University Hospital, Stockholm, Sweden

William F. Vann, Jr. and A. Diane Baker
1 Department of Pediatric Dentistry, School of Dentistry, University of North Carolina at Chapel Hill, Chapel Hill, NC, United States of America

Jessica Y. Lee
Department of Pediatric Dentistry, School of Dentistry, University of North Carolina at Chapel Hill, Chapel Hill, NC, United States of America
Department of Health Policy and Management, UNC Gillings School of Global Public Health, University of North Carolina at Chapel Hill, Chapel Hill, NC, United States of America

R. Gary Rozier
Department of Health Policy and Management, UNC Gillings School of Global Public Health, University of North Carolina at Chapel Hill, Chapel Hill, NC, United States of America

Kimon Divaris
Department of Pediatric Dentistry, School of Dentistry, University of North Carolina at Chapel Hill, Chapel Hill, NC, United States of America
Department of Epidemiology, UNC Gillings School of Global Public Health, University of North Carolina at Chapel Hill, Chapel Hill, NC, United States of America

Darren A. DeWalt
School of Medicine and Cecil G. Sheps Center for Health Services Research, University of North Carolina at Chapel Hill, Chapel Hill, NC, United States of America

Ziya Gizlice
Center for Health Promotion and Disease Prevention, University of North Carolina at Chapel Hill, Chapel Hill, NC, United States of America

Dodi Safari and Miftahuddin Majid Khoeri
Eijkman Institute for Molecular Biology, Jakarta, Indonesia

Nia Kurniati
Department of Child Health, Dr. Cipto Mangunkusumo Hospital/Faculty of Medicine Universitas Indonesia, Jakarta, Indonesia

Lia Waslia
Eijkman Oxford Clinical Research Unit, Jakarta, Indonesia

Tiara Putri
Faculty of Biology, Gajah Mada University, Yogyakarta, Indonesia

Debby Bogaert and Krzysztof Trzciński
Department of Pediatric Immunology and Infectious Diseases, Wilhelmina's Children Hospital, University Medical Center Utrecht, Utrecht, the Netherlands

Elizabeth Orton
Lecturer and Specialty Registrar in Public Health, Division of Primary Care, University Park, University of Nottingham, Nottingham United Kingdom

Denise Kendrick
Professor of Primary Care Research, Division of Primary Care, University Park, University of Nottingham, Nottingham United Kingdom

Joe West
Clinical Associate Professor and Reader in Epidemiology; Consultant Gastroenterologist, Division of Epidemiology and Public Health, Nottingham City Hospital, University of Nottingham, Nottingham, United Kingdom

Laila J. Tata
Associate Professor in Epidemiology, Division of Epidemiology and Public Health, Nottingham City Hospital, University of Nottingham, Nottingham, United Kingdom

Sarah Siddiqui, Shilpi Chattopadhyay, Md. Salman Akhtar, Mohammad Zeeshan Najm and Syed Akhtar Husain
Department of Biotechnology, Jamia Millia Islamia, New Delhi, India

S. V. S. Deo and N. K. Shukla
Department of Surgical Oncology, All India Institute of Medical Sciences, New Delhi, India

Elizabeth M. Miller
Department of Anthropology, University of South Florida, Tampa, Florida, United States of America

Matthew R. Markovetz
Department of Chemical and Petroleum Engineering, Swanson School of Engineering, University of Pittsburgh, Pittsburgh, PA, United States of America,

Timothy E. Corcoran
Department of Chemical and Petroleum Engineering, Swanson School of Engineering, University of Pittsburgh, Pittsburgh, PA, United States of America
Pulmonary Allergy and Critical Care Medicine, University of Pittsburgh, Pittsburgh, PA, United States of America
Department of Bioengineering, Swanson School of Engineering, University of Pittsburgh, Pittsburgh, PA, United States of America

Landon W. Locke, Michael M. Myerburg and Joseph M. Pilewski
Pulmonary Allergy and Critical Care Medicine, University of Pittsburgh, Pittsburgh, PA, United States of America,

Robert S. Parker
Department of Chemical and Petroleum Engineering, Swanson School of Engineering, University of Pittsburgh, Pittsburgh, PA, United States of America
McGowan Institute of Regenerative Medicine, University of Pittsburgh, Pittsburgh, PA, United States of America
Clinical Research, Investigation, and Systems Modeling of Acute Illness (CRISMA) Laboratories, University of Pittsburgh, Pittsburgh, PA, United States of America
University of Pittsburgh Cancer Institute, University of Pittsburgh, Pittsburgh, PA, United States of America

Index